Cortical Development: Neurogenesis and Neurological Disorders

Cortical Development: Neurogenesis and Neurological Disorders

Editor: Oliva Novak

AMERICAN
MEDICAL PUBLISHERS
www.americanmedicalpublishers.com

AMERICAN
MEDICAL PUBLISHERS
www.americanmedicalpublishers.com

Cataloging-in-Publication Data

Cortical development : neurogenesis and neurological disorders / edited by Oliva Novak.
p. cm.
Includes bibliographical references and index.
ISBN 979-8-88740-023-5
1. Developmental neurobiology. 2. Nervous system--Diseases. 3. Neocortex--Growth.
4. Developmental neurophysiology. 5. Neurophysiology. I. Novak, Oliva.
QP363.5 .C67 2023
612.8--dc23

American Medical Publishers,
41 Flatbush Avenue,
1st Floor, New York,
NY 11217, USA

ISBN 979-8-88740-023-5 (Hardback)

Contents

Preface

Every book is initially just a concept; it takes months of research and hard work to give it the final shape in which the readers receive it. In its early stages, this book also went through rigorous reviewing. The notable contributions made by experts from across the globe were first molded into patterned chapters and then arranged in a sensibly sequential manner to bring out the best results.

Cortical development is generally referred to as the process through which cerebral cortex is formed in mammals. The development of the cerebral cortex is crucial and necessitates complicated sequential processes which must be precisely orchestrated. The specific connectivity, identity and laminar positioning of each single cortical neuron are determined by the timing and localization of neuronal progenitor proliferation and neuronal migration. Variations in any of these organized series of events, whether caused by environmental factors or genetic mutations, leads to defined brain pathologies commonly referred as malformations of cortical development (MCDs). They are known as the major cause of intellectual disability and drug-resistant epilepsy. In these varied group of disorders, macroscopic variations in the brain structure can be identified and possibly subtend a general restructuring of neuronal circuits. This book is compiled in such a manner, that it will provide in-depth knowledge about the neurogenesis and neurological disorders with respect to cortical development. Researchers and students in this field will be assisted by it.

It has been my immense pleasure to be a part of this project and to contribute my years of learning in such a meaningful form. I would like to take this opportunity to thank all the people who have been associated with the completion of this book at any step.

Editor

1

Crosstalk between Intracellular and Extracellular Signals Regulating Interneuron Production, Migration and Integration into the Cortex

Elise Peyre[1,2†], *Carla G. Silva*[1,2†] *and Laurent Nguyen*[1,2,3*]

[1] *GIGA-Neurosciences, University of Liège, Liège, Belgium,* [2] *Interdisciplinary Cluster for Applied Genoproteomics (GIGA-R), University of Liège, Liège, Belgium,* [3] *Wallon Excellence in Lifesciences and Biotechnology, University of Liège, Liège, Belgium*

***Correspondence:**
Laurent Nguyen,
GIGA-Neurosciences, Quartier Hôpital, University of Liège, Tour B36, Avenue Hippocrate 15, 4000 Liège, Belgium
lnguyen@ulg.ac.be

†These authors have contributed equally to this work.

During embryogenesis, cortical interneurons are generated by ventral progenitors located in the ganglionic eminences of the telencephalon. They travel along multiple tangential paths to populate the cortical wall. As they reach this structure they undergo intracortical dispersion to settle in their final destination. At the cellular level, migrating interneurons are highly polarized cells that extend and retract processes using dynamic remodeling of microtubule and actin cytoskeleton. Different levels of molecular regulation contribute to interneuron migration. These include: (1) Extrinsic guidance cues distributed along migratory streams that are sensed and integrated by migrating interneurons; (2) Intrinsic genetic programs driven by specific transcription factors that grant specification and set the timing of migration for different subtypes of interneurons; (3) Adhesion molecules and cytoskeletal elements/regulators that transduce molecular signalings into coherent movement. These levels of molecular regulation must be properly integrated by interneurons to allow their migration in the cortex. The aim of this review is to summarize our current knowledge of the interplay between microenvironmental signals and cell autonomous programs that drive cortical interneuron porduction, tangential migration, and intergration in the developing cerebral cortex.

Keywords: interneurons, cortex, migration, progenitors, nucleokinesis, branching

Introduction

During mouse embryogenesis, cortical interneurons (cINs) are generated in the ventral subpallium. Distinct proliferative regions can be identified in this area, including the lateral ganglionic eminence (LGE), the medial ganglionic eminence (MGE), the caudal ganglionic eminence (CGE) and the preoptic area (POA). While the MGE, CGE and POA contribute to the generation of cortical interneurons (cINs) (Flames et al., 2007; Rubin et al., 2010), the LGE is mostly involved in striatal and olfactory bulb histogenesis (Yun et al., 2003). These distinct subpallial regions differ

Abbreviations: CGE, caudal ganglionic eminence; cIN, cortical interneuron; CP, cortical plate; CR, calretinin; dMGE, dorsal medial ganglionic eminence; F-actine, fibrilar actine; G-actine, globular actine; IP, intermediate progenitor; IZ, intermediate zone; LGE, lateral ganglionic eminence; MGE, medial ganglionic eminence; MT, microtubule; MZ, marginal zone; NPY, neuropeptide Y; POA, preoptic areo; PTM, post-translational modification; PV, parvalbumin; SAP, subapical progenitor; SNP, short neuroal precursor; SP, subplate; SST, somatostatin; SVZ, subventricular zone; VIP, vasointestinal peptide; vMGE, ventral medial ganglionic eminence; VZ, ventricular zone.

in progenitor domain composition and in the ability to generate IN subtypes characterized by specific networks of transcription factors. In addition to genetic programs, diffusing molecules also participate in shaping the timing, space and specificity of cIN subtype production. Indeed, at the earlier stages of corticogenesis, molecules acting as mitogens and morphogens induce genetic programs eventually leading to the expansion of proliferative regions, specification and maturation of cINs. In rodents, cINs migrate long distances to reach their final destination. Again, they are under control of genetic programs and signaling cascades triggered by extracellular cues that work together to produce a synchronized, harmonious and directed movement toward the cortex. At the cellular level, these informations are integrated and translated by the cytoskeleton into appropriate cellular behavior. After settling at their final location, cINs integrate and organize in coherent networks. Here we will review the current understanding of how genetic programs intermingle with extracellular signaling pathways to achieve the production, migration and network integration of INs in the cortex.

The exact number of cIN subtypes remains debated, mainly due to the diversity in their morphological, molecular and functional properties (Petilla Interneuron Nomenclature et al., 2008). In this review, a simplified nomenclature combining molecular and physiological properties of cINs will be used. According to this nomenclature (Gelman and Marin, 2010), the large variety of cIN subtypes will fall in one of four major groups: (a) fast spiking, parvalbumin (PV)-expressing cINs; (b) burst spiking or adapting non-fast spiking somatostatin (SST)-expressing cINs; (c) non-fast spiking and fast adapting calretinin (CR)- and/or vasointestinal peptide (VIP)-expressing cINs; (d) rapidly adapting neuropeptide Y (NPY)- and/or reelin-expressing cINs. Most studies discussed here used rodents as experimental model. They have been useful in the understanding of the physiopathology underlying cortical interneuron development. We will finalize by giving example of how these findings fit with what starts being known about the production, migration and cortical integration of GABAergic neurons in primate and human.

Generation and Specification of Cortical Interneurons

Role of Morphogens in Establishing Ventral Identity

MGE histogenesis starts at around embryonic day (E) 9, followed by the generation of LGE at E10 and CGE at E11 (Smart, 1976). GEs histogenesis requires a complex interplay between morphogens and transcription factors to ventralize the structure and promote IN production. Sonic hedgehog (SHH) and fibroblast growth factors (FGFs) contribute to the dorso-ventral patterning and subpallium development (Jessell, 2000; Briscoe and Ericson, 2001; Ingham and McMahon, 2001). *Shh* is widely expressed in the prospective MGE by E9 and by E12 its expression spreads to the mantle zone of the MGE and POA (Echelard et al., 1993). Cell responsiveness to SHH greatly depends on the action of the transcription factors of the GLI family that can, in their constitutively cleaved forms, act as transcriptional repressors in the absence of SHH signaling. Conversely if uncleaved, they function as transcriptional activators in the presence of SHH (Bai et al., 2004; Pan et al., 2006). The current understanding postulates that SHH signaling is required to counteract GLI3 repressor activity therefore contributing to the positioning of the dorsoventral boundary (**Figure 1**). At early stages of brain development, SHH prevents dorsalization of the ventral telencephalon, allowing the subsequent formation of the GEs. This is in contrast with the role of GLI proteins in the spinal cord where these factors act as activators by directly promoting ventral patterning (Rallu et al., 2002; Bai et al., 2004). Downstream effectors of SHH signaling are also required for ventral development. They include smoothened, the low-density lipoprotein receptor-related protein 2 (LRP2) or megalin and the multifunctional transmembrane protein Cdo (Fuccillo et al., 2004; Spoelgen et al., 2005; Zhang et al., 2006). In *Shh* knockout mouse models, rescue of the ventral telencephalon by compound *Gli3* removal gives the indication that other genes might act independently or downstream of *Shh* (Rallu et al., 2002). Several studies provide evidence that FGFs act downstream of SHH and can directly induce ventral gene expression in dorsal telencephalic explants when SHH signaling is inhibited (Aoto et al., 2002; Ohkubo et al., 2002; Kuschel et al., 2003; Gutin et al., 2006; Rash and Grove, 2007). Since SHH promotes *Fgf* expression (Martynoga et al., 2005), FGFs are considered mandatory effectors of SHH signaling (**Figure 1**). The forkhead G1 factor (FOXG1) is the main generator of direct ventralization within the forming ventral telencephalon as it induces expression of *Fgf8* (Martynoga et al., 2005) in the MGE or *FGF15* in the CGE (Borello et al., 2008). *Foxg1* acts in concert with FGF signaling, forming a positive feedback loop (Shimamura et al., 1995; Martynoga et al., 2005). *Foxg1* expression is independent of the direct action of SHH but impaired in the absence of *Shh* due to the increased repressor activity of GLI3 (Rash and Grove, 2007).

Transcription Factors acting in Concert with Morphogens in the MGE

The MGE contributes to the production of 50–60% of the total population of cINs in the mouse (Pleasure et al., 2000; Butt et al., 2005; Wonders and Anderson, 2006). On top of the hierarchical MGE SHH- and FGF-dependent organizers is *Nkx2-1* transcription factor (Sussel et al., 1999; Gutin et al., 2006; Storm et al., 2006; Fogarty et al., 2007; Xu et al., 2008, 2010). *Nkx2-1* itself maintains *Shh* expression within the early MGE, a process depending on FoxA2/HNF-3β transcription factor (Sussel et al., 1999) (**Figure 1**). Moreover, early removal of *Nkx2.1* from MGE progenitors re-specifies INs into early LGE medium spiny neuron identity, while its late removal leads to acquisition of CGE IN profile (Butt et al., 2008). *Nkx2*-1 is no longer detected in mice that lack expression of both *Fgfr1* and *Fgfr2* (Gutin et al., 2006). The analysis of the expression of several transcription factors within the ventricular zone (VZ) of the MGE have led to the proposal that this region can be compartmentalized into five different progenitor domains (Flames et al., 2007). The dorsal region of the MGE (dMGE) preferentially gives rise to somatostatin (SST)-expressing cINs. In contrast, the ventral part of the MGE (vMGE) was shown to mostly generate paravalbulin (PV)-expressing cINs.

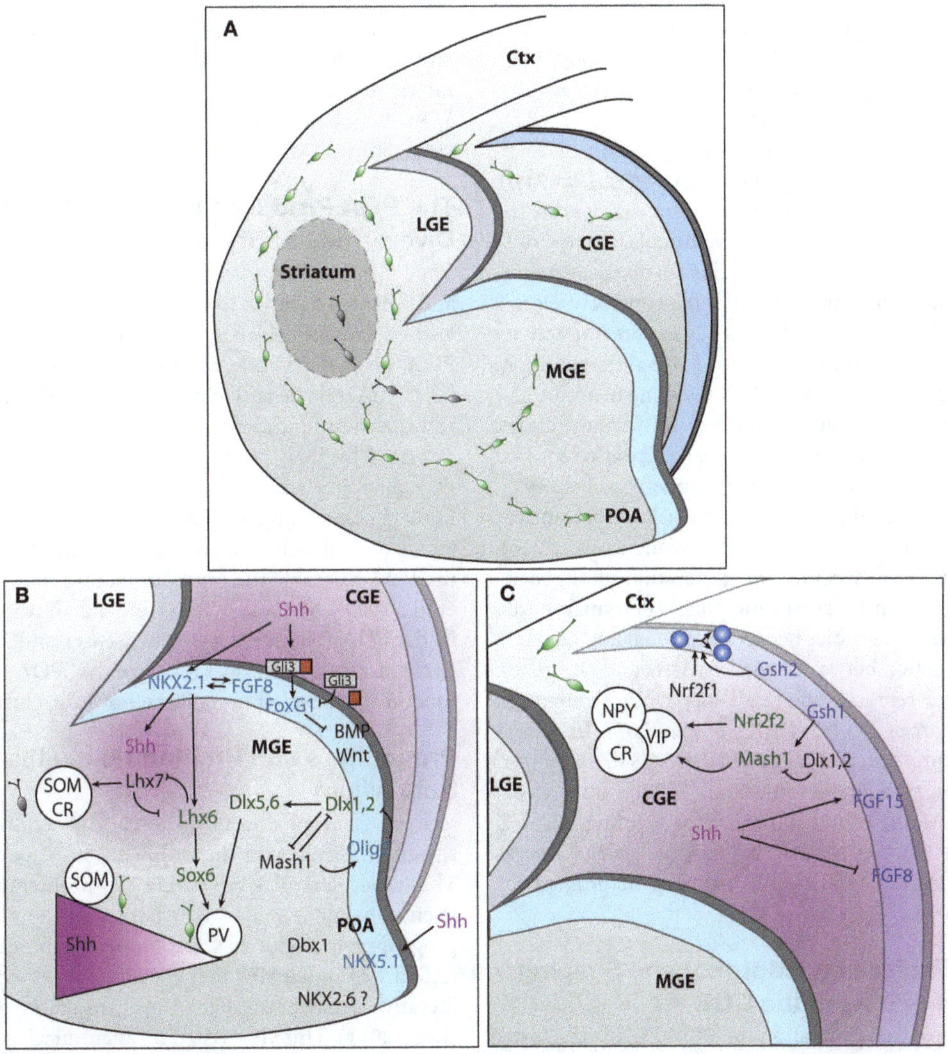

FIGURE 1 | Genetic regulation of cINs production in the different compartments of the subpallium. (A) Representation of the developing mouse brain with the different subpallium structures and interneurons migration routes. **(B)** Signaling cascades regulating cIN production and specification, in the MGE and POA. **(C)** Signaling cascades regulating cIN production and specification, in the CGE. The two main sources of SHH, ventricles and mantle zone, are depicted in purple.

Since *Nkx2-1* expression promotes the specification of both SST and PV cIN subtypes, it was suggested that the SHH gradient determines the final fate of interneurons. High levels of SHH signaling would favor the generation of SST-expressing cINs at the expenses of PV-expressing cINs (Xu et al., 2010). Consistently, high expression levels of SHH effectors were found in the dMGE (Wonders et al., 2008). More recently, it was demonstrated that neurons from the mantle zone are an additional source of SHH (Flandin et al., 2011). They play a relevant role in maintaining a high SHH gradient in the dMGE, far away from the VZ. SHH production by mantle neurons was shown to require expression of *Lhx6* (Flandin et al., 2011), a direct target of *Nkx2-1*, also implicated in PV or SST fate acquisition. In the absence of *Lhx6*, NPY fate was promoted at the expenses of PV or SST (Liodis et al., 2007; Zhao et al., 2008). It was also shown that disruption of the gene encoding *FGF receptor 1* (*Fgfr1*) lead to a loss of *Lhx6* and *Lhx8(7)* expression, both necessary for the formation of MGE-derived INs (Fragkouli et al., 2005; Gutin et al., 2006; Liodis et al., 2007) and maturation of PV-cINs (Smith et al., 2014). Other genes act downstream of or in concert with *Nkx2-1*. For example, high levels of *Lhx8(7)* expression shifts the fate of cINs toward globus pallidus GABAergic neurons and into cholinergic INs from the striatum (Zhao et al., 2003; Fragkouli et al., 2005). *Sox6* expression is required for the generation of the appropriate number of PV and SST INs as demonstrated in studies using *germline* and conditional knockout mice (Azim et al., 2009; Batista-Brito et al., 2009). In these mice models, a concomitant increase of NPY cINs was observed (Azim et al., 2009; Batista-Brito et al., 2009). *Sox6* acts downstream *Lhx6* and is expressed continuously within the MGE from postmitotic progenitor stage until adulthood and is implicated in the placement and maturation of PV and ST cINs (Batista-Brito et al., 2009). *Dlx* genes also contribute to cINs specification and maturation. *Dlx* genes expression is temporally regulated, following the sequence: *Dlx2, Dlx1, Dlx5, and Dlx6* (Liu et al., 1997; Eisenstat et al., 1999). *Dlx1/2* gene seems to be particularly important for the acquisition of SST, calretinin (CR), NPY and reelin fates (Cobos et al., 2005) as its absence leads to an abnormal expression of cortical markers in the ventral telencephalon (Long et al., 2009a,b). The expression of a wide range of transcription factors in the MGE progenitors from the VZ and subventricular zone (SVZ) as well as non-transcription factor proteins involved in migration and cortical integration are also under the control of *Dlx1/2* (Long et al., 2009a). For example, *Dlx1/2* has a repressor activity over *Arx* transcription factor, required for MGE differentiation. In their absence, cIN migration is blocked, resulting in accumulation of cells in the GEs and reduced numbers of INs in the cortex (Colombo et al., 2007). In addition, *Dlx1/2* genes are also required for the delayed expression of *Dlx5/6* genes (Anderson et al., 1997; Yun et al., 2002; Long et al., 2009b), particularly important for the establishment of PV subtype identity (Wang et al., 2010). Furthermore, *Dlx1/2* tightly control the generation of oligodendrocytes in the forebrain by repressing *Olig2* (Petryniak et al., 2007). More precisely, the choice between neuronal and glial fate involves cross-regulation between *Mash1* or *Acsl1* and *Dlx* genes. *Mash1* binds to and represses the regulatory DNA elements in the intergenic region of *Dlx1/2* (Parras et al., 2007). In *Mash1* mutants, *Dlx1/2* expression is expanded in the VZ/SVZ (Casarosa et al., 1999; Horton et al., 1999; Yun et al., 2002; Poitras et al., 2007). Conversely *Mash1* expression is increased in the VZ/SVZ of *Dlx1/2* mutants (Yun et al., 2002). Thus, the role of *Mash1* consists in restricting the number of *Dlx*-expressing progenitors (Petryniak et al., 2007).

Transcription Factors and Morphogens Shaping the Generation of cINs in the CGE

CGE contributes to the generation of 30–40% of all cortical interneurons. Several studies have demonstrated that CGE derived interneurons acquire either a CR and/or VIP (Pleasure et al., 2000; Butt et al., 2005) or reelin identity (Miyoshi et al., 2010). *Gsh* or *Gsx* homeobox TFs act at the top of the genetic network involved in CGE cell specification (**Figure 1**). *Gsh2* is particularly relevant for the generation of CR bipolar cINs (Xu et al., 2010). Interestingly, *Gsh1* and *Gsh2* are co-expressed but have antagonist functions within the CGE, *Gsh2* promoting progenitor state and *Gsh1* promoting neuronal differentiation (Pei et al., 2011). Interestingly, the control of the choice between proliferation and differentiation by *Gsh* genes seems to involve the downstream target *Mash1* (Fode et al., 2000). In *Mash1* loss of function there is premature differentiation of progenitors located in the SVZ and precocious expression of *Dlx* genes (Casarosa et al., 1999; Yun et al., 2002), downstream effectors. On the other hand, overexpression of *Mash1* contributes to cell type specification (Fode et al., 2000). *Dlx1* and *Dlx2* are co-expressed in subsets of progenitor cells and contribute to cell maturation by downregulating *Gsh2/Mash1* (Yun et al., 2002). Other CGE transcription factors include *Nrf2f1and Nrf2f2 or Couptf1* and *Couptf2*, respectively, as well as *SP8*. These genes are however not exclusive from CGE, as they have been identified in the dMGE and POA (Lodato et al., 2011a). *Nrf2f1* is required for proper progenitor proliferation and necessary for generation of interneuron diversity in the cortex (Lodato et al., 2011a). *Nrf2f2* is important for directing interneurons through a caudal migratory path (Cai et al., 2013). *SP8* function in the hierarchy of CGE specification/maturation is yet unknown (Ma et al., 2012).

The POA Produces a Reduced Number of Diverse cIN Subtypes

The POA is the most ventral region of the developing subpallium and it has been shown to generate around 10% of GABAergic INs. Using a Cre line driven by *Nkx5-1* or *Hmx3*, a gene exclusive from POA, gives rise to a small population (around 4%) of multipolar GABAergic cells (Gelman et al., 2009). Another 5% of total INs is also produced by progenitors present in this region, characterized by their expression of the transcription factor Dbx1. Fate mapping and *in utero* transplantation demonstrated that POA generates diverse cINs subtypes (Gelman et al., 2011). In terms of molecular markers expression, the cells generated by the POA resemble the ones originating from the CGE (Gelman et al., 2009). *Shh* and *Nkx2-1* but not *Lhx6* are also expressed in the POA (Flames et al., 2007). *Dbx1* and *Nkx6-2* are respectively markers of the dorsal and ventral POA (see **Figure 1**). The function of these genes remains, however, elusive.

Progenitors and Proliferation in the Ventral Subpallium

Ventral telencephalon expansion and generation of a great diversity of cINs relies on the proliferation of pools of progenitors. The molecular rules governing cell proliferation in the ventral telencephalon as well as the characterization of the distinct cIN progenitor behavior has just started to be unveiled. For some time it was anticipated that GE progenitors would display a proliferative behavior similar to progenitors in the cerebral cortex (Ross, 2011). This view relied on anatomical and cumulative bromodeoxyuridine (BrdU) experiments. These studies were important as they served identifying both VZ and SVZ as two distinct proliferative compartments (Sheth and Bhide, 1997). The lack of selective markers for the SVZ and the superposition of proliferating and migrating cINs hampered for some time detailed studies aiming at characterizing the cellular biology of cell division of ventral progenitors. Improvement of molecular tools and imaging techniques overcame these limitations. For example, an elegant study by Brown and colleagues used a clonal approach to understand how cINs were generated within these regions. Low concentration of retrovirus expressing GFP was injected in the ventricle of E11 embryos. In order to specifically infect INs progenitor cells, the virus entry receptor was expressed under the control of *Nkx2*-1 (Brown et al., 2011). They found that cINs are produced as spatially organized clonal units and clonally related INs form spatially isolated cluster in the neocortex. They identified the presence of radial glia (RG) in the VZ of MGE and POA that undergo interkinetic nuclear migration and divide asymmetrically in the VZ to self-renew and produce intermediate progenitors (IPs) or differentiating cINs. Using time-lapse microscopy, Pilz et al. (2013) proposed a more complex hierarchical classification for ventral progenitors. RG cells sit at the base of this classification and divide asymmetrically to generate both an amplifying and a self-renewal branch. These cells give rise to short neural precursors (SNPs). Both RG and SNPs generate subapical progenitors (SAPs) which in turn divide to produce basal radial glia (bRG) or basal progenitors (BPs). Basal radial glia and BPs contribute to the great SVZ expansion. *Mash1* levels were shown to control the numbers of SAPs (Pilz et al., 2013). Although this study was performed in the LGE, such hierarchical complexity might be expected for the entirety of the ventral telencephalon.

Molecular Regulation of Ventral Proliferation

Studies performed by Vidaki et al. (2012) showed that classical proteins displaying a role in dorsal proliferation, such as Ras-related C3 botulinum toxin substrate 1 (Rac1), are also important regulators of *Nkx2-1*-expressing MGE progenitor division. In the absence of Rac1, cyclin D proteins levels are reduced and similarly low levels of Retinoblastoma (Rb) phosphorylation is detected. Cortical interneuron progenitors are thus blocked from completing cell cycle (halted in G1 phase) and accumulate in the GEs. Interestingly, the lack of *cyclin D2* in SVZ progenitors lead to the production of lower number of PV but not SST cIN subtypes (Glickstein et al., 2007a,b, 2009), suggesting that cell division and cell fate acquisition are linked events (Glickstein et al., 2007b; Ross, 2011). Rb family proteins and the closely related protein p107, play a role in cell proliferation by regulating the activity of E2F transcription factors, notably E2F4 a transcription repressor (Trimarchi and Lees, 2002). Deficiency of E2F4 expression impairs the self-renewal of neuronal precursor cells (Ruzhynsky et al., 2007) and results in loss of ventral telencephalic structures. The underlying mechanism involves a dramatic loss of *Shh*, *Nkx2-1*, and *Dlx2* expression.

Acting extracellularly, morphogens such as SHH and FGFs can also potentially act as mitogens (Hebert and Fishell, 2008). SHH-mediated proliferation is regulated in space and time (Blaess et al., 2006). If progenitors are exposed to SHH during the peak of neurogenesis, it will enhance proliferation, whereas exposure during the post-neurogenic period maintains cells in the undifferentiated state (Rowitch et al., 1999). Downstream effectors of SHH regulating the cell cycle are N-*myc* (Kenney et al., 2003), *cyclin D1* (Kenney and Rowitch, 2000), *E2f1* and *E2f2* (Oliver et al., 2003). The induction of N-*myc* occurs through GLI proteins and its stabilization depends on phosphatidylinositol-3-kinase (PI3-K) (Kenney et al., 2004; Sjostrom et al., 2005). FGFs control cell cycle length mainly during G1 phase. In a cell culture model, addition of FGF2 results in G1 phase shortening and an increase in the number of proliferative divisions by E14-E16 (Lukaszewicz et al., 2002). *In vivo*, *Fgf8* controls ventral telencephalon size mainly in rostral regions (Storm et al., 2006). This effect mainly relied on the control over progenitor survival (Storm et al., 2006). Deletion of *Fgf3* in addition to *Fgf8* further decreased the telencephalic size, indicating that both genes act in synergy (Theil et al., 2008). *Fgf15* controls progenitor differentiation at earlier developmental stages by promoting cell cycle shortening and exit, an effect opposite of what was observed at later stages (Borello et al., 2008). Neurotransmitter receptors are another class of diffusible molecules that control cell proliferation in the developing telencephalon (Cameron et al., 1998; Nguyen et al., 2001; Owens and Kriegstein, 2002a,b). cIN precursors and progenitors appear to be sources of gamma aminobutyric acid (GABA) (Bellion and Metin, 2005). Indeed, the extracellular GABA concentrations in the GEs may be as high as 0.5 μM (Cuzon et al., 2006). Proliferating cIN precursors also display detectable levels of GABA synthetizing enzymes and functional $GABA_B$ receptors (Maric et al., 2001) as well as GABA and chloride transporters (Laurie et al., 1992; Ma and Barker, 1995). Glutamate is also present in the telencephalic germinal zones where it acts as mitogen. In the cortex, both GABA and glutamate where shown to decrease proliferation in the SVZ probably by reducing DNA synthesis as a consequence of membrane depolarization and Ca^{2+} increase (LoTurco et al., 1995; Haydar et al., 2000), in opposition to what was observed on VZ progenitors (Haydar et al., 2000). Glutamate actions were found to be diverse and depend on the glutamate receptor subtype involved in the signaling. For example, DNA synthesis inhibition occurs when α-amino-3-hydroxy-5-méthylisoazol-4-propionate (AMPA)/ kainate (KA) receptors are activated (LoTurco et al., 1995). N-methyl-D-aspartate (NMDA) receptor-dependent signaling instead promotes proliferation of striatal neural progenitors (Sadikot et al., 1998; Luk et al., 2003). The ERK (Extracellular Signal-Regulated Kinase)-PI3K pathway is triggered downstream NMDA receptor activation to control proliferation of striatal progenitors (Luk et al., 2003). Variation in glutamate concentration (Haydar et al., 2000) and interaction between glutamate receptor-mediated and growth factors-mediates signaling pathways (Dobbertin et al., 2000) might further contribute for a differential responsiveness of distinct progenitors. The action of morphogens and/or mitogens can be disrupted by many environmental agents and by epigenetic modifications during the period of corticogenesis. It is thus of utmost interest to fully characterize the signaling cascades triggering ventral proliferation.

Migration of Cortical Interneurons

During development, cINs migrate over long distances to reach the cortex and settle within cortical layers. Migrating cINs are highly polarized cells harboring a branched and dynamic leading process that terminates in a growth cone-like structure. They also possess a membrane protrusion at the rear of the cell called trailing process. While migrating, cINs display a stereotyped cyclic movement (**Figure 2A**). First, there is an extension of branches emanating from the leading process and as one of the branches stabilizes, a transient swelling forms close to the cell body where the centrosome and Golgi apparatus are displaced (Bellion et al., 2005). Then, cINs move forward by sudden and fast nuclear translocation into the swelling, an event called nucleokinesis. The jumping behavior of cINs characterizes its migration pattern and distinguishes it from the treadmill-like movement observed in a large range of cells. Finally, the trailing process is retracted and the cycle repeats. cINs can significantly change the direction of migration by inverting polarity, the trailing process extending and becoming the new leading process while the older leading process undergoes retraction (Nadarajah

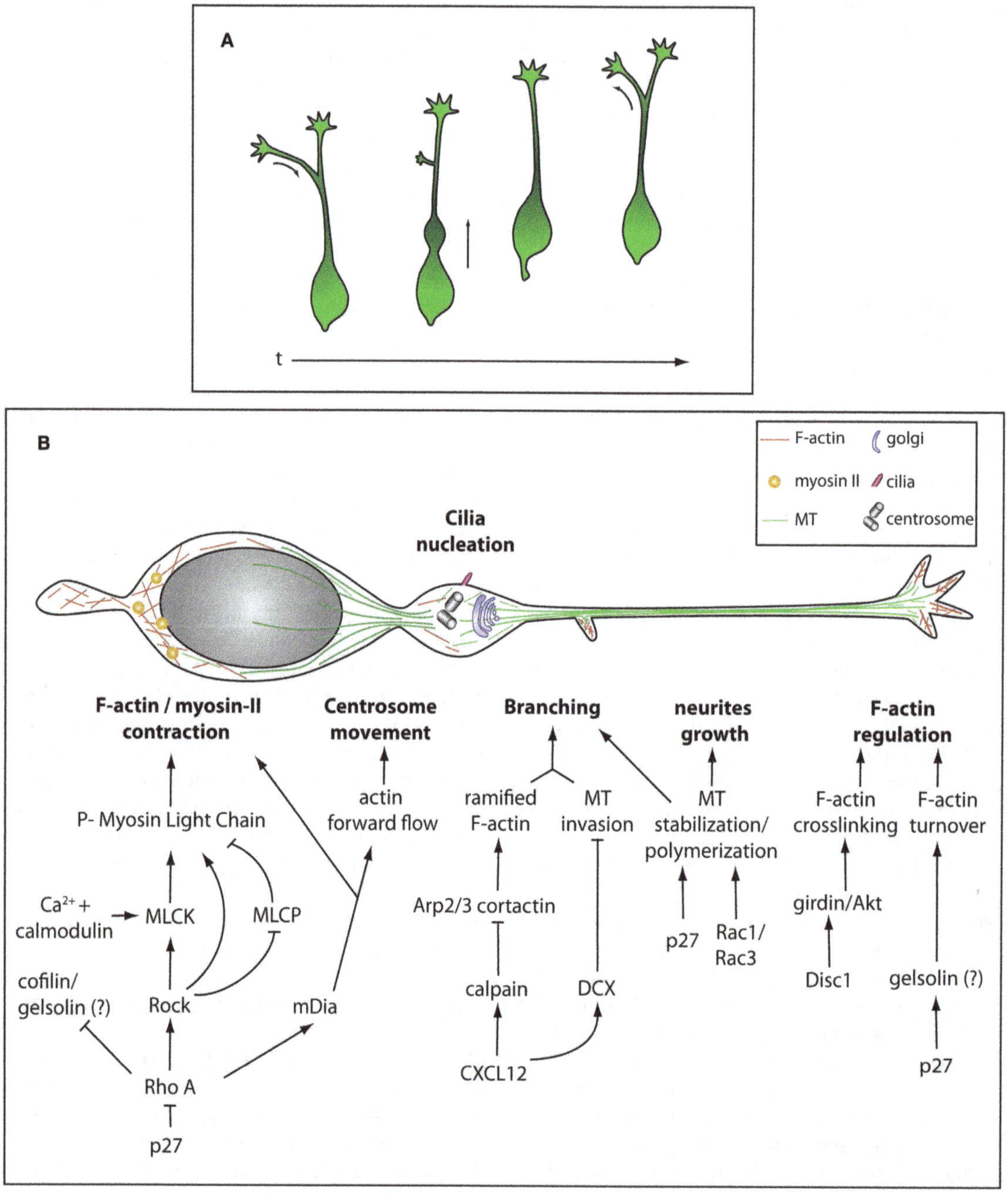

FIGURE 2 | Morphological remodeling during cIN migration and cytoskeleton regulation. (A) Different stereotypical morphologies during of cIN migration over time. **(B)** Representation of the cytoskeleton and some cellular components of a migrating cIN. Cytoskeleton-regulating cascades are represented in specific cellular compartments, not meaning they are exclusive to these different compartments.

et al., 2002) (**Figure 2A**). All these dynamic phases heavily rely on cytoskeleton remodeling.

Molecular Regulation of the Cytoskeleton in Migrating cINs

cINs Migration and Nucleokinesis

In cINs, a microtubule (MT) "cage" surrounds the nucleus and a large array of MTs connects this structure to the centrosome (Tanaka et al., 2004; Higginbotham and Gleeson, 2007; Godin et al., 2012) (**Figure 2B**). MTs are nucleated ahead of the nucleus to guide centrosome movement and docking to the cell membrane. At the membrane, the mother centriole is then able to grow a cilium allowing the cell to sense extracellular signals such as SHH (Baudoin et al., 2012). It was previously considered that the MT network was responsible for generating forces required for nucleokinesis, through dynein-dynactin directed motor movement. This type of MT-generated forces has been described for migration of projection neurons and cerebellar granule cells where MT-associated proteins Lissencephaly-1 (Lis-1) and Doublecortine (DCX) couple MT to the nucleus (Tanaka et al., 2004; Nasrallah et al., 2006; Tsai et al., 2007). Similarly, cINs depleted for Lis-1 show a reduced rate of migration (McManus et al., 2004). It was however demonstrated *in vitro* that the chemical destabilization of the MT network does not completely abolish nucleokinesis (Schaar and McConnell, 2005; Baudoin et al., 2008; Martini and Valdeolmillos, 2010). Instead, acto-myosin contractibility is necessary for nuclear movement, as shown by experiments in which non-muscle myosin-II-mediated contraction was blocked (Bellion et al., 2005; Schaar and McConnell, 2005; Baudoin et al., 2008; Martini and Valdeolmillos, 2010). Myosin-II is enriched behind the nucleus during nuclear translocation, where F-actin also shows a strong accumulation (Bellion et al., 2005; Schaar and McConnell, 2005; Martini and Valdeolmillos, 2010) (**Figure 2B**). Acto-myosin cytoskeleton is also necessary to promote centrosome separation from the nucleus upon swelling formation and for the dynamic remodeling of growth cones (Metin et al., 2006). Altogether, this strongly suggests that the forward movement occurring during nucleokinesis arises from pushing forces generated by acto-myosin contraction at the rear of the nucleus, together with limited MT- generated pulling forces (He et al., 2010; Steinecke et al., 2014a). Although well studied in the context of radial migration of projection neurons, the molecular cascade regulating acto-myosin cytoskeleton during tangential migration is not as well described. In many cell types the Rho family GTPases including Rho, Rac, and cell division control protein 42 homolog (CDC42) have been implicated in the regulation of acto-myosin contractility (reviewed in Heasman and Ridley, 2008; Govek et al., 2011). In cINs, modification of RhoA activation levels by loss of function of its inhibitor p27Kip1 leads to migration defects (Besson et al., 2004) due to myosin-II hyperactivation (Godin et al., 2012). Active RhoA, in its GTP bound state, regulates migration by activating the downstream kinase Rho-associated protein kinase (ROCK) and mDia but also by inhibiting cofilin, an actin severing enzyme (Kawauchi et al., 2006; Nguyen et al., 2006; Godin et al., 2012). ROCK promotes acto-myosin contraction using different mechanisms. It can directly phosphorylate Myosin Light Chain (MLC), inhibit Myosin Light Chain Phosphatase (MLCP) or activate Myosin Light Chain Kinase (MLCK) (Amano et al., 1996; Chrzanowska-Wodnicka and Burridge, 1996; Kimura et al., 1996; Ishizaki et al., 1997). MLCK activation leads to acto-myosin contraction by phosphorylating MLC. MLCK activity is modulated by its cofactor calmodulin, a calcium-activated protein (Gallagher et al., 1997). mDia is an actin nucleator that helps producing long filaments of actin fibers (Higashida et al., 2004) (**Figure 2B**). Interestingly, mutant mice for *mDia1* show impaired tangential migration, but no defects in radial cortical dispersion. In this animal model the anterograde actin flow that moves the centrosome forward as well as F-actin accumulation at the rear of the nucleus are impaired. In contrast, actin dynamics in the growth cone is normal (Shinohara et al., 2012). This argues for a differential regulation of cytoskeleton-generated forces in different subcellular compartments where ROCK and mDia cooperate to grant proper acto-myosin dynamics during cIN migration. F-actin turnover is a crucial parameter in acto-myosin dynamics as inhibition of F-actin severing was shown to stabilize the leading process and can lead to cell migration arrest (Chai et al., 2009a,b). In INs, partial inactivation of cofilin in mice lacking *p27* does not result in strong accumulation of F-actin, suggesting that F-actin severing can be mediated by redundant mechanisms, for example by the action of gelsolin (Godin et al., 2012) (**Figure 2B**).

cINs Leading Process, Branching, and Growth Cone Regulation

cINs navigate in their environment using a branched leading-process bearing dynamic growth cones. When a chemo-repulsive cue is sensed, the growth cone collapses and the branch is consequently retracted. In parallel, another branch is stabilized and it determines the new direction of migration (Martini et al., 2009). Leading process branching requires the coordination of both acto-myosin and MT networks. During this process a new membrane protrusion is formed thanks to the underlying ramified F-actin meshwork organized by cortactin and Actin-related proteins 2/3 (Arp2/3) (Spillane et al., 2011; Lysko et al., 2014). Then, invasion by unbundled and freely spreading MTs stabilizes the protrusion and allow the emergence of the branch. Recent evidence shows that fine-tuning of cIN branching is negatively regulated by CXCL12 or SDF-1 (Lysko et al., 2014). Binding of CXCL12 to its receptor CXCR4, results in decreased levels of cAMP and de-repression of calpain and DCX expression. This intracellular signaling has a double effect on the cytoskeleton: generation of straight F-actin fibers by calpain-mediated proteolysis of cortactin and MT bundling by DCX. Membrane protrusions are thus less likely to form in the absence of a branched actin meshwork and be stabilized by bundled MTs. Accordingly, hyperbranching is observed in cINs lacking *DCX* (Kappeler et al., 2006; Friocourt et al., 2007; Lysko et al., 2014) (**Figure 2B**). Proper regulation of MT dynamics is also essential for cIN tangential migration as neurite growth is depending on the establishment of new MT-networks. For example, in *p27kip1* mutant, neurite growth defects are observed and cannot be fully rescued by modulating the acto-myosin contraction mediated by the RhoA pathway (Godin et al., 2012). Interestingly it was shown that p27kip1 acts also as a MT-associated protein (MAP) thanks to its proline-rich domain that promotes MT polymerization both *in vivo* and *in vitro*. This indicates that MT polymerization is an essential parameter in modulating neurite growth and migration properties of cINs (Godin et al., 2012). Similarly, the establishment of a long leading process also requires MT stabilization. In *Rac1/Rac3* mutant mice, migrating cINs show a hyper-branched phenotype similar to the one observed in *Dcx* knockout mice as well as a reduced leading process length. This is also accompanied by MTs harboring less post-translational modifications (PTMs), frequent on stable and long-lived MTs. The phenotype was partially rescued by treating the cells with taxol, a MT stabilizing agent, indicating that establishment of a correct migration needs a minimal amount of stable MTs (Tivodar et al., 2014) (**Figure 2B**). Growth cone shape is modulated by both MT polymerization that generates pushing forces on the plasma membrane and by acto-myosin network underlying pulling forces on the leading edge.

Actin undergoes polymerization and depolymerisation activity and acto-myosin contraction leads to the generation of an actin retrograde flow. The balance between these two networks will either allow growth or retraction of the leading process (Martini et al., 2009). Behind the leading edge, interactions between cell surface and migration substrate together with actin retrograde flow generate traction forces. Importantly, sectioning the leading tip or locally inhibiting acto-myosin contraction halts nucleokinesis, highlighting the role of this region in force generation (He et al., 2010). Actin cytoskeleton is regulated at the leading edge by Discl and cINs deficient for this protein accumulate less F-actin together with less phosphorylated Girders of Actin filaments (girdin) and Protein kinase B (Akt), crosslinkers of actin filaments (Steinecke et al., 2014a). Girdin targeting to to the leading tip requires interaction with Discl (Steinecke et al., 2014a). Mice mutant for *Discl* or *Lis1*, display decreased level of acetylation, a marker of stable MTs in the growth cone. This suggests that stable bundles of MTs are not properly entering this structure and are important to grant the proper shape to the growth cone (Gopal et al., 2010; Steinecke et al., 2014a) (**Figure 2B**).

cINs Migration Substrate

Adhesion to a migration substrate allows cINs to generate acto-myosin forces as well as to organize cellular polarization and directionality. cINs seem to use cell-cell interaction to migrate along bundles of fibers of the corticofugal system invading the GEs (Metin and Godement, 1996). TAG-1 or contactin-2, a member of the immunoglobulin superfamily expressed by the corticofugal axons was proposed to mediate cell-cell contact between migrating cINs and corticofugal fibers as inhibition of TAG-1 leads to a strong reduction of cIN migration *in vitro* (Denaxa et al., 2001). However, *in vivo* TAG-1 does not play a role during migration cINs (Denaxa et al., 2005). In cINs, proteins displaying a role in adhesion such as talin, paxilin or Focal Adhesion Kinases (FAKs) are also calpain substrates (Franco and Huttenlocher, 2005). Calpain inhibition reduces migration speed despite the increased levels of F-actin (Lysko et al., 2014), implying that local adhesion turnover by cleavage is primordial for correct migration. Finally, N-cadherin, a homophilic cell adhesion molecule has been shown to be necessary during tangential migration (Luccardini et al., 2013). N-cadherin not only promotes cINs motility *in vitro* and *in vivo,* likely by promoting adhesion through the acto-myosin cytoskeleton (Giannone et al., 2009) but also contributes to the polarity maintenance. N-cadherin inhibition unable the centrosome/Golgi apparatus to enter the swelling and contributes to local defects of Myosin II contraction at the nuclear rear (Luccardini et al., 2013). Cell adhesion molecules play a relevant role for cINs migration as they are at the interface between the extracellular environment and the cytoskeleton.

Migration of cINs: Extracellular Cues Guide cINs Movement

To allow proper directionality, integration of extracellular signaling is paramount. The extracellular cues are received by exploring the local environment thanks to stochastic branching of the leading process, and relevant cues are transduced at the level of cytoskeleton to grant the proper response of the cell: either extension of a new leading process is the right direction and/or retraction of existing branches (Britto et al., 2009). The first stage in which cINs are challenged by extracellular cues occurs within the GEs. During the differentiation process, newborn cINs need to be displaced from the VZ and SVZ and be driven toward the exit of the GEs. Two types of signaling drive the movement of cINs away from GEs. One has a chemo-repulsive effect to steer the cells in the good direction and the other stimulates cellular motility to enhance migration.

Chemo-Repulsion within the GEs

Regarding the mechanisms mediating repulsion of INs from GEs, similarities were found with general mechanisms implicated in axonal guidance. Using a paradigm of *in vitro* brain slice preparation, Ephrin-A5/EphA4R interaction was shown to be necessary to control the repulsion response of cINs. The guidance molecule Ephrin-A5 is abundant in the VZ and cINs express the Ephrin receptor EphA4 (EphA4R) (Zimmer et al., 2008). In absence of Ephrin-A5, cINs were found ectopically invading the VZ, a phenotype rescued when the slices were treated with recombinant Ephrin-A5 (Zimmer et al., 2008). EphA4R-mediated forward signaling is also used by cINs to avoid migration toward the ventral region of the subpallium (Zimmer et al., 2011) as it also binds Ephrin-B3 present in the MGE and POA. It is noteworthy that EphA4R also promotes cIN migration trough EphrinA2 reverse signaling (Steinecke et al., 2014b). EphA signaling is integrated at the cellular level to remodel the actin cytoskeleton and steer cells in the right direction. Although little is known about the intracellular cascades downstream EphA4 in cINs, it generally acts in neurons through regulation of RhoA to stimulate growth cone collapse (Wahl et al., 2000). Moreover, in cINs, Src family kinases (SFKs) have been implicated in this process. Indeed, SFK inhibition results in the loss of Ephrin-A5/EphA4 repulsion (Zimmer et al., 2008). In mouse, four redundant SFKs have been identified (Thomas and Brugge, 1997) and they have been linked to the phosphorylation of numerous targets. They control the Rho family GTPase (Kullander and Klein, 2002) and inactivate cortactin (Huang et al., 1997; Weaver et al., 2001) resulting in decreased activity of Arp 2/3, actin filament breakdown and growth cone collapse (Weed and Parsons, 2001). Slit/Robo is another signaling pathway mediating chemo-repulsion in GEs and cINs express Roundabout homolog 1 (Robo1) (Bagri et al., 2002; Marillat et al., 2002), a receptor recognizing the ligands Slit homolog 1 and 2 (Slit1 and 2). These ligands and Robo1 are found in a complementary expression pattern in the VZ (Marin et al., 2002), and it was first thought that Robo/Slit signaling was at play to push cINs away from the VZ. However, mice deficient for *Slit1/2* do not show cIN migration defects (Marin et al., 2003). Instead, the lack of Slit ligands or removal of *Robo1* leads to aberrant striatal invasion by cINs (Andrews et al., 2006; Hernandez-Miranda et al., 2011). This indicates that on the way toward the GEs exit, cINs face a second set of signaling molecules that refine their migratory routes through the LGE, and around the forming striatum. It was previously shown that the striatum is a strong repulsive structure for cINs thanks to the expression of class 3 semaphorins: Sema3A and Sema3F (Marin et al., 2001). The effect of semaphorins is mediated in cINs by neuropilin (Nrps) and Plexin receptors. Sema3A transduces signal specifically trough Nrp1 and PlexinA1 receptors (McKinsey et al., 2013) and Robo1 modulate semaphorin-neuropilin/plexin expression levels (Hernandez-Miranda et al., 2011). It is noteworthy that Nrp1 is present exclusively in cINs so that they respond to the repulsive signals secreted by the striatum. *Nrp1* expression depends on the transcription factor Sip1 involved in *Nkx2-1* down-regulation and *Nkx2-1* is a *Nrp1* repressor (McKinsey et al., 2013). On the contrary, striatal INs generated by the same progenitors as cINs, do not express Nrp1 as they maintain highs levels of *Nkx2*.1 (Marin et al., 2000; Butt et al., 2008; Nobrega-Pereira et al., 2008). Since the signaling pathway downstream of Sema3A is highly conserved, although not directly studied in cINs, it is anticipated that similar mechanisms are at play in these cells. Sema3A signaling regulates actin-dependent growth cone collapse trough RhoA, ROCK and LIM Kinase (LIMK) activation to eventually phosphorylate cofilin and inhibits F-actin turnover (Aizawa et al., 2001; Causeret et al., 2004). RhoA activation also leads to increased actin contractibility (Zhang et al., 2003). In the axon growth cone, a crosstalk between actin and MT cytoskeletons has been observed as retrograde F-actin flow on filopodia can displace distal position of MTs (Schaefer et al., 2002). Sema3A signaling could also directly regulate MT dynamics by inducing double phosphorylation of Collapsin Response Mediator Protein 2 (CRMP2) by Glycogen Synthase Kinase 3B (GSK3B) and Cyclin-dependent Kinase 5 (CdK5). The double phosphorylated state of CRMP2 reduces its tubulin affinity and overexpression of the phospho- mutant CRMP2 decreases Sema3A-induced growth cone collapse (Uchida et al., 2005).

Migration of cINs: Motogenic Factors

Newly produced cINs are stimulated by diffusible molecules to enhance movement and migration. A wide range of factors, including neurotrophins and neurotransmitters (NTs), were found to increase cINs motility *in vitro* (Heng et al., 2007). Demonstration came from experiments in which recombinant Brain Derived Neurotrophic Factor (BDNF) or Neurotrophin-4 (NT4) where applied to organotypic slice cultures (Polleux et al., 2002). BDNF- or NT4 effects are mediated by the Tyrosin Kinase B Receptor (TrkBR) (Polleux et al., 2002). Downstream signaling likely involves PI3K and the modulation of actin cytoskeleton. However this effect was observed *in vitro* but not in mouse mutant for *TrkB* where number and position of cINs are unchanged (Jones et al., 1994; Polleux et al., 2002; Sanchez-Huertas and Rico, 2011). *In vivo*, neurotrophin-mediated signaling promoting cINs motility was also linked to the action of Glial Cell-Derived Neurotrophic Factor (GDNF), binding and activating GDNF Family Receptor α1 (GFRα1). GDNF-mediated effects did not result from expression of Rearranged During Transfection (RET) or Neural Cell Adhesion Molecule (NCAM), two classical co-receptor signaling molecules (Pozas and Ibanez, 2005; Canty et al., 2009). The downstream signaling involves a matrix-bound form of GDNF and syndecan-3. This interaction then activates SFK to promote neurite outgrowth. GDNF may thus promote cell migration by acting on the actin cytoskeleton via SFK and cortactin pathway (Yoneda and Couchman, 2003; Bespalov et al., 2011). Since *GFRα1* mutant mice shows perturbations in cINs regionalization and subtype differentiation, GDNF might have additional functions beyond modulating cINs motility (Pozas and Ibanez, 2005; Canty et al., 2009). The hepatocyte growth factor/scatter factor (HGF/SF) and its receptor MET were also reported to have a potent motogenic action on cINs *in vitro*. Mutant mouse for the *urokinase-type plasminogen activator receptor* (*uPAR*) that cleaves and releases the active form of HGF/SF (Powell et al., 2001) or mutant mice for *MET* (Eagleson et al., 2011) shows a decreased number of cINs in the cortex. The cell-autonomous effect of HGF/SF-mediated signaling was later questioned since MET is not found to be expressed in cINs *in vivo* but is rather found in projection neurons and their axonal fibers (Eagleson et al., 2011). Several NTs/neuromodulators have also been implicated in cINs migration. Ambient GABA is found in high concentration in the MGE and in the cortical migration streams (Cuzon et al., 2006). cINs express $GABA_A$ and $GABA_B$ receptors and as a result of an inverted chloride gradient, they respond to GABA by membrane depolarization (Owens et al., 1999) that triggers opening of L-type voltage-sensitive Ca^{2+} channels and induces Ca^{2+} transients (Bortone and Polleux, 2009). Antagonizing $GABA_A$ receptor function prevents cINs from crossing the cortico-striatal barrier, leading to their accumulation at the pallial/subpallial boundary. Conversely, in experiments where exogenous GABA or diazepam are added to brain organotypic slices, a higher number of cINs were found exiting the GEs (Cuzon et al., 2006). Similarly, Glycine $\alpha 2$ receptor is also regulating cIN migration and in particular nucleokinesis by fine tuning acto-myosin II contraction (Avila et al., 2013). Activation of GlyRs by glycine leads to Ca^{2+} transients due to opening of voltage-gated Ca^{2+} channels and GlyRs $\alpha 2$ loss of function impairs cINs migration in the cortex. Glutamate signaling through AMPARs, located on the plasma membrane of migrating cINs also induces membrane depolarization and sodium influx (Metin et al., 2000; Manent et al., 2006). Blockade of AMPARs decreases cortical and hippocampal invasion by INs (Manent et al., 2006; Bortone and Polleux, 2009). Membrane depolarization and Ca^{2+} transients are thought to stimulate cINs motility as calmodulin bound to Ca^{2+} ions can interact and activate MLCK. In turn, MLCK phosphorylates Myosin Light chain II on serine 19 and promotes acto-myosin contraction (Metin et al., 2000; Bortone and Polleux, 2009). Another example is the motogenic effect mediated by dopamine. Ambient dopamine is secreted in the GEs and close to the lateral VZ by projecting thalamo-striatal axons in the neo-striatum. Dopamine receptors D_1 and D_2 are expressed by cINs and have opposite effects on migration (Ohtani et al., 2003). When selectively blocked, D_1R induces activation of D_2R and impedes migration. This indicates that D_1R has migration promoting action and conversely D_2R is rather a migration stop signal. Other ubiquitous signaling molecules such as adenosine have also been implicated in the modulation of cINs migration. However the underlying mechanisms are still unknown (Silva et al., 2013).

Migration of cINs: Chemo-Attraction Toward the Cortex

As cortical INs are steered away from the VZ/SVZ and around the striatum, they are simultaneously attracted toward the cortex by other molecules to cross the cortico-striatal junction and invade the pallium. Neuregulin-1 (Nrgl) is a strong attractant for cINs and can have both short and long-range effects depending on the isoform recruited. CRD-Nrgl, is membrane bound and acts on neighboring cells. It is mainly expressed by LGE cells and contributes to the formation of a permissive migration corridor for cINs. It is sensed by cINs as they probe their environment and inhibition of their branching behavior leads to a decreased ability to follow Nrg-1 gradient (Martini et al., 2009). The downstream signaling involves recruitment and activation of associated tyrosine kinases related to the epidermal growth factor (EGF) receptor ErbB4. Lg-Nrgl is a diffusible form expressed by the cortex that can act as a long-range attractant to guide cells toward the cortical regions as they exit the LGE. *In vivo*, the loss of either *Nrg-1* or *ErbB4* causes migration defects and reduces the number of INs in the cortex (Yau et al., 2003; Flames et al., 2004; Neddens and Buonanno, 2010). At the cellular level, the presence of a Nrg-1 gradient does not prompt cINs to reorient an existing branch but rather to sprout a new leading process in the direction and at an angle corresponding to highest concentration of the attractant. The signaling events downstream ErbB4 have not been completely characterized in cINs, but they seem to be ROCK-independent (Martini et al., 2009). Thanks to its tyrosine kinase activity, ErbB4 can activate several distinct signaling pathways including the ras/raf/MAPK or the PI3 kinase pathway (Scaltriti and Baselga, 2006). In ErbB4 can be cleaved in its intracellular domain and be targeted to the nucleus (Ni et al., 2001). Interestingly, ErbBs can also phosphorylate β-catenin and modulate Cadherin signaling pathways involved in actin cytoskeleton remodeling (Hazan and Norton, 1998; Behrens, 1999; Al Moustafa et al., 2002). Moreover, other signaling molecules participate to the attraction of cINs toward the cortex. For example, CXCL12 is secreted by proliferating cortical cells from SVZ and IZ and is an attractant molecule for migrating cINs (Tiveron et al., 2006; Stumm et al., 2007).

Migration of cINs: The Choice of the Migratory Route

Cortical invasion does not occur in a stochastic manner as cINs integrate and move in migratory streams. At earlier stages of cortical development, two streams can be identified in the pallium: one called intermediate zone (IZ) stream and located above the VZ/SVZ surface (Nadarajah et al., 2002) and the other positioned at the level of the marginal zone (MZ) and called MZ stream (Lavdas et al., 1999). Between E15 and E16, a third subplate (SP) stream forms between the IZ and MZ streams. Other routes have also been identified, for example a caudally directed stream arising from the CGE (Yozu et al., 2005). Although not depending on their birth place (MGE, CGE or POA), the choice of the migratory route by cINs does not seem to be random (Miyoshi and Fishell, 2011). Evidence comes from the observation that populations of cINs migrating along the different cortical streams do not show the same gene expression profile as revealed by microarray analysis on micro-dissected Gad67+ positive cells isolated from either IZ or MZ streams (Antypa et al., 2011). Some population-specific genes, such as Cdh8, Plxndl, Sema5a, Robo 1 and 2 or the reelin receptor Dabl, play key roles in neuronal migration.

Moreover *in vivo* experimental approaches have also shed light on intrinsic cellular component that are implicated in cINs sorting between the different migration routes. For example, it was found that mutations in the *Rb* gene unable cINs to enter the MZ stream and redirects them to the IZ stream (Ferguson et al., 2005). This effect is cell autonomous as suggested by cINs transplantation experiments made on wild-type organotypic brain slices. A similar phenotype was found to be linked to glycine receptor α2 subunit (Glyα2R), present on the plasma membrane of migrating cINs. Activation of Glyα2R opens voltage-gated Ca^{2+} channel (Avila et al., 2013). Extracellular cues seem to indeed play a relevant role in sorting cINs trough the different migration stream. Mutation of both Netrinl and α3β1 integrin, in the cells serving as migration substrate for cINs, gives rise to major migration defects in the MZ stream (Stanco et al., 2009). Finally GABA signaling, in addition to its migration promoting role, seems to be also implicated in the choice of the migratory route during cortical migration. Upon selective blockade of metabotropic $GABA_BR$, cINs where found to be displaced from the MZ and CP stream toward the VZ/SVZ compartments (Lopez-Bendito et al., 2003).

Migration of cINs: Molecular Regulation Controlling the Timing of Cortical Invasion

In the streams, tangentially migrating cINs do not invade the cortical plate (CP) and this process is coordinated with projection neurons migrating radially to form the cortical layers. Avoidance of the CP do not require repulsive cues coming from the projection neurons but rather the formation of a permissive corridor in the MZ and IZ thanks to chemokine signaling. CXCL12 is secreted by proliferating cortical cells from SVZ and IZ and it is a strong attractant molecule for migrating cINs (Daniel et al., 2005; Tiveron et al., 2006; Lopez-Bendito et al., 2008). Two receptors for this chemokine were identified in interneurons, CXCR4 and CXCR7 (Tiveron et al., 2006; Lopez-Bendito et al., 2008; Wang et al., 2011) and they signal through different downstream cascades. CXCR4 signals through Gα(i/o) while CXCR7 transduces independently on heterodymeric G proteins (Wang et al., 2011). In immature MGE neurons, CXCR7 acts as potent activator of MAP kinase signaling required for ERK1/2 phosphorylation (Wang et al., 2011). *Cxcr7* expression in the cortical plate expression follows a dorsoventral gradient, opposite to *Cxcl12* gradient in the SVZ. It was proposed that CXCR7 may lower the concentration of CXCL12 in the CP, generating a gradient from MZ and SVZ to the CP. A gradient of CXCL12 would be important for the regulation of cortical invasion (Wang et al., 2011). Indeed, disruption of CXCR4 or CXCR7 function results in premature exit of cINs from their migratory streams and perturbs their laminar and regional distribution within the neocortex (Li et al., 2008; Lopez-Bendito et al., 2008; Tanaka et al., 2010).

Integration OF cINs into Cortical Assemblies

Cortical neurogenesis generates a six-layered cortex and cortical neurons distribute within these layers in an age-dependent manner, deep layers being generated before upper layers. Neurons sharing the same layers exhibit similar patterns of connectivity (Dantzker and Callaway, 2000). The cortex is also organized vertically and cells sharing the same cortical column will be linked by extrinsic connectivity (Mountcastle, 1997). Interneurons have to integrate into cortical circuits in order to fit in these two patterns of organization. Two studies have shown that clonally related cINs are preferentially consigned to specific cortical layers or columns (Brown et al., 2011; Ciceri et al., 2013). cINs generated by clonally-related progenitors are however diverse as they express markers of distinct subtypes. Furthermore, cINs from the same cardinal class are able to form connections with a variety of synaptic partners (Kepecs and Fishell, 2014). From their birthdates, the first interneurons populating the cortex are generated in the MGE and express PV, SST or CR/SST (Butt et al., 2005; Wonders and Anderson, 2006). The second wave of cortical invasion generated by the CGE produces INs expressing VIP, CR/VIP, calbindin (CB) or choline acetyltransferase (ChAT) and NPY, (Yozu et al., 2004; Miyoshi et al., 2010). While pioneer cINs populate the cortex in an inside-out mode following the pattern of cortical integration of projection neurons (Miller, 1985; Fairen et al., 1986; Valcanis and Tan, 2003; Rymar and Sadikot, 2007), late-migrating cINs instead concentrate in supragranular layers, independently of their birthdate (Xu et al., 2004; Rymar and Sadikot, 2007; Miyoshi et al., 2010). Since the birthdate and birthplace are not general predictors of the final specification and lamination of cINs, the mechanisms determining the proper and site-specific integration of INs in the developing cortex need to be clarified. This raises the question whether intrinsic and/or extrinsic factors determine the cortical integration and lamination.

Intrinsic Factors Regulating cINs Integration into Cortical Layers

There is evidence that a maturational program exists and the behavior of cINs, at a given developmental stage, depends on their cellular age. In the cortical streams, cINs generated at different developmental stages co-exist and they exit the migratory streams at different time points even if the signaling regulating the exit from the streams is the same. Thus, cINs born earlier invade the cortical place before late-born interneurons (Lopez-Bendito et al., 2008). Further evidence supports this concept of intrinsic regulation. For example, it was found that the motility of interneurons in cortical slices gradually decreases as development proceeds and is almost abolished by the end of the first postnatal week (Inamura et al., 2012). Accordingly, late-born cINs transplanted in younger embryos settle in deep layers instead of occupying the expected superficial layers (Pla et al., 2006). The mechanisms explaining intrinsic regulation of neuronal migration remain elusive. It was suggested that the frequency of Ca^{2+} transients is reduced as the neuron completes its migratory program (Kumada and Komuro, 2004). Other studies proposed that the intrinsic regulation of motility might be linked to the expression of the potassium-chloride transporter KCC2. KCC2 could modulate cINs motility by reverting the chloride potential and thus reducing membrane depolarization upon $GABA_A$ receptor activation to serve as a stop signal for migration (Bortone and Polleux, 2009; Inamura et al., 2012). This is in agreement with the observation that cINs up-regulate KCC2 chloride transporter as soon as they exit the tangential mode of migration and start their radial sorting in the cortex (Miyoshi and Fishell, 2011). Cell autonomous regulation also contributes to the survival of interneurons as they invade the cortical plate. Transplantation experiments revealed that many cINs undergo programmed cell death *in vivo* between postnatal day (P) 7 and P11. When transplanted in older cortices, younger cINs die by apoptosis later than resident cINs (Southwell et al., 2012).

Extrinsic Factors Regulating cINs Integration into Cortical Layers

Regional distribution of cINs seems also depending on extrinsic signaling. Elegant studies suggested, in the last past years, that molecular cues released by projection neurons contribute to the establishment of the laminar distribution of cINs (Hevner et al., 2004; Pla et al., 2006; Yabut et al., 2007; Lodato et al., 2011b). The works from Hevner (Hevner et al., 2004), Pla (Pla et al., 2006), and Yabut (Yabut et al., 2007) using the *reeler* mouse model showed that cINs distribution within the cortex mostly results from the aberrant organization of cortical layers rather than the loss of reelin signaling transduction in cINs. The subsequent work from Lodato et al. (2011b) further support this hypothesis. *Fezf2* mutant mice lack sub-cerebral projection neurons, while all other projection neurons are normally produced. They show that *Fezf2* depletion does not impair cINs specification but rather the lack of subcerebral projection neurons non-autonomously impairs the proper distribution of SST, PV but not CR cINs subtype. Delayed overexpression of *Fezf2* in *Fezf2* null mice leads to the production of ectopically located clusters of subcerebral projection neurons. Many cINs invade these aggregates while the number of INs recruited depends on the size of the ectopic aggregates. Local excitatory and inhibitory signals may also influence the final positioning of INs (De Marco Garcia et al., 2011; Lyons et al., 2012; McKinsey et al., 2013). For example, it was shown that attenuating the activity of specific cIN populations affects the migration and morphologic development of cIN (De Marco Garcia et al., 2011). A number of activity-dependent genes specifically expressed by cINs have been identified. These include *Dlx1, Elmo1, and Mef2c.* Moreover the observation that voltage-gated Ca^{2+} influx may induce *de novo* gene expression opens the possibility that local activity might regulate direct region-specific differentiation and maturation of INs (De Marco Garcia et al., 2011; West and Greenberg, 2011). Additional evidence came from studies showing that MGE-derived interneurons are able to integrate in pathological neural circuits (Martinez-Cerdeno et al., 2010; Braz et al., 2012).

Conclusion

The recognition that many neurologic disorders such as schizophrenia, epilepsy and autism have components related to cIN development greatly prompted advances in this field. Postmortem analysis of the human brain and studies performed in primates strongly support the idea that human and primate cINs are produced in both dorsal and ventral regions (Fertuzinhos et al., 2009; Hansen et al., 2013; Ma et al., 2013). These studies have been instrumental to highlight the differences and similarities between in cINs generation across species, acknowledging more similarities than initially expected. These findings have given more credit to studies performed in rodents, designed to understand the genetic and molecular regulation underlying human pathology. For example, in the case of schizophrenia, *NRG1* and *ERB4* as well as DISC1 have been identified as susceptibility genes in human (Millar et al., 2000a,b; Corvin et al., 2004; Marin, 2012). Studies performed in rodents established a coherent outline of the biological causes of this human disease (Flames et al., 2004; Fazzari et al., 2010). How developmental perturbations of cINs lead to a specific brain disorder remains unclear although it has been proposed to depend, to some extent, on the cIN subtype affected (Marin, 2012). Thus, understanding the role of different classes of cINs and the neuro-circuitry they modulate will be relevant for unraveling the genetic causes of human diseases and to propose effective therapeutic approaches.

In the last decades, important advancements were made in the understanding of how INs are generated and function into networks. However, the fine regulation of cIN development might not be explained merely by genetic programs and extracellular signaling. Indeed, a fully new dimension of regulation, including post-transcriptional and post-translational modifications (PTMs) might be at play during corticogenesis. Post-transcriptional and PTMs can oppose or reinforce genetically-encoded and/or extrinsically-mediated signaling. A recent study explored the role of miRNA in distinct aspects of cINs development (Tuncdemir et al., 2014). In this study, *Dicer*, an enzyme required for miRNA processing and maturation was genetically deleted from MGE-derived cINs. Interestingly, the loss of miRNAs had no effect on cell proliferation and initiation of tangential migration but affected the transition from tangential to radial migration as well as modified the survival and maturation of cINs. Upon *Dicer* knockdown there was a precocious expression of cINs markers such as *SST, GAD65 and NPY* and at a later stage. MGE-derived cells failed to express markers of their subtype identity. PV-expressing cINs seem particularly affected by the absence of miRNAs. Furthermore, a different profile of gene expression related to differentiation, cellular interaction and survival was found in *Dicer* knockout mice. The role of miRNA signaling was also recently tested in a mouse model of schizophrenia and bipolar disorder (Toritsuka et al., 2013). This study showed a direct link between the 22q11 micro deletion and defects in cortical and hippocampal interneuron migration, relying on functional abnormalities in CXCR4/CXCL12 signaling. Mechanistically, Toritsuka et al. (2013) demonstrate the pivotal role of *DiGeorge syndrome critical region gene 8* (*Dgcr8*)-mediated in miR-200a regulation necessary for the maintenance of CXCR4 levels. PTMs occur in most proteins and often contribute to their functions and subcellular behaviors. Not many studies were developed to investigate the contribution of PTMs on brain development but there is evidence that they can regulate different aspects of cIN development. For example, it was demonstrated that acylation of SHH N-terminus changes its efficacy as a signaling molecule and greatly enhances its ability to ventralize early LGE progenitors (Kohtz et al., 2001). A C-terminal cholesterol modification has also been identified on SHH relevant for SHH tethering to the cell surface (Porter et al., 1996). At the functional level, these PTMs were showed to be primordial in determining SHH "short range" or "long range" function (Burke et al., 1999). Another example is the polysialylation of the neural cell adhesion molecule (PSA-NCAM), important to control the timing of the perisomatic GABAergic synapse maturation in the mouse cortex (Di Cristo et al., 2007). Di Cristo and colleagues showed that premature removal of PSA in the visual cortex resulted in precocious maturation of perisomatic innervation by PV basket cINs. Interestingly, polysialytransferases have been implicated in schizophrenia (Arai et al., 2006; Tao et al., 2007; Isomura et al., 2011). In light of this, it seems highly pertinent to pursue on understanding how genes, signaling molecules and environment communicate to shape brain development and function.

Acknowledgments

LN is a Research Associate and CG a postdoctoral fellow at the Belgian National Fund for Scientific Research (F.R.S-F.N.R.S.). EP is a postdoctoral fellow. LN is funded by grants from the F.R.S.-F.N.R.S., the Fonds Léon Fredericq, the Fondation Médicale Reine Elisabeth, and the Belgian Science Policy (IAP-VII network P7/20). LN and EP are funded by a grant from Actions de Recherche Concertée (ARC11/16-01). Some scientific projects in the Nguyen are funded by the Walloon excellence in lifesciences and biotechnology (WELBIO).

References

Aizawa, H., Wakatsuki, S., Ishii, A., Moriyama, K., Sasaki, Y., Ohashi, K., et al. (2001). Phosphorylation of cofilin by LIM-kinase is necessary for semaphorin 3A-induced growth cone collapse. *Nat. Neurosci.* 4, 367–373. doi: 10.1038/86011

Al Moustafa, A. E., Yen, L., Benlimame, N., and Alaoui-Jamali, M. A. (2002). Regulation of E-cadherin/catenin complex patterns by epidermal growth factor receptor modulation in human lung cancer cells. *Lung Cancer* 37, 49–56. doi: 10.1016/S0169-5002(02)00025-9

Amano, M., Ito, M., Kimura, K., Fukata, Y., Chihara, K., Nakano, T., et al. (1996). Phosphorylation and activation of myosin by Rho-associated kinase (Rho-kinase). *J. Biol. Chem.* 271, 20246–20249.

Anderson, S. A., Eisenstat, D. D., Shi, L., and Rubenstein, J. L. (1997). Interneuron migration from basal forebrain to neocortex: dependence on Dlx genes. *Science* 278, 474–476.

Andrews, W., Liapi, A., Plachez, C., Camurri, L., Zhang, J., Mori, S., et al. (2006). Robo1 regulates the development of major axon tracts and interneuron migration in the forebrain. *Development* 133, 2243–2252. doi: 10.1242/dev.02379

Antypa, M., Faux, C., Eichele, G., Parnavelas, J. G., and Andrews, W. D. (2011). Differential gene expression in migratory streams of cortical interneurons. *Eur. J. Neurosci.* 34, 1584–1594. doi: 10.1111/j.1460-9568.2011.07896.x

Aoto, K., Nishimura, T., Eto, K., and Motoyama, J. (2002). Mouse GLI3 regulates Fgf8 expression and apoptosis in the developing neural tube, face, and limb bud. *Dev. Biol.* 251, 320–332. doi: 10.1006/dbio.2002.0811

Arai, M., Yamada, K., Toyota, T., Obata, N., Haga, S., Yoshida, Y., et al. (2006). Association between polymorphisms in the promoter region of the sialyltransferase 8B (SIAT8B) gene and schizophrenia. *Biol. Psychiatry* 59, 652–659. doi: 10.1016/j.biopsych.2005.08.016

Avila, A., Vidal, P. M., Dear, T. N., Harvey, R. J., Rigo, J. M., and Nguyen, L. (2013). Glycine receptor alpha2 subunit activation promotes cortical interneuron migration. *Cell Rep.* 4, 738–750. doi: 10.1016/j.celrep.2013.07.016

Azim, E., Jabaudon, D., Fame, R. M., and Macklis, J. D. (2009). SOX6 controls dorsal progenitor identity and interneuron diversity during neocortical development. *Nat. Neurosci.* 12, 1238–1247. doi: 10.1038/nn.2387

Bagri, A., Marin, O., Plump, A. S., Mak, J., Pleasure, S. J., Rubenstein, J. L., et al. (2002). Slit proteins prevent midline crossing and determine the dorsoventral position of major axonal pathways in the mammalian forebrain. *Neuron* 33, 233–248. doi: 10.1016/S0896-6273(02)00561-5

Bai, C. B., Stephen, D., and Joyner, A. L. (2004). All mouse ventral spinal cord patterning by hedgehog is Gli dependent and involves an activator function of Gli3. *Dev. Cell* 6, 103–115. doi: 10.1016/S1534-5807(03)00394-0

Batista-Brito, R., Rossignol, E., Hjerling-Leffler, J., Denaxa, M., Wegner, M., Lefebvre, V., et al. (2009). The cell-intrinsic requirement of Sox6 for cortical interneuron development. *Neuron* 63, 466–481. doi: 10.1016/j.neuron.2009.08.005

Baudoin, J. P., Alvarez, C., Gaspar, P., and Metin, C. (2008). Nocodazole-induced changes in microtubule dynamics impair the morphology and directionality of migrating medial ganglionic eminence cells. *Dev. Neurosci.* 30, 132–143. doi: 10.1159/000109858

Baudoin, J. P., Viou, L., Launay, P. S., Luccardini, C., Espeso Gil, S., Kiyasova, V., et al. (2012). Tangentially migrating neurons assemble a primary cilium that promotes their reorientation to the cortical plate. *Neuron* 76, 1108–1122. doi: 10.1016/j.neuron.2012.10.027

Behrens, J. (1999). Cadherins and catenins: role in signal transduction and tumor progression. *Cancer Metastasis Rev.* 18, 15–30.

Bellion, A., and Metin, C. (2005). Early regionalisation of the neocortex and the medial ganglionic eminence. *Brain Res. Bull.* 66, 402–409. doi: 10.1016/j.brainresbull.2005.07.010

Bellion, A., Baudoin, J. P., Alvarez, C., Bornens, M., and Metin, C. (2005). Nucleokinesis in tangentially migrating neurons comprises two alternating phases: forward migration of the Golgi/centrosome associated with centrosome splitting and myosin contraction at the rear. *J. Neurosci.* 25, 5691–5699. doi: 10.1523/JNEUROSCI.1030-05.2005

Bespalov, M. M., Sidorova, Y. A., Tumova, S., Ahonen-Bishopp, A., Magalhaes, A. C., Kulesskiy, E., et al. (2011). Heparan sulfate proteoglycan syndecan-3 is a novel receptor for GDNF, neurturin, and artemin. *J. Cell Biol.* 192, 153–169. doi: 10.1083/jcb.201009136

Besson, A., Gurian-West, M., Schmidt, A., Hall, A., and Roberts, J. M. (2004). p27Kip1 modulates cell migration through the regulation of RhoA activation. *Genes Dev.* 18, 862–876. doi: 10.1101/gad.1185504

Blaess, S., Corrales, J. D., and Joyner, A. L. (2006). Sonic hedgehog regulates Gli activator and repressor functions with spatial and temporal precision in the mid/hindbrain region. *Development* 133, 1799–1809. doi: 10.1242/dev.02339

Borello, U., Cobos, I., Long, J. E., McWhirter, J. R., Murre, C., and Rubenstein, J. L. (2008). FGF15 promotes neurogenesis and opposes FGF8 function during neocortical development. *Neural Dev.* 3:17. doi: 10.1186/1749-8104-3-17

Bortone, D., and Polleux, F. (2009). KCC2 expression promotes the termination of cortical interneuron migration in a voltage-sensitive calcium-dependent manner. *Neuron* 62, 53–71. doi: 10.1016/j.neuron.2009.01.034

Braz, J. M., Sharif-Naeini, R., Vogt, D., Kriegstein, A., Alvarez-Buylla, A., Rubenstein, J. L., et al. (2012). Forebrain GABAergic neuron precursors integrate into adult spinal cord and reduce injury-induced neuropathic pain. *Neuron* 74, 663–675. doi: 10.1016/j.neuron.2012.02.033

Briscoe, J., and Ericson, J. (2001). Specification of neuronal fates in the ventral neural tube. *Curr. Opin. Neurobiol.* 11, 43–49. doi: 10.1016/S0959-4388(00)00172-0

Britto, J. M., Johnston, L. A., and Tan, S. S. (2009). The stochastic search dynamics of interneuron migration. *Biophys. J.* 97, 699–709. doi: 10.1016/j.bpj.2009.04.064

Brown, K. N., Chen, S., Han, Z., Lu, C. H., Tan, X., Zhang, X. J., et al. (2011). Clonal production and organization of inhibitory interneurons in the neocortex. *Science* 334, 480–486. doi: 10.1126/science.1208884

Burke, R., Nellen, D., Bellotto, M., Hafen, E., Senti, K. A., Dickson, B. J., et al. (1999). Dispatched, a novel sterol-sensing domain protein dedicated to the release of cholesterol-modified hedgehog from signaling cells. *Cell* 99, 803–815.

Butt, S. J., Fuccillo, M., Nery, S., Noctor, S., Kriegstein, A., Corbin, J. G., et al. (2005). The temporal and spatial origins of cortical interneurons predict their physiological subtype. *Neuron* 48, 591–604. doi: 10.1016/j.neuron.2005.09.034

Butt, S. J., Sousa, V. H., Fuccillo, M. V., Hjerling-Leffler, J., Miyoshi, G., Kimura, S., et al. (2008). The requirement of Nkx2-1 in the temporal specification of cortical interneuron subtypes. *Neuron* 59, 722–732. doi: 10.1016/j.neuron.2008.07.031

Cai, Y., Zhang, Q., Wang, C., Zhang, Y., Ma, T., Zhou, X., et al. (2013). Nuclear receptor COUP-TFII-expressing neocortical interneurons are derived from the medial and lateral/caudal ganglionic eminence and define specific subsets of mature interneurons. *J. Comp. Neurol.* 521, 479–497. doi: 10.1002/cne.23186

Cameron, H. A., Hazel, T. G., and McKay, R. D. (1998). Regulation of neurogenesis by growth factors and neurotransmitters. *J. Neurobiol.* 36, 287–306.

Canty, A. J., Dietze, J., Harvey, M., Enomoto, H., Milbrandt, J., and Ibanez, C. F. (2009). Regionalized loss of parvalbumin interneurons in the cerebral cortex of mice with deficits in GFRalpha1 signaling. *J. Neurosci.* 29, 10695–10705. doi: 10.1523/JNEUROSCI.2658-09.2009

Casarosa, S., Fode, C., and Guillemot, F. (1999). Mash1 regulates neurogenesis in the ventral telencephalon. *Development* 126, 525–534.

Causeret, F., Hidalgo-Sanchez, M., Fort, P., Backer, S., Popoff, M. R., Gauthier-Rouviere, C., et al. (2004). Distinct roles of Rac1/Cdc42 and Rho/Rock for axon outgrowth and nucleokinesis of precerebellar neurons toward netrin 1. *Development* 131, 2841–2852. doi: 10.1242/dev.01162

Chai, X., Forster, E., Zhao, S., Bock, H. H., and Frotscher, M. (2009a). Reelin acts as a stop signal for radially migrating neurons by inducing phosphorylation of n-cofilin at the leading edge. *Commun. Integr. Biol.* 2, 375–377. doi: 10.4161/cib.2.4.8614

Chai, X., Forster, E., Zhao, S., Bock, H. H., and Frotscher, M. (2009b). Reelin stabilizes the actin cytoskeleton of neuronal processes by inducing n-cofilin phosphorylation at serine3. *J. Neurosci.* 29, 288–299. doi: 10.1523/JNEUROSCI.2934-08.2009

Chrzanowska-Wodnicka, M., and Burridge, K. (1996). Rho-stimulated contractility drives the formation of stress fibers and focal adhesions. *J. Cell Biol.* 133, 1403–1415.

Ciceri, G., Dehorter, N., Sols, I., Huang, Z. J., Maravall, M., and Marin, O. (2013). Lineage-specific laminar organization of cortical GABAergic interneurons. *Nat. Neurosci.* 16, 1199–1210. doi: 10.1038/nn.3485

Cobos, I., Calcagnotto, M. E., Vilaythong, A. J., Thwin, M. T., Noebels, J. L., Baraban, S. C., et al. (2005). Mice lacking Dlx1 show subtype-specific loss of interneurons, reduced inhibition and epilepsy. *Nat. Neurosci.* 8, 1059–1068. doi: 10.1038/nn1499

Colombo, E., Collombat, P., Colasante, G., Bianchi, M., Long, J., Mansouri, A., et al. (2007). Inactivation of Arx, the murine ortholog of the X-linked lissencephaly with ambiguous genitalia gene, leads to severe disorganization of the ventral telencephalon with impaired neuronal migration and differentiation. *J. Neurosci.* 27, 4786–4798. doi: 10.1523/JNEUROSCI.0417-07.2007

Corvin, A., Nangle, J. M., and Gill, M. (2004). Schizophrenia susceptibility genes: recent discoveries and new challenges. *Ir. Med. J.* 97, 70–72.

Cuzon, V. C., Yeh, P. W., Cheng, Q., and Yeh, H. H. (2006). Ambient GABA promotes cortical entry of tangentially migrating cells derived from the medial ganglionic eminence. *Cereb. Cortex* 16, 1377–1388. doi: 10.1093/cercor/bhj084

Daniel, D., Rossel, M., Seki, T., and Konig, N. (2005). Stromal cell-derived factor-1 (SDF-1) expression in embryonic mouse cerebral cortex starts in the intermediate zone close to the pallial-subpallial boundary and extends progressively towards the cortical hem. *Gene Expr. Patterns* 5, 317–322. doi: 10.1016/j.modgep.2004.10.007

Dantzker, J. L., and Callaway, E. M. (2000). Laminar sources of synaptic input to cortical inhibitory interneurons and pyramidal neurons. *Nat. Neurosci.* 3, 701–707. doi: 10.1038/76656

De Marco Garcia, N. V., Karayannis, T., and Fishell, G. (2011). Neuronal activity is required for the development of specific cortical interneuron subtypes. *Nature* 472, 351–355. doi: 10.1038/nature09865

Denaxa, M., Chan, C. H., Schachner, M., Parnavelas, J. G., and Karagogeos, D. (2001). The adhesion molecule TAG-1 mediates the migration of cortical interneurons from the ganglionic eminence along the corticofugal fiber system. *Development* 128, 4635–4644.

Denaxa, M., Kyriakopoulou, K., Theodorakis, K., Trichas, G., Vidaki, M., Takeda, Y., et al. (2005). The adhesion molecule TAG-1 is required for proper migration of the superficial migratory stream in the medulla but not of cortical interneurons. *Dev. Biol.* 288, 87–99. doi: 10.1016/j.ydbio.2005.09.021

Di Cristo, G., Chattopadhyaya, B., Kuhlman, S. J., Fu, Y., Belanger, M. C., Wu, C. Z., et al. (2007). Activity-dependent PSA expression regulates inhibitory maturation and onset of critical period plasticity. *Nat. Neurosci.* 10, 1569–1577. doi: 10.1038/nn2008

Dobbertin, A., Gervais, A., Glowinski, J., and Mallat, M., (2000). Activation of ionotropic glutamate receptors reduces the production of transforming growth factor-beta2 by developing neurons. *Eur. J. Neurosci.* 12, 4589–4593. doi: 10.1046/j.0953-816X.2000.01354.x

Eagleson, K. L., Campbell, D. B., Thompson, B. L., Bergman, M. Y., and Levitt, P. (2011). The autism risk genes MET and PLAUR differentially impact cortical development. *Autism Res.* 4, 68–83. doi: 10.1002/aur.172

Echelard, Y., Epstein, D. J., St-Jacques, B., Shen, L., Mohler, J., McMahon, J. A., et al. (1993). Sonic hedgehog, a member of a family of putative signaling molecules, is implicated in the regulation of CNS polarity. *Cell* 75, 1417–1430.

Eisenstat, D. D., Liu, J. K., Mione, M., Zhong, W., Yu, G., Anderson, S. A., et al. (1999). DLX-1, DLX-2, and DLX-5 expression define distinct stages of basal forebrain differentiation. *J. Comp. Neurol.* 414, 217–237.

Fairen, A., Cobas, A., and Fonseca, M. (1986). Times of generation of glutamic acid decarboxylase immunoreactive neurons in mouse somatosensory cortex. *J. Comp. Neurol.* 251, 67–83. doi: 10.1002/cne.902510105

Fazzari, P., Paternain, A. V., Valiente, M., Pla, R., Lujan, R., Lloyd, K., et al. (2010). Control of cortical GABA circuitry development by Nrg1 and ErbB4 signalling. *Nature* 464, 1376–1380. doi: 10.1038/nature08928

Ferguson, K. L., McClellan, K. A., Vanderluit, J. L., McIntosh, W. C., Schuurmans, C., Polleux, F., et al. (2005). A cell-autonomous requirement for the cell cycle regulatory protein, Rb, in neuronal migration. *EMBO J.* 24, 4381–4391. doi: 10.1038/sj.emboj.7600887

Fertuzinhos, S., Krsnik, Z., Kawasawa, Y. I., Rasin, M. R., Kwan, K. Y., Chen, J. G., et al. (2009). Selective depletion of molecularly defined cortical interneurons in human holoprosencephaly with severe striatal hypoplasia. *Cereb. Cortex* 19, 2196–2207. doi: 10.1093/cercor/bhp009

Flames, N., Long, J. E., Garratt, A. N., Fischer, T. M., Gassmann, M., Birchmeier, C., et al. (2004). Short- and long-range attraction of cortical GABAergic interneurons by neuregulin-1. *Neuron* 44, 251–261. doi: 10.1016/j.neuron.2004.09.028

Flames, N., Pla, R., Gelman, D. M., Rubenstein, J. L., Puelles, L., and Marin, O. (2007). Delineation of multiple subpallial progenitor domains by the combinatorial expression of transcriptional codes. *J. Neurosci.* 27, 9682–9695. doi: 10.1523/JNEUROSCI.2750-07.2007

Flandin, P., Zhao, Y., Vogt, D., Jeong, J., Long, J., Potter, G., et al. (2011). Lhx6 and Lhx8 coordinately induce neuronal expression of Shh that controls the generation of interneuron progenitors. *Neuron* 70, 939–950. doi: 10.1016/j.neuron.2011.04.020

Fode, C., Ma, Q., Casarosa, S., Ang, S. L., Anderson, D. J., and Guillemot, F. (2000). A role for neural determination genes in specifying the dorsoventral identity of telencephalic neurons. *Genes Dev.* 14, 67–80. doi: 10.1101/gad.14.1.67

Fogarty, M., Grist, M., Gelman, D., Marin, O., Pachnis, V., and Kessaris, N. (2007). Spatial genetic patterning of the embryonic neuroepithelium generates GABAergic interneuron diversity in the adult cortex. *J. Neurosci.* 27, 10935–10946. doi: 10.1523/JNEUROSCI.1629-07.2007

Fragkouli, A., Hearn, C., Errington, M., Cooke, S., Grigoriou, M., and Bliss, T. (2005). Loss of forebrain cholinergic neurons and impairment in spatial learning and memory in LHX7-deficient mice. *Eur. J. Neurosci.* 21, 2923–2938. doi: 10.1111/j.1460-9568.2005.04141.x

Franco, S. J., and Huttenlocher, A. (2005). Regulating cell migration: calpains make the cut. *J. Cell Sci.* 118, 3829–3838. doi: 10.1242/jcs.02562

Friocourt, G., Liu, J. S., Antypa, M., Rakic, S., Walsh, C. A., and Parnavelas, J. G. (2007). Both doublecortin and doublecortin-like kinase play a role in cortical interneuron migration. *J. Neurosci.* 27, 3875–3883. doi: 10.1523/JNEUROSCI.4530-06.2007

Fuccillo, M., Rallu, M., McMahon, A. P., and Fishell, G. (2004). Temporal requirement for hedgehog signaling in ventral telencephalic patterning. *Development* 131, 5031–5040. doi: 10.1242/dev.01349

Gallagher, P. J., Herring, B. P., and Stull, J. T. (1997). Myosin light chain kinases. *J. Muscle Res. Cell Motil.* 18, 1–16.

Gelman, D. M., and Marin, O. (2010). Generation of interneuron diversity in the mouse cerebral cortex. *Eur. J. Neurosci.* 31, 2136–2141. doi: 10.1111/j.1460-9568.2010.07267.x

Gelman, D. M., Martini, F. J., Nobrega-Pereira, S., Pierani, A., Kessaris, N., and Marin, O. (2009). The embryonic preoptic area is a novel source of cortical GABAergic interneurons. *J. Neurosci.* 29, 9380–9389. doi: 10.1523/JNEUROSCI.0604-09.2009

Gelman, D., Griveau, A., Dehorter, N., Teissier, A., Varela, C., Pla, R., et al. (2011). A wide diversity of cortical GABAergic interneurons derives from the embryonic preoptic area. *J. Neurosci.* 31, 16570–16580. doi: 10.1523/JNEUROSCI.4068-11.2011

Giannone, G., Mege, R. M., and Thoumine, O. (2009). Multi-level molecular clutches in motile cell processes. *Trends Cell Biol.* 19, 475–486. doi: 10.1016/j.tcb.2009.07.001

Glickstein, S. B., Alexander, S., and Ross, M. E. (2007a). Differences in cyclin D2 and D1 protein expression distinguish forebrain progenitor subsets. *Cereb. Cortex* 17, 632–642. doi: 10.1093/cercor/bhk008

Glickstein, S. B., Moore, H., Slowinska, B., Racchumi, J., Suh, M., Chuhma, N., et al. (2007b). Selective cortical interneuron and GABA deficits in cyclin D2-null mice. *Development* 134, 4083–4093. doi: 10.1242/dev.008524

Glickstein, S. B., Monaghan, J. A., Koeller, H. B., Jones, T. K., and Ross, M. E. (2009). Cyclin D2 is critical for intermediate progenitor cell proliferation in the embryonic cortex. *J. Neurosci.* 29, 9614–9624. doi: 10.1523/JNEUROSCI.2284-09.2009

Godin, J. D., Thomas, N., Laguesse, S., Malinouskaya, L., Close, P., Malaise, O., et al. (2012). p27(Kip1) is a microtubule-associated protein that promotes microtubule polymerization during neuron migration. *Dev. Cell* 23, 729–744. doi: 10.1016/j.devcel.2012.08.006

Gopal, P. P., Simonet, J. C., Shapiro, W., and Golden, J. A. (2010). Leading process branch instability in Lis1+/- nonradially migrating interneurons. *Cereb. Cortex* 20, 1497–1505. doi: 10.1093/cercor/bhp211

Govek, E. E., Hatten, M. E., and Van Aelst, L. (2011). The role of Rho GTPase proteins in CNS neuronal migration. *Dev. Neurobiol.* 71, 528–553. doi: 10.1002/dneu.20850

Gutin, G., Fernandes, M., Palazzolo, L., Paek, H., Yu, K., Ornitz, D. M., et al. (2006). FGF signalling generates ventral telencephalic cells independently of SHH. *Development* 133, 2937–2946. doi: 10.1242/dev.02465

Hansen, D. V., Lui, J. H., Flandin, P., Yoshikawa, K., Rubenstein, J. L., Alvarez-Buylla, A., et al. (2013). Non-epithelial stem cells and cortical interneuron production in the human ganglionic eminences. *Nat. Neurosci.* 16, 1576–1587. doi: 10.1038/nn.3541

Haydar, T. F., Wang, F., Schwartz, M. L., and Rakic, P. (2000). Differential modulation of proliferation in the neocortical ventricular and subventricular zones. *J. Neurosci.* 20, 5764–5774.

Hazan, R. B., and Norton, L. (1998). The epidermal growth factor receptor modulates the interaction of E-cadherin with the actin cytoskeleton. *J. Biol. Chem.* 273, 9078–9084.

He, M., Zhang, Z. H., Guan, C. B., Xia, D., and Yuan, X. B. (2010). Leading tip drives soma translocation via forward F-actin flow during neuronal migration. *J. Neurosci.* 30, 10885–10898. doi: 10.1523/JNEUROSCI.0240-10.2010

Heasman, S. J., and Ridley, A. J. (2008). Mammalian Rho GTPases: new insights into their functions from *in vivo* studies. *Nat. Rev. Mol. Cell Biol.* 9, 690–701. doi: 10.1038/nrm2476

Hebert, J. M., and Fishell, G. (2008). The genetics of early telencephalon patterning: some assembly required. *Nat. Rev. Neurosci.* 9, 678–685. doi: 10.1038/nrn2463

Heng, J. I., Moonen, G., and Nguyen, L. (2007). Neurotransmitters regulate cell migration in the telencephalon. *Eur. J. Neurosci.* 26, 537–546. doi: 10.1111/j.1460-9568.2007.05694.x

Hernandez-Miranda, L. R., Cariboni, A., Faux, C., Ruhrberg, C., Cho, J. H., Cloutier, J. F., et al. (2011). Robo1 regulates semaphorin signaling to guide the migration of cortical interneurons through the ventral forebrain. *J. Neurosci.* 31, 6174–6187. doi: 10.1523/JNEUROSCI.5464-10.2011

Hevner, R. F., Daza, R. A., Englund, C., Kohtz, J., and Fink, A. (2004). Postnatal shifts of interneuron position in the neocortex of normal and reeler mice: evidence for inward radial migration. *Neuroscience* 124, 605–618. doi: 10.1016/j.neuroscience.2003.11.033

Higashida, C., Miyoshi, T., Fujita, A., Oceguera-Yanez, F., Monypenny, J., Andou, Y., et al. (2004). Actin polymerization-driven molecular movement of mDia1 in living cells. *Science* 303, 2007–2010. doi: 10.1126/science.1093923

Higginbotham, H. R., and Gleeson, J. G. (2007). The centrosome in neuronal development. *Trends Neurosci.* 30, 276–283. doi: 10.1016/j.tins.2007.04.001

Horton, S., Meredith, A., Richardson, J. A., and Johnson, J. E. (1999). Correct coordination of neuronal differentiation events in ventral forebrain requires the bHLH factor MASH1. *Mol. Cell. Neurosci.* 14, 355–369. doi: 10.1006/mcne.1999.0791

Huang, C., Ni, Y., Wang, T., Gao, Y., Haudenschild, C. C., and Zhan, X. (1997). Down-regulation of the filamentous actin cross-linking activity of cortactin by Src-mediated tyrosine phosphorylation. *J. Biol. Chem.* 272, 13911–13915.

Inamura, N., Kimura, T., Tada, S., Kurahashi, T., Yanagida, M., Yanagawa, Y., et al. (2012). Intrinsic and extrinsic mechanisms control the termination of cortical interneuron migration. *J. Neurosci.* 32, 6032–6042. doi: 10.1523/JNEUROSCI.3446-11.2012

Ingham, P. W., and McMahon, A. (2001). P. Hedgehog signaling in animal development: paradigms and principles. *Genes Dev.* 15, 3059–3087. doi: 10.1101/gad.938601

Ishizaki, T., Naito, M., Fujisawa, K., Maekawa, M., Watanabe, N., Saito, Y., et al. (1997). p160ROCK, a Rho-associated coiled-coil forming protein kinase, works downstream of Rho and induces focal adhesions. *FEBS Lett.* 404, 118–124.

Isomura, R., Kitajima, K., and Sato, C. (2011). Structural and functional impairments of polysialic acid by a mutated polysialyltransferase found in schizophrenia. *J. Biol. Chem.* 286, 21535–21545. doi: 10.1074/jbc.M111.221143

Jessell, T. M. (2000). Neuronal specification in the spinal cord: inductive signals and transcriptional codes. *Nat. Rev. Genet.* 1, 20–29. doi: 10.1038/35049541

Jones, K. R., Farinas, I., Backus, C., and Reichardt, L. F. (1994). Targeted disruption of the BDNF gene perturbs brain and sensory neuron development but not motor neuron development. *Cell* 76, 989–999.

Kappeler, C., Saillour, Y., Baudoin, J. P., Tuy, F. P., Alvarez, C., Houbron, C., et al. (2006). Branching and nucleokinesis defects in migrating interneurons derived from doublecortin knockout mice. *Hum. Mol. Genet.* 15, 1387–1400. doi: 10.1093/hmg/ddl062

Kawauchi, T., Chihama, K., Nabeshima, Y., and Hoshino, M. (2006). Cdk5 phosphorylates and stabilizes p27kip1 contributing to actin organization and cortical neuronal migration. *Nat. Cell Biol.* 8, 17–26. doi: 10.1038/ncb1338

Kenney, A. M., and Rowitch, D. H. (2000). Sonic hedgehog promotes G(1) cyclin expression and sustained cell cycle progression in mammalian neuronal precursors. *Mol. Cell. Biol.* 20, 9055–9067. doi: 10.1128/MCB.20.23.9055-9067.2000

Kenney, A. M., Cole, M. D., and Rowitch, D. H. (2003). Nmyc upregulation by sonic hedgehog signaling promotes proliferation in developing cerebellar granule neuron precursors. *Development* 130, 15–28. doi: 10.1242/dev.00182

Kenney, A. M., Widlund, H. R., and Rowitch, D. H. (2004). Hedgehog and PI-3 kinase signaling converge on Nmyc1 to promote cell cycle progression in cerebellar neuronal precursors. *Development* 131, 217–228. doi: 10.1242/dev.00891

Kepecs, A., and Fishell, G. (2014). Interneuron cell types are fit to function. *Nature* 505, 318–326. doi: 10.1038/nature12983

Kimura, K., Ito, M., Amano, M., Chihara, K., Fukata, Y., Nakafuku, M., et al. (1996). Regulation of myosin phosphatase by Rho and Rho-associated kinase (Rho-kinase). *Science* 273, 245–248.

Kohtz, J. D., Lee, H. Y., Gaiano, N., Segal, J., Ng, E., Larson, T., et al. (2001). N-terminal fatty-acylation of sonic hedgehog enhances the induction of rodent ventral forebrain neurons. *Development* 128, 2351–2363.

Kullander, K., and Klein, R. (2002). Mechanisms and functions of Eph and ephrin signalling. *Nat. Rev. Mol. Cell Biol.* 3, 475–486. doi: 10.1038/nrm856

Kumada, T., and Komuro, H. (2004). Completion of neuronal migration regulated by loss of Ca(2+) transients. *Proc. Natl. Acad. Sci. U.S.A.* 101, 8479–8484. doi: 10.1073/pnas.0401000101

Kuschel, S., Ruther, U., and Theil, T. (2003). A disrupted balance between Bmp/Wnt and Fgf signaling underlies the ventralization of the Gli3 mutant telencephalon. *Dev. Biol.* 260, 484–495. doi: 10.1016/S0012-1606(03)00252-5

Laurie, D. J., Wisden, W., and Seeburg, P. H. (1992). The distribution of thirteen GABAA receptor subunit mRNAs in the rat brain. III. Embryonic and postnatal development. *J. Neurosci.* 12, 4151–4172.

Lavdas, A. A., Grigoriou, M., Pachnis, V., and Parnavelas, J. G. (1999). The medial ganglionic eminence gives rise to a population of early neurons in the developing cerebral cortex. *J. Neurosci.* 19, 7881–7888.

Li, G., Adesnik, H., Li, J., Long, J., Nicoll, R. A., Rubenstein, J. L., et al. (2008). Regional distribution of cortical interneurons and development of inhibitory tone are regulated by Cxcl12/Cxcr4 signaling. *J. Neurosci.* 28, 1085–1098. doi: 10.1523/JNEUROSCI.4602-07.2008

Liodis, P., Denaxa, M., Grigoriou, M., Akufo-Addo, C., Yanagawa, Y., and Pachnis, V. (2007). Lhx6 activity is required for the normal migration and specification of cortical interneuron subtypes. *J. Neurosci.* 27, 3078–3089. doi: 10.1523/JNEUROSCI.3055-06.2007

Liu, J. K., Ghattas, I., Liu, S., Chen, S., and Rubenstein, J. L. (1997). Dlx genes encode DNA-binding proteins that are expressed in an overlapping and sequential pattern during basal ganglia differentiation. *Dev. Dyn.* 210, 498–512. doi: 10.1002/(SICI)1097-0177(199712)210:4<498::AID-AJA12>3.0.CO;2-3

Lodato, S., Tomassy, G. S., De Leonibus, E., Uzcategui, Y. G., Andolfi, G., Armentano, M., et al. (2011a). Loss of COUP-TFI alters the balance between caudal ganglionic eminence- and medial ganglionic eminence-derived cortical interneurons and results in resistance to epilepsy. *J. Neurosci.* 31, 4650–4662. doi: 10.1523/JNEUROSCI.6580-10.2011

Lodato, S., Rouaux, C., Quast, K. B., Jantrachotechatchawan, C., Studer, M., Hensch, T. K., et al. (2011b). Excitatory projection neuron subtypes control the distribution of local inhibitory interneurons in the cerebral cortex. *Neuron* 69, 763–779. doi: 10.1016/j.neuron.2011.01.015

Long, J. E., Cobos, I., Potter, G. B., and Rubenstein, J. L. (2009a). Dlx1&2 and Mash1 transcription factors control MGE and CGE patterning and differentiation through parallel and overlapping pathways. *Cereb. Cortex* 19(Suppl. 1), i96–i106. doi: 10.1093/cercor/bhp045

Long, J. E., Swan, C., Liang, W. S., Cobos, I., Potter, G. B., and Rubenstein, J. L. (2009b). Dlx1&2 and Mash1 transcription factors control striatal patterning and differentiation through parallel and overlapping pathways. *J. Comp. Neurol.* 512, 556–572. doi: 10.1002/cne.21854

Lopez-Bendito, G., Lujan, R., Shigemoto, R., Ganter, P., Paulsen, O., and Molnar, Z. (2003). Blockade of GABA(B) receptors alters the tangential migration of cortical neurons. *Cereb. Cortex* 13, 932–942. doi: 10.1093/cercor/13.9.932

Lopez-Bendito, G., Sanchez-Alcaniz, J. A., Pla, R., Borrell, V., Pico, E., Valdeolmillos, M., et al. (2008). Chemokine signaling controls intracortical migration and final distribution of GABAergic interneurons. *J. Neurosci.* 28, 1613–1624. doi: 10.1523/JNEUROSCI.4651-07.2008

LoTurco, J. J., Owens, D. F., Heath, M. J., Davis, M. B., and Kriegstein, A. R. (1995). GABA and glutamate depolarize cortical progenitor cells and inhibit DNA synthesis. *Neuron* 15, 1287–1298.

Luccardini, C., Hennekinne, L., Viou, L., Yanagida, M., Murakami, F., Kessaris, N., et al. (2013). N-cadherin sustains motility and polarity of future cortical interneurons during tangential migration. *J. Neurosci.* 33, 18149–18160. doi: 10.1523/JNEUROSCI.0593-13.2013

Luk, K. C., Kennedy, T. E., and Sadikot, A. F. (2003). Glutamate promotes proliferation of striatal neuronal progenitors by an NMDA receptor-mediated mechanism. *J. Neurosci.* 23, 2239–2250.

Lukaszewicz, A., Savatier, P., Cortay, V., Kennedy, H., and Dehay, C. (2002). Contrasting effects of basic fibroblast growth factor and neurotrophin 3 on cell cycle kinetics of mouse cortical stem cells. *J. Neurosci.* 22, 6610–6622.

Lyons, M. R., Schwarz, C. M., and West, A. E. (2012). Members of the myocyte enhancer factor 2 transcription factor family differentially regulate Bdnf transcription in response to neuronal depolarization. *J. Neurosci.* 32, 12780–12785. doi: 10.1523/JNEUROSCI.0534-12.2012

Lysko, D. E., Putt, M., and Golden, J. A. (2014). SDF1 reduces interneuron leading process branching through dual regulation of actin and microtubules. *J. Neurosci.* 34, 4941–4962. doi: 10.1523/JNEUROSCI.4351-12.2014

Ma, W., and Barker, J. L. (1995). Complementary expressions of transcripts encoding GAD67 and GABAA receptor alpha 4, beta 1, and gamma 1 subunits in the proliferative zone of the embryonic rat central nervous system. *J. Neurosci.* 15, 2547–2560.

Ma, T., Zhang, Q., Cai, Y., You, Y., Rubenstein, J. L., and Yang, Z. (2012). A subpopulation of dorsal lateral/caudal ganglionic eminence-derived neocortical interneurons expresses the transcription factor Sp8. *Cereb. Cortex* 22, 2120–2130. doi: 10.1093/cercor/bhr296

Ma, T., Wang, C., Wang, L., Zhou, X., Tian, M., Zhang, Q., et al. (2013). Subcortical origins of human and monkey neocortical interneurons. *Nat. Neurosci.* 16, 1588–1597. doi: 10.1038/nn.3536

Manent, J. B., Jorquera, I., Ben-Ari, Y., Aniksztejn, L., and Represa, A. (2006). Glutamate acting on AMPA but not NMDA receptors modulates the migration of hippocampal interneurons. *J. Neurosci.* 26, 5901–5909. doi: 10.1523/JNEUROSCI.1033-06.2006

Maric, D., Liu, Q. Y., Maric, I., Chaudry, S., Chang, Y. H., Smith, S. V., et al. (2001). GABA expression dominates neuronal lineage progression in the embryonic rat neocortex and facilitates neurite outgrowth via GABA(A) autoreceptor/Cl- channels. *J. Neurosci.* 21, 2343–2360.

Marillat, V., Cases, O., Nguyen-Ba-Charvet, K. T., Tessier-Lavigne, M., Sotelo, C., and Chedotal, A. (2002). Spatiotemporal expression patterns of slit and robo genes in the rat brain. *J. Comp. Neurol.* 442, 130–155. doi: 10.1002/cne.10068

Marin, O. (2012). Interneuron dysfunction in psychiatric disorders. *Nat. Rev. Neurosci.* 13, 107–120. doi: 10.1038/nrn3155

Marin, O., Anderson, S. A., and Rubenstein, J. L. (2000). Origin and molecular specification of striatal interneurons. *J. Neurosci.* 20, 6063–6076.

Marin, O., Yaron, A., Bagri, A., Tessier-Lavigne, M., and Rubenstein, J. L. (2001). Sorting of striatal and cortical interneurons regulated by semaphorin-neuropilin interactions. *Science* 293, 872–875. doi: 10.1126/science.1061891

Marin, O., Baker, J., Puelles, L., and Rubenstein, J. L. (2002). Patterning of the basal telencephalon and hypothalamus is essential for guidance of cortical projections. *Development* 129, 761–773.

Marin, O., Plump, A. S., Flames, N., Sanchez-Camacho, C., Tessier-Lavigne, M., and Rubenstein, J. L. (2003). Directional guidance of interneuron migration to the cerebral cortex relies on subcortical Slit1/2-independent repulsion and cortical attraction. *Development* 130, 1889–1901. doi: 10.1242/dev.00417

Martinez-Cerdeno, V., Noctor, S. C., Espinosa, A., Ariza, J., Parker, P., Orasji, S., et al. (2010). Embryonic MGE precursor cells grafted into adult rat striatum integrate and ameliorate motor symptoms in 6-OHDA-lesioned rats. *Cell Stem Cell* 6, 238–250. doi: 10.1016/j.stem.2010.01.004

Martini, F. J., and Valdeolmillos, M. (2010). Actomyosin contraction at the cell rear drives nuclear translocation in migrating cortical interneurons. *J. Neurosci.* 30, 8660–8670. doi: 10.1523/JNEUROSCI.1962-10.2010

Martini, F. J., Valiente, M., Lopez Bendito, G., Szabo, G., Moya, F., Valdeolmillos, M., et al. (2009). Biased selection of leading process branches mediates chemotaxis during tangential neuronal migration. *Development* 136, 41–50. doi: 10.1242/dev.025502

Martynoga, B., Morrison, H., Price, D. J., and Mason, J. O. (2005). Foxg1 is required for specification of ventral telencephalon and region-specific regulation of dorsal telencephalic precursor proliferation and apoptosis. *Dev. Biol.* 283, 113–127. doi: 10.1016/j.ydbio.2005.04.005

McKinsey, G. L., Lindtner, S., Trzcinski, B., Visel, A., Pennacchio, L. A., Huylebroeck, D., et al. (2013). Dlx1&2-dependent expression of Zfhx1b (Sip1, Zeb2) regulates the fate switch between cortical and striatal interneurons. *Neuron* 77, 83–98. doi: 10.1016/j.neuron.2012.11.035

McManus, M. F., Nasrallah, I. M., Pancoast, M. M., Wynshaw-Boris, A., and Golden, J. A. (2004). Lis1 is necessary for normal non-radial migration of inhibitory interneurons. *Am. J. Pathol.* 165, 775–784. doi: 10.1016/S0002-9440(10)63340-8

Metin, C., and Godement, P. (1996). The ganglionic eminence may be an intermediate target for corticofugal and thalamocortical axons. *J. Neurosci.* 16, 3219–3235.

Metin, C., Denizot, J. P., and Ropert, N. (2000). Intermediate zone cells express calcium-permeable AMPA receptors and establish close contact with growing axons. *J. Neurosci.* 20, 696–708.

Metin, C., Baudoin, J. P., Rakic, S., and Parnavelas, J. G. (2006). Cell and molecular mechanisms involved in the migration of cortical interneurons. *Eur. J. Neurosci.* 23, 894–900. doi: 10.1111/j.1460-9568.2006.04630.x

Millar, J. K., Christie, S., Semple, C. A., and Porteous, D. J. (2000a). Chromosomal location and genomic structure of the human translin-associated factor X gene (TRAX; TSNAX) revealed by intergenic splicing to DISC1, a gene disrupted by a translocation segregating with schizophrenia. *Genomics* 67, 69–77. doi: 10.1006/geno.2000.6239

Millar, J. K., Wilson-Annan, J. C., Anderson, S., Christie, S., Taylor, M. S., Semple, C. A., et al. (2000b). Disruption of two novel genes by a translocation co-segregating with schizophrenia. *Hum. Mol. Genet.* 9, 1415–1423. doi: 10.1093/hmg/9.9.1415

Miller, M. W. (1985). Cogeneration of retrogradely labeled corticocortical projection and GABA-immunoreactive local circuit neurons in cerebral cortex. *Brain Res.* 355, 187–192.

Miyoshi, G., and Fishell, G. (2011). GABAergic interneuron lineages selectively sort into specific cortical layers during early postnatal development. *Cereb. Cortex* 21, 845–852. doi: 10.1093/cercor/bhq155

Miyoshi, G., Hjerling-Leffler, J., Karayannis, T., Sousa, V. H., Butt, S. J., Battiste, J., et al. (2010). Genetic fate mapping reveals that the caudal ganglionic eminence produces a large and diverse population of superficial cortical interneurons. *J. Neurosci.* 30, 1582–1594. doi: 10.1523/JNEUROSCI.4515-09.2010

Mountcastle, V. B. (1997). The columnar organization of the neocortex. *Brain* 120(Pt 4), 701–722.

Nadarajah, B., Alifragis, P., Wong, R. O., and Parnavelas, J. G. (2002). Ventricle-directed migration in the developing cerebral cortex. *Nat. Neurosci.* 5, 218–224. doi: 10.1038/nn813

Nasrallah, I. M., McManus, M. F., Pancoast, M. M., Wynshaw-Boris, A., and Golden, J. A. (2006). Analysis of non-radial interneuron migration dynamics and its disruption in Lis1+/- mice. *J. Comp. Neurol.* 496, 847–858. doi: 10.1002/cne.20966

Neddens, J., and Buonanno, A. (2010). Selective populations of hippocampal interneurons express ErbB4 and their number and distribution is altered in ErbB4 knockout mice. *Hippocampus* 20, 724–744. doi: 10.1002/hipo.20675

Nguyen, L., Rigo, J. M., Rocher, V., Belachew, S., Malgrange, B., Rogister, B., et al. (2001). Neurotransmitters as early signals for central nervous system development. *Cell Tissue Res.* 305, 187–202. doi: 10.1007/s004410000343

Nguyen, L., Besson, A., Heng, J. I., Schuurmans, C., Teboul, L., Parras, C., et al. (2006). p27kip1 independently promotes neuronal differentiation and migration in the cerebral cortex. *Genes Dev.* 20, 1511–1524. doi: 10.1101/gad.377106

Ni, C. Y., Murphy, M. P., Golde, T. E., and Carpenter, G. (2001). gamma -Secretase cleavage and nuclear localization of ErbB-4 receptor tyrosine kinase. *Science* 294, 2179–2181. doi: 10.1126/science.1065412

Nobrega-Pereira, S., Kessaris, N., Du, T., Kimura, S., Anderson, S. A., and Marin, O. (2008). Postmitotic Nkx2-1 controls the migration of telencephalic interneurons by direct repression of guidance receptors. *Neuron* 59, 733–745. doi: 10.1016/j.neuron.2008.07.024

Ohkubo, Y., Chiang, C., and Rubenstein, J. L. (2002). Coordinate regulation and synergistic actions of BMP4, SHH and FGF8 in the rostral prosencephalon regulate morphogenesis of the telencephalic and optic vesicles. *Neuroscience* 111, 1–17. doi: 10.1016/S0306-4522(01)00616-9

Ohtani, N., Goto, T., Waeber, C., and Bhide, P. G. (2003). Dopamine modulates cell cycle in the lateral ganglionic eminence. *J. Neurosci.* 23, 2840–2850.

Oliver, T. G., Grasfeder, L. L., Carroll, A. L., Kaiser, C., Gillingham, C. L., Lin, S. M., et al. (2003). Transcriptional profiling of the Sonic hedgehog response: a critical role for N-myc in proliferation of neuronal precursors. *Proc. Natl. Acad. Sci. U.S.A.* 100, 7331–7336. doi: 10.1073/pnas.0832317100

Owens, D. F., and Kriegstein, A. R. (2002a). Is there more to GABA than synaptic inhibition? *Nat. Rev. Neurosci.* 3, 715–727. doi: 10.1038/nrn919

Owens, D. F., and Kriegstein, A. R. (2002b). Developmental neurotransmitters? *Neuron* 36, 989–991. doi: 10.1016/S0896-6273(02)01136-4

Owens, D. F., Liu, X., and Kriegstein, A. R. (1999). Changing properties of GABA(A) receptor-mediated signaling during early neocortical development. *J. Neurophysiol.* 82, 570–583.

Pan, Y., Bai, C. B., Joyner, A. L., and Wang, B. (2006). Sonic hedgehog signaling regulates Gli2 transcriptional activity by suppressing its processing and degradation. *Mol. Cell. Biol.* 26, 3365–3377. doi: 10.1128/MCB.26.9.3365-3377.2006

Parras, C. M., Hunt, C., Sugimori, M., Nakafuku, M., Rowitch, D., and Guillemot, F. (2007). The proneural gene Mash1 specifies an early population of telencephalic oligodendrocytes. *J. Neurosci.* 27, 4233–4242. doi: 10.1523/JNEUROSCI.0126-07.2007

Pei, Z., Wang, B., Chen, G., Nagao, M., Nakafuku, M., and Campbell, K. (2011). Homeobox genes Gsx1 and Gsx2 differentially regulate telencephalic progenitor maturation. *Proc. Natl. Acad. Sci. U.S.A.* 108, 1675–1680. doi: 10.1073/pnas.1008824108

Petilla Interneuron Nomenclature, G., Ascoli, G. A., Alonso-Nanclares, L., Anderson, S. A., Barrionuevo, G., Benavides-Piccione, R., et al. (2008). Petilla terminology: nomenclature of features of GABAergic interneurons of the cerebral cortex. *Nat. Rev. Neurosci.* 9, 557–568. doi: 10.1038/nrn2402

Petryniak, M. A., Potter, G. B., Rowitch, D. H., and Rubenstein, J. L. (2007). Dlx1 and Dlx2 control neuronal versus oligodendroglial cell fate acquisition in the developing forebrain. *Neuron* 55, 417–433. doi: 10.1016/j.neuron.2007.06.036

Pilz, G. A., Shitamukai, A., Reillo, I., Pacary, E., Schwausch, J., Stahl, R., et al. (2013). Amplification of progenitors in the mammalian telencephalon includes a new radial glial cell type. *Nat. Commun.* 4:2125. doi: 10.1038/ncomms3125

Pla, R., Borrell, V., Flames, N., and Marin, O. (2006). Layer acquisition by cortical GABAergic interneurons is independent of Reelin signaling. *J. Neurosci.* 26, 6924–6934. doi: 10.1523/JNEUROSCI.0245-06.2006

Pleasure, S. J., Anderson, S., Hevner, R., Bagri, A., Marin, O., Lowenstein, D. H., et al. (2000). Cell migration from the ganglionic eminences is required for the development of hippocampal GABAergic interneurons. *Neuron* 28, 727–740. doi: 10.1016/S0896-6273(00)00149-5

Poitras, L., Ghanem, N., Hatch, G., and Ekker, M. (2007). The proneural determinant MASH1 regulates forebrain Dlx1/2 expression through the I12b intergenic enhancer. *Development* 134, 1755–1765. doi: 10.1242/dev.02845

Polleux, F., Whitford, K. L., Dijkhuizen, P. A., Vitalis, T., and Ghosh, A. (2002). Control of cortical interneuron migration by neurotrophins and PI3-kinase signaling. *Development* 129, 3147–3160.

Porter, J. A., Young, K. E., and Beachy, P. A. (1996). Cholesterol modification of hedgehog signaling proteins in animal development. *Science* 274, 255–259.

Powell, E. M., Mars, W. M., and Levitt, P. (2001). Hepatocyte growth factor/scatter factor is a motogen for interneurons migrating from the ventral to dorsal telencephalon. *Neuron* 30, 79–89. doi: 10.1016/S0896-6273(01)00264-1

Pozas, E., and Ibanez, C. F. (2005). GDNF and GFRalpha1 promote differentiation and tangential migration of cortical GABAergic neurons. *Neuron* 45, 701–713. doi: 10.1016/j.neuron.2005.01.043

Rallu, M., Machold, R., Gaiano, N., Corbin, J. G., McMahon, A. P., and Fishell, G. (2002). Dorsoventral patterning is established in the telencephalon of mutants lacking both Gli3 and Hedgehog signaling. *Development* 129, 4963–4974.

Rash, B. G., and Grove, E. A. (2007). Patterning the dorsal telencephalon: a role for sonic hedgehog? *J. Neurosci.* 27, 11595–11603. doi: 10.1523/JNEUROSCI.3204-07.2007

Ross, M. E. (2011). Cell cycle regulation and interneuron production. *Dev. Neurobiol.* 71, 2–9. doi: 10.1002/dneu.20823

Rowitch, D. H., S-Jacques, B., Lee, S. M., Flax, J. D., Snyder, E. Y., and McMahon, A. P. (1999). Sonic hedgehog regulates proliferation and inhibits differentiation of CNS precursor cells. *J. Neurosci.* 19, 8954–8965.

Rubin, A. N., Alfonsi, F., Humphreys, M. P., Choi, C. K., Rocha, S. F., and Kessaris, N. (2010). The germinal zones of the basal ganglia but not the septum generate GABAergic interneurons for the cortex. *J. Neurosci.* 30, 12050–12062. doi: 10.1523/JNEUROSCI.6178-09.2010

Ruzhynsky, V. A., McClellan, K. A., Vanderluit, J. L., Jeong, Y., Furimsky, M., Park, D. S., et al. (2007). Cell cycle regulator E2F4 is essential for the development of the ventral telencephalon. *J. Neurosci.* 27, 5926–5935. doi: 10.1523/JNEUROSCI.1538-07.2007

Rymar, V. V., and Sadikot, A. F. (2007). Laminar fate of cortical GABAergic interneurons is dependent on both birthdate and phenotype. *J. Comp. Neurol.* 501, 369–380. doi: 10.1002/cne.21250

Sadikot, A. F., Burhan, A. M., Belanger, M. C., and Sasseville, R. (1998). NMDA receptor antagonists influence early development of GABAergic interneurons in the mammalian striatum. *Brain Res. Dev. Brain Res.* 105, 35–42.

Sanchez-Huertas, C., and Rico, B. (2011). CREB-Dependent Regulation of GAD65 Transcription by BDNF/TrkB in Cortical Interneurons. *Cereb. Cortex* 21, 777–788. doi: 10.1093/cercor/bhq150

Scaltriti, M., and Baselga, J. (2006). The epidermal growth factor receptor pathway: a model for targeted therapy. *Clin. Cancer Res.* 12, 5268–5272. doi: 10.1158/1078-0432.CCR-05-1554

Schaar, B. T., and McConnell, S. K. (2005). Cytoskeletal coordination during neuronal migration. *Proc. Natl. Acad. Sci. U.S.A.* 102, 13652–13657. doi: 10.1073/pnas.0506008102

Schaefer, A. W., Kabir, N., and Forscher, P. (2002). Filopodia and actin arcs guide the assembly and transport of two populations of microtubules with unique dynamic parameters in neuronal growth cones. *J. Cell Biol.* 158, 139–152. doi: 10.1083/jcb.200203038

Sheth, A. N., and Bhide, P. G. (1997). Concurrent cellular output from two proliferative populations in the early embryonic mouse corpus striatum. *J. Comp. Neurol.* 383, 220–230.

Shimamura, K., Hartigan, D. J., Martinez, S., Puelles, L., and Rubenstein, J. L. (1995). Longitudinal organization of the anterior neural plate and neural tube. *Development* 121, 3923–3933.

Shinohara, R., Thumkeo, D., Kamijo, H., Kaneko, N., Sawamoto, K., Watanabe, K., et al. (2012). A role for mDia, a Rho-regulated actin nucleator, in tangential migration of interneuron precursors. *Nat. Neurosci.* 15, 373–380, S371–S372. doi: 10.1038/nn.3020

Silva, C. G., Metin, C., Fazeli, W., Machado, N. J., Darmopil, S., Launay, P. S., et al. (2013). Adenosine receptor antagonists including caffeine alter fetal brain development in mice. *Sci. Transl. Med.* 5:197ra104. doi: 10.1126/scitranslmed.3006258

Sjostrom, S. K., Finn, G., Hahn, W. C., Rowitch, D. H., and Kenney, A. M. (2005). The Cdk1 complex plays a prime role in regulating N-myc phosphorylation and turnover in neural precursors. *Dev. Cell* 9, 327–338. doi: 10.1016/j.devcel.2005.07.014

Smart, I. H. (1976). A pilot study of cell production by the ganglionic eminences of the developing mouse brain. *J. Anat.* 121, 71–84.

Smith, K. M., Maragnoli, M. E., Phull, P. M., Tran, K. M., Choubey, L., and Vaccarino, F. M. (2014). Fgfr1 inactivation in the mouse telencephalon results in impaired maturation of interneurons expressing parvalbumin. *PLoS ONE* 9:e103696. doi: 10.1371/journal.pone.0103696

Southwell, D. G., Paredes, M. F., Galvao, R. P., Jones, D. L., Froemke, R. C., Sebe, J. Y., et al. (2012). Intrinsically determined cell death of developing cortical interneurons. *Nature* 491, 109–113. doi: 10.1038/nature11523

Spillane, M., Ketschek, A., Jones, S. L., Korobova, F., Marsick, B., Lanier, L., et al. (2011). The actin nucleating Arp2/3 complex contributes to the formation of axonal filopodia and branches through the regulation of actin patch precursors to filopodia. *Dev. Neurobiol.* 71, 747–758. doi: 10.1002/dneu.20907

Spoelgen, R., Hammes, A., Anzenberger, U., Zechner, D., Andersen, O. M., Jerchow, B., et al. (2005). LRP2/megalin is required for patterning of the ventral telencephalon. *Development* 132, 405–414. doi: 10.1242/dev.01580

Stanco, A., Szekeres, C., Patel, N., Rao, S., Campbell, K., Kreidberg, J. A., et al. (2009). Netrin-1-alpha3beta1 integrin interactions regulate the migration of interneurons through the cortical marginal zone. *Proc. Natl. Acad. Sci. U.S.A.* 106, 7595–7600. doi: 10.1073/pnas.0811343106

Steinecke, A., Gampe, C., Nitzsche, F., and Bolz, J. (2014a). DISC1 knockdown impairs the tangential migration of cortical interneurons by affecting the actin cytoskeleton. *Front. Cell. Neurosci.* 8:190. doi: 10.3389/fncel.2014.00190

Steinecke, A., Gampe, C., Zimmer, G., Rudolph, J., and Bolz, J. (2014b). EphA/ephrin A reverse signaling promotes the migration of cortical interneurons from the medial ganglionic eminence. *Development* 141, 460–471. doi: 10.1242/dev.101691

Storm, E. E., Garel, S., Borello, U., Hebert, J. M., Martinez, S., McConnell, S. K., et al. (2006). Dose-dependent functions of Fgf8 in regulating telencephalic patterning centers. *Development* 133, 1831–1844. doi: 10.1242/dev.02324

Stumm, R., Kolodziej, A., Schulz, S., Kohtz, J. D., and Hollt, V. (2007). Patterns of SDF-1alpha and SDF-1gamma mRNAs, migration pathways, and phenotypes of CXCR4-expressing neurons in the developing rat telencephalon. *J. Comp. Neurol.* 502, 382–399. doi: 10.1002/cne.21336

Sussel, L., Marin, O., Kimura, S., and Rubenstein, J. L. (1999). Loss of Nkx2.1 homeobox gene function results in a ventral to dorsal molecular respecification within the basal telencephalon: evidence for a transformation of the pallidum into the striatum. *Development* 126, 3359–3370.

Tanaka, T., Serneo, F. F., Higgins, C., Gambello, M. J., Wynshaw-Boris, A., and Gleeson, J. G. (2004). Lis1 and doublecortin function with dynein to mediate coupling of the nucleus to the centrosome in neuronal migration. *J. Cell Biol.* 165, 709–721. doi: 10.1083/jcb.200309025

Tanaka, D. H., Mikami, S., Nagasawa, T., Miyazaki, J., Nakajima, K., and Murakami, F. (2010). CXCR4 is required for proper regional and laminar distribution of cortical somatostatin-, calretinin-, and neuropeptide Y-expressing GABAergic interneurons. *Cereb. Cortex* 20, 2810–2817. doi: 10.1093/cercor/bhq027

Tao, R., Li, C., Zheng, Y., Qin, W., Zhang, J., Li, X., et al. (2007). Positive association between SIAT8B and schizophrenia in the Chinese Han population. *Schizophr. Res.* 90, 108–114. doi: 10.1016/j.schres.2006.09.029

Theil, T., Dominguez-Frutos, E., and Schimmang, T. (2008). Differential requirements for Fgf3 and Fgf8 during mouse forebrain development. *Dev. Dyn.* 237, 3417–3423. doi: 10.1002/dvdy.21765

Thomas, S. M., and Brugge, J. S. (1997). Cellular functions regulated by Src family kinases. *Annu. Rev. Cell Dev. Biol.* 13, 513–609. doi: 10.1146/annurev.cellbio.13.1.513

Tiveron, M. C., Rossel, M., Moepps, B., Zhang, Y. L., Seidenfaden, R., Favor, J., et al. (2006). Molecular interaction between projection neuron precursors and invading interneurons via stromal-derived factor 1 (CXCL12)/CXCR4 signaling in the cortical subventricular zone/intermediate zone. *J. Neurosci.* 26, 13273–13278. doi: 10.1523/JNEUROSCI.4162-06.2006

Tivodar, S., Kalemaki, K., Kounoupa, Z., Vidaki, M., Theodorakis, K., Denaxa, M., et al. (2014). Rac-GTPases regulate microtubule stability and axon growth of cortical GABAergic interneurons. *Cereb. Cortex.* doi: 10.1093/cercor/bhu037. [Epub ahead of print].

Toritsuka, M., Kimoto, S., Muraki, K., Landek-Salgado, M. A., Yoshida, A., Yamamoto, N., et al. (2013). Deficits in microRNA-mediated Cxcr4/Cxcl12 signaling in neurodevelopmental deficits in a 22q11 deletion syndrome mouse model. *Proc. Natl. Acad. Sci. U.S.A.* 110, 17552–17557. doi: 10.1073/pnas.1312661110

Trimarchi, J. M., and Lees, J. A. (2002). Sibling rivalry in the E2F family. *Nat. Rev. Mol. Cell Biol.* 3, 11–20. doi: 10.1038/nrm714

Tsai, J. W., Bremner, K. H., and Vallee, R. B. (2007). Dual subcellular roles for LIS1 and dynein in radial neuronal migration in live brain tissue. *Nat. Neurosci.* 10, 970–979. doi: 10.1038/nn1934

Tuncdemir, S. N., Fishell, G., and Batista-Brito, R. (2014). miRNAs are essential for the survival and maturation of cortical interneurons. *Cereb. Cortex.* doi: 10.1093/cercor/bht426. [Epub ahead of print].

Uchida, Y., Ohshima, T., Sasaki, Y., Suzuki, H., Yanai, S., Yamashita, N., et al. (2005). Semaphorin3A signalling is mediated via sequential Cdk5 and GSK3beta phosphorylation of CRMP2: implication of common phosphorylating mechanism underlying axon guidance and Alzheimer's disease. *Genes Cells* 10, 165–179. doi: 10.1111/j.1365-2443.2005.00827.x

Valcanis, H., and Tan, S. S. (2003). Layer specification of transplanted interneurons in developing mouse neocortex. *J. Neurosci.* 23, 5113–5122.

Vidaki, M., Tivodar, S., Doulgeraki, K., Tybulewicz, V., Kessaris, N., Pachnis, V., et al. (2012). Rac1-dependent cell cycle exit of MGE precursors and GABAergic interneuron migration to the cortex. *Cereb. Cortex* 22, 680–692. doi: 10.1093/cercor/bhr145

Wahl, S., Barth, H., Ciossek, T., Aktories, K., and Mueller, B. K. (2000). Ephrin-A5 induces collapse of growth cones by activating Rho and Rho kinase. *J. Cell Biol.* 149, 263–270.

Wang, Y., Dye, C. A., Sohal, V., Long, J. E., Estrada, R. C., Roztocil, T., et al. (2010). Dlx5 and Dlx6 regulate the development of parvalbumin-expressing cortical interneurons. *J. Neurosci.* 30, 5334–5345. doi: 10.1523/JNEUROSCI.5963-09.2010

Wang, Y., Li, G., Stanco, A., Long, J. E., Crawford, D., Potter, G. B., et al. (2011). CXCR4 and CXCR7 have distinct functions in regulating interneuron migration. *Neuron* 69, 61–76. doi: 10.1016/j.neuron.2010.12.005

Weaver, A. M., Karginov, A. V., Kinley, A. W., Weed, S. A., Li, Y., Parsons, J. T., et al. (2001). Cortactin promotes and stabilizes Arp2/3-induced actin filament network formation. *Curr. Biol.* 11, 370–374.

Weed, S. A., and Parsons, J. T. (2001). Cortactin: coupling membrane dynamics to cortical actin assembly. *Oncogene* 20, 6418–6434. doi: 10.1038/sj.onc.1204783

West, A. E., and Greenberg, M. E. (2011). Neuronal activity-regulated gene transcription in synapse development and cognitive function. *Cold Spring Harb Perspect Biol* 3. doi: 10.1101/cshperspect.a005744

Wonders, C. P., and Anderson, S. A. (2006). The origin and specification of cortical interneurons. *Nat. Rev. Neurosci.* 7, 687–696. doi: 10.1038/nrn1954

Wonders, C. P., Taylor, L., Welagen, J., Mbata, I. C., Xiang, J. Z., and Anderson, S. A. (2008). A spatial bias for the origins of interneuron subgroups within the medial ganglionic eminence. *Dev. Biol.* 314, 127–136. doi: 10.1016/j.ydbio.2007.11.018

Xu, Q., Cobos, I., De La Cruz, E., Rubenstein, J. L., and Anderson, S. A. (2004). Origins of cortical interneuron subtypes. *J. Neurosci.* 24, 2612–2622. doi: 10.1523/JNEUROSCI.5667-03.2004

Xu, Q., Tam, M., and Anderson, S. A. (2008). Fate mapping Nkx2.1-lineage cells in the mouse telencephalon. *J. Comp. Neurol.* 506, 16–29. doi: 10.1002/cne.21529

Xu, Q., Guo, L., Moore, H., Waclaw, R. R., Campbell, K., and Anderson, S. A. (2010). Sonic hedgehog signaling confers ventral telencephalic progenitors with distinct cortical interneuron fates. *Neuron* 65, 328–340. doi: 10.1016/j.neuron.2010.01.004

Yabut, O., Renfro, A., Niu, S., Swann, J. W., Marin, O., and D'Arcangelo, G. (2007). Abnormal laminar position and dendrite development of interneurons in the reeler forebrain. *Brain Res.* 1140, 75–83. doi: 10.1016/j.brainres.2005.09.070

Yau, H. J., Wang, H. F., Lai, C., and Liu, F. C. (2003). Neural development of the neuregulin receptor ErbB4 in the cerebral cortex and the hippocampus: preferential expression by interneurons tangentially migrating from the ganglionic eminences. *Cereb. Cortex* 13, 252–264.

Yoneda, A., and Couchman, J. R. (2003). Regulation of cytoskeletal organization by syndecan transmembrane proteoglycans. *Matrix Biol.* 22, 25–33.

Yozu, M., Tabata, H., and Nakajima, K. (2004). Birth-date dependent alignment of GABAergic neurons occurs in a different pattern from that of non-GABAergic neurons in the developing mouse visual cortex. *Neurosci. Res.* 49, 395–403. doi: 10.1016/j.neures.2004.05.005

Yozu, M., Tabata, H., and Nakajima, K. (2005). The caudal migratory stream: a novel migratory stream of interneurons derived from the caudal ganglionic eminence in the developing mouse forebrain. *J. Neurosci.* 25, 7268–7277. doi: 10.1523/JNEUROSCI.2072-05.2005

Yun, K., Fischman, S., Johnson, J., Hrabe de Angelis, M., Weinmaster, G., and Rubenstein, J. L. (2002). Modulation of the notch signaling by Mash1 and Dlx1/2 regulates sequential specification and differentiation of progenitor cell types in the subcortical telencephalon. *Development* 129, 5029–5040.

Yun, K., Garel, S., Fischman, S., and Rubenstein, J. L. (2003). Patterning of the lateral ganglionic eminence by the Gsh1 and Gsh2 homeobox genes regulates striatal and olfactory bulb histogenesis and the growth of axons through the basal ganglia. *J. Comp. Neurol.* 461, 151–165. doi: 10.1002/cne.10685

Zhang, X. F., Schaefer, A. W., Burnette, D. T., Schoonderwoert, V. T., and Forscher, P. (2003). Rho-dependent contractile responses in the neuronal growth cone are independent of classical peripheral retrograde actin flow. *Neuron* 40, 931–944.

Zhang, W., Kang, J. S., Cole, F., Yi, M. J., and Krauss, R. S. (2006). Cdo functions at multiple points in the Sonic Hedgehog pathway, and Cdo-deficient mice accurately model human holoprosencephaly. *Dev. Cell* 10, 657–665. doi: 10.1016/j.devcel.2006.04.005

Zhao, Y., Marin, O., Hermesz, E., Powell, A., Flames, N., Palkovits, M., et al. (2003). The LIM-homeobox gene Lhx8 is required for the development of many cholinergic neurons in the mouse forebrain. *Proc. Natl. Acad. Sci. U.S.A.* 100, 9005–9010. doi: 10.1073/pnas.1537759100

Zhao, Y., Flandin, P., Long, J. E., Cuesta, M. D., Westphal, H., and Rubenstein, J. L. (2008). Distinct molecular pathways for development of telencephalic interneuron subtypes revealed through analysis of Lhx6 mutants. *J. Comp. Neurol.* 510, 79–99. doi: 10.1002/cne.21772

Zimmer, G., Garcez, P., Rudolph, J., Niehage, R., Weth, F., Lent, R., et al. (2008). Ephrin-A5 acts as a repulsive cue for migrating cortical interneurons. *Eur. J. Neurosci.* 28, 62–73. doi: 10.1111/j.1460-9568.2008.06320.x

Zimmer, G., Rudolph, J., Landmann, J., Gerstmann, K., Steinecke, A., Gampe, C., et al. (2011). Bidirectional ephrinB3/EphA4 signaling mediates the segregation of medial ganglionic eminence- and preoptic area-derived interneurons in the deep and superficial migratory stream. *J. Neurosci.* 31, 18364–18380. doi: 10.1523/JNEUROSCI.4690-11.2011

2

MCPH1: A Window into Brain Development and Evolution

Jeremy N. Pulvers[1]*, Nathalie Journiac*[2,3]*, Yoko Arai*[4] *and Jeannette Nardelli*[2,3]*

[1] Sydney Medical Program, University of Sydney, Sydney, Australia, [2] U1141 Inserm, Paris, France, [3] Université Paris Diderot, Sorbonne Paris Cité, UMRS 1141, Paris, France, [4] Institut Jacques Monod, CNRS UMR 7592, Université Paris Diderot, Sorbonne Paris Cité, Paris, France

Correspondence:
Jeannette Nardelli, U1141 Inserm, Hôpital Robert Debré, 48 Blvd Sérurier, 75019 Paris, France

The development of the mammalian cerebral cortex involves a series of mechanisms: from patterning, progenitor cell proliferation and differentiation, to neuronal migration. Many factors influence the development of the cerebral cortex to its normal size and neuronal composition. Of these, the mechanisms that influence the proliferation and differentiation of neural progenitor cells are of particular interest, as they may have the greatest consequence on brain size, not only during development but also in evolution. In this context, causative genes of human autosomal recessive primary microcephaly, such as *ASPM* and *MCPH1*, are attractive candidates, as many of them show positive selection during primate evolution. *MCPH1* causes microcephaly in mice and humans and is involved in a diverse array of molecular functions beyond brain development, including DNA repair and chromosome condensation. Positive selection of *MCPH1* in the primate lineage has led to much insight and discussion of its role in brain size evolution. In this review, we will present an overview of *MCPH1* from these multiple angles, and whilst its specific role in brain size regulation during development and evolution remain elusive, the pieces of the puzzle will be discussed with the aim of putting together the full picture of this fascinating gene.

Keywords: MCPH1, microcephaly, brain development, brain evolution, mouse models, human

Introduction: *MCPH1* in Brain Development and Evolution

The study of mammalian neurogenesis and cortical development stands at a fascinating intersection between neuroscience, cell biology, developmental biology, genetics, and evolutionary biology (Molnár et al., 2014; Paridaen and Huttner, 2014; Sun and Hevner, 2014). The studies of the genes that cause autosomal recessive primary microcephaly (MCPH) are exemplary of this exciting synthesis of research fields (Woods et al., 2005; Kaindl et al., 2010; Gilmore and Walsh, 2013). One of the causative genes of this condition, *MCPH1* (syn. *BRIT1*, *Microcephalin*), plays a role in brain development (Jackson et al., 1998, 2002), DNA damage repair (Xu et al., 2004; Lin et al., 2005; Peng et al., 2009), chromosome condensation (Neitzel et al., 2002; Trimborn et al., 2004; Yamashita et al., 2011), cancer (Chaplet et al., 2006; Rai et al., 2006; Richardson et al., 2011), germline function (Liang et al., 2010), and has also provided insights into brain evolution (Evans et al., 2004, 2005; Wang and Su, 2004; Ponting and Jackson, 2005). Many unanswered questions remain on this multifaceted gene, such as how the lack of *MCPH1* leads to microcephaly, its molecular mechanisms in neurogenesis, and the key question of its role in the evolution of brain size.

The development of the cerebral cortex begins with formation and patterning of the neural tube (Lumsden and Krumlauf, 1996; Rubenstein et al., 1998; Copp et al., 2003), which is followed by the amplification of neuroepithelial cells, the primary neural progenitor cells, and their subsequent differentiation into downstream progenitors and neurons, or "neurogenesis" (Götz and Huttner, 2005; Paridaen and Huttner, 2014; Sun and Hevner, 2014). A constellation of processes follows to form a fully developed cerebral cortex, including neuronal migration (Sidman and Rakic, 1973; Nadarajah and Parnavelas, 2002; Marín and Rubenstein, 2003), axon guidance (Tessier-Lavigne and Goodman, 1996; Dickson, 2002) and synaptogenesis (Garner et al., 2002; Waites et al., 2005). In the context of brain development and evolution, the embryonic development of the mammalian cerebral cortex (neocortex) is the subject of prime interest, being the seat of higher brain functions, and has powerful implications for primate and human evolution (Rakic, 2009; Clowry et al., 2010).

Investigations into cortical malformations give profound insight into not only developmental and molecular mechanisms, but also provide a platform to investigate the evolution of brain size and function (Walsh, 1999; Mochida and Walsh, 2001; Sun and Hevner, 2014). Amongst these conditions, congenital microcephaly of genetic etiology is of particular interest, as they allow the dissection of fundamental molecular and developmental mechanisms. Interestingly, these mechanisms may be affected in congenital microcephaly linked to environmental intrauterine insults, such as viral infections (Cheeran et al., 2009), alcohol, or other extrinsic cues, exemplified by the finding that *Mcph1*, the mouse ortholog of human *MCPH1*, was shown to be down-regulated in a mouse model of microcephaly induced by early embryonic exposure to a VIP (vasoactive intestinal peptide) antagonist (Passemard et al., 2011). *MCPH1* may be a common denominator in the pathway causing microcephaly, encompassing the spectrum of both environmental and genetic forms of microcephaly. Therefore, given its implication in diverse molecular and cellular mechanisms during brain development, investigating *MCPH1* function is of particular interest. Here, an overview of the key issues relating to the function of *MCPH1* in brain development and evolution will be reviewed.

Autosomal Recessive Primary Microcephaly (MCPH)

Microcephaly is the clinical finding of a small brain, typically measured by head circumference (HC), compared to the population mean values of the age, sex, and ethnicity of the individual (Woods, 2004; Kaindl et al., 2010; Woods and Parker, 2013). HC, or more specifically occipito-frontal circumference (OFC) is commonly used as a surrogate measure of brain size (Woods et al., 2005); head size being a readily measurable approximation of brain size, and thus the terms microcephaly (small head) and microencephaly (small brain) are generally interchangeable (Gilmore and Walsh, 2013). An OFC of three standard deviations below the age- and sex-matched means (<−3 SD) is commonly accepted as a clinical definition of microcephaly (Woods and Parker, 2013). Furthermore, microcephaly is subdivided into primary and secondary microcephaly (Qazi and Reed, 1973). Primary microcephaly (microcephaly *vera*) is generally defined as being present at birth, with no obvious abnormalities other than gross brain size (Mochida and Walsh, 2001), and has a variety of genetic and non-genetic causes such as infections (Woods and Parker, 2013), prenatal radiation exposure (Plummer, 1952; Wood et al., 1967), and prenatal alcohol exposure (Ouellette et al., 1977; Spohr et al., 1993). Secondary microcephaly is generally defined as manifesting after birth (Woods and Parker, 2013). From the perspective of investigating brain development, the distinction between primary and secondary microcephaly is key, as primary microcephaly is likely to be related to neurogenesis, and secondary microcephaly may involve any of the downstream processes post-neurogenesis (Woods, 2004; Woods et al., 2005). Furthermore, microcephaly of genetic etiology, or autosomal recessive primary microcephaly, allows the detailed dissection of the relevant molecular mechanisms. The pathological defect in primary microcephaly is likely to fall temporally within the neurogenic interval and spatially within the neural progenitor cell compartment, making it ideal for the investigation of the regulation of brain size. However, in this context it is important to note that neuronal death due to alterations in diverse aspects of neuronal differentiation (including but not limited to neuronal migration and maturation) cannot be excluded, and may also account for the decrease in brain size seen in primary microcephaly. The main challenge in this regard is to determine how the alteration of these different processes at multiple stages of cortical development, ultimately impacts the final brain size.

Autosomal recessive primary microcephaly (MCPH) is a genetically heterogeneous condition (Mochida and Walsh, 2001), with 12 or more causative genes identified, all of which produce a clinically indistinguishable phenotype. The loci are numbered MCPH1 to MCPH12 (Kaindl, 2014), and the genes identified in this order are: *MCPH1* (Jackson et al., 1998, 2002), *WDR62* (Roberts et al., 1999; Nicholas et al., 2010), *CDK5RAP2* (Moynihan et al., 2000; Bond et al., 2005), *CASC5* (Jamieson et al., 1999; Genin et al., 2012), *ASPM* (Jamieson et al., 2000; Pattison et al., 2000; Bond et al., 2002), *CENPJ* (Leal et al., 2003; Bond et al., 2005), *STIL* (Kumar et al., 2009), *CEP135* (Hussain et al., 2012), *CEP152* (Guernsey et al., 2010), *ZNF335* (Yang et al., 2012), *PHC1* (Awad et al., 2013), and *CDK6* (Hussain et al., 2013). Mutations in *CEP63* have also been identified as causing primary microcephaly (Sir et al., 2011). *ASPM* (*MCPH5*) is reported as being the most common locus for MCPH, with *WDR62* (*MCPH2*) being the second, followed by *MCPH1* and the other loci being rarer causes of MCPH (Roberts et al., 2002; Darvish et al., 2010; Nicholas et al., 2010; Sajid Hussain et al., 2013).

It has long been noted that the MCPH genes are all related to the mitotic spindle or centrosome (Bond and Woods, 2006; Bettencourt-Dias et al., 2011), and most MCPH proteins are located at the centrosome or spindle. However the more recently identified genes do not appear to be related to these functions, such as *PHC1* which plays a role in chromatin remodeling and DNA repair (Awad et al., 2013). It is interesting to note that MCPH1 traverses multiple functions related to: transcription activation (Yang et al., 2008), mitotic spindle and centrosome (Gruber et al., 2011), and DNA damage repair (Zhou et al., 2013), which raises a possible link between DNA repair and microcephaly. Although the hitherto known functions of the MCPH genes are linked to the cell cycle, the fact that the loss-of-function mutation of only one gene is sufficient to cause microcephaly excludes the possibility of functional redundancy. Nevertheless, such exclusion does not rule out genetic interactions between MCPH genes. Further investigations of the spatio-temporal expression patterns of these genes during cortical development and a detailed assessment of the neurodevelopmental defects occurring in MCPH patients and mouse model mutants will be necessary to answer the question of a crosstalk between MCPH genes, and the identity of a common centrosome- or spindle-related mechanism regulating brain size (Bond and Woods, 2006).

Genetics of *MCPH1*

MCPH1 was the first locus identified for MCPH, initially mapped to 8p22-pter (Jackson et al., 1998). The gene was later identified and the protein was named Microcephalin (Jackson et al., 2002). A feature unique to primary microcephaly caused by mutations in *MCPH1* are defects in chromosome condensation, specifically premature chromosome condensation (PCC) in early G2-phase, and delayed decondensation post-mitosis (Trimborn et al., 2006). This condition was originally named PCC syndrome (Neitzel et al., 2002); however mutations in *MCPH1* were later identified, and PCC and primary microcephaly caused by mutations in *MCPH1* were found to be allelic disorders (Trimborn et al., 2004). PCC is detected in cytogenetic preparations, as a high proportion of prophase-like cells and poor quality metaphase G-banding (Trimborn et al., 2004). PCC is a pathognomonic feature of *MCPH1*, being absent in all other mutations of MCPH genes. Another autosomal recessive condition characterized by microcephaly with additional craniofacial features and mitotic and chromosomal defects (Tommerup et al., 1993), was later found to also be caused by mutations in *MCPH1* (Farooq et al., 2010). *MCPH1* was also identified independently in a screen for transcriptional repressors of hTERT (catalytic subunit of human telomerase) and named *BRIT1*, BRCT-repeat inhibitor of hTERT expression (Lin and Elledge, 2003), which was later shown to be the same gene as *MCPH1* (Lin et al., 2005). Taken together, these molecular features of *MCPH1* collectively reveal that the gene is implicated in diverse processes that are crucial not only for proper brain development, but also for the maintenance of genome integrity (Liang et al., 2010).

MCPH1 Protein Structure and Function

In human and mouse (*Mus musculus*), the *MCPH1* coding sequence contains 14 exons, distributed across 200 kb of genomic DNA. The protein contains three BRCT (**BRC**A1 **C-T**erminal) domains (**Figures 1, 2**), which were first described in BRCA proteins and mediate protein-protein interactions (Koonin et al., 1996; Huyton et al., 2000). One domain is located at the N-terminal side of the MCPH1 protein (BRCT1), and a tandem of two domains spans the C-terminal sequence (BRCT2/3). These domains are predicted to be crucial for function (Jeffers et al., 2008) and may be differentially involved in the diverse roles of MCPH1 by mediating interactions with distinct partners. In line with this notion, repeats of BRCT domains, such as BRCT2/3, have been shown to preferentially interact with phosphorylated residues (Woods et al., 2012).

A number of studies have reported on MCPH1 interaction partners and differential functions of the N-terminal BRCT1 domain, and the more C-terminal BRCT2/3 domains (**Figure 1**). Two regions of human MCPH1: an N-terminal fragment containing BRCT1 (residues 1–195), and a central fragment (residues 381–435) interact with different subunits of condensin II to regulate chromosome condensation (Yamashita et al., 2011). The N-terminal sequence (residues 1–48) was shown to be necessary to recruit BAF170, a component of the chromatin remodeling complex SWI/SNF, to relax chromatin for DNA repair (Peng et al., 2009). This suggests a possible role of MCPH1 in chromatin conformation. BRCT2/3 domains have been shown to bind to E2F1 to form a complex able to transactivate BRCA1 and CHK1 (Yang et al., 2008). Interactions between MCPH1 BRCT2/3 domains and Cdc27, a subunit of the anaphase-promoting complex (Singh et al., 2012b), and a phosphorylated domain of H2A.X have also been reported (Singh et al., 2012a). On the other hand, a truncated MCPH1 protein lacking BRCT2/3, is able to complement the defective chromosome condensation in human MCPH1-deficient cells (Gavvovidis et al., 2012), indicating that these domains are dispensable for this function. Molecular interactions between MCPH1 and partners may likely be regulated by post-translational modifications. In line with this notion, Ser322 phosphorylation of MCPH1 by ATR is required for TopBP1 recruitment and sustained ATR signaling for DNA repair (Zhang et al., 2014). Further mechanistic dissection of the functions of BRCT1 and BRCT2/3 domains will allow a better definition of the different molecular and biochemical mechanisms impaired by *MCPH1* mutations.

Human *MCPH1* Mutations

A large number of homozygous mutations in *MCPH1* causing primary microcephaly have been identified (**Table 1; Figures 1, 2**). These include large deletions of exons (Garshasbi et al., 2006; Darvish et al., 2010; Pfau et al., 2013), single base-pair insertions and deletions (Trimborn et al., 2004; Darvish et al., 2010; Sajid Hussain et al., 2013), nonsense mutations (Jackson et al., 2002; Farooq et al., 2010; Hosseini et al., 2012), missense mutations (Trimborn et al., 2005; Darvish et al., 2010; Leung et al., 2011; Ghani-Kakhki et al., 2012), and one splice site mutation (Darvish et al., 2010). Interestingly, all missense mutations identified so far are located in exons 2 or 3 (**Table 1; Figure 1**), which is within the N-terminal BRCT domain (BRCT1; see previous section on MCPH1 protein). The missense mutations all lead to non-conservative changes in an amino acid residue: threonine to arginine (c.80C>G, p.Thr27Arg) which is polar uncharged to positively charged (Trimborn et al., 2005), histidine to glutamine (c.147C>G, p.His49Gln) which is positively charged to polar uncharged (Darvish et al., 2010), serine to leucine (c.215C>T, p.Ser72Leu) which is polar uncharged to non-polar (Darvish et al., 2010; Ghani-Kakhki et al., 2012), and tryptophan to arginine (c.223T>C, p.Trp75Arg) which is non-polar aromatic to positively charged (Ghani-Kakhki et al., 2012). These mutated residues are highly conserved during evolution, Thr27 being conserved in orthologs of *MCPH1* in mammals and amphibians (Trimborn et al., 2005). Ser72 and Trp75 are conserved in all vertebrates and *Drosophila*, and these two residues are also conserved in BRCT domains of *BRCA1* (Ghani-Kakhki et al., 2012). In one case a homozygous double mutation in consecutive codons (c.149T>G, c.151A>G; p.Val50Gly, p.Ile51Val) was found, which leads to conservative residue changes (both non-polar to non-polar); however still within the N-terminal BRCT domain. Molecular and biochemical studies of full-length MCPH1 proteins harboring these various amino acid changes may be a powerful tool in correlating *MCPH1* genotype and molecular function with phenotype.

As previously noted for *ASPM* (Nicholas et al., 2009), correlations between mutation and phenotype, such as the severity of microcephaly, could not be established so far

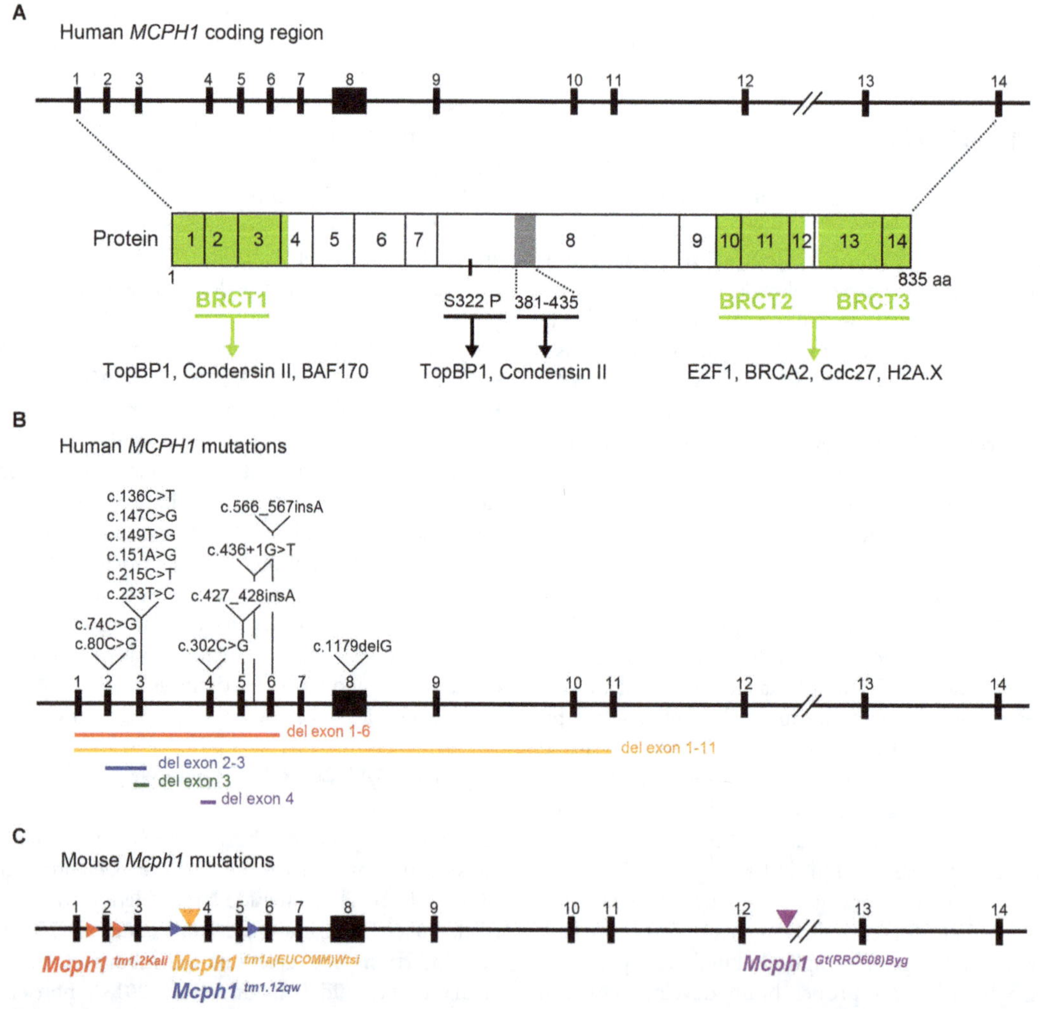

FIGURE 1 | Schematic of MCPH1 gene and protein domain structures and the positions of reported mutations in humans and mice. **(A)** Schematic of *MCPH1* gene intron-exon structure (upper) and protein domain structures (lower), which are highly conserved between mouse and human. The *MCPH1* coding sequence includes 14 exons shown as black rectangles numbered from 1–14. The three BRCT domains are shaded in green. Factors interacting with the BRCT domains are indicated below each domain. A domain including residues 381–435 in exon 8 and interacting with condensin II is shaded gray, and the phosphorylation site Ser322 (S322P) important for TopBP1 recruitment is also shown. **(B)** Reported mutations in *MCPH1* causing primary microcephaly are indicated on the gene schematic (see **Table 1**; **Figure 2** for amino acid changes). The extent of the deletions is indicated as colored bars below the gene structure. **(C)** Schematic of the four reported *Mcph1* mutations in mice (see also **Table 2**). For targeted deletions, the triangles overlaid on the intron flanks the exons that were targeted for deletion, with the allele name indicated by the same color below. For the gene trap mutation and knockout-first allele, the site of the insertion is indicated by a triangle above the intron, with the corresponding allele name in the same color.

```
Human   ------MAAPILKDVVAYVEVWSSNGTENYSKTFTTQLVDMGAKVSKTFNKQVTHVIFKD
Mouse   MEASGGVGGAFLKDVVAYVEVWSSKGTENYSRTFAKQLEDMGATVSKTLNKQVTHVIFKD

Human   GYQSTWDKAQKRGVKLVSVLWVEKCRTAGAHIDESLFPAANMNEHLSSLIKKKRKCMQPK
Mouse   GYQSTWDKAQKTGAKLVSVLWVEKCRMAGALVDESLFPAVNTDEHLPNLSRKKHKCMQPK

Human   DFNFKTPENDKRFQKKFEKMAKELQRQKTNLDDDVPILLFESNGSLIYTPTIEINSSHHS
Mouse   DFILKTPENDKRLQKKFEKMAEELQRQKAALDDDVPVLLFESPRSLVYSSPV-------N

Human   AMEKRLQEMKEKRENLSPTSSQMIQQSHDNPSNSLCEAPLNISRDTLCSDEYFAGGLHSS
Mouse   VMKRRLQDMKEKRENLSPTSSQMLEQSQQNPCVSLFETSLNISHQPLSSDESFASGSHSS

Human   FDDLCGNSGCGNQERKLEGSINDIKSDVCISSLVLKANNIHSSPSFTHLDKSSPQKFLSN
Mouse   FGDSC-----GDQERKLGRSANEMTTVTCPSSPVLRASSFYGSASPNHLRQPRPQKAPDS

Human   LSKEEINLQRNIAGKVVTPDQKQAAGMSQETFEEKYRLSPTLSSTKGHLLIHSRPRSSSV
Mouse   PSKESINCQKDATGAVADSERKQAAGVSQGVPDEKLCLSPTMSIIEEHQVRL-GPKNSSA

Human   KRKRVSHGSHSPPKEKCKRKRSTRRSIMPRLQLCRSEDRLQHVAGPALEALSCGESSYDD
Mouse   KRKRAADLGSSP-KGKLKKRY--KRKSALAIQLFKSDQSPPSTIRLIPGTPDVEASSYED

Human   YFSPDNLKERYSENLPPESQLPSSPAQLSCRSLSKKERTSIFEMSDFSCVGKKTRTVDIT
Mouse   YFSPDNLKERNSERLPPEAQQLASPSLFHCRGLSKWERRNMLEMCDFTCIGEKHRSISSI

Human   NFTAKTISSPRKTGNGEGRATSSCVTS---APEEALRCCRQAGK---EDACPEGNGFSY
Mouse   SDLISKSASSLEKPVKEEVNTASTCLLLVETSANDSPGLCSQPGPQLRDDTGPEGSSHPD

Human   TIEDPALPKGHDDDLTPLEGSLEEMKEAVGLKSTQNKGTTSKISNSSEGEAQSEHEPCFI
Mouse   T------LSSSAHHITPLKGNSTETRDPGDGKGSPKEGSTPPASASPEDEV-HICNLSLG

Human   VDCNMETSTEEKENLPGGYSGSVKNRPTRHDVLDDSCDGFKDLIKPHEELKKSGRGKKPT
Mouse   EDCNVEKSVEEKENIATGYSESVKNGPGRPDPSDSSCTGL---VRPQQKPKKSEKEEKPT

Human   RTLVMTSMPSEKQNVVIQVVDKLKGFSIAPDVCETTTHVLSGKPLRTLNVLLGIARGCWV
        RTLVMTSMPSEKQTLIIQVVSTLKGFSFAPEVCETTTHVLVGKSARTLNVLMGIARGCWI

Human   LSYDWVLWSLELGHWISEEPFELSHHFPAAPLCRSECHLSAGPYRGTLFADQPAMFVSPA
Mouse   LSYEWVLLSLELGHWISEEPFELSETFPAAPICRLERHLSTQQYQGTLFANQPKMFIAPA

Human   SSPPVAKLCELVHLCGGRVSQVPRQASIVIGPYSGKKKATVKYLSEKWVLDSITQHKVCA
Mouse   SSPPRAKLCELVLLCGGQVSPAPQLASLIIGPYKGKKKARIQYLSEKWVLDSITQHKICD

Human   PENYLLSQ
Mouse   FNNYQLLQ
```

FIGURE 2 | ClustalX alignment of human MCPH1 and mouse Mcph1 proteins. Conserved amino acids are shown in bold characters. Blue upper lines indicate BRCT domains, and red underlines indicate nuclear localization signals (Gavvovidis et al., 2012). Amino acid residues mutated in microcephaly (either nonsense or missense; see **Table 1**; **Figure 1**) are in red.

(**Table 1**). One notable exception is the p.Thr27Arg missense mutation, which shows only a mild microcephaly (–2.4 SD at birth), and the fraction of prophase-like cells being only marginally higher than controls (Trimborn et al., 2005; Ghani-Kakhki et al., 2012). Meta-analysis of genotype and phenotype correlations are hampered however by the rarity of patients with *MCPH1* mutations, and by the fact that the HC data is reported at birth in some cases (Trimborn et al., 2005) but often at older ages for others, and often only a range of HCs are shown for multiple individuals within a family (Darvish et al., 2010). Similarly, PCC is often reported qualitatively (Pfau et al., 2013), without a careful quantification of prophase-like cells as seen in other studies (Ghani-Kakhki et al., 2012). Molecular studies comparing the activities of the mutant proteins may aid in answering some of these questions (Leung et al., 2011), and will provide powerful clues in understanding the mechanisms of MCPH1.

Mouse Models of *Mcph1* Deficiency: Microcephaly Phenotype

A number of mouse models for *Mcph1* loss-of-function have been reported (**Table 2**; **Figure 1**). These mutant mouse lines have been successful in recapitulating the features of primary microcephaly and PCC caused by mutations in *MCPH1* in humans. The first study demonstrating a microcephaly phenotype in a *Mcph1* null mutant mouse model (Gruber et al., 2011) was generated by targeted deletion of *Mcph1* exon 4–5 ($Mcph1^{tm1.1Zqw}$). A follow-up study of this mouse model was reported by the same group (Zhou et al., 2013). In homozygous $Mcph1^{tm1.1Zqw}$ mutant mice, the size of the newborn mouse brain was visibly smaller, and brain weight was also reduced, fulfilling the criteria of human primary microcephaly at a gross anatomical level. Histological examination of the newborn brains revealed an approximate 20% reduction in both the radial thickness and the lateral extent of the neocortex. The *Mcph1* mutant brain at embryonic day (E) 13.5 was reported as reduced, and the cortical wall was thinner at E15.5 (Gruber et al., 2011), implying an early defect. Interestingly, in adult mutant mice, the anterior portion of the brain (defined in this case as the olfactory bulb, cerebrum, and thalamus) showed a more significant reduction compared to the remaining posterior portion. Moreover, histological examination of the cerebellum at post-natal day (P) 21 was reportedly normal suggesting that *MCPH1* may not be required for the development of the cerebellar cortex (Zhou et al., 2013).

Importantly, *MCPH1* mutant mice were also reported to have an approximate 20% reduction in body weight (at P0, P21, and P180; i.e., at birth, weaning, and adult) and the proportion of brain weight to body weight showed no significant difference compared to controls (Zhou et al., 2013). Short stature is a variable feature of human *MCPH1* and is seen in some patients (Trimborn et al., 2004). However, a proportionate reduction in both brain and body weight, raises questions of the specificity of *Mcph1* as a sole brain size regulator, at least in the mouse model. In another mouse model, a *Mcph1* null mutant generated by a targeted deletion of exon 2 ($Mcph1^{tm1.2Kali}$), growth retardation was also found, also showing an approximate 20% reduction in weight; however brain weights were not reported in this study (Liang et al., 2010). The answer to the question of a specific effect of Mcph1 on brain size, rather than an effect on overall body size, will require the analysis of mouse conditional mutants, with specific inactivation in the brain or in the neocortex. In contrast, reported mouse models of *ASPM* show a specific reduction in brain weight, with no or minimal reduction in body weight (Pulvers et al., 2010; Fujimori et al., 2014).

Two other mouse models of *Mcph1* have been reported, one generated from gene trap ES cells (Skarnes et al., 2004), and another harboring a knockout-first allele (Skarnes et al.,

TABLE 1 | Reported mutations in *MCPH1* causing autosomal recessive primary microcephaly.

Mutation	Protein	Exon	HC	Reference
del exon 1–6	?	1–6	−3 SD	Garshasbi et al. (2006), Darvish et al. (2010)
del exon 1–11	?	1–11	−3 SD (birth) <−5 SD (10 m)	Pfau et al. (2013)
c.74C>G	p.Ser25Ter	2	−5 to −10 SD	Jackson et al. (2002)
c.80C>G	p.Thr27Arg	2	−2.4 SD (birth) −3 SD (6 yr)	Trimborn et al. (2005)
del exon 2–3	?	2–3	−6 to −8 SD	Darvish et al. (2010)
del exon 3	?	3	−6 to −10 SD	Darvish et al. (2010)
c.136C>T	p.Gln46Ter	3	<−4 SD	Hosseini et al. (2012)
c.147C>G	p.His49Gln	3	−7 to −9 SD	Darvish et al. (2010)
c.149T>G; c.151A>G	p.Val50Gly; p.Ile51Val	3	<0.4th centile	Leung et al. (2011)
c.215C>T	p.Ser72Leu	3	−6 to −7 SD −3.5 SD (birth)	Darvish et al. (2010), Ghani-Kakhki et al. (2012)
c.223T>C	p.Trp75Arg	3	−5.7 SD (birth)	Ghani-Kakhki et al. (2012)
del exon 4	?	4	−10 to −11 SD	Darvish et al. (2010)
c.302C>G	p.Ser101Ter	4	?	Farooq et al. (2010)
c.427_428insA	p.Thr143Asnfs	5	−8 to −10 SD	Trimborn et al. (2004)
c.436 + 1G>T	Splice mut.	Intr. 5	−9 SD	Darvish et al. (2010)
c.566_567insA	p.Asn189fs	6	−6 SD	Darvish et al. (2010)
c.1179delG	p.Arg393Serfs	8	−8 to −10 SD	Sajid Hussain et al. (2013)

The genotype, predicted effect on protein ("?" if unknown or not described), the exon containing the mutation, standard deviation (SD) of the head circumference (HC), and the reference are shown. All mutations are homozygous.

TABLE 2 | Summary of mouse models of human *MCPH1*.

Genotype/gene product	Phenotype	Reference
Mcph1$^{Gt(RRO608)Byg}$ Hypomorphic mutation Gene trap between exons 12–13 Predicted to lack C-term 97aa Residual *wt* transcript detected	Body weight normal Brain/body weight normal Brain volume normal (MRI) Defective chromosome condensation Shortened lifespan; fertility normal	Trimborn et al. (2010)
Mcph1$^{tm1.2Kali}$ Targeted deletion of exon 2 Null mutation	Growth retardation IR hypersensitivity Smaller testis and ovary; infertile Spermatogenesis defects No ovarian follicles *Hom* born at lower than Mendelian ratio	Liang et al. (2010)
Mcph1$^{tm1.1Zqw}$ Targeted deletion of exon 4–5 Null mutation	Brain weight reduced (∼20%) Growth retardation (∼20%) Brain/body weight normal Reduction of neocortex in radial and lateral dimensions; cerebellum normal Neural progenitor apoptosis and increased cell cycle exit; deviation of progenitor mitotic cleavage plane Smaller testis and ovary; infertile	Gruber et al. (2011), Zhou et al. (2013)
Mcph1$^{tm1a(EUCOMM)Wtsi}$ Hypomorphic mutation Knockout-first allele Insertion between exons 3–4 Residual *wt* transcript detected	Brain weight reduced (∼15%) Growth normal *Hom* born at lower than Mendelian ratio Infertile Hearing impairment	Chen et al. (2013)

Genotypes of mouse Mcph1 mutations, the phenotypes of the mice, and the references are shown. Allele names obtained from Mouse Genome Informatics (MGI:2443308). MRI, magnetic resonance imaging; IR, ionizing radiation; Hom, homozygous mutant; wt, wildtype.

2011). The model containing a gene trap vector between exons 12–13 (*Mcph1*$^{Gt(RRO608)Byg}$), which leads to a protein lacking only the most C-terminal BRCT3 domain, showed normal body and brain weight, however did exhibit the

PCC phenotype (Trimborn et al., 2010). The knockout-first allele mouse model with an insertion between exons 3–4 ($Mcph1^{tm1a(EUCOMM)Wtsi}$) showed brain weight reduction (~15%); however there was no evidence of growth retardation (Chen et al., 2013). Both of these *Mcph1* models are hypomorphic mutants with detectable residual wild-type transcript, and it is thus difficult to interpret these phenotypes and compare them to the other *Mcph1* null mutants and human *MCPH1* patients.

Mouse Models of *Mcph1* Deficiency: Non-Brain Phenotypes

A number of other phenotypes have been reported in the *Mcph1* mutant mice (**Table 2**). Infertility has been observed in the two null mutants (Liang et al., 2010; Gruber et al., 2011; Zhou et al., 2013) and one of the hypomorphic mutants (Chen et al., 2013). Phenotypes were observed in both spermatogenesis and in the ovary (Liang et al., 2010). Germline phenotypes have also been reported for mouse models of *ASPM* (Pulvers et al., 2010; Fujimori et al., 2014). This raises the important question of whether infertility, or testicular or ovarian atrophy, is seen in human primary microcephaly. So far no cases have been reported and the relationship between primary microcephaly and infertility in humans remains an interesting question, as it may provide clues to the mechanism of the gene, and also raises the possibility that the function of MCPH1 in the germline may have been the target of positive selection in the primate lineage (Woods et al., 2006; Dobson-Stone et al., 2007; Timpson et al., 2007).

In one of the *Mcph1* hypomorphic mutants ($Mcph1^{Gt(RRO608)Byg}$), homozygous mice exhibited a shortened lifespan, specifically a significant difference in survival after 65 weeks of age (Trimborn et al., 2010). This observation of decreased overall survival in *Mcph1* homozygous mutants was replicated in the $Mcph1^{tm1.2Kali}$ null mutant, which manifests an increased cancer susceptibility (Liang et al., 2014). This difference in survival was not reported in the other mutants (Gruber et al., 2011; Chen et al., 2013; Zhou et al., 2013); however as the difference becomes apparent when mice are older, a shortened lifespan may have been overlooked. This raises the question of whether patients with primary microcephaly exhibit a shortened lifespan, independent of other comorbidities that may be exacerbated by the associated mental retardation. Epidemiological studies may be difficult due to the rarity of MCPH. However, one post-mortem case report of a 77-year old with primary microcephaly exists (McCreary et al., 1996) and another study reports on MCPH patients ranging to their 70 s (Darvish et al., 2010) indicating that the condition is compatible with normal lifespan.

Another interesting phenotype of *Mcph1* mutant mice reported in two studies (Liang et al., 2010; Chen et al., 2013) is a significantly reduced proportion of homozygous mice (10~15% vs. the expected normal 25% Mendelian ratio) born from intercrossing of heterozygous *Mcph1* mutant mice. This indicates the possibility of an embryonic lethal phenotype of varying penetrance caused by homozygous mutations in *Mcph1*.

MCPH1 and Neurogenesis

The vastly complex cerebral cortex has its developmental origin in the germinal zone, or ventricular zone (VZ), of the dorsal telencephalon of the neural tube (Götz and Huttner, 2005). The VZ is composed of neuroepithelial cells, which line along the ventricles of the embryonic brain vesicles and spinal cord, and serve as the primary progenitor cells of all neural cells of the central nervous system. Neuroepithelial cells exhibit typical epithelial cell characteristics, such as apical-basal polarity (Chenn et al., 1998), and its nuclei undergo a unique movement in the apical-basal axis correlated with the cell cycle, termed interkinetic nuclear migration (Sauer, 1935; Taverna and Huttner, 2010; Kosodo, 2012), which gives the tissue a pseudostratified histological appearance, and thus its classification as a pseudostratified epithelium. Neuroepithelial cells, or neural progenitor cells, initially proliferate to expand the progenitor pool, and later commence differentiative divisions into downstream progenitors and neurons (Paridaen and Huttner, 2014), the process of neurogenesis.

In cortical development, the lateral dimension of the laminar structure is largely dictated by the expansion of neural progenitor cells or proliferative units, and the radial dimension is a result of the extent of neurogenesis subsequent to progenitor proliferation within an ontogenetic column or radial-unit (Rakic, 1988, 1995, 2009). This framework allows the dissection of cortical phenotypes, where a reduction in the lateral dimension is likely a deficit in the initial progenitor pool and its subsequent proliferative expansion, and a reduction in the radial dimension may be caused by a reduced capacity for neurogenesis, shortening of the neurogenic interval, or neuronal loss. Conceptually, an analysis distinguishing the radial and lateral dimensions is useful in phenotypic dissection of mutant mice to further clarify their respective impact on the final neurogenic outcome.

Mcph1 inactivation has an impact on both lateral and radial dimensions (Gruber et al., 2011; Zhou et al., 2013). These characteristics have been related to a loss of progenitors and to a specific decrease in upper layer neuron output, possibly due to premature progenitor exhaustion. They appear to result from the deficiency of two distinct *Mcph1* functions: the control of the centrosome cycle through the Chk1-Cdc25 pathway, and DNA damage repair. The relative contribution of each deficiency in this progenitor loss has not been addressed and will require further studies. Likewise, it will be interesting to address whether the aforementioned participation of Mcph1 in chromatin conformation during DNA repair could also be important for chromatin conformation with regards to progenitor fate determination during neurogenesis. In line with this notion, competitive interactions between BAF170 and BAF155 with Pax6 have been shown to play an important role in the choice between cell cycle maintenance vs. differentiation (Tuoc et al., 2013). Interestingly, mutations of several BAF genes, including BAF170 and BAF155, have been reported to be involved in brain disorders (Ronan et al., 2013), and it will be interesting to further explore how interactions between BAF and MCPH1 proteins impact brain size and function.

The full interpretation of the defects reported for *Mcph1* mutant mice is hampered by the lack of detailed information on the pattern of Mcph1 expression during cortical development, such as the temporal dynamics of gene activation, the cell types expressing the gene and the sub-cellular localization of the Mcph1 protein. It remains thus difficult to establish a direct link between the described phenotypes and gene function. Moreover, gaining insight into the spatio-temporal mode of *MCPH1* expression in mouse and human will also allow the delineation of how the function of the gene may have diverged between both species. In particular, it will be interesting to determine if *MCPH1*, along with other MCPH genes, are expressed in the OSVZ (outer subventricular zone) progenitors (Smart et al., 2002), and eventually how the MCPH genes may impact the proliferation rate and division mode of these progenitors, which are considered to be involved in the expansion of the surface area of the neocortex (Lui et al., 2011; Betizeau et al., 2013; Sun and Hevner, 2014).

MCPH1 and Brain Evolution

Ever since the identification of *MCPH* genes, there has been intense interest in their possible roles in the evolution of brain size (Evans et al., 2004; Wang and Su, 2004; Ponting and Jackson, 2005; Woods et al., 2005). Microcepaly (primary microcephaly, or microcephaly *vera*) has long been the subject of evolutionary interest, and is commonly described in the literature as an atavistic (or "throwback") condition, a reversion to an ancestral form (Mochida and Walsh, 2001; Gilbert et al., 2005; Ponting and Jackson, 2005; Vallender et al., 2008). In fact, microcephaly was already proposed in the mid-19th centrury by Carl Vogt to be the reappearance of an ancestral primate (Komai et al., 1955; Richardson, 2011). Much of the intrigue and fascination of research into *MCPH* genes has been fueled by the remarkable phenotype of primary microcephay: a significant and specific reduction in brain size with the absence of other neurological and non-neurological abnormalities (Woods et al., 2005). However, as little is known about the actual disturbance in cortical structure and cytoarchitecture in *MCPH*, and since the neuroanatomy of ancestral primates and hominids may forever remain in the realm of speculation and extrapolation from the comparison of extant species (Holloway, 1968; Rilling and Insel, 1999; Falk et al., 2000), parallels between the pathological condition of microcephaly, and the evolutionary change in primate brain size must be made with caution. Moreover, *MCPH* cannot be described as "atavistic" in genetic terms, as all mutations identifyed so far, whether they result in loss-of-function or the truncated MCPH1 protein has a toxic effect, are mutations predicted to cause gene dysfunction, not a reversal to an ancestral sequence (Gilbert et al., 2005). However, the MCPH phenotype does provide insight into a cell biological mechanism of brain size regulation, which may indeed have been involved in primate brain evolution (Bond and Woods, 2006; Fish et al., 2008; Thornton and Woods, 2009; Sun and Hevner, 2014).

Intriguinly, *Mcph1* loss of function in mice primarily affects the number of upper-layer neurons (Zhou et al., 2013), which are very important for intra-cortical connections and are involved in higher cognitive functions. The output of these neurons has increased during evolution correlating with increasing complexity of cognitive functions, as observed in humans and primates (DeFelipe et al., 2002; Molnar et al., 2006; Fame et al., 2011). The participation of *MCPH* genes in the development of upper-layer neurons (Lizarraga et al., 2010; Yang et al., 2012; Zhou et al., 2013) may thus represent a major clue for understanding the evolution of brain size and function.

Regarding studies on the evolution of *MCPH* genes, interest has generally centered on (i) the possibility of genetic variations in these genes being directly involved in brain size regulation during primate and human evolution; or (ii) through the analysis of the function of these genes a molecular mechanism or pathway regulating brain size may be identified.

MCPH1: Positive Selection and Polymorphisms

With regards to variations in *MCPH1*, studies have focussed on either the analysis of positive (or Darwinian) selection of *MCPH1* in extant primate species, or through the analysis of polymophisms in human populations. Positive selection in the context of protein evolution can be studied by the analysis of the ratio of non-synonymous (K_a) to synonymous (K_s) changes in DNA sequence (Yang and Bielawski, 2000; Hurst, 2002), and has commonly been used in investigating the link between brain development and evolution (Dorus et al., 2004; Gilbert et al., 2005). Briefly, since synonymous mutations in codons do not change amino acid sequence and therefore do not alter the biochemical properties of the protein, they are assumed to be selectively neutral and reflect the neutral mutation rate. Non-synonymous mutations on the other hand, alters the amino acid sequence which may in turn alter protein function, which more commonly would lead to gene dysfunction and an evolutionary disadvantage, and rarely may confer a gain-of-function or an evolutionary advantage (Woods et al., 2005). Therefore a non-synonymous/synonymous substitution ratio (K_a/K_s or dN/dS) of >1 can be interpreted as evidence for positive selection. Utilizing these methods, *MCPH1* was found to exhibit positive selection in the primate lineage, specifically from the common ancestor of great apes and humans (Evans et al., 2004; Wang and Su, 2004). Another study which investigated four microcephaly genes across 21 species of anthropoid primates identified positive selection correlating with neonatal and adult brain size for *ASPM* and *CDK5RAP2*, but interestingly not for *MCPH1* and *CENPJ* (Montgomery et al., 2011). Positive selection of *MCPH1* was also identified in cetaceans, which was however also not associated with variations in brain size (McGowen et al., 2011). Examination of positive selection of microcephaly genes across 33 eutherian mammal species revealed signs of positive selection of *MCPH1* across non-primate mammals, however *MCPH1* did not correlate with neonatal brain size (Montgomery and Mundy, 2014). How *MCPH1* may be involved in brain size regulation more broadly across vertebrates and whether variations show any correlations between gyrencephalic vs. non-gyrencephalic species remains an interesting question.

A large number of non-pathogenetic mutations or polymorphisms in *MCPH1* are known, particularly in exon 8 and 13 (Scala et al., 2010). One of which, c.940G>C (p.Asp314His, non-conservative missense from negatively to positively charged, exon 8; rs930557), has received much attention. This polymorphism which is diagnostic for a haplotype with the derived C allele, designated as haplogroup D, has a relatively young coalescence age (i.e., time to single ancestral copy) of 37,000 years, however with a high population frequency worldwide, indicating strong positive selection among anatomically modern humans (Evans et al., 2005). Further analysis on the origin of haplogroup D indicated its divergence 1.1 million years ago from the human lineage and subsequent introgression of this derived allele into human populations 37,000 years ago, possibly due to interbreeding between humans and an archaic *homo* species, which was speculated as Neanderthals (Evans et al., 2006). Although Neanderthals were suggested as the possible archaic *homo* (Hawks et al., 2008), subsequent sequencing of *MCPH1* of Neanderthals revealed the non-D (ancestral) haplotype (Green et al., 2010; Lari et al., 2010).

A large number of studies have attempted at identifying associations between *MCPH1* haplogroup D and a variety of brain-related phenotypes. In short, no associations have been identified with regards to HC, brain size by MRI, IQ or mental retardation (Woods et al., 2006; Dobson-Stone et al., 2007; Mekel-Bobrov et al., 2007; Rushton et al., 2007; Timpson et al., 2007; Bates et al., 2008; Maghirang-Rodriguez et al., 2009). One study identified an association with the population freqency of haplogroup D and linguistic tone (Dediu and Ladd, 2007), although a later study showed that the derived allele is not associated with lexical tone perception (Wong et al., 2012).

The derived allele of another *MCPH1* polymorphism, c.2282T>C (p.Val761Ala, conservative missense from non-polar to non-polar, exon 13; rs1057090), was associated with an increase in cranial volume in Chinese males, but not females (Wang et al., 2008). Non-exonic common variants in *MCPH1* have been associated with brain size and cortical surface area in females (Rimol et al., 2010), and another study has investigated *MCPH* genes and their association with sexual dimorphism in brain size in primates (Montgomery and Mundy, 2013). Mechanistically, how *MCPH1* may contribute to sexually-dimorphic brain phenotypes remains unclear.

Key questions remain as to whether *MCPH1* did play a role in the evolution of brain size in the primate lineage, and whether common variants of *MCPH1* in human populations today are associated with any structural or functional brain phenotype. In light of the phenotypic data from mouse models (Liang et al., 2010; Trimborn et al., 2010; Gruber et al., 2011; Chen et al., 2013; Zhou et al., 2013) which implicate *MCPH1* in a number of other non-nervous systems, notably the germline, positive selection in primates and humans may not be due to adaptive changes in brain size or function (Woods et al., 2006; Dobson-Stone et al., 2007; Timpson et al., 2007). In this context it is interesting to note that a large scale study of human and chimpanzee orthologs for evidence of positive selection revealed a large number of genes involved in tumor suppression, apoptosis, and spermatogenesis (Nielsen et al., 2005); functions where *MCPH1* may play a major role. Interestingly, two *MCPH1* polymorphisms have been associated with breast cancer risk (Jo et al., 2013), which further stresses the need of examining non-nervous system phenotypes in the context of *MCPH1* evolution and also in primary microcephaly patients.

MCPH1 Evolution: From a Cell Biological Perspective

Cortical development in rodents and primates share many features, however there are a number of important differences relevant for brain size evolution. A key difference and one that is of relevance to *MCPH1*, is the mechanisms which regulate the production of progenitors in the OSVZ, the germinal compartment which has enlarged strikingly in primates and humans and is considered as the seat of the evolutionary expansion of neocortical surface area (Smart et al., 2002; Lui et al., 2011; Sun and Hevner, 2014). The analysis and comparison of these differences in progenitor cell types and lineage relationships, germinal layer cytoarchitecture, and cell biological mechanisms will help in constructing a model of mammalian brain evolution from a developmental and cell biological perspective (Fish et al., 2008; Rakic, 2009; Fietz and Huttner, 2011; Lui et al., 2011; Sun and Hevner, 2014). Another clue recently emerged is the importance of DNA repair pathways, revealed by a preferential effect of mutations of genes implicated in such pathways, including *MCPH1*, on neural progenitors (Gilmore and Walsh, 2013). This suggests the existence of a specific cross-talk between DNA repair pathways and primary cell cycle functions in these progenitors, which might have become more critical during evolution. Integrating these molecular findings with genetics and evolutionary biology will be a powerful approach in investigating brain size evolution (Enard, 2014).

With regards to *MCPH1*, some studies have taken this approach in investigating its function in brain size evolution. One study identified an E2F1 binding motif in the *MCPH1* promoter region, which is specific to primates and absent in mice and other vetebrates (Shi and Su, 2012). E2F1 is a transcription factor regulating genes involved in cell cycle and apoptosis (Ginsberg, 2002), and interestingly MCPH1 is involved in transcriptional regulation of several DNA repair, checkpoint and apoptosis genes, via interaction with E2F1 (Yang et al., 2008). Another study performed a cell line assay comparing human and rhesus macaque MCPH1 protein and its affects on down-stream gene expression, and found that human-specific amino acid changes in MCPH1 led to differences in expression of three downstream genes involved in cell cycle regulation and apoptosis (Shi et al., 2013). These studies go beyond correlating genetic changes with brain size, and attempt to experimentally test the hypothesis that *MCPH1* is an important gene in brain size evolution. Futher approaches may be to generate humanized and primatized mice expressing human and other primate *MCPH1* (Pulvers et al., 2010), or the use of cerebral organoids (Lancaster et al., 2013), an *in vitro* model of human cortical development, where microcephaly-causing mutations in humans and primate-specific variants in *MCPH1* can be investigated in detail in a system amenable to experimentation (Enard, 2014). Gene expression profiling studies aimed at identifying pathways dependent on *MCPH1* in mouse and human, as well as the characterization of molecular partners for both the mouse and human proteins, will provide major clues on the molecular mechanisms involving MCPH1 and its role in the evolution of brain size. Much may be learnt regarding the role of MCPH genes in brain size evolution, from constructing developmental and cell biological tools for analyzing evolutionary questions.

MCPH1 is well-positioned as a candidate gene for understanding the mechanisms of brain size evolution, as it is related not only to the other primary microcephaly genes with regards to its phenotype, but also harbors the same BRCT domains as *BRCA1*, which has also been shown to be important for brain development (Pulvers and Huttner, 2009; Pao et al., 2014) and shows positive selection in the primate linage (Huttley et al., 2000; Lou et al., 2014).

Conclusions

Advances in medical genetics have greatly enhanced our understanding of the origins of many brain and nervous system development disorders; microcephaly in particular. Nevertheless, the molecular and cellular processes underlying such disorders remain poorly understood, and gaining insight into the pathological mechanisms has remained as a major challenge in developmental neurobiology. In this respect, microcephaly of genetic etiology represents a valuable context for the study of the mechanisms that control the final neurogenic output, and by extension to animal models, to assess how these mechanisms have been adjusted and modulated during evolution along with the remarkable expansion of brain size. So far, interests have focused mainly on aspects related to cell division and proliferation; however the pathological mechanisms associated with microcephaly may prove to be more complex and multifactorial. In line with this notion, *MCPH1* appears to assume multifaceted functions, including but not limited to: brain development (Jackson et al., 1998, 2002), DNA damage repair (Xu et al., 2004; Lin et al., 2005; Peng et al., 2009), chromosome condensation (Neitzel et al., 2002; Trimborn et al., 2004; Yamashita et al., 2011), cancer (Chaplet et al., 2006; Rai et al., 2006; Richardson et al., 2011), and germline function (Liang et al., 2010), as reviewed here and elsewhere (Venkatesh and Suresh, 2014). Further comparative expression and functional studies in different species, including primates, will prove to be highly informative in further delineating the molecular and genetic networks controlled by *MCPH1*, and how they may have been tuned or co-opted to participate in the expansion of brain size. Such progress in the understanding of fundamental developmental mechanisms of the brain is expected to have a valuable impact not only in the understanding of clinical conditions such as microcephaly, but also to answer one of the most enduring questions in biology: *the evolution of brain size.*

Acknowledgments

We are grateful to Pierre Gressens for critical reading of the manuscript. JN and NJ were supported by Inserm, University Paris 7 Denis Diderot, Grace de Monaco and Roger de Spoelberch Foundations, ARC (Association pour la Recherche sur le Cancer); and YA by ARC, FRM (Fondation pour la Recherche Médicale) and JSPS (Japan Society for the Promotion of Science).

References

Awad, S., Al-Dosari, M. S., Al-Yacoub, N., Colak, D., Salih, M. A., Alkuraya, F. S., et al. (2013). Mutation in PHC1 implicates chromatin remodeling in primary microcephaly pathogenesis. *Hum. Mol. Genet.* 22, 2200–2213. doi: 10.1093/hmg/ddt072

Bates, T. C., Luciano, M., Lind, P. A., Wright, M. J., Montgomery, G. W., and Martin, N. G. (2008). Recently-derived variants of brain-size genes ASPM, MCPH1, CDK5RAP and BRCA1 not associated with general cognition, reading or language. *Intelligence* 36, 689–693. doi: 10.1016/j.intell.2008.04.001

Betizeau, M., Cortay, V., Patti, D., Pfister, S., Gautier, E., Bellemin-Ménard, A., et al. (2013). Precursor diversity and complexity of lineage relationships in the outer subventricular zone of the primate. *Neuron* 80, 442–457. doi: 10.1016/j.neuron.2013.09.032

Bettencourt-Dias, M., Hildebrandt, F., Pellman, D., Woods, G., and Godinho, S. A. (2011). Centrosomes and cilia in human disease. *Trends Genet.* 27, 307–315. doi: 10.1016/j.tig.2011.05.004

Bond, J., Roberts, E., Mochida, G. H., Hampshire, D. J., Scott, S., Askham, J. M., et al. (2002). ASPM is a major determinant of cerebral cortical size. *Nat. Genet.* 32, 316–320. doi: 10.1038/ng995

Bond, J., Roberts, E., Springell, K., Lizarraga, S. B., Scott, S., Higgins, J., et al. (2005). A centrosomal mechanism involving CDK5RAP2 and CENPJ controls brain size. *Nat. Genet.* 37, 353–355. doi: 10.1038/ng1539

Bond, J., and Woods, C. G. (2006). Cytoskeletal genes regulating brain size. *Curr. Opin. Cell Biol.* 18, 95–101. doi: 10.1016/j.ceb.2005.11.004

Chaplet, M., Rai, R., Jackson-Bernitsas, D., Li, K., and Lin, S. Y. (2006). BRIT1/MCPH1: a guardian of genome and an enemy of tumors. *Cell Cycle* 5, 2579–2583. doi: 10.4161/cc.5.22.3471

Cheeran, M. C., Lokensgard, J. R., and Schleiss, M. R. (2009). Neuropathogenesis of congenital cytomegalovirus infection: disease mechanisms and prospects for intervention. *Clin. Microbiol. Rev.* 22, 99–126, Table of Contents. doi: 10.1128/CMR.00023-08

Chen, J., Ingham, N., Clare, S., Raisen, C., Vancollie, V. E., Ismail, O., et al. (2013). Mcph1-deficient mice reveal a role for MCPH1 in otitis media. *PLoS One* 8:e58156. doi: 10.1371/journal.pone.0058156

Chenn, A., Zhang, Y. A., Chang, B. T., and McConnell, S. K. (1998). Intrinsic polarity of mammalian neuroepithelial cells. *Mol. Cell. Neurosci.* 11, 183–193. doi: 10.1006/mcne.1998.0680

Clowry, G., Molnár, Z., and Rakic, P. (2010). Renewed focus on the developing human neocortex. *J. Anat.* 217, 276–288. doi: 10.1111/j.1469-7580.2010.01281.x

Copp, A. J., Greene, N. D., and Murdoch, J. N. (2003). The genetic basis of mammalian neurulation. *Nat. Rev. Genet.* 4, 784–793. doi: 10.1038/nrg1181

Darvish, H., Esmaeeli-Nieh, S., Monajemi, G. B., Mohseni, M., Ghasemi-Firouzabadi, S., Abedini, S. S., et al. (2010). A clinical and molecular genetic study of 112 Iranian families with primary microcephaly. *J. Med. Genet.* 47, 823–828. doi: 10.1136/jmg.2009.076398

Dediu, D., and Ladd, D. R. (2007). Linguistic tone is related to the population frequency of the adaptive haplogroups of two brain size genes, ASPM and Microcephalin. *Proc. Natl. Acad. Sci. U S A* 104, 10944–10949. doi: 10.1073/pnas.0610848104

DeFelipe, J., Alonso-Nanclares, L., and Arellano, J. I. (2002). Microstructure of the neocortex: comparative aspects. *J. Neurocytol.* 31, 299–316. doi: 10.1023/A:1024130211265

Dickson, B. J. (2002). Molecular mechanisms of axon guidance. *Science* 298, 1959–1964. doi: 10.1126/science.1072165

Dobson-Stone, C., Gatt, J. M., Kuan, S. A., Grieve, S. M., Gordon, E., Williams, L. M., et al. (2007). Investigation of MCPH1 G37995C and ASPM A44871G polymorphisms and brain size in a healthy cohort. *Neuroimage* 37, 394–400. doi: 10.1016/j.neuroimage.2007.05.011

Dorus, S., Vallender, E. J., Evans, P. D., Anderson, J. R., Gilbert, S. L., Mahowald, M., et al. (2004). Accelerated evolution of nervous system genes in the origin of Homo sapiens. *Cell* 119, 1027–1040. doi: 10.1016/j.cell.2004.11.040

Enard, W. (2014). Comparative genomics of brain size evolution. *Front. Hum. Neurosci.* 8:345. doi: 10.3389/fnhum.2014.00345

Evans, P. D., Anderson, J. R., Vallender, E. J., Choi, S. S., and Lahn, B. T. (2004). Reconstructing the evolutionary history of microcephalin, a gene controlling human brain size. *Hum. Mol. Genet.* 13, 1139–1145. doi: 10.1093/hmg/ddh126

Evans, P. D., Gilbert, S. L., Mekel-Bobrov, N., Vallender, E. J., Anderson, J. R., Vaez-Azizi, L. M., et al. (2005). Microcephalin, a gene regulating brain size, continues to evolve adaptively in humans. *Science* 309, 1717–1720. doi: 10.1126/science.1113722

Evans, P. D., Mekel-Bobrov, N., Vallender, E. J., Hudson, R. R., and Lahn, B. T. (2006). Evidence that the adaptive allele of the brain size gene microcephalin introgressed into Homo sapiens from an archaic Homo lineage. *Proc. Natl. Acad. Sci. U S A* 103, 18178–18183. doi: 10.1073/pnas.0606966103

Falk, D., Redmond, J. C. Jr., Guyer, J., Conroy, C., Recheis, W., Weber, G. W., et al. (2000). Early hominid brain evolution: a new look at old endocasts. *J. Hum. Evol.* 38, 695–717. doi: 10.1006/jhev.1999.0378

Fame, R. M., MacDonald, J. L., and Macklis, J. D. (2011). Development, specification and diversity of callosal projection neurons. *Trends Neurosci.* 34, 41–50. doi: 10.1016/j.tins.2010.10.002

Farooq, M., Baig, S., Tommerup, N., and Kjaer, K. W. (2010). Craniosynostosis-microcephaly with chromosomal breakage and other abnormalities is caused by a truncating MCPH1 mutation and is allelic to premature chromosomal condensation syndrome and primary autosomal recessive microcephaly type 1. *Am. J. Med. Genet. A* 152A, 495–497. doi: 10.1002/ajmg.a.33234

Fietz, S. A., and Huttner, W. B. (2011). Cortical progenitor expansion, self-renewal and neurogenesis-a polarized perspective. *Curr. Opin. Neurobiol.* 21, 23–35. doi: 10.1016/j.conb.2010.10.002

Fish, J. L., Dehay, C., Kennedy, H., and Huttner, W. B. (2008). Making bigger brains-the evolution of neural-progenitor-cell division. *J. Cell Sci.* 121, 2783–2793. doi: 10.1242/jcs.023465

Fujimori, A., Itoh, K., Goto, S., Hirakawa, H., Wang, B., Kokubo, T., et al. (2014). Disruption of Aspm causes microcephaly with abnormal neuronal differentiation. *Brain Dev.* 36, 661–669. doi: 10.1016/j.braindev.2013.10.006

Garner, C. C., Zhai, R. G., Gundelfinger, E. D., and Ziv, N. E. (2002). Molecular mechanisms of CNS synaptogenesis. *Trends Neurosci.* 25, 243–251. doi: 10.1016/s0166-2236(02)02152-5

Garshasbi, M., Motazacker, M. M., Kahrizi, K., Behjati, F., Abedini, S. S., Nieh, S. E., et al. (2006). SNP array-based homozygosity mapping reveals MCPH1 deletion in family with autosomal recessive mental retardation and mild microcephaly. *Hum. Genet.* 118, 708–715. doi: 10.1007/s00439-005-0104-y

Gavvovidis, I., Rost, I., Trimborn, M., Kaiser, F. J., Purps, J., Wiek, C., et al. (2012). A novel MCPH1 isoform complements the defective chromosome condensation of human MCPH1-deficient cells. *PLoS One* 7:e40387. doi: 10.1371/journal.pone.0040387

Genin, A., Desir, J., Lambert, N., Biervliet, M., Van Der Aa, N., Pierquin, G., et al. (2012). Kinetochore KMN network gene CASC5 mutated in primary microcephaly. *Hum. Mol. Genet.* 21, 5306–5317. doi: 10.1093/hmg/dds386

Ghani-Kakhki, M., Robinson, P. N., Morlot, S., Mitter, D., Trimborn, M., Albrecht, B., et al. (2012). Two missense mutations in the primary autosomal recessive microcephaly gene MCPH1 disrupt the function of the highly conserved N-terminal BRCT domain of microcephalin. *Mol. Syndromol.* 3, 6–13. doi: 10.1159/000338975

Gilbert, S. L., Dobyns, W. B., and Lahn, B. T. (2005). Genetic links between brain development and brain evolution. *Nat. Rev. Genet.* 6, 581–590. doi: 10.1038/nrg1634

Gilmore, E. C., and Walsh, C. A. (2013). Genetic causes of microcephaly and lessons for neuronal development. *Wiley Interdiscip. Rev. Dev. Biol.* 2, 461–478. doi: 10.1002/wdev.89

Ginsberg, D. (2002). E2F1 pathways to apoptosis. *FEBS Lett.* 529, 122–125. doi: 10.1016/s0014-5793(02)03270-2

Götz, M., and Huttner, W. B. (2005). The cell biology of neurogenesis. *Nat. Rev. Mol. Cell Biol.* 6, 777–788. doi: 10.1038/nrm1739

Green, R. E., Krause, J., Briggs, A. W., Maricic, T., Stenzel, U., Kircher, M., et al. (2010). A draft sequence of the Neandertal genome. *Science* 328, 710–722. doi: 10.1126/science.1188021

Gruber, R., Zhou, Z., Sukchev, M., Joerss, T., Frappart, P. O., and Wang, Z. Q. (2011). MCPH1 regulates the neuroprogenitor division mode by coupling the centrosomal cycle with mitotic entry through the Chk1-Cdc25 pathway. *Nat. Cell Biol.* 13, 1325–1334. doi: 10.1038/ncb2342

Guernsey, D. L., Jiang, H., Hussin, J., Arnold, M., Bouyakdan, K., Perry, S., et al. (2010). Mutations in centrosomal protein CEP152 in primary microcephaly families linked to MCPH4. *Am. J. Hum. Genet.* 87, 40–51. doi: 10.1016/j.ajhg.2010.06.003

Hawks, J., Cochran, G., Harpending, H. C., and Lahn, B. T. (2008). A genetic legacy from archaic Homo. *Trends Genet.* 24, 19–23. doi: 10.1016/j.tig.2007.10.003

Holloway, R. L. Jr. (1968). The evolution of the primate brain: some aspects of quantitative relations. *Brain Res.* 7, 121–172. doi: 10.1016/0006-8993(68)90094-2

Hosseini, M. M., Tonekaboni, S. H., Papari, E., Bahman, I., Behjati, F., Kahrizi, K., et al. (2012). A novel mutation in MCPH1 gene in an Iranian family with primary microcephaly. *J. Pak. Med. Assoc.* 62, 1244–1247.

Hurst, L. D. (2002). The K_a/K_s ratio: diagnosing the form of sequence evolution. *Trends Genet.* 18, 486–487. doi: 10.1016/s0168-9525(02)02722-1

Hussain, M. S., Baig, S. M., Neumann, S., Nürnberg, G., Farooq, M., Ahmad, I., et al. (2012). A truncating mutation of CEP135 causes primary microcephaly and disturbed centrosomal function. *Am. J. Hum. Genet.* 90, 871–878. doi: 10.1016/j.ajhg.2012.03.016

Hussain, M. S., Baig, S. M., Neumann, S., Peche, V. S., Szczepanski, S., Nürnberg, G., et al. (2013). CDK6 associates with the centrosome during mitosis and is mutated in a large Pakistani family with primary microcephaly. *Hum. Mol. Genet.* 22, 5199–5214. doi: 10.1093/hmg/ddt374

Huttley, G. A., Easteal, S., Southey, M. C., Tesoriero, A., Giles, G. G., McCredie, M. R., et al. (2000). Adaptive evolution of the tumour suppressor BRCA1 in humans and chimpanzees. Australian breast cancer family study. *Nat. Genet.* 25, 410–413. doi: 10.1038/78092

Huyton, T., Bates, P. A., Zhang, X., Sternberg, M. J., and Freemont, P. S. (2000). The BRCA1 C-terminal domain: structure and function. *Mutat. Res.* 460, 319–332. doi: 10.1016/s0921-8777(00)00034-3

Jackson, A. P., Eastwood, H., Bell, S. M., Adu, J., Toomes, C., Carr, I. M., et al. (2002). Identification of microcephalin, a protein implicated in determining the size of the human brain. *Am. J. Hum. Genet.* 71, 136–142. doi: 10.1086/341283

Jackson, A. P., McHale, D. P., Campbell, D. A., Jafri, H., Rashid, Y., Mannan, J., et al. (1998). Primary autosomal recessive microcephaly (MCPH1) maps to chromosome 8p22-pter. *Am. J. Hum. Genet.* 63, 541–546. doi: 10.1086/301966

Jamieson, C. R., Fryns, J. P., Jacobs, J., Matthijs, G., and Abramowicz, M. J. (2000). Primary autosomal recessive microcephaly: MCPH5 maps to 1q25–q32. *Am. J. Hum. Genet.* 67, 1575–1577. doi: 10.1086/316909

Jamieson, C. R., Govaerts, C., and Abramowicz, M. J. (1999). Primary autosomal recessive microcephaly: homozygosity mapping of MCPH4 to chromosome 15. *Am. J. Hum. Genet.* 65, 1465–1469. doi: 10.1086/302640

Jeffers, L. J., Coull, B. J., Stack, S. J., and Morrison, C. G. (2008). Distinct BRCT domains in Mcph1/Brit1 mediate ionizing radiation-induced focus formation and centrosomal localization. *Oncogene* 27, 139–144. doi: 10.1038/sj.onc.1210595

Jo, Y. H., Kim, H. O., Lee, J., Lee, S. S., Cho, C. H., Kang, I. S., et al. (2013). MCPH1 protein expression and polymorphisms are associated with risk of breast cancer. *Gene* 517, 184–190. doi: 10.1016/j.gene.2012.12.088

Kaindl, A. M. (2014). Autosomal recessive primary microcephalies (MCPH). *Eur. J. Paediatr. Neurol.* 18, 547–548. doi: 10.1016/j.ejpn.2014.03.010

Kaindl, A. M., Passemard, S., Kumar, P., Kraemer, N., Issa, L., Zwirner, A., et al. (2010). Many roads lead to primary autosomal recessive microcephaly. *Prog. Neurobiol.* 90, 363–383. doi: 10.1016/j.pneurobio.2009.11.002

Komai, T., Kishimoto, K., and Ozaki, Y. (1955). Genetic study of microcephaly based on Japanese material. *Am. J. Hum. Genet.* 7, 51–65.

Koonin, E. V., Altschul, S. F., and Bork, P. (1996). BRCA1 protein products ... Functional motifs ... *Nat. Genet.* 13, 266–268. doi: 10.1038/ng0796-266

Kosodo, Y. (2012). Interkinetic nuclear migration: beyond a hallmark of neurogenesis. *Cell. Mol. Life Sci.* 69, 2727–2738. doi: 10.1007/s00018-012-0952-2

Kumar, A., Girimaji, S. C., Duvvari, M. R., and Blanton, S. H. (2009). Mutations in STIL, encoding a pericentriolar and centrosomal protein, cause primary microcephaly. *Am. J. Hum. Genet.* 84, 286–290. doi: 10.1016/j.ajhg.2009.01.017

Lancaster, M. A., Renner, M., Martin, C. A., Wenzel, D., Bicknell, L. S., Hurles, M. E., et al. (2013). Cerebral organoids model human brain development and microcephaly. *Nature* 501, 373–379. doi: 10.1038/nature12517

Lari, M., Rizzi, E., Milani, L., Corti, G., Balsamo, C., Vai, S., et al. (2010). The microcephalin ancestral allele in a Neanderthal individual. *PLoS One* 5:e10648. doi: 10.1371/journal.pone.0010648

Leal, G. F., Roberts, E., Silva, E. O., Costa, S. M., Hampshire, D. J., and Woods, C. G. (2003). A novel locus for autosomal recessive primary microcephaly (MCPH6) maps to 13q12.2. *J. Med. Genet.* 40, 540–542. doi: 10.1136/jmg.40.7.540

Leung, J. W., Leitch, A., Wood, J. L., Shaw-Smith, C., Metcalfe, K., Bicknell, L. S., et al. (2011). SET nuclear oncogene associates with microcephalin/MCPH1 and regulates chromosome condensation. *J. Biol. Chem.* 286, 21393–21400. doi: 10.1074/jbc.M110.208793

Liang, Y., Gao, H., Lin, S. Y., Goss, J. A., Du, C., and Li, K. (2014). Mcph1/Brit1 deficiency promotes genomic instability and tumor formation in a mouse model. *Oncogene* doi: 10.1038/onc.2014.367. [Epub ahead of print].

Liang, Y., Gao, H., Lin, S. Y., Peng, G., Huang, X., Zhang, P., et al. (2010). BRIT1/MCPH1 is essential for mitotic and meiotic recombination DNA repair and maintaining genomic stability in mice. *PLoS Genet.* 6:e1000826. doi: 10.1371/journal.pgen.1000826

Lin, S. Y., and Elledge, S. J. (2003). Multiple tumor suppressor pathways negatively regulate telomerase. *Cell* 113, 881–889. doi: 10.1016/s0092-8674(03)00430-6

Lin, S. Y., Rai, R., Li, K., Xu, Z. X., and Elledge, S. J. (2005). BRIT1/MCPH1 is a DNA damage responsive protein that regulates the Brca1-Chk1 pathway, implicating checkpoint dysfunction in microcephaly. *Proc. Natl. Acad. Sci. U S A* 102, 15105–15109. doi: 10.1073/pnas.0507722102

Lizarraga, S. B., Margossian, S. P., Harris, M. H., Campagna, D. R., Han, A. P., Blevins, S., et al. (2010). Cdk5rap2 regulates centrosome function and chromosome segregation in neuronal progenitors. *Development* 137, 1907–1917. doi: 10.1242/dev.040410

Lou, D. I., McBee, R. M., Le, U. Q., Stone, A. C., Wilkerson, G. K., Demogines, A. M., et al. (2014). Rapid evolution of BRCA1 and BRCA2 in humans and other primates. *BMC Evol. Biol.* 14:155. doi: 10.1186/1471-2148-14-155

Lui, J. H., Hansen, D. V., and Kriegstein, A. R. (2011). Development and evolution of the human neocortex. *Cell* 146, 18–36. doi: 10.1016/j.cell.2011.06.030

Lumsden, A., and Krumlauf, R. (1996). Patterning the vertebrate neuraxis. *Science* 274, 1109–1115. doi: 10.1126/science.274.5290.1109

Maghirang-Rodriguez, R., Archie, J. G., Schwartz, C. E., and Collins, J. S. (2009). The c.940G variant of the Microcephalin (MCPH1) gene is not associated with microcephaly or mental retardation. *Am. J. Med. Genet. A* 149A, 622–625. doi: 10.1002/ajmg.a.32721

Marín, O., and Rubenstein, J. L. (2003). Cell migration in the forebrain. *Annu. Rev. Neurosci.* 26, 441–483. doi: 10.1146/annurev.neuro.26.041002.131058

McCreary, B. D., Rossiter, J. P., and Robertson, D. M. (1996). Recessive (true) microcephaly: a case report with neuropathological observations. *J. Intellect. Disabil. Res.* 40(Pt. 1), 66–70. doi: 10.1111/j.1365-2788.1996.tb00604.x

McGowen, M. R., Montgomery, S. H., Clark, C., and Gatesy, J. (2011). Phylogeny and adaptive evolution of the brain-development gene microcephalin (MCPH1) in cetaceans. *BMC Evol. Biol.* 11:98. doi: 10.1186/1471-2148-11-98

Mekel-Bobrov, N., Posthuma, D., Gilbert, S. L., Lind, P., Gosso, M. F., Luciano, M., et al. (2007). The ongoing adaptive evolution of ASPM and Microcephalin is not explained by increased intelligence. *Hum. Mol. Genet.* 16, 600–608. doi: 10.1093/hmg/ddl487

Mochida, G. H., and Walsh, C. A. (2001). Molecular genetics of human microcephaly. *Curr. Opin. Neurol.* 14, 151–156. doi: 10.1097/00019052-200104000-00003

Molnár, Z., Kaas, J. H., de Carlos, J. A., Hevner, R. F., Lein, E., and Němec, P. (2014). Evolution and development of the mammalian cerebral cortex. *Brain Behav. Evol.* 83, 126–139. doi: 10.1159/000357753

Molnar, Z., Metin, C., Stoykova, A., Tarabykin, V., Price, D. J., Francis, F., et al. (2006). Comparative aspects of cerebral cortical development. *Eur. J. Neurosci.* 23, 921–934. doi: 10.1111/j.1460-9568.2006.04611.x

Montgomery, S. H., Capellini, I., Venditti, C., Barton, R. A., and Mundy, N. I. (2011). Adaptive evolution of four microcephaly genes and the evolution of brain size in anthropoid primates. *Mol. Biol. Evol.* 28, 625–638. doi: 10.1093/molbev/msq237

Montgomery, S. H., and Mundy, N. I. (2013). Microcephaly genes and the evolution of sexual dimorphism in primate brain size. *J. Evol. Biol.* 26, 906–911. doi: 10.1111/jeb.12091

Montgomery, S. H., and Mundy, N. I. (2014). Microcephaly genes evolved adaptively throughout the evolution of eutherian mammals. *BMC Evol. Biol.* 14:120. doi: 10.1186/1471-2148-14-120

Moynihan, L., Jackson, A. P., Roberts, E., Karbani, G., Lewis, I., Corry, P., et al. (2000). A third novel locus for primary autosomal recessive microcephaly maps to chromosome 9q34. *Am. J. Hum. Genet.* 66, 724–727. doi: 10.1086/302777

Nadarajah, B., and Parnavelas, J. G. (2002). Modes of neuronal migration in the developing cerebral cortex. *Nat. Rev. Neurosci.* 3, 423–432. doi: 10.1038/nrn845

Neitzel, H., Neumann, L. M., Schindler, D., Wirges, A., Tonnies, H., Trimborn, M., et al. (2002). Premature chromosome condensation in humans associated with microcephaly and mental retardation: a novel autosomal recessive condition. *Am. J. Hum. Genet.* 70, 1015–1022. doi: 10.1086/339518

Nicholas, A. K., Khurshid, M., Desir, J., Carvalho, O. P., Cox, J. J., Thornton, G., et al. (2010). WDR62 is associated with the spindle pole and is mutated in human microcephaly. *Nat. Genet.* 42, 1010–1014. doi: 10.1038/ng.682

Nicholas, A. K., Swanson, E. A., Cox, J. J., Karbani, G., Malik, S., Springell, K., et al. (2009). The molecular landscape of ASPM mutations in primary microcephaly. *J. Med. Genet.* 46, 249–253. doi: 10.1136/jmg.2008.062380

Nielsen, R., Bustamante, C., Clark, A. G., Glanowski, S., Sackton, T. B., Hubisz, M. J., et al. (2005). A scan for positively selected genes in the genomes of humans and chimpanzees. *PLoS Biol.* 3:e170. doi: 10.1371/journal.pbio.0030170

Ouellette, E. M., Rosett, H. L., Rosman, N. P., and Weiner, L. (1977). Adverse effects on offspring of maternal alcohol abuse during pregnancy. *N. Engl. J. Med.* 297, 528–530. doi: 10.1056/nejm197709082971003

Pao, G. M., Zhu, Q., Perez-Garcia, C. G., Chou, S. J., Suh, H., Gage, F. H., et al. (2014). Role of BRCA1 in brain development. *Proc. Natl. Acad. Sci. U S A* 111, E1240–E1248. doi: 10.1073/pnas.1400783111

Paridaen, J. T., and Huttner, W. B. (2014). Neurogenesis during development of the vertebrate central nervous system. *EMBO Rep.* 15, 351–364. doi: 10.1002/embr.201438447

Passemard, S., El Ghouzzi, V., Nasser, H., Verney, C., Vodjdani, G., Lacaud, A., et al. (2011). VIP blockade leads to microcephaly in mice via disruption of Mcph1-Chk1 signaling. *J. Clin. Invest.* 121, 3071–3087. doi: 10.1172/JCI43824

Pattison, L., Crow, Y. J., Deeble, V. J., Jackson, A. P., Jafri, H., Rashid, Y., et al. (2000). A fifth locus for primary autosomal recessive microcephaly maps to chromosome 1q31. *Am. J. Hum. Genet.* 67, 1578–1580. doi: 10.1086/316910

Peng, G., Yim, E. K., Dai, H., Jackson, A. P., Burgt, I., Pan, M. R., et al. (2009). BRIT1/MCPH1 links chromatin remodelling to DNA damage response. *Nat. Cell Biol.* 11, 865–872. doi: 10.1038/ncb1895

Pfau, R. B., Thrush, D. L., Hamelberg, E., Bartholomew, D., Botes, S., Pastore, M., et al. (2013). MCPH1 deletion in a newborn with severe microcephaly and premature chromosome condensation. *Eur. J. Med. Genet.* 56, 609–613. doi: 10.1016/j.ejmg.2013.09.007

Plummer, G. (1952). Anomalies occurring in children exposed in utero to the atomic bomb in Hiroshima. *Pediatrics* 10, 687–693.

Ponting, C., and Jackson, A. P. (2005). Evolution of primary microcephaly genes and the enlargement of primate brains. *Curr. Opin. Genet. Dev.* 15, 241–248. doi: 10.1016/j.gde.2005.04.009

Pulvers, J. N., Bryk, J., Fish, J. L., Wilsch-Bräuninger, M., Arai, Y., Schreier, D., et al. (2010). Mutations in mouse Aspm (abnormal spindle-like microcephaly associated) cause not only microcephaly but also major defects in the germline. *Proc. Natl. Acad. Sci. U S A* 107, 16595–16600. doi: 10.1073/pnas.1010494107

Pulvers, J. N., and Huttner, W. B. (2009). Brca1 is required for embryonic development of the mouse cerebral cortex to normal size by preventing apoptosis of early neural progenitors. *Development* 136, 1859–1868. doi: 10.1242/dev.033498

Qazi, Q. H., and Reed, T. E. (1973). A problem in diagnosis of primary versus secondary microcephaly. *Clin. Genet.* 4, 46–52. doi: 10.1111/j.1399-0004.1973.tb01121.x

Rai, R., Dai, H., Multani, A. S., Li, K., Chin, K., Gray, J., et al. (2006). BRIT1 regulates early DNA damage response, chromosomal integrity and cancer. *Cancer Cell* 10, 145–157. doi: 10.1016/j.ccr.2006.07.002

Rakic, P. (1988). Specification of cerebral cortical areas. *Science* 241, 170–176. doi: 10.1126/science.3291116

Rakic, P. (1995). Radial versus tangential migration of neuronal clones in the developing cerebral cortex. *Proc. Natl. Acad. Sci. U S A* 92, 11323–11327. doi: 10.1073/pnas.92.25.11323

Rakic, P. (2009). Evolution of the neocortex: a perspective from developmental biology. *Nat. Rev. Neurosci.* 10, 724–735. doi: 10.1038/nrn2719

Richardson, S. S. (2011). Race and IQ in the postgenomic age: the microcephaly case. *Biosocieties* 6, 420–446. doi: 10.1057/biosoc.2011.20

Richardson, J., Shaaban, A. M., Kamal, M., Alisary, R., Walker, C., Ellis, I. O., et al. (2011). Microcephalin is a new novel prognostic indicator in breast cancer associated with BRCA1 inactivation. *Breast Cancer Res. Treat.* 127, 639–648. doi: 10.1007/s10549-010-1019-4

Rilling, J. K., and Insel, T. R. (1999). The primate neocortex in comparative perspective using magnetic resonance imaging. *J. Hum. Evol.* 37, 191–223. doi: 10.1006/jhev.1999.0313

Rimol, L. M., Agartz, I., Djurovic, S., Brown, A. A., Roddey, J. C., Kähler, A. K., et al. (2010). Sex-dependent association of common variants of microcephaly genes with brain structure. *Proc. Natl. Acad. Sci. U S A* 107, 384–388. doi: 10.1073/pnas.0908454107

Roberts, E., Hampshire, D. J., Pattison, L., Springell, K., Jafri, H., Corry, P., et al. (2002). Autosomal recessive primary microcephaly: an analysis of locus heterogeneity and phenotypic variation. *J. Med. Genet.* 39, 718–721. doi: 10.1136/jmg.39.10.718

Roberts, E., Jackson, A. P., Carradice, A. C., Deeble, V. J., Mannan, J., Rashid, Y., et al. (1999). The second locus for autosomal recessive primary microcephaly (MCPH2) maps to chromosome 19q13.1–13.2. *Eur. J. Hum. Genet.* 7, 815–820. doi: 10.1038/sj.ejhg.5200385

Ronan, J. L., Wu, W., and Crabtree, G. R. (2013). From neural development to cognition: unexpected roles for chromatin. *Nat. Rev. Genet.* 14, 347–359. doi: 10.1038/nrg3413

Rubenstein, J. L., Shimamura, K., Martinez, S., and Puelles, L. (1998). Regionalization of the prosencephalic neural plate. *Annu. Rev. Neurosci.* 21, 445–477. doi: 10.1146/annurev.neuro.21.1.445

Rushton, J. P., Vernon, P. A., and Bons, T. A. (2007). No evidence that polymorphisms of brain regulator genes Microcephalin and ASPM are associated with general mental ability, head circumference or altruism. *Biol. Lett.* 3, 157–160. doi: 10.1098/rsbl.2006.0586

Sajid Hussain, M., Marriam Bakhtiar, S., Farooq, M., Anjum, I., Janzen, E., Reza Toliat, M., et al. (2013). Genetic heterogeneity in Pakistani microcephaly families. *Clin. Genet.* 83, 446–451. doi: 10.1111/j.1399-0004.2012.01932.x

Sauer, F. C. (1935). Mitosis in the neural tube. *J. Comp. Neurol.* 62, 377–405. doi: 10.1002/cne.900620207

Scala, I., Titomanlio, L., Del Giudice, E., Passemard, S., Figliuolo, C., Annunziata, P., et al. (2010). Absence of microcephalin gene mutations in a large cohort of non-consanguineous patients with autosomal recessive primary microcephaly. *Am. J. Med. Genet. A* 152A, 2882–2885. doi: 10.1002/ajmg.a.33672

Shi, L., Li, M., Lin, Q., Qi, X., and Su, B. (2013). Functional divergence of the brain-size regulating gene MCPH1 during primate evolution and the origin of humans. *BMC Biol.* 11:62. doi: 10.1186/1741-7007-11-62

Shi, L., and Su, B. (2012). Identification and functional characterization of a primate-specific E2F1 binding motif regulating MCPH1 expression. *FEBS J.* 279, 491–503. doi: 10.1111/j.1742-4658.2011.08441.x

Sidman, R. L., and Rakic, P. (1973). Neuronal migration, with special reference to developing human brain: a review. *Brain Res.* 62, 1–35. doi: 10.1016/0006-8993(73)90617-3

Singh, N., Basnet, H., Wiltshire, T. D., Mohammad, D. H., Thompson, J. R., Heroux, A., et al. (2012a). Dual recognition of phosphoserine and phosphotyrosine in histone variant H2A.X by DNA damage response protein MCPH1. *Proc. Natl. Acad. Sci. U S A* 109, 14381–14386. doi: 10.1073/pnas.1212366109

Singh, N., Wiltshire, T. D., Thompson, J. R., Mer, G., and Couch, F. J. (2012b). Molecular basis for the association of microcephalin (MCPH1) protein with the cell division cycle protein 27 (Cdc27) subunit of the anaphase-promoting complex. *J. Biol. Chem.* 287, 2854–2862. doi: 10.1074/jbc.M111.307868

Sir, J. H., Barr, A. R., Nicholas, A. K., Carvalho, O. P., Khurshid, M., Sossick, A., et al. (2011). A primary microcephaly protein complex forms a ring around parental centrioles. *Nat. Genet.* 43, 1147–1153. doi: 10.1038/ng.971

Skarnes, W. C., Rosen, B., West, A. P., Koutsourakis, M., Bushell, W., Iyer, V., et al. (2011). A conditional knockout resource for the genome-wide study of mouse gene function. *Nature* 474, 337–342. doi: 10.1038/nature10163

Skarnes, W. C., von Melchner, H., Wurst, W., Hicks, G., Nord, A. S., Cox, T., et al. (2004). A public gene trap resource for mouse functional genomics. *Nat. Genet.* 36, 543–544. doi: 10.1038/ng0604-543

Smart, I. H., Dehay, C., Giroud, P., Berland, M., and Kennedy, H. (2002). Unique morphological features of the proliferative zones and postmitotic compartments of the neural epithelium giving rise to striate and extrastriate cortex in the monkey. *Cereb. Cortex* 12, 37–53. doi: 10.1093/cercor/12.1.37

Spohr, H. L., Willms, J., and Steinhausen, H. C. (1993). Prenatal alcohol exposure and long-term developmental consequences. *Lancet* 341, 907–910. doi: 10.1016/0140-6736(93)91207-3

Sun, T., and Hevner, R. F. (2014). Growth and folding of the mammalian cerebral cortex: from molecules to malformations. *Nat. Rev. Neurosci.* 15, 217–232. doi: 10.1038/nrn3707

Taverna, E., and Huttner, W. B. (2010). Neural progenitor nuclei IN motion. *Neuron* 67, 906–914. doi: 10.1016/j.neuron.2010.08.027

Tessier-Lavigne, M., and Goodman, C. S. (1996). The molecular biology of axon guidance. *Science* 274, 1123–1133. doi: 10.1126/science.274.5290.1123

Thornton, G. K., and Woods, C. G. (2009). Primary microcephaly: do all roads lead to Rome? *Trends Genet.* 25, 501–510. doi: 10.1016/j.tig.2009.09.011

Timpson, N., Heron, J., Smith, G. D., and Enard, W. (2007). Comment on papers by Evans et al. and Mekel-Bobrov et al. on evidence for positive selection of MCPH1 and ASPM. *Science* 317:1036a. doi: 10.1126/science.1141705

Tommerup, N., Mortensen, E., Nielsen, M. H., Wegner, R. D., Schindler, D., and Mikkelsen, M. (1993). Chromosomal breakage, endomitosis, endoreduplication and hypersensitivity toward radiomimetric and alkylating agents: a possible new autosomal recessive mutation in a girl with craniosynostosis and microcephaly. *Hum. Genet.* 92, 339–346. doi: 10.1007/bf01247331

Trimborn, M., Bell, S. M., Felix, C., Rashid, Y., Jafri, H., Griffiths, P. D., et al. (2004). Mutations in microcephalin cause aberrant regulation of chromosome condensation. *Am. J. Hum. Genet.* 75, 261–266. doi: 10.1086/422855

Trimborn, M., Ghani, M., Walther, D. J., Dopatka, M., Dutrannoy, V., Busche, A., et al. (2010). Establishment of a mouse model with misregulated chromosome condensation due to defective Mcph1 function. *PLoS One* 5:e9242. doi: 10.1371/journal.pone.0009242

Trimborn, M., Richter, R., Sternberg, N., Gavvovidis, I., Schindler, D., Jackson, A. P., et al. (2005). The first missense alteration in the MCPH1 gene causes autosomal recessive microcephaly with an extremely mild cellular and clinical phenotype. *Hum. Mutat.* 26:496. doi: 10.1002/humu.9382

Trimborn, M., Schindler, D., Neitzel, H., and Hirano, T. (2006). Misregulated chromosome condensation in MCPH1 primary microcephaly is mediated by condensin II. *Cell Cycle* 5, 322–326. doi: 10.4161/cc.5.3.2412

Tuoc, T. C., Boretius, S., Sansom, S. N., Pitulescu, M. E., Frahm, J., Livesey, F. J., et al. (2013). Chromatin regulation by BAF170 controls cerebral cortical size and thickness. *Dev. Cell* 25, 256–269. doi: 10.1016/j.devcel.2013.04.005

Vallender, E. J., Mekel-Bobrov, N., and Lahn, B. T. (2008). Genetic basis of human brain evolution. *Trends Neurosci.* 31, 637–644. doi: 10.1016/j.tins.2008.08.010

Venkatesh, T., and Suresh, P. S. (2014). Emerging roles of MCPH1: expedition from primary microcephaly to cancer. *Eur J. Cell Biol.* 93, 98–105. doi: 10.1016/j.ejcb.2014.01.005

Waites, C. L., Craig, A. M., and Garner, C. C. (2005). Mechanisms of vertebrate synaptogenesis. *Annu. Rev. Neurosci.* 28, 251–274. doi: 10.1146/annurev.neuro.27.070203.144336

Walsh, C. A. (1999). Genetic malformations of the human cerebral cortex. *Neuron* 23, 19–29. doi: 10.1016/s0896-6273(00)80749-7

Wang, J. K., Li, Y., and Su, B. (2008). A common SNP of MCPH1 is associated with cranial volume variation in Chinese population. *Hum. Mol. Genet.* 17, 1329–1335. doi: 10.1093/hmg/ddn021

Wang, Y. Q., and Su, B. (2004). Molecular evolution of microcephalin, a gene determining human brain size. *Hum. Mol. Genet.* 13, 1131–1137. doi: 10.1093/hmg/ddh127

Wong, P. C., Chandrasekaran, B., and Zheng, J. (2012). The derived allele of ASPM is associated with lexical tone perception. *PLoS One* 7:e34243. doi: 10.1371/journal.pone.0034243

Wood, J. W., Johnson, K. G., and Omori, Y. (1967). In utero exposure to the Hiroshima atomic bomb. An evaluation of head size and mental retardation: twenty years later. *Pediatrics* 39, 385–392.

Woods, C. G. (2004). Human microcephaly. *Curr. Opin. Neurobiol.* 14, 112–117. doi: 10.1016/j.conb.2004.01.003

Woods, C. G., Bond, J., and Enard, W. (2005). Autosomal recessive primary microcephaly (MCPH): a review of clinical, molecular and evolutionary findings. *Am. J. Hum. Genet.* 76, 717–728. doi: 10.1086/429930

Woods, R. P., Freimer, N. B., De Young, J. A., Fears, S. C., Sicotte, N. L., Service, S. K., et al. (2006). Normal variants of Microcephalin and ASPM do not account for brain size variability. *Hum. Mol. Genet.* 15, 2025–2029. doi: 10.1093/hmg/ddl126

Woods, N. T., Mesquita, R. D., Sweet, M., Carvalho, M. A., Li, X., Liu, Y., et al. (2012). Charting the landscape of tandem BRCT domain-mediated protein interactions. *Sci. Signal.* 5:rs6. doi: 10.1126/scisignal.2002255

Woods, C. G., and Parker, A. (2013). Investigating microcephaly. *Arch. Dis. Child.* 98, 707–713. doi: 10.1136/archdischild-2012-302882

Xu, X., Lee, J., and Stern, D. F. (2004). Microcephalin is a DNA damage response protein involved in regulation of CHK1 and BRCA1. *J. Biol. Chem.* 279, 34091–34094. doi: 10.1074/jbc.c400139200

Yamashita, D., Shintomi, K., Ono, T., Gavvovidis, I., Schindler, D., Neitzel, H., et al. (2011). MCPH1 regulates chromosome condensation and shaping as a composite modulator of condensin II. *J. Cell Biol.* 194, 841–854. doi: 10.1083/jcb.201106141

Yang, Y. J., Baltus, A. E., Mathew, R. S., Murphy, E. A., Evrony, G. D., Gonzalez, D. M., et al. (2012). Microcephaly gene links trithorax and REST/NRSF to control neural stem cell proliferation and differentiation. *Cell.* 151, 1097–1112. doi: 10.1016/j.cell.2012.10.043

Yang, Z., and Bielawski, J. P. (2000). Statistical methods for detecting molecular adaptation. *Trends Ecol. Evol.* 15, 496–503. doi: 10.1016/s0169-5347(00)01994-7

Yang, S. Z., Lin, F. T., and Lin, W. C. (2008). MCPH1/BRIT1 cooperates with E2F1 in the activation of checkpoint, DNA repair and apoptosis. *EMBO Rep.* 9, 907–915. doi: 10.1038/embor.2008.128

Zhang, B., Wang, E., Dai, H., Shen, J., Hsieh, H. J., Lu, X., et al. (2014). Phosphorylation of the BRCA1 C terminus (BRCT) repeat inhibitor of hTERT (BRIT1) protein coordinates TopBP1 protein recruitment and amplifies ataxia telangiectasia-mutated and Rad3-related (ATR) Signaling. *J. Biol. Chem.* 289, 34284–34295. doi: 10.1074/jbc.m114.587113

Zhou, Z. W., Tapias, A., Bruhn, C., Gruber, R., Sukchev, M., and Wang, Z. Q. (2013). DNA damage response in microcephaly development of MCPH1 mouse model. *DNA Repair (Amst)* 12, 645–655. doi: 10.1016/j.dnarep.2013.04.017

3

Neurophysiology of the Developing Cerebral Cortex: What We Have Learned and What We Need to Know

*Heiko J. Luhmann**

Institute of Physiology, University Medical Center Mainz, Mainz, Germany

Correspondence:
Heiko J. Luhmann
luhmann@uni-mainz.de

This review article aims to give a brief summary on the novel technologies, the challenges, our current understanding, and the open questions in the field of the neurophysiology of the developing cerebral cortex in rodents. In the past, *in vitro* electrophysiological and calcium imaging studies on single neurons provided important insights into the function of cellular and subcellular mechanism during early postnatal development. In the past decade, neuronal activity in large cortical networks was recorded in pre- and neonatal rodents *in vivo* by the use of novel high-density multi-electrode arrays and genetically encoded calcium indicators. These studies demonstrated a surprisingly rich repertoire of spontaneous cortical and subcortical activity patterns, which are currently not completely understood in their functional roles in early development and their impact on cortical maturation. Technological progress in targeted genetic manipulations, optogenetics, and chemogenetics now allow the experimental manipulation of specific neuronal cell types to elucidate the function of early (transient) cortical circuits and their role in the generation of spontaneous and sensory evoked cortical activity patterns. Large-scale interactions between different cortical areas and subcortical regions, characterization of developmental shifts from synchronized to desynchronized activity patterns, identification of transient circuits and hub neurons, role of electrical activity in the control of glial cell differentiation and function are future key tasks to gain further insights into the neurophysiology of the developing cerebral cortex.

Keywords: cerebral cortex, neurophysiology, development, rodent, methods

INTRODUCTION—WHAT ARE OUR TOOLS?

In the last decade life sciences has shown a tremendous progress in developing and improving novel technologies. In cellular neurophysiology classical electrophysiological recording techniques and cellular imaging methods are very successfully combined with new tools in molecular biology and genetics to gain deeper insights into the function of single neurons and defined neuronal networks. Using the powerful Patch-seq technique, whole-cell patch-clamp recordings can be combined with morphological reconstructions, immunohistochemistry, and single-cell RNA-sequencing (scRNA-seq) to perform a multidimensional characterization of a single cell and to correlate the gene expression profile with its structural and functional properties (Cadwell et al., 2017; Scala et al., 2021). When combined with retrograde labeling, information on the projection patterns of single neurons can be added (Peng et al., 2021). Laser capture microdissection allows the transcriptomic characterization of subcellular compartments, such as soma vs. dendrite (Perez et al., 2021). Paired recordings from synaptically connected neurons combined with precise 3D reconstructions of the cells' morphology provided very detailed information on the function of local neuronal networks, e.g., a cortical column (Feldmeyer et al., 2018). With the vitro multi-patch approach 10–15 neurons can be simultaneously patch-clamp recorded, intracellularly labeled and subsequently analyzed in their synaptic connectivity (Peng et al., 2019). Functional connectivity maps at a larger scale, but with less temporal and spatial precision, can be obtained in brain slices with caged glutamate laser-scanning photostimulation (Meng et al., 2020).

Beside these advances in *in vitro* neurophysiology, *in vivo* recording, and stimulation techniques became also very powerful. Two-photon microscopy can be used to accomplish whole-cell membrane potential recordings of fluorescently labeled and genetically defined neurons in awake head-fixed mice while performing specific behavioral tasks (Petersen, 2017). Juxtacellular stimulation and recording of single cells in head-fixed or freely moving rats allows to study the role of single neurons in cognition and behavior (Houweling and Brecht, 2008; Tang et al., 2014). The number of simultaneously recorded neurons increased over the last decade from a few hundreds to a few thousands (Steinmetz et al., 2019; Perez-Prieto and Delgado-Restituto, 2021) and we may soon approach the neurophysiologist's dream (or nightmare?) to "concurrently record electrical spikes from every neuron in a mammalian brain" (Kleinfeld et al., 2019). To reach this aim, close cooperations with other scientific fields are already on-going (Jun et al., 2017; Garcia-Etxarri and Yuste, 2021). Material sciences and electronic engineering will foster the development of biocompatible multi-electrode arrays with very high number of electrodes, which can be used for recordings of single units and focal electrical stimulation (Jun et al., 2017; Kleinfeld et al., 2019; Perez-Prieto and Delgado-Restituto, 2021). Recently, chronic single unit recordings could be obtained from freely moving rats over up to 4 months with Neuropixel electrodes (Luo et al., 2020). These technological developments will also have an impact on experimental and clinical approaches of deep brain stimulation and brain-machine interfaces.

In the last decade subcellular, cellular, meso-scale, and large-scale imaging methods also showed tremendous technological progress. Genetically encoded calcium indicators, mostly from the GCaMP family, are powerful tools to monitor neuronal activity in small networks up to large-scale dynamics in behaving animals (Cardin et al., 2020; Linden et al., 2021; Ren and Komiyama, 2021). The large majority of these *in vivo* studies are restricted to upper neocortical regions because of technical limitations (Yang and Yuste, 2017). However, red-shifted fluorescent calcium indicators (Tischbirek et al., 2017) and three-photon microscopy (Takasaki et al., 2019) now enables imaging of deep cortical layers with single-cell resolution. Longitudinal calcium imaging from cortical and also deep brain structures can be obtained in freely behaving mice with the (wireless) miniature fluorescence microscope (miniScope) technology (Barbera et al., 2019; Zhang et al., 2019), which also allows recording of neuronal activity at single-cell resolution. Recently high-resolution two-photon calcium imaging of both cortical hemispheres have been performed in awake head-fixed mice (Barson et al., 2020; Cardin et al., 2020). This powerful method allows for the first time the analysis of the entire cortical mantle with cellular resolution. However, calcium imaging still has a number of disadvantages when compared to cellular neurophysiology. Electrophysiological recordings with sub-millisecond resolution provides high temporal information on the spiking output of the neuron, whereas calcium imaging cannot directly monitor the output, but rather monitors the increase in $[Ca^{2+}]_i$ following (subthreshold) synaptic activation and internal state changes (West et al., 2001). A recent study in the visual cortex of awake mice using the genetically encoded calcium indicator GCaMP6f and extracellular recordings with silicon probes demonstrated the advantages and disadvantages of both methods (Siegle et al., 2021). While electrophysiological recordings showed a higher fraction of units with stimulus-driven activity, GCaMP6f calcium imaging revealed a higher selectivity (sharper tuning) among responsive neurons. Another *in vivo* study in the visual cortex of awake transgenic mice expressing GCaMP6s or GCaMP6f demonstrated that $<10\%$ and 20–30%, respectively, of isolated single spikes were detectable with calcium imaging (Huang et al., 2021). Critical assessment of calcium imaging data (Rupprecht et al., 2021) and the development of new calcium indicators with fast kinetics (such as jGCaMP8) may solve some of these problems (Zhang et al., 2021).

Subthreshold synaptic inputs are very difficult to detect with somatic calcium signals. Genetically encoded voltage indicators (GEVIs) can monitor subthreshold transmembrane potential dynamics *in vitro* and *in vivo* (Bando et al., 2019). The classical voltage-sensitive dyes developed over the last 30 years were most valuable in elucidating cortical function (Grinvald et al., 2016). The GEVIs have the advantage that they can be targeted to specific cell types and when combined with 2-photon excitation allows imaging of membrane potential dynamics with single-cell resolution in the cerebral cortex *in vivo* (Bando et al., 2019). GEVIs can be also used at the subcellular level, e.g., to study action potential generation at the axon initial segment or transmitter release at the presynaptic terminal (Panzera and Hoppa, 2019).

Beside this progress in cellular electrophysiological and imaging techniques a number of novel genetic and molecular biological methods became most valuable tools to manipulate gene expression and activity of defined single cells during distinct time points of development. Targeted gene delivery via *in vivo* (e.g., *in utero*) electroporation (De Vry et al., 2010), directed genetic manipulations by CRISPR-based technology (Kampmann, 2020), viral tools for specific cell and circuit manipulation (Vormstein-Schneider et al., 2020), Designer Receptors Exclusively Activated by Designer Drugs (DREADD)-based chemogenetic tools (Roth, 2016), and optogenetics (Deisseroth, 2015) are used to activate or silence specific neurons. Some of these methods, especially optogenetics, become even more powerful when combined with *in vivo* targeted whole-cell recordings in behaving animals (Gasselin et al., 2021) or with miniScope technology in freely moving mice (de Groot et al., 2020).

These impressive methodological developments offer the chance to booster interdisciplinary cooperations between experts in cellular electrophysiology, molecular biology, and biostatistics or biomathematicians, and as in the past, physicists are always welcome. Does that mean that the times, that a cellular neurophysiologist is sitting for 6–12 h alone at his/her *in vitro* or *in vivo* set-up, obtaining all relevant data on-line and analyzing the data with rather simple statistics and mathematics programs is over?

The next three sections will focus on the cellular neurophysiology of the developing cerebral cortex in rodents. Since the function of individual neurons is not only determined by its intrinsic properties, but also by its synaptic inputs, early cortical network activity will be also briefly discussed.

THE CHALLENGES OF STUDYING THE NEUROPHYSIOLOGY OF THE DEVELOPING CEREBRAL CORTEX IN RODENTS

Everybody who studies the cellular and network properties of the cerebral cortex in newborn rodents faces a number of challenges. In mice and rats (and in many other mammals such as ferrets), the cerebral cortex at birth has not yet reached its mature six-layered structure. Neurons are still migrating to their final location in layer (L) 2 and L3, perhaps even L4, and these layers are formed until postnatal day (P) 2–3. This migration process, as neuronal proliferation and differentiation (for review Uhlen et al., 2015), is controlled by spontaneous intracellular calcium transients (Bando et al., 2016). Thus, the neocortical network of a newborn rodent changes its layered architecture on a daily basis!

This add-on process in neocortical layering is accompanied by the reorganization of an early transient cortical network, which at birth consists of the marginal zone (later L1), the cortical plate (later L2–L6) and the subplate (for review Kanold and Luhmann, 2010; Hoerder-Suabedissen and Molnár, 2015). At late embryonic and early postnatal stage thalamocortical afferents form functional glutamatergic synapses with subplate neurons, which play important roles in synaptic plasticity and synchronized network activity of the developing cortical network (for review Colonnese and Phillips, 2018; López-Bendito, 2018; Luhmann et al., 2018; Molnár et al., 2020). Between P1 and P2, these thalamocortical fibers disconnect from the subplate and innervate their final targets in L4 and L5/6. Another transient thalamocortical circuit is assembled by infragranular somatostatin (SST) expressing interneurons which innervate parvalbumin (PV) and pyramidal neurons. This early thalamocortical-intracortical circuit disappears by the end of the first postnatal week and is important for the development of thalamic feedforward inhibition via PV interneurons (Tuncdemir et al., 2016). Using transgenic mouse lines Marques-Smith et al. identified in the neonatal mouse somatosensory a transient and activity-dependent early reciprocal circuit cortex between L5b SST-positive interneurons and L4 spiny stellate cells (Marques-Smith et al., 2016). Thus, the newborn rodent cortex exhibits a number of transient circuits and changes its thalamic activation pattern within 3–4 days.

Beside subplate cells, other neocortical neurons also fulfill important roles in early cortical development and are only transiently present during peri-/neonatal stages. Cajal-Retzius neurons in the marginal zone/L1 control a number of important developmental processes and mostly disappear by programmed cell death (apoptosis) during the first postnatal days after termination of neuronal migration (Causeret et al., 2021). Beside subplate and Cajal-Retzius neurons, glutamatergic and GABAergic neurons also die to a large extent by apoptosis during the first postnatal week (with a peak at ~P7) (Causeret et al., 2018). Notably, this apoptosis process is strongly regulated by electrical activity (Blanquie et al., 2017; Riva et al., 2019). Beside the activity-dependent control in overall cell number, the axonal and dendritic morphology and synaptic connectivity of single cortical neurons is also regulated by early activity (Callaway and Borrell, 2011; Malyshevskaya et al., 2013; Grant et al., 2016) (for review Leighton and Lohmann, 2016). Defined subpopulations of GABAergic interneurons control spontaneous cortical activity patterns and play central roles in the early postnatal development of the cerebral cortex (Leighton et al., 2021). During the first two postnatal week, vasocative-intestinal-peptide and somatostatin interneurons undergo developmental transitions in their cortical function and their processing of sensory information (Kastli et al., 2020). Well-connected early generated interneurons with relatively mature electrophysiological and morphological properties exert a strong influence on cortical activity and ablation of these neurons disturbs spontaneous activity and inhibitory synapse formation (Wang et al., 2019). Using longitudinal *in vivo* calcium imaging of somatosensory cortical activity in non-anesthetized mouse pups, Duan et al. convincely demonstrated that developmental network patterns in interneurons and pyramidal cells are essential for the assembly of neocortical circuits and for the control of interneurons' cell death (Duan et al., 2020). Using *in vivo* imaging in the developing mouse barrel cortex, Modol et al. show that PV interneurons form transient periphery-driven and experience-dependent patches of correlated activity (Modol et al., 2020). Embryonic disturbances in interneuron generation and cortical network integration cause a transient dysfunction with long-term behavioral consequences (Magno et al., 2021). Thus, during the first two postnatal weeks the rodent cerebral cortex is characterized by the deconstruction of transient neuronal networks and simultaneously by the construction of its characteristic six-layered, columnar architecture, intracortical microcircuits, corticothalamic connections, and corticocortical connections.

Spontaneous and sensory evoked activity, monitored by calcium imaging *in vivo*, has been not only observed in neurons of the developing cerebral cortex (Rochefort et al., 2009; Yuryev et al., 2018), but also in astrocytes (Wang et al., 2006). In the embryonic ventricular zone spontaneous calcium waves propagate through radial glia cells and modulate proliferation (Weissman et al., 2004). Astrocytes in newborn mouse neocortical slices reveal spontaneous ultraslow (~2 per hour) and very long (~8 min) sodium fluctuations that are largely restricted to the first postnatal week (Felix et al., 2019). The mechanisms underlying this slow activity and its functional role are currently unknown. Spontaneous activity controls myelination since oligodendrocytes preferentially myelinate electrically active axons via axo-glial interactions leading to local calcium rises in glial cell processes (Wake et al., 2015). *In vitro* data indicate that patterned neuronal activity promotes the survival of oligodendrocytes (Gary et al., 2012) and that GABA released from inhibitory neurons controls myelination and internode length thereby tuning the conduction velocity (Hamilton et al., 2017). Vice versa, oligodendrocyte precursor cells not only respond to, but also modulate neuronal network function, demonstrating a bidirectional glia-neuron cross-talk (Sakry et al., 2014).

This developmental reorganization in cortical structure is accompanied by four neurophysiological processes, which have a strong impact on early cortical function and development. As in the hippocampus (Ben-Ari, 2014), the cerebral cortex also shows a developmental shift in GABA action from depolarizing/excitatory to hyperpolarizing/inhibitory (for review Kirmse et al., 2018; Kilb, 2020). This shift in GABA action differs between *in vitro* and *in vivo* preparations as shown by optogenetic studies (Valeeva et al., 2016). Electrophysiological differences between *in vitro* and *in vivo* preparations have been further reported following the deletion of NKCC1, the primary chloride inward transporter (Graf et al., 2021). *In vivo* reports (Kirmse et al., 2015; Murata and Colonnese, 2020) and modeling studies (Lombardi et al., 2021) provide a more complex picture of the developmental shift in GABA action, especially when on-going spatiotemporal interactions between GABAergic and glutamatergic inputs are taken into account (for review Kilb, 2021). It is not the aim of this short review to summarize the current data on this topic, but it is well-accepted that the intracellular chloride concentration is regulated by development, various molecular factors, and neuronal activity (Kaila et al., 2014; Watanabe and Fukuda, 2015; Virtanen et al., 2020, 2021). Thus, the action and function of the important neurotransmitter GABA, and also glycine and taurine (for review Kilb and Fukuda, 2017), changes dramatically during the first postnatal week in rodent cortex!

The second developmental change in cortical function is the transition from electrical coupling via gap junctions to mostly chemical synaptic transmission (Valiullina et al., 2016; Yao et al., 2016). During embryonic and early postnatal development, gap junctions play important roles in various developmental processes (Allene and Cossart, 2010; Niculescu and Lohmann, 2014). Yu et al. found strong electrical coupling between clonally related excitatory neurons in columnar manner forming the functional template of ontogenetic columns (Yu et al., 2012). Lineage-related electrical coupling has been also demonstrated between interneurons of the same subtype over an extended period of time and across a range of distances (Zhang et al., 2017). At later stages electrical synapses may interact with chemical synapses (Pereda, 2014). Neonatal connexin 26 removal impairs neocortical development and leads to elevated anxiety (Su et al., 2017). With maturation intercellular communication via gap junctions largely disappears during the second postnatal week and remains restricted to specific cell types, mostly interneurons (Connors, 2017), or cell compartments as axo-axonal coupling (Traub et al., 2004). Thus, intercellular functional interactions shift from electrical coupling to chemical synaptic transmission!

The third developmental change in cortical function is the transition from highly synchronized network activity during the late prenatal/early postnatal period to a more desynchronized state at later stages. Using two-photon calcium imaging of the barrel cortex *in vivo*, Mizuno et al. demonstrated that during the first postnatal week L4 neurons within one barrel show synchronized spontaneous activity (Mizuno et al., 2018). This patchwork activity pattern disappeared during the second postnatal week when L4 neurons fired asynchronously within one barrel. Several spontaneous network activity patterns (cortical early network oscillations, spindle bursts/delta brushes, early gamma oscillations, cortical giant depolarizing potentials, spontaneous activity transients, and others) have been characterized in the neonatal cerebral cortex of various mammalian species, from mouse to human (Colonnese and Khazipov, 2012; Luhmann et al., 2016; Luhmann and Khazipov, 2018; Molnár et al., 2020). For some of these patterns, the subplate and other transient cortical circuits play a central role (Kanold and Luhmann, 2010; Colonnese and Phillips, 2018; Luhmann et al., 2018). Beside these developmental changes in the pattern of spontaneous activity, cortical processing of sensory evoked activity undergoes a similar transition from bursting in pre- and neonatal stages to continuous "adult-like" activity during further development (Colonnese et al., 2010). Thus, during early development the neocortex shifts from a highly synchronized to a more desynchronized state!

The fourth developmental change in cortical function is the gradual innervation of the cortical layers by ascending neuromodulatory systems, such as the cholinergic, serotonergic, dopaminergic, and the noradrenergic system. Although the subplate receives functional neuromodulatory inputs already at early stages (Hanganu and Luhmann, 2004; Dupont et al., 2006; Hanganu et al., 2009), cortical layers 2 to 6 are only gradually innervated in an inside first—out side last sequence (Calarco and Robertson, 1995; Mechawar and Descarries, 2001). The emergence of the neuromodulatory inputs accompanies the developmental switch from bursting to continuous desynchronized activity (Colonnese et al., 2010) and the developmental changes in vigilance states and active movements (Mukherjee et al., 2017; Dooley et al., 2020; Glanz et al., 2021). Thus, these neuromodulatory systems have a progressively stronger influence on spontaneous and sensory evoked cortical function during the early postnatal period.

These dramatic structural and functional changes in the rodent developing cortex represent a major problem for everybody studying early neocortical development in mice and rats, because one should not (or better cannot) merge data from different postnatal days. The neocortex of a P0 mouse is different from that of a P1 mouse, and that differs from a P2 mouse! In a careful and detailed study, one should either focus on one single postnatal day (Mojtahedi et al., 2021) or form groups that differ in age not more than 1–2 days (Yang et al., 2009; Shen and Colonnese, 2016).

NEUROPHYSIOLOGY OF THE DEVELOPING CEREBRAL CORTEX: WHAT WE HAVE LEARNED

Although recording techniques from freely moving rodents are important and become increasingly more powerful, such recordings from newborn rodents are only of limited value, because newborn mice and rats do not actively move so much during the first 10 postnatal days (van der Bourg et al., 2017). However, newborn rodents are exposed to a variety of sensory stimuli (e.g., from the proprioceptive and probably vestibular system) and from passive interactions with the mother and littermates. Sensory feedback from passive stimulation by littermates trigger cortical activity (Akhmetshina et al., 2016). Furthermore, spontaneous self-generated movements (myoclonic twitches) can be already observed very early and play an important role in the development of the sensorimotor system (Inacio et al., 2016; Dooley et al., 2020; Gomez et al., 2021). Head-fixation of newborn rodents allows simultaneous recordings of large-scale neuronal activity and spontaneous movements of the animal's snout including the whiskers, the forelimbs, hindlimbs, and the tail using electromyography (EMG) or multiple video camera monitoring (Dooley and Blumberg, 2018; Glanz et al., 2021; Gomez et al., 2021). Neuronal structures involved in the generation or modulation of spontaneous movements in newborns can be studied with imaging or multi-electrodes recording techniques. Central pattern generator (CPG) networks in spinal cord, brainstem, thalamus, motor cortex, and also cerebellum are of pivotal interest (Colonnese and Khazipov, 2012; Blumberg et al., 2013; Luhmann et al., 2016) and as many brain regions as possible should be recorded simultaneously in awake animals. CPGs and motor-related networks may trigger spontaneous movements, which subsequently activate the sensory system, thereby promoting the spatio-temporal binding of developing neuronal networks in the sensory-motor system. In the somatosensory and motor cortex of newborn rodents spindle burst and gamma oscillations mediate this binding process (Khazipov et al., 2004, 2013; Yang et al., 2009, 2013; Minlebaev et al., 2011; An et al., 2014; Luhmann and Khazipov, 2018; Dooley et al., 2020; Glanz et al., 2021).

Spindle burst and gamma oscillatory activity has been also demonstrated in the visual cortex of rodents before eye opening (Ackman and Crair, 2014; Colonnese and Phillips, 2018). Spindle bursts in the visual cortex are triggered by retinal bursts (Hanganu et al., 2006; Colonnese and Khazipov, 2010) and are modulated by the cholinergic system (Hanganu et al., 2006; Ackman et al., 2012). Spontaneous activity generated in the cochlea before hearing onset controls the development of central auditory pathways (Tritsch et al., 2007; Wang et al., 2015), but the function of spindle bursts and gamma oscillations in the auditory cortex of newborn rodents is less clear as compared to those in the visual and somatosensory system.

Nested gamma spindle bursts have been demonstrated in the prefrontal–hippocampal network of the neonatal rat (Brockmann et al., 2011; Bitzenhofer et al., 2015) and cholinergic projections facilitate this oscillatory coupling by activation of muscarinic acetylcholine receptors (Janiesch et al., 2011). In neonatal mice optogenetic activation of channelrhodopsin-expressing pyramidal neurons in L2/3, but not L5/6, of the prefrontal cortex boost oscillatory activity in beta–gamma frequency bands (Bitzenhofer et al., 2017).

In summary, spontaneous and sensory evoked activity pattern recorded in sensory, motor and prefrontal cortex of newborn rodents share many similarities and most likely fulfill similar functions. It is not surprising that these activity patterns also occur in the cerebral cortex of preterm human babies, when the cortex resembles in its structure and function the cortex of a newborn rodent (Colonnese et al., 2010; Luhmann and Fukuda, 2020). The activity patterns recorded in different cortical areas of preterm human babies are termed spindle bursts, delta brushes, *tracé discontinue, tracé alternant*, and spontaneous activity transients (SAT) (Vanhatalo and Kaila, 2006; Milh et al., 2007; Colonnese et al., 2010; Chipaux et al., 2013; Koolen et al., 2016) and serve as biomarkers for the cognitive and motor development of the child (Iyer et al., 2015; Tokariev et al., 2019; Moghadam et al., 2021).

Over the last decade we got deeper insights into the functional roles of these early cortical activity patterns. During embryonic stages spontaneous activity arising from the thalamus regulates coordinate cortical sensory area patterning and drives the emergence of functional cortical maps (Moreno-Juan et al., 2017; Anton-Bolanos et al., 2018, 2019; Martini et al., 2021). In newborn rodent cortex spontaneous and sensory evoked cortical activity often locally synchronizes column-like networks resembling early topographic cortical maps (Yang et al., 2013; Kummer et al., 2016). At perinatal stage this columnar cortical activity ("columnar burst," Colonnese et al., 2010) is mediated by the activation of a local network in the subplate (Dupont et al., 2006; Hanganu et al., 2009). Removal of the subplate in the neonatal rat barrel cortex reduces spindle burst activity and prevents the development of the thalamocortical barrel field patterning (Tolner et al., 2012). Li et al. have demonstrated that not only the development of barrel-related columns, but also the emergence of L4 depends on early activity, specifically on glutamate released from thalamocortical afferents (Li et al., 2013).

In a number of elegant studies Hanganu-Opatz and coworkers demonstrated how genetic or experimentally induced manipulations in the oscillatory network activity in neonatal prefrontal cortex results in long-term functional and behavioral deficits (Chini and Hanganu-Opatz, 2021). In a mouse model of mental disorders, Chini et al. demonstrated an early-emerging prefrontal network dysfunction that subsequently gives rise to cognitive deficits. They show that this deficiency can be rescued by minocycline administration, thus identifying a potential biomarker (Chini et al., 2020). Bitzenhofer et al. manipulated early activity in the prefrontal cortex of neonatal mice, resulting in disruption of coordinated patterns of electrical activity, excitation-inhibition imbalance, and impaired cognitive abilities at adult age. Thus, prefrontal activity during development is critical for adult network function and behavioral performance (Bitzenhofer et al., 2021).

THE OPEN QUESTIONS AND FUTURE TASKS

This last section provides a personal viewpoint on the open questions and tasks that should be addressed in the third decade of the 21st century to gain further insights into the neurophysiology of the developing cerebral cortex. If possible, these studies should be performed *in vivo* in non-anesthetized animals.

1) Study with cell resolution recording and imaging techniques the large-scale interactions between different cortical areas (sensory, association, prefrontal, motor) and subcortical regions in pre- and early postnatal development. What are the underlying mechanisms of local vs. global interactions and what are their functions? Define the relationship and the role of local vs. propagating activity.
2) Identify at different developmental stages the interactions between spontaneous, movement related and sensory evoked activity. Characterize the developmental shift from synchronized to desynchronized network activity in sensory, prefrontal, and motor system including subcortical regions.
3) What is the functional role of early cortical activity patterns in shaping the pre- and early postnatal cortex at micro- (e.g., spines), meso- (e.g., microcircuitry), and macroscale (e.g., cortico-cortical connections)?
4) Determine the dynamic spatio-temporal action of GABA and glycine during earliest (prenatal) stages of development under non-anesthetized *in vivo* conditions and by the use of non-invasive techniques?
5) Characterize the role of neuromodulators (e.g., acetylcholine, noradrenaline, serotonin) on cortical neurophysiology at different developmental stages.
6) Define and elucidate the emergence of cognitive functions, e.g., learning and memory, spatial navigation, social interactions.
7) Characterize the role of distinct populations of early generated GABAergic interneurons (Wang et al., 2019) and identify and manipulate hub neurons in developing neocortical networks (cf. hub neurons in immature hippocampal networks Bonifazi et al., 2009; Picardo et al., 2011; Bocchio et al., 2020).
8) In their seminal review article Connors and Gutnick described in the rodent cerebral cortex three distinct functional cell types based on their intrinsic firing pattern (Connors and Gutnick, 1990): regular spiking, fast spiking and bursting neurons. Over the last 30 years we learned that cortical neurons, especially interneurons, can be subdivided into many more cell type classes (DeFelipe et al., 2013). A recent single-cell transcriptomic analysis of the mouse primary motor cortex identified over 56 neuronal cell types (Yao et al., 2021). Kriegstein and coworkers recently characterized 138 neocortical cell type clusters throughout the second trimester of human development and demonstrated that "gene-expression patterns are highly dynamic across cortical regions" and "borders between clusters are fluid" (Bhaduri et al., 2021). Since it is well-established that the firing pattern of neocortical neurons *in vivo* is strongly regulated by the action of modulatory systems (Steriade, 2001a), cell classifications based on firing patterns may be also more "fluid" as estimated by experimental protocols used in mostly *in vitro* slice preparations. Thus, cell type classifications in (developing) cerebral cortex should take technical limitations (c.f. Steriade, 2001b) and dynamic changes into account.
9) Identify the mechanisms and the functional role of activity-dependent interactions between neurons and astrocytes, oligodendrocytes, radial glia, and microglia in perinatal cortex. How do certain spontaneous activity patterns promote myelination (for review Zuchero and Barres, 2013)? How does neuronal activity influence the development of the tri-partite synapse (for review Dallerac et al., 2018) and "quad-partite" synapse including microglia (for review Schafer et al., 2013)?
10) Characterize the neuro-glia-vessel communication in perinatal cortex (Segarra et al., 2018) and identify a potential role of early spontaneous and sensory evoked activity in cortical vascularization and development of the blood-brain barrier (Whiteus et al., 2013).
11) Critically evaluate the use of rodent models in understanding early cortical development in humans (Luhmann and Fukuda, 2020) and whether rodents fulfill criteria to study preclinical manifestations of human diseases (Al Dahhan et al., 2019).
12) Organoids may become most valuable models for early cortical development in humans (Trujillo et al., 2019; Chan et al., 2021). However, it needs to be studied whether important cortical circuits present in pre- and neonatal human cortex are also present in organoids (e.g., the fetal subplate circuits Kostovic, 2020; Kostovic et al., 2021). Further, it remains to be studied in more detail whether the spontaneous activity patterns present in pre- and neonatal human cortex (Stjerna et al., 2012; Omidvarnia et al., 2014; Koolen et al., 2016) can be also demonstrated in human organoids.
13) Complement experimental studies with computational modeling of neocortical circuit development (Richter and Gjorgjieva, 2017; Shenoy and Kao, 2021).
14) The Introduction gave a brief overview on the recent technological developments. However, as Frégnac stated in his review we may face "dangers of letting technology-driven—rather than concept-driven—strategies shape the future industrialization of neuroscience through the rapid emergence of very-large-scale data-mining initiatives" (Frégnac, 2017).

AUTHOR CONTRIBUTIONS

The author confirms being the sole contributor of this work and has approved it for publication.

REFERENCES

Ackman, J. B., Burbridge, T. J., and Crair, M. C. (2012). Retinal waves coordinate patterned activity throughout the developing visual system. *Nature*, 490, 219–225. doi: 10.1038/nature11529

Ackman, J. B., and Crair, M. C. (2014). Role of emergent neural activity in visual map development. *Curr. Opin. Neurobiol.* 24, 166–175. doi: 10.1016/j.conb.2013.11.011

Akhmetshina, D., Nasretdinov, A., Zakharov, A., Valeeva, G., and Khazipov, R. (2016). The nature of the sensory input to the neonatal rat barrel cortex. *J. Neurosci.* 36, 9922–9932. doi: 10.1523/JNEUROSCI.1781-16.2016

Al Dahhan, N. Z., De Felice, F. G., and Munoz, D. P. (2019). Potentials and pitfalls of cross-translational models of cognitive impairment. *Front. Behav. Neurosci.* 13:48. doi: 10.3389/fnbeh.2019.00048

Allene, C., and Cossart, R. (2010). Early NMDA receptor-driven waves of activity in the developing neocortex: physiological or pathological network oscillations? *J. Physiol.* 588, 83–91. doi: 10.1113/jphysiol.2009.178798

An, S., Kilb, W., and Luhmann, H. J. (2014). Sensory-evoked and spontaneous gamma and spindle bursts in neonatal rat motor cortex. *J. Neurosci.* 34, 10870–10883. doi: 10.1523/JNEUROSCI.4539-13.2014

Anton-Bolanos, N., Espinosa, A., and López-Bendito, G. (2018). Developmental interactions between thalamus and cortex: a true love reciprocal story. *Curr. Opin. Neurobiol.* 52, 33–41. doi: 10.1016/j.conb.2018.04.018

Anton-Bolanos, N., Sempere-Ferrandez, A., Guillamon-Vivancos, T., Martini, F. J., Perez-Saiz, L., Gezelius, H., et al. (2019). Prenatal activity from thalamic neurons governs the emergence of functional cortical maps in mice. *Science* 364, 987–990. doi: 10.1126/science.aav7617

Bando, Y., Irie, K., Shimomura, T., Umeshima, H., Kushida, Y., Kengaku, M., et al. (2016). Control of spontaneous Ca2+ transients is critical for neuronal maturation in the developing neocortex. *Cerebral Cortex* 26, 106–117. doi: 10.1093/cercor/bhu180

Bando, Y., Sakamoto, M., Kim, S., Ayzenshtat, I., and Yuste, R. (2019). Comparative evaluation of genetically encoded voltage indicators. *Cell Rep.* 26, 802–813 e804. doi: 10.1016/j.celrep.2018.12.088

Barbera, G., Liang, B., Zhang, L., Li, Y., and Lin, D. T. (2019). A wireless miniScope for deep brain imaging in freely moving mice. *J. Neurosci. Methods* 323, 56–60. doi: 10.1016/j.jneumeth.2019.05.008

Barson, D., Hamodi, A. S., Shen, X., Lur, G., Constable, R. T., Cardin, J. A., et al. (2020). Simultaneous mesoscopic and two-photon imaging of neuronal activity in cortical circuits. *Nat. Methods* 17, 107–113. doi: 10.1038/s41592-019-0625-2

Ben-Ari, Y. (2014). The GABA excitatory/inhibitory developmental sequence: a personal journey. *Neuroscience* 279, 187–219. doi: 10.1016/j.neuroscience.2014.08.001

Bhaduri, A., Sandoval-Espinosa, C., Otero-Garcia, M., Oh, I., Yin, R., Eze, U. C., et al. (2021). An atlas of cortical arealization identifies dynamic molecular signatures. *Nature* 598, 200–204. doi: 10.1038/s41586-021-03910-8

Bitzenhofer, S. H., Ahlbeck, J., Wolff, A., Wiegert, J. S., Gee, C. E., Oertner, T. G., et al. (2017). Layer-specific optogenetic activation of pyramidal neurons causes beta-gamma entrainment of neonatal networks. *Nat. Commun.* 8:14563. doi: 10.1038/ncomms14563

Bitzenhofer, S. H., Pöpplau, J. A., Chini, M., Marquardt, A., and Hanganu-Opatz, I. L. (2021). A transient developmental increase in prefrontal activity alters network maturation and causes cognitive dysfunction in adult mice. *Neuron* 109, 1350–1364 e1356. doi: 10.1016/j.neuron.2021.02.011

Bitzenhofer, S. H., Sieben, K., Siebert, K. D., Spehr, M., and Hanganu-Opatz, I. L. (2015). Oscillatory activity in developing prefrontal networks results from theta-gamma-modulated synaptic inputs. *Cell Rep.* 11, 486–497. doi: 10.1016/j.celrep.2015.03.031

Blanquie, O., Kilb, W., Sinning, A., and Luhmann, H. J. (2017). Homeostatic interplay between electrical activity and neuronal apoptosis in the developing neocortex. *Neuroscience* 358, 190–200. doi: 10.1016/j.neuroscience.2017.06.030

Blumberg, M. S., Marques, H. G., and Iida, F. (2013). Twitching in sensorimotor development from sleeping rats to robots. *Curr. Biol.* 23, R532–R537. doi: 10.1016/j.cub.2013.04.075

Bocchio, M., Gouny, C., Angulo-Garcia, D., Toulat, T., Tressard, T., Quiroli, E., et al. (2020). Hippocampal hub neurons maintain distinct connectivity throughout their lifetime. *Nat. Commun.* 11:4559. doi: 10.1038/s41467-020-18432-6

Bonifazi, P., Goldin, M., Picardo, M. A., Jorquera, I., Cattani, A., Bianconi, G., et al. (2009). GABAergic hub neurons orchestrate synchrony in developing hippocampal networks. *Science* 326, 1419–1424. doi: 10.1126/science.1175509

Brockmann, M. D., Poschel, B., Cichon, N., and Hanganu-Opatz, I. L. (2011). Coupled oscillations mediate directed interactions between prefrontal cortex and hippocampus of the neonatal rat. *Neuron* 71, 332–347. doi: 10.1016/j.neuron.2011.05.041

Cadwell, C. R., Scala, F., Li, S., Livrizzi, G., Shen, S., Sandberg, R., et al. (2017). Multimodal profiling of single-cell morphology, electrophysiology, and gene expression using Patch-seq. *Nat. Protoc.* 12, 2531–2553. doi: 10.1038/nprot.2017.120

Calarco, C. A., and Robertson, R. T. (1995). Development of basal forebrain projections to visual cortex: DiI studies in rat. *J. Comp. Neurol.* 354, 608–626. doi: 10.1002/cne.903540409

Callaway, E. M., and Borrell, V. (2011). Developmental sculpting of dendritic morphology of layer 4 neurons in visual cortex: influence of retinal input. *J. Neurosci.* 31, 7456–7470. doi: 10.1523/JNEUROSCI.5222-10.2011

Cardin, J. A., Crair, M. C., and Higley, M. J. (2020). Mesoscopic imaging: shining a wide light on large-scale neural dynamics. *Neuron* 108, 33–43. doi: 10.1016/j.neuron.2020.09.031

Causeret, F., Coppola, E., and Pierani, A. (2018). Cortical developmental death: selected to survive or fated to die. *Curr. Opin. Neurobiol.* 53, 35–42. doi: 10.1016/j.conb.2018.04.022

Causeret, F., Moreau, M. X., Pierani, A., and Blanquie, O. (2021). The multiple facets of Cajal-Retzius neurons. *Development* 148:dev199409. doi: 10.1242/dev.199409

Chan, W. K., Fetit, R., Griffiths, R., Marshall, H., Mason, J. O., and Price, D. J. (2021). Using organoids to study human brain development and evolution. *Dev. Neurobiol.* 81, 608–622. doi: 10.1002/dneu.22819

Chini, M., and Hanganu-Opatz, I. L. (2021). Prefrontal cortex development in health and disease: lessons from rodents and humans. *Trends Neurosci.* 44, 227–240. doi: 10.1016/j.tins.2020.10.017

Chini, M., Popplau, J. A., Lindemann, C., Carol-Perdiguer, L., Hnida, M., Oberlander, V., et al. (2020). Resolving and rescuing developmental miswiring in a mouse model of cognitive impairment. *Neuron* 105, 60–74 e67. doi: 10.1016/j.neuron.2019.09.042

Chipaux, M., Colonnese, M. T., Mauguen, A., Fellous, L., Mokhtari, M., Lezcano, O., et al. (2013). Auditory stimuli mimicking ambient sounds drive temporal "Delta-Brushes" in premature infants. *Plos ONE* 8:e79028. doi: 10.1371/journal.pone.0079028

Colonnese, M., and Khazipov, R. (2012). Spontaneous activity in developing sensory circuits: implications for resting state fMRI. *Neuroimage* 62, 2212–2221. doi: 10.1016/j.neuroimage.2012.02.046

Colonnese, M. T., Kaminska, A., Minlebaev, M., Milh, M., Bloem, B., Lescure, S., et al. (2010). A conserved switch in sensory processing prepares developing neocortex for vision. *Neuron* 67, 480–498. doi: 10.1016/j.neuron.2010.07.015

Colonnese, M. T., and Khazipov, R. (2010). "Slow activity transients" in infant rat visual cortex: a spreading synchronous oscillation patterned by retinal waves. *J. Neurosci.* 30, 4325–4337. doi: 10.1523/JNEUROSCI.4995-09.2010

Colonnese, M. T., and Phillips, M. A. (2018). Thalamocortical function in developing sensory circuits. *Curr. Opin. Neurobiol.* 52, 72–79. doi: 10.1016/j.conb.2018.04.019

Connors, B. W. (2017). Synchrony and so much more: diverse roles for electrical synapses in neural circuits. *Dev. Neurobiol.* 77, 610–624. doi: 10.1002/dneu.22493

Connors, B. W., and Gutnick, M. J. (1990). Intrinsic firing patterns of diverse neocortical neurons. *Trends Neurosci.* 13, 99–104. doi: 10.1016/0166-2236(90)90185-D

Dallerac, G., Zapata, J., and Rouach, N. (2018). Versatile control of synaptic circuits by astrocytes: where, when and how? *Nat. Rev. Neurosci.* 19, 729–743. doi: 10.1038/s41583-018-0080-6

de Groot, A., van den Boom, B. J., van Genderen, R. M., Coppens, J., van Veldhuijzen, J., Bos, J., et al. (2020). NINscope, a versatile miniscope for multi-region circuit investigations. *Elife* 9:e49987. doi: 10.7554/eLife.49987

De Vry, J., Martinez-Martinez, P., Losen, M., Temel, Y., Steckler, T., Steinbusch, H. W., et al. (2010). *In vivo* electroporation of the central nervous system: a non-viral approach for targeted gene delivery. *Prog. Neurobiol.* 92, 227–244. doi: 10.1016/j.pneurobio.2010.10.001

DeFelipe, J., Lopez-Cruz, P. L., Benavides-Piccione, R., Bielza, C., Larranaga, P., Anderson, S., et al. (2013). New insights into the classification and nomenclature of cortical GABAergic interneurons. *Nat. Rev. Neurosci.* 14, 202–216. doi: 10.1038/nrn3444

Deisseroth, K. (2015). Optogenetics: 10 years of microbial opsins in neuroscience. *Nat. Neurosci.* 18, 1213–1225. doi: 10.1038/nn.4091

Dooley, J. C., and Blumberg, M. S. (2018). Developmental 'awakening' of primary motor cortex to the sensory consequences of movement. *Elife* 7:e41841. doi: 10.7554/eLife.41841

Dooley, J. C., Glanz, R. M., Sokoloff, G., and Blumberg, M. S. (2020). Self-generated whisker movements drive state-dependent sensory input to developing barrel cortex. *Curr. Biol.* 30, 2404–2410 e2404. doi: 10.1016/j.cub.2020.04.045

Duan, Z. R. S., Che, A., Chu, P., Modol, L., Bollmann, Y., Babij, R., et al. (2020). GABAergic restriction of network dynamics regulates interneuron survival in the developing cortex. *Neuron* 105, 75–92 e75. doi: 10.1016/j.neuron.2019.10.008

Dupont, E., Hanganu, I. L., Kilb, W., Hirsch, S., and Luhmann, H. J. (2006). Rapid developmental switch in the mechanisms driving early cortical columnar networks. *Nature* 439, 79–83. doi: 10.1038/nature04264

Feldmeyer, D., Qi, G., Emmenegger, V., and Staiger, J. F. (2018). Inhibitory interneurons and their circuit motifs in the many layers of the barrel cortex. *Neuroscience* 368, 132–151. doi: 10.1016/j.neuroscience.2017.05.027

Felix, L., Ziemens, D., Seifert, G., and Rose, C. R. (2019). Spontaneous Ultraslow Na(+) fluctuations in the neonatal mouse brain. *Cells* 9:102. doi: 10.3390/cells9010102

Frégnac, Y. (2017). Big data and the industrialization of neuroscience: aa safe roadmap for understanding the brain? *Science* 358, 470–477. doi: 10.1126/science.aan8866

Garcia-Etxarri, A., and Yuste, R. (2021). Time for NanoNeuro. *Nat. Methods* 18, 1287–1293. doi: 10.1038/s41592-021-01270-9

Gary, D. S., Malone, M., Capestany, P., Houdayer, T., and McDonald, J. W. (2012). Electrical stimulation promotes the survival of oligodendrocytes in mixed cortical cultures. *J. Neurosci. Res.* 90, 72–83. doi: 10.1002/jnr.22717

Gasselin, C., Hohl, B., Vernet, A., Crochet, S., and Petersen, C. C. H. (2021). Cell-type-specific nicotinic input disinhibits mouse barrel cortex during active sensing. *Neuron* 109, 778–787 e773. doi: 10.1016/j.neuron.2020.12.018

Glanz, R. M., Dooley, J. C., Sokoloff, G., and Blumberg, M. S. (2021). Sensory coding of limb kinematics in motor cortex across a key developmental transition. *J Neurosci* 41, 6905–6918. doi: 10.1523/JNEUROSCI.0921-21.2021

Gomez, L. J., Dooley, J. C., Sokoloff, G., and Blumberg, M. S. (2021). Parallel and serial sensory processing in developing primary somatosensory and motor cortex. *J. Neurosci.* 41, 3418–3431. doi: 10.1523/JNEUROSCI.2614-20.2021

Graf, J., Zhang, C., Marguet, S. L., Herrmann, T., Flossmann, T., Hinsch, R., et al. (2021). A limited role of NKCC1 in telencephalic glutamatergic neurons for developing hippocampal network dynamics and behavior. *Proc. Natl. Acad. Sci. U.S.A.* 118:e2014784118. doi: 10.1073/pnas.201478 4118

Grant, E., Hoerder-Suabedissen, A., and Molnár, Z. (2016). The regulation of corticofugal fiber targeting by retinal inputs. *Cereb. Cortex* 26, 1336–1348. doi: 10.1093/cercor/bhv315

Grinvald, A., Omer, D. B., Sharon, D., Vanzetta, I., and Hildesheim, R. (2016). Voltage-sensitive dye imaging of neocortical activity. *Cold Spring Harb. Protoc.* 2016 pdb.top089367 doi: 10.1101/pdb.top089367

Hamilton, N. B., Clarke, L. E., Arancibia-Carcamo, I. L., Kougioumtzidou, E., Matthey, M., Karadottir, R., et al. (2017). Endogenous GABA controls oligodendrocyte lineage cell number, myelination, and CNS internode length. *Glia* 65, 309–321. doi: 10.1002/glia.23093

Hanganu, I. L., Ben-Ari, Y., and Khazipov, R. (2006). Retinal waves trigger spindle bursts in the neonatal rat visual cortex. *J. Neurosci.* 26, 6728–6736. doi: 10.1523/JNEUROSCI.0752-06.2006

Hanganu, I. L., and Luhmann, H. J. (2004). Functional nicotinic acetylcholine receptors on subplate neurons in neonatal rat somatosensory cortex. *J. Neurophysiol.* 92, 189–198. doi: 10.1152/jn.00010.2004

Hanganu, I. L., Okabe, A., Lessmann, V., and Luhmann, H. J. (2009). Cellular mechanisms of subplate-driven and cholinergic input-dependent network activity in the neonatal rat somatosensory cortex. *Cereb. Cortex* 19, 89–105. doi: 10.1093/cercor/bhn061

Hoerder-Suabedissen, A., and Molnár, Z. (2015). Development, evolution and pathology of neocortical subplate neurons. *Nat. Rev. Neurosci.* 16, 133–146. doi: 10.1038/nrn3915

Houweling, A. R., and Brecht, M. (2008). Behavioural report of single neuron stimulation in somatosensory cortex. *Nature* 451, 65–68. doi: 10.1038/nature06447

Huang, L., Ledochowitsch, P., Knoblich, U., Lecoq, J., Murphy, G. J., Reid, R. C., et al. (2021). Relationship between simultaneously recorded spiking activity and fluorescence signal in GCaMP6 transgenic mice. *Elife* 10:e51675. doi: 10.7554/eLife.51675

Inacio, A. R., Nasretdinov, A., Lebedeva, J., and Khazipov, R. (2016). Sensory feedback synchronizes motor and sensory neuronal networks in the neonatal rat spinal cord. *Nat. Commun.* 7:13060. doi: 10.1038/ncomms13060

Iyer, K. K., Roberts, J. A., Hellstrom-Westas, L., Wikström, S., Hansen-Pupp, I., Ley, D., et al. (2015). Cortical burst dynamics predict clinical outcome early in extremely preterm infants. *Brain* 138, 2206–2218. doi: 10.1093/brain/awv129

Janiesch, P. C., Krüger, H. S., Pöschel, B., and Hanganu-Opatz, I. L. (2011). Cholinergic control in developing prefrontal-hippocampal networks. *J. Neurosci.* 31, 17955–17970. doi: 10.1523/JNEUROSCI.2644-11.2011

Jun, J. J., Steinmetz, N. A., Siegle, J. H., Denman, D. J., Bauza, M., Barbarits, B., et al. (2017). Fully integrated silicon probes for high-density recording of neural activity. *Nature* 551, 232–236. doi: 10.1038/nature24636

Kaila, K., Price, T. J., Payne, J. A., Puskarjov, M., and Voipio, J. (2014). Cation-chloride cotransporters in neuronal development, plasticity and disease. *Nat. Rev. Neurosci.* 15, 637–654. doi: 10.1038/nrn3819

Kampmann, M. (2020). CRISPR-based functional genomics for neurological disease. *Nat. Rev. Neurol.* 16, 465–480. doi: 10.1038/s41582-020-0373-z

Kanold, P. O., and Luhmann, H. J. (2010). The subplate and early cortical circuits. *Annu. Rev. Neurosci.* 33, 23–48. doi: 10.1146/annurev-neuro-060909-153244

Kastli, R., Vighagen, R., van der Bourg, A., Argunsah, A. O., Iqbal, A., Voigt, F. F., et al. (2020). Developmental divergence of sensory stimulus representation in cortical interneurons. *Nat. Commun.* 11:5729. doi: 10.1038/s41467-020-19427-z

Khazipov, R., Minlebaev, M., and Valeeva, G. (2013). Early gamma oscillations. *Neuroscience* 250, 240–252. doi: 10.1016/j.neuroscience.2013.07.019

Khazipov, R., Sirota, A., Leinekugel, X., Holmes, G. L., Ben-Ari, Y., and Buzsáki, G. (2004). Early motor activity drives spindle bursts in the developing somatosensory cortex. *Nature* 432, 758–761. doi: 10.1038/nature03132

Kilb, W. (2020). "The relation between neuronal chloride transporter activities, GABA inhibition, and neuronal activity," in *Neuronal Chloride Transporters in Health and Disease*, ed X. Tang (London: Elsevier), 43–57. doi: 10.1016/B978-0-12-815318-5.00003-0

Kilb, W. (2021). When are depolarizing GABAergic responses excitatory? *Front. Mol. Neurosci.* 14:747835. doi: 10.3389/fnmol.2021.747835

Kilb, W., and Fukuda, A. (2017). Taurine as an essential neuromodulator during perinatal cortical development. *Front. Cell. Neurosci.* 11:328. doi: 10.3389/fncel.2017.00328

Kirmse, K., Hübner, C. A., Isbrandt, D., Witte, O. W., and Holthoff, K. (2018). GABAergic transmission during brain development: multiple effects at multiple stages. *Neuroscientist* 24, 36–53. doi: 10.1177/1073858417701382

Kirmse, K., Kummer, M., Kovalchuk, Y., Witte, O. W., Garaschuk, O., and Holthoff, K. (2015). GABA depolarizes immature neurons and inhibits network activity in the neonatal neocortex *in vivo*. *Nat. Commun.* 6:7750. doi: 10.1038/ncomms8750

Kleinfeld, D., Luan, L., Mitra, P. P., Robinson, J. T., Sarpeshkar, R., Shepard, K., et al. (2019). Can one concurrently record electrical spikes from every neuron in a mammalian brain? *Neuron* 103, 1005–1015. doi: 10.1016/j.neuron.2019.08.011

Koolen, N., Dereymaeker, A., Räsänen, O., Jansen, K., Vervisch, J., Matic, V., et al. (2016). Early development of synchrony in cortical activations in the human. *Neuroscience* 322, 298–307. doi: 10.1016/j.neuroscience.2016.02.017

Kostovic, I. (2020). The enigmatic fetal subplate compartment forms an early tangential cortical nexus and provides the framework for construction of cortical connectivity. *Prog. Neurobiol.* 194:101883. doi: 10.1016/j.pneurobio.2020.101883

Kostovic, I., Rados, M., Kostovic-Srzentic, M., and Krsnik, Z. (2021). Fundamentals of the development of connectivity in the human fetal brain in late gestation: from 24 weeks gestational age to term. *J. Neuropathol. Exp. Neurol.* 80, 393–414. doi: 10.1093/jnen/nlab024

Kummer, M., Kirmse, K., Zhang, C., Haueisen, J., Witte, O. W., and Holthoff, K. (2016). Column-like Ca(2+) clusters in the mouse neonatal neocortex revealed by three-dimensional two-photon Ca(2+) imaging *in vivo*. *Neuroimage* 138, 64–75. doi: 10.1016/j.neuroimage.2016.05.050

Leighton, A. H., Cheyne, J. E., Houwen, G. J., Maldonado, P. P., De Winter, F., Levelt, C. N., et al. (2021). Somatostatin interneurons restrict cell recruitment to retinally driven spontaneous activity in the developing cortex. *Cell Rep.* 36:109316. doi: 10.1016/j.celrep.2021.109316

Leighton, A. H., and Lohmann, C. (2016). The wiring of developing sensory circuits-from patterned spontaneous activity to synaptic plasticity mechanisms. *Front. Neural Circuits* 10:71. doi: 10.3389/fncir.2016.00071

Li, H., Fertuzinhos, S., Mohns, E., Hnasko, T. S., Verhage, M., Edwards, R., et al. (2013). Laminar and columnar development of barrel cortex relies on thalamocortical neurotransmission. *Neuron* 79, 970–986. doi: 10.1016/j.neuron.2013.06.043

Linden, N. J., Tabuena, D. R., Steinmetz, N. A., Moody, W. J., Brunton, S. L., and Brunton, B. W. (2021). Go with the FLOW: visualizing spatiotemporal dynamics in optical widefield calcium imaging. *J. R. Soc. Interface* 18:20210523. doi: 10.1098/rsif.2021.0523

Lombardi, A., Jedlicka, P., Luhmann, H. J., and Kilb, W. (2021). Coincident glutamatergic depolarizations enhance GABAA receptor-dependent Cl- influx in mature and suppress Cl- efflux in immature neurons. *PLoS Comput. Biol.* 17:e1008573. doi: 10.1371/journal.pcbi.1008573

López-Bendito, G. (2018). Development of the thalamocortical interactions: past, present and future. *Neuroscience* 385, 67–74. doi: 10.1016/j.neuroscience.2018.06.020

Luhmann, H. J., and Fukuda, A. (2020). Can we understand human brain development from experimental studies in rodents? *Pediatr. Int.* 62, 1139–1144. doi: 10.1111/ped.14339

Luhmann, H. J., and Khazipov, R. (2018). Neuronal activity patterns in the developing barrel cortex. *Neuroscience* 368, 256–267. doi: 10.1016/j.neuroscience.2017.05.025

Luhmann, H. J., Kirischuk, S., and Kilb, W. (2018). The superior function of the subplate in early neocortical development. *Front. Neuroanat.* 12:97. doi: 10.3389/fnana.2018.00097

Luhmann, H. J., Sinning, A., Yang, J. W., Reyes-Puerta, V., Stüttgen, M. C., Kirischuk, S., et al. (2016). Spontaneous neuronal activity in developing neocortical networks: from single cells to large-scale interactions. *Front. Neural Circuits* 10:40. doi: 10.3389/fncir.2016.00040

Luo, T. Z., Bondy, A. G., Gupta, D., Elliott, V. A., Kopec, C. D., and Brody, C. D. (2020). An approach for long-term, multi-probe Neuropixels recordings in unrestrained rats. *Elife* 9:e59716. doi: 10.7554/eLife.59716

Magno, L., Asgarian, Z., Pendolino, V., Velona, T., Mackintosh, A., Lee, F., et al. (2021). Transient developmental imbalance of cortical interneuron subtypes presages long-term changes in behavior. *Cell Rep.* 35:109249. doi: 10.1016/j.celrep.2021.109249

Malyshevskaya, O., Shiraishi, Y., Kimura, F., and Yamamoto, N. (2013). Role of electrical activity in horizontal axon growth in the developing cortex: a time-lapse study using optogenetic stimulation. *PLoS ONE* 8:e82954. doi: 10.1371/journal.pone.0082954

Marques-Smith, A., Lyngholm, D., Kaufmann, A. K., Stacey, J. A., Hoerder-Suabedissen, A., Becker, E. B. E., et al. (2016). A transient translaminar GABAergic interneuron circuit connects thalamocortical recipient layers in neonatal somatosensory cortex. *Neuron* 89, 536–549. doi: 10.1016/j.neuron.2016.01.015

Martini, F. J., Guillamon-Vivancos, T., Moreno-Juan, V., Valdeolmillos, M., and López-Bendito, G. (2021). Spontaneous activity in developing thalamic and cortical sensory networks. *Neuron* 109, 2519–2534. doi: 10.1016/j.neuron.2021.06.026

Mechawar, N., and Descarries, L. (2001). The cholinergic innervation develops early and rapidly in the rat cerebral cortex: a quantitative immunocytochemical study. *Neuroscience* 108, 555–567. doi: 10.1016/S0306-4522(01)00389-X

Meng, X., Solarana, K., Bowen, Z., Liu, J., Nagode, D. A., Sheikh, A., et al. (2020). Transient subgranular hyperconnectivity to L2/3 and enhanced pairwise correlations during the critical period in the mouse auditory cortex. *Cereb. Cortex* 30, 1914–1930. doi: 10.1093/cercor/bhz213

Milh, M., Kaminska, A., Huon, C., Lapillonne, A., Ben-Ari, Y., and Khazipov, R. (2007). Rapid cortical oscillations and early motor activity in premature human neonate. *Cereb. Cortex* 17, 1582–1594. doi: 10.1093/cercor/bhl069

Minlebaev, M., Colonnese, M., Tsintsadze, T., Sirota, A., and Khazipov, R. (2011). Early gamma oscillations synchronize developing thalamus and cortex. *Science* 334, 226–229. doi: 10.1126/science.1210574

Mizuno, H., Ikezoe, K., Nakazawa, S., Sato, T., Kitamura, K., and Iwasato, T. (2018). Patchwork-type spontaneous activity in neonatal barrel cortex layer 4 transmitted via thalamocortical projections. *Cell Rep.* 22, 123–135. doi: 10.1016/j.celrep.2017.12.012

Modol, L., Bollmann, Y., Tressard, T., Baude, A., Che, A., Duan, Z. R. S., et al. (2020). Assemblies of perisomatic GABAergic neurons in the developing barrel cortex. *Neuron* 105, 93–105e104. doi: 10.1016/j.neuron.2019.10.007

Moghadam, S. M., Pinchefsky, E., Tse, I., Marchi, V., Kohonen, J., Kauppila, M., et al. (2021). Building an open source classifier for the neonatal EEG background: a systematic feature-based approach from expert scoring to clinical visualization. *Front. Hum. Neurosci.* 15:675154. doi: 10.3389/fnhum.2021.675154

Mojtahedi, N., Kovalchuk, Y., Bottcher, A., and Garaschuk, O. (2021). Stable behavioral state-specific large scale activity patterns in the developing cortex of neonates. *Cell Calcium* 98:102448. doi: 10.1016/j.ceca.2021.102448

Molnár, Z., Luhmann, H. J., and Kanold, P. O. (2020). Transient cortical circuits match spontaneous and sensory-driven activity during development. *Science* 370:eabb2153. doi: 10.1126/science.abb2153

Moreno-Juan, V., Filipchuk, A., Anton-Bolanos, N., Mezzera, C., Gezelius, H., Andres, B., et al. (2017). Prenatal thalamic waves regulate cortical area size prior to sensory processing. *Nat. Commun.* 8:14172. doi: 10.1038/ncomms14172

Mukherjee, D., Yonk, A. J., Sokoloff, G., and Blumberg, M. S. (2017). Wakefulness suppresses retinal wave-related neural activity in visual cortex. *J. Neurophysiol.* 118, 1190–1197. doi: 10.1152/jn.00264.2017

Murata, Y., and Colonnese, M. T. (2020). GABAergic interneurons excite neonatal hippocampus *in vivo*. *Sci. Adv.* 6:eaba1430. doi: 10.1126/sciadv.aba1430

Niculescu, D., and Lohmann, C. (2014). Gap junctions in developing thalamic and neocortical neuronal networks. *Cereb. Cortex* 24, 3097–3106. doi: 10.1093/cercor/bht175

Omidvarnia, A., Fransson, P., Metsaranta, M., and Vanhatalo, S. (2014). Functional bimodality in the brain networks of preterm and term human newborns. *Cereb. Cortex* 24, 2657–2668. doi: 10.1093/cercor/bht120

Panzera, L. C., and Hoppa, M. B. (2019). Genetically encoded voltage indicators are illuminating subcellular physiology of the axon. *Front. Cell. Neurosci.* 13:52. doi: 10.3389/fncel.2019.00052

Peng, H., Xie, P., Liu, L., Kuang, X., Wang, Y., Qu, L., et al. (2021). Morphological diversity of single neurons in molecularly defined cell types. *Nature* 598, 174–181. doi: 10.1038/s41586-021-03941-1

Peng, Y., Mittermaier, F. X., Planert, H., Schneider, U. C., Alle, H., and Geiger, J. R. P. (2019). High-throughput microcircuit analysis of individual human brains through next-generation multineuron patch-clamp. *Elife* 8:e48178. doi: 10.7554/eLife.48178

Pereda, A. E. (2014). Electrical synapses and their functional interactions with chemical synapses. *Nat. Rev. Neurosci.* 15, 250–263. doi: 10.1038/nrn3708

Perez, J. D., Dieck, S. T., Alvarez-Castelao, B., Tushev, G., Chan, I. C., and Schuman, E. M. (2021). Subcellular sequencing of single neurons reveals the dendritic transcriptome of GABAergic interneurons. *Elife* 10:e63092. doi: 10.7554/eLife.63092

Perez-Prieto, N., and Delgado-Restituto, M. (2021). Recording strategies for high channel count, densely spaced microelectrode arrays. *Front. Neurosci.* 15:681085. doi: 10.3389/fnins.2021.681085

Petersen, C. C. H. (2017). Whole-cell recording of neuronal membrane potential during behavior. *Neuron* 95, 1266–1281. doi: 10.1016/j.neuron.2017.06.049

Picardo, M. A., Guigue, P., Bonifazi, P., Batista-Brito, R., Allene, C., Ribas, A., et al. (2011). Pioneer GABA cells comprise a subpopulation of hub neurons in the developing hippocampus. *Neuron* 71, 695–709. doi: 10.1016/j.neuron.2011.06.018

Ren, C., and Komiyama, T. (2021). Characterizing cortex-wide dynamics with wide-field calcium imaging. *J. Neurosci.* 41, 4160–4168. doi: 10.1523/JNEUROSCI.3003-20.2021

Richter, L. M., and Gjorgjieva, J. (2017). Understanding neural circuit development through theory and models. *Curr. Opin. Neurobiol.* 46, 39–47. doi: 10.1016/j.conb.2017.07.004

Riva, M., Genescu, I., Habermacher, C., Orduz, D., Ledonne, F., Rijli, F. M., et al. (2019). Activity-dependent death of transient Cajal-Retzius neurons is required for functional cortical wiring. *Elife* 8:e50503. doi: 10.7554/eLife.50503

Rochefort, N. L., Garaschuk, O., Milos, R. I., Narushima, M., Marandi, N., Pichler, B., et al. (2009). Sparsification of neuronal activity in the visual cortex at eye-opening. *Proc. Natl. Acad. Sci. U.S.A.* 106, 15049–15054. doi: 10.1073/pnas.0907660106

Roth, B. L. (2016). DREADDs for neuroscientists. *Neuron* 89, 683–694. doi: 10.1016/j.neuron.2016.01.040

Rupprecht, P., Carta, S., Hoffmann, A., Echizen, M., Blot, A., Kwan, A. C., et al. (2021). A database and deep learning toolbox for noise-optimized, generalized spike inference from calcium imaging. *Nat. Neurosci.* 24, 1324–1337. doi: 10.1101/2020.08.31.272450

Sakry, D., Neitz, A., Singh, J., Frischknecht, R., Marongiu, D., Biname, F., et al. (2014). Oligodendrocyte precursor cells modulate the neuronal network by activity-dependent ectodomain cleavage of glial NG2. *PLoS Biol.* 12:e1001993. doi: 10.1371/journal.pbio.1001993

Scala, F., Kobak, D., Bernabucci, M., Bernaerts, Y., Cadwell, C. R., Castro, J. R., et al. (2021). Phenotypic variation of transcriptomic cell types in mouse motor cortex. *Nature* 598, 144–150. doi: 10.1038/s41586-020-2907-3

Schafer, D. P., Lehrman, E. K., and Stevens, B. (2013). The "quad-partite" synapse: microglia-synapse interactions in the developing and mature CNS. *Glia* 61, 24–36. doi: 10.1002/glia.22389

Segarra, M., Aburto, M. R., Cop, F., Llao-Cid, C., Hartl, R., Damm, M., et al. (2018). Endothelial Dab1 signaling orchestrates neuro-glia-vessel communication in the central nervous system. *Science* 361:eaao2861. doi: 10.1126/science.aao2861

Shen, J., and Colonnese, M. T. (2016). Development of activity in the mouse visual cortex. *J. Neurosci.* 36, 12259–12275. doi: 10.1523/JNEUROSCI.1903-16.2016

Shenoy, K. V., and Kao, J. C. (2021). Measurement, manipulation and modeling of brain-wide neural population dynamics. *Nat. Commun.* 12:633. doi: 10.1038/s41467-020-20371-1

Siegle, J. H., Ledochowitsch, P., Jia, X., Millman, D. J., Ocker, G. K., Caldejon, S., et al. (2021). Reconciling functional differences in populations of neurons recorded with two-photon imaging and electrophysiology. *Elife* 10:e69068. doi: 10.7554/eLife.69068

Steinmetz, N. A., Zatka-Haas, P., Carandini, M., and Harris, K. D. (2019). Distributed coding of choice, action and engagement across the mouse brain. *Nature* 576, 266–273. doi: 10.1038/s41586-019-1787-x

Steriade, M. (2001a). Impact of network activities on neuronal properties in corticothalamic systems. *J. Neurophysiol.* 86, 1–39. doi: 10.1152/jn.2001.86.1.1

Steriade, M. (2001b). *The Intact and Sliced Brain.* Cambridge: MIT Press. doi: 10.7551/mitpress/3822.001.0001

Stjerna, S., Voipio, J., Metsaranta, M., Kaila, K., and Vanhatalo, S. (2012). Preterm EEG: a multimodal neurophysiological protocol. *J. Visual. Exp.* 18:3774. doi: 10.3791/3774

Su, X., Chen, J. J., Liu, L. Y., Huang, Q., Zhang, L. Z., Li, X. Y., et al. (2017). Neonatal CX26 removal impairs neocortical development and leads to elevated anxiety. *Proc. Natl. Acad. Sci. U.S.A.* 114, 3228–3233. doi: 10.1073/pnas.1613237114

Takasaki, K. T., Tsyboulski, D., and Waters, J. (2019). Dual-plane 3-photon microscopy with remote focusing. *Biomed. Opt. Express* 10, 5585–5599. doi: 10.1364/BOE.10.005585

Tang, Q. S., Brecht, M., and Burgalossi, A. (2014). Juxtacellular recording and morphological identification of single neurons in freely moving rats. *Nat. Protoc.* 9, 2369–2381. doi: 10.1038/nprot.2014.161

Tischbirek, C. H., Birkner, A., and Konnerth, A. (2017). *In vivo* deep two-photon imaging of neural circuits with the fluorescent Ca2+ indicator Cal-590. *J. Physiol.* 595, 3097–3105. doi: 10.1113/JP272790

Tokariev, A., Roberts, J. A., Zalesky, A., Zhao, X., Vanhatalo, S., Breakspear, M., et al. (2019). Large-scale brain modes reorganize between infant sleep states and carry prognostic information for preterms. *Nat. Commun.* 10:2619. doi: 10.1038/s41467-019-10467-8

Tolner, E. A., Sheikh, A., Yukin, A. Y., Kaila, K., and Kanold, P. O. (2012). Subplate neurons promote spindle bursts and thalamocortical patterning in the neonatal rat somatosensory cortex. *J. Neurosci.* 32, 692–702. doi: 10.1523/JNEUROSCI.1538-11.2012

Traub, R. D., Bibbig, A., LeBeau, F. E., Buhl, E. H., and Whittington, M. A. (2004). Cellular mechanisms of neuronal population oscillations in the hippocampus *in vitro*. *Annu. Rev. Neurosci.* 27, 247–278. doi: 10.1146/annurev.neuro.27.070203.144303

Tritsch, N. X., Yi, E., Gale, J. E., Glowatzki, E., and Bergles, D. E. (2007). The origin of spontaneous activity in the developing auditory system. *Nature* 450, 50–55. doi: 10.1038/nature06233

Trujillo, C. A., Gao, R., Negraes, P. D., Gu, J., Buchanan, J., Preissl, S., et al. (2019). Complex oscillatory waves emerging from cortical organoids model early human brain network development. *Cell Stem Cell* 25, 558–569 e557. doi: 10.1016/j.stem.2019.08.002

Tuncdemir, S. N., Wamsley, B., Stam, F. J., Osakada, F., Goulding, M., Callaway, E. M., et al. (2016). Early somatostatin interneuron connectivity mediates the maturation of deep layer cortical circuits. *Neuron* 89, 521–535. doi: 10.1016/j.neuron.2015.11.020

Uhlen, P., Fritz, N., Smedler, E., Malmersjo, S., and Kanatani, S. (2015). Calcium signaling in neocortical development. *Dev. Neurobiol.* 75, 360–368. doi: 10.1002/dneu.22273

Valeeva, G., Tressard, T., Mukhtarov, M., Baude, A., and Khazipov, R. (2016). An optogenetic approach for investigation of excitatory and inhibitory network GABA actions in mice expressing Channelrhodopsin-2 in GABAergic neurons. *J. Neurosci.* 36, 5961–5973. doi: 10.1523/JNEUROSCI.3482-15.2016

Valiullina, F., Akhmetshina, D., Nasretdinov, A., Mukhtarov, M., Valeeva, G., Khazipov, R., et al. (2016). Developmental changes in electrophysiological properties and a transition from electrical to chemical coupling between excitatory layer 4 neurons in the rat barrel cortex. *Front. Neural Circuits* 10:1. doi: 10.3389/fncir.2016.00001

van der Bourg, A., Yang, J. W., Reyes-Puerta, V., Laurenczy, B., Wieckhorst, M., Stüttgen, M. C., et al. (2017). Layer-specific refinement of sensory coding in developing mouse barrel cortex. *Cereb. Cortex* 27, 4835–4850. doi: 10.1093/cercor/bhw280

Vanhatalo, S., and Kaila, K. (2006). Development of neonatal EEG activity: from phenomenology to physiology. *Semin. Fetal Neonatal Med.* 11, 471–478. doi: 10.1016/j.siny.2006.07.008

Virtanen, M. A., Uvarov, P., Hübner, C. A., and Kaila, K. (2020). NKCC1, an elusive molecular target in brain development: making sense of the existing data. *Cells* 9:2607. doi: 10.3390/cells9122607

Virtanen, M. A., Uvarov, P., Mavrovic, M., Poncer, J. C., and Kaila, K. (2021). The multifaceted roles of KCC2 in cortical development. *Trends Neurosci.* 44, 378–392. doi: 10.1016/j.tins.2021.01.004

Vormstein-Schneider, D., Lin, J. D., Pelkey, K. A., Chittajallu, R., Guo, B., Arias-Garcia, M. A., et al. (2020). Viral manipulation of functionally distinct interneurons in mice, non-human primates and humans. *Nat. Neurosci.* 23, 1629–1636. doi: 10.1101/808170

Wake, H., Ortiz, F. C., Woo, D. H., Lee, P. R., Angulo, M. C., and Fields, R. D. (2015). Nonsynaptic junctions on myelinating glia promote preferential myelination of electrically active axons. *Nature Commun.* 6:7844. doi: 10.1038/ncomms8844

Wang, C. Z., Ma, J., Xu, Y. Q., Jiang, S. N., Chen, T. Q., Yuan, Z. L., et al. (2019). Early-generated interneurons regulate neuronal circuit formation during early postnatal development. *Elife* 8:e44649. doi: 10.7554/eLife.44649

Wang, H. C., Lin, C. C., Cheung, R., Zhang-Hooks, Y., Agarwal, A., Ellis-Davies, G., et al. (2015). Spontaneous activity of cochlear hair cells triggered by fluid secretion mechanism in adjacent support cells. *Cell* 163, 1348–1359. doi: 10.1016/j.cell.2015.10.070

Wang, X., Lou, N., Xu, Q., Tian, G. F., Peng, W. G., Han, X., et al. (2006). Astrocytic Ca2+ signaling evoked by sensory stimulation *in vivo*. *Nat. Neurosci.* 9, 816–823. doi: 10.1038/nn1703

Watanabe, M., and Fukuda, A. (2015). Development and regulation of chloride homeostasis in the central nervous system. *Front. Cell. Neurosci.* 9:371. doi: 10.3389/fncel.2015.00371

Weissman, T. A., Riquelme, P. A., Ivic, L., Flint, A. C., and Kriegstein, A. R. (2004). Calcium waves propagate through radial glial cells and modulate proliferation in the developing neocortex. *Neuron* 43, 647–661. doi: 10.1016/j.neuron.2004.08.015

West, A. E., Chen, W. G., Dalva, M. B., Dolmetsch, R. E., Kornhauser, J. M., Shaywitz, A. J., et al. (2001). Calcium regulation of neuronal gene expression. *Proc. Natl. Acad. Sci. U.S.A.* 98, 11024–11031. doi: 10.1073/pnas.191352298

Whiteus, C., Freitas, C., and Grutzendler, J. (2013). Perturbed neural activity disrupts cerebral angiogenesis during a postnatal critical period. *Nature* 505, 407–411. doi: 10.1038/nature12821

Yang, J. W., An, S., Sun, J. J., Reyes-Puerta, V., Kindler, J., Berger, T., et al. (2013). Thalamic network oscillations synchronize ontogenetic columns in the newborn rat barrel cortex. *Cereb. Cortex* 23, 1299–1316. doi: 10.1093/cercor/bhs103

Yang, J. W., Hanganu-Opatz, I. L., Sun, J. J., and Luhmann, H. J. (2009). Three patterns of oscillatory activity differentially synchronize developing neocortical networks *in vivo. J. Neurosci.* 29, 9011–9025. doi: 10.1523/JNEUROSCI.5646-08.2009

Yang, W., and Yuste, R. (2017). *In vivo* imaging of neural activity. *Nat. Methods* 14, 349–359. doi: 10.1038/nmeth.4230

Yao, X. H., Wang, M., He, X. N., He, F., Zhang, S. Q., Lu, W., et al. (2016). Electrical coupling regulates layer 1 interneuron microcircuit formation in the neocortex. *Nat. Commun.* 7:12229. doi: 10.1038/ncomms12229

Yao, Z., Liu, H., Xie, F., Fischer, S., Adkins, R. S., Aldridge, A. I., et al. (2021). A transcriptomic and epigenomic cell atlas of the mouse primary motor cortex. *Nature* 598, 103–110. doi: 10.1038/s41586-021-03500-8

Yu, Y. C., He, S. J., Chen, S., Fu, Y. H., Brown, K. N., Yao, X. H., et al. (2012). Preferential electrical coupling regulates neocortical lineage-dependent microcircuit assembly. *Nature* 486, 113–U139. doi: 10.1038/nature10958

Yuryev, M., Andriichuk, L., Leiwe, M., Jokinen, V., Carabalona, A., and Rivera, C. (2018). *In vivo* two-photon imaging of the embryonic cortex reveals spontaneous ketamine-sensitive calcium activity. *Sci. Rep.* 8:16059. doi: 10.1038/s41598-018-34410-x

Zhang, L., Liang, B., Barbera, G., Hawes, S., Zhang, Y., Stump, K., et al. (2019). Miniscope GRIN lens system for calcium imaging of neuronal activity from deep brain structures in behaving animals. *Curr. Protoc. Neurosci.* 86:e56. doi: 10.1002/cpns.56

Zhang, X. J., Li, Z., Han, Z., Sultan, K. T., Huang, K., and Shi, S. H. (2017). Precise inhibitory microcircuit assembly of developmentally related neocortical interneurons in clusters. *Nat. Commun.* 8:16091. doi: 10.1038/ncomms16091

Zhang, Y., Rózsa, M., Liang, Y., Bushey, D., Wei, Z., Zheng, J., et al. (2021). Fast and sensitive GCaMP calcium indicators for imaging neural populations. *BioRxiv* PPR417430. doi: 10.1101/2021.11.08.467793

Zuchero, J. B., and Barres, B. A. (2013). Intrinsic and extrinsic control of oligodendrocyte development. *Curr. Opin. Neurobiol.* 23, 914–920. doi: 10.1016/j.conb.2013.06.005

4

Cortical Interneurons Migrating on a Pure Substrate of N-Cadherin Exhibit Fast Synchronous Centrosomal and Nuclear Movements and Reduced Ciliogenesis

Camilla Luccardini[1,2,3†], *Claire Leclech*[1,2,3], *Lucie Viou*[1,2,3], *Jean-Paul Rio*[1,2,3†] *and Christine Métin*[1,2,3*]

[1] *INSERM, UMR-S839, Paris, France,* [2] *Sorbonne Universités, UPMC University Paris 06, UMR-S839, Paris, France,* [3] *Institut du Fer à Moulin, Paris, France*

Correspondence:
Christine Métin,
INSERM, UMR-S839, 17 Rue du Fer À Moulin, 75005 Paris, France
christine.metin@inserm.fr

†*Present address:*
Camilla Luccardini,
Université Claude Bernard Lyon 1, CGphiMC UMR CNRS 5534, Villeurbanne 69622, France
camilla.luccardini@univ-lyon1.fr;
Jean-Paul Rio,
Institut du Cerveau et de la Moelle Epinière ICM-INSERM U 1127, Hôpital de la Pitié-Salpêtrière 47, Bd de L'Hôpital 75013 Paris, France
jean-paul.rio@icm-institute.org

The embryonic development of the cortex involves a phase of long distance migration of interneurons born in the basal telencephalon. Interneurons first migrate tangentially and then reorient their trajectories radially to enter the developing cortex. We have shown that migrating interneurons can assemble a primary cilium, which maintains the centrosome to the plasma membrane and processes signals to control interneuron trajectory (Baudoin et al., 2012). In the developing cortex, N-cadherin is expressed by migrating interneurons and by cells in their migratory pathway. N-cadherin promotes the motility and maintains the polarity of tangentially migrating interneurons (Luccardini et al., 2013). Because N-cadherin is an important factor that regulates the migration of medial ganglionic eminence (MGE) cells *in vivo*, we further characterized the motility and polarity of MGE cells on a substrate that only comprises this protein. MGE cells migrating on a N-cadherin substrate were seven times faster than on a laminin substrate and two times faster than on a substrate of cortical cells. A primary cilium was much less frequently observed on MGE cells migrating on N-cadherin than on laminin. Nevertheless, the mature centriole (MC) frequently docked to the plasma membrane in MGE cells migrating on N-cadherin, suggesting that plasma membrane docking is a basic feature of the centrosome in migrating MGE cells. On the N-cadherin substrate, centrosomal and nuclear movements were remarkably synchronous and the centrosome remained near the nucleus. Interestingly, MGE cells with cadherin invalidation presented centrosomal movements no longer coordinated with nuclear movements. In summary, MGE cells migrating on a pure substrate of N-cadherin show fast, coordinated nuclear and centrosomal movements, and rarely present a primary cilium.

Keywords: migration, cortical interneuron, cytoskeleton, primary cilium, N-cadherin, electron microscopy, videomicroscopy

Introduction

Cell migration, including neuronal migration, is described as a repetitive process comprising several steps (Ridley et al., 2003; Valiente and Marín, 2010): (i) cell polarization; (ii) leading process elongation; (iii) leading process stabilization through the formation of adherent junctions and/or adhesive contacts; (iv) forward displacement of organelles by forces anchored on adhesion sites; and (v) tail retraction. The whole process involves the capability of migrating cells to polarize and to interact with cues in their environment. Although adhesive interactions play a crucial role in cell migration, their role in the migration of embryonic neurons is not fully understood (Solecki, 2012). Recent studies have demonstrated a major role of N-cadherin mediated cell-cell adhesion in the radial migration of principal cortical neurons in the mouse embryo (Kawauchi et al., 2010; Franco et al., 2011; Jossin and Cooper, 2011). They showed that N-cadherin recycling controls the adhesion of migrating neurons to the radial glia, and that N-cadherin-mediated adhesion functionally interacts with the reelin signaling pathway to control transition steps at the beginning and at the end of the radial migration. Another study in young post-mitotic cortical neurons showed that N-cadherin enrichment at one pole determines the orientation of the polarity axis of the cell, on which the nucleus and centrosome thereafter position (Gärtner et al., 2012). Whether centrosome positioning organizes cell polarity or stabilizes a polarized organization resulting from interactions with extrinsic cues, is unclear in migrating cells of which the centrosome is most often positioned in front of the nucleus (Ueda et al., 1997; Solecki et al., 2004; Higginbotham and Gleeson, 2007; Yanagida et al., 2012).

In the developing forebrain, cortical GABAergic interneurons migrate long distances from the medial ganglionic eminence (MGE) and caudal ganglionic eminence (CGE) where they originate, to the cortex where they settle among principal cells and further differentiate (Anderson et al., 1997; Wichterle et al., 1999; Nery et al., 2002; Butt et al., 2005; Wonders and Anderson, 2006; Flames et al., 2007; Fogarty et al., 2007; Miyoshi et al., 2010). Maintaining the same direction of migration during a long journey toward their final target, is thus crucial for MGE and CGE cells (Marín et al., 2010). In a previous study, we examined whether N-cadherin contributed to the long distance migration of cortical interneurons, as previously demonstrated for precerebellar neurons (Taniguchi et al., 2006). We showed that N-cadherin ablation or invalidation in MGE cells delay the tangential migration of MGE cells and alter their capacity to colonize the cortical plate (Luccardini et al., 2013). Analyses in a co-culture model showed that MGE cells with N-cadherin invalidation exhibit reduced migration speed and abnormal cell directionality because nuclear movements frequently reversed.

N-cadherin is a homophilic cell-cell adhesion protein largely expressed by telencephalic cells on which MGE cells migrate *in vivo* (Kadowaki et al., 2007). To further understand how N-cadherin contributes to the motility and directionality of migrating MGE cells, we have compared the migration of MGE cells on a pure substrate of N-cadherin, on a pure substrate of laminin that also influences cell migration and polarization (Kawauchi, 2012; Solecki, 2012), and on a substrate of cortical cells on which MGE cells exhibit their "*in vivo*-like" migration cycle. MGE cells migrated faster on the N-cadherin substrate than on any other substrate, and did not aggregate to each other. We have recently shown that the centrosome of MGE cells migrating on cortical cells can dock to the plasma membrane and assemble a primary cilium able to collect extrinsic information (Baudoin et al., 2012; Métin and Pedraza, 2014). We show here that the proportion of MGE cells with a primary cilium was strongly decreased on the N-cadherin substrate as compared with the proportion of ciliated MGE cells on the laminin substrate or on the substrate of cortical cells. Ultrastructural analyses surprisingly revealed that the mature centriole (MC) that assembles and anchors the primary cilium at the cell surface, docked to the plasma membrane at the same frequency in MGE cells cultured on N-cadherin, which rarely assemble a primary cilium, and in MGE cells cultured on cortical cells, which frequently assemble a primary cilium. In MGE cells migrating on the N-cadherin substrate, centrosomal and nuclear movements were fast and synchronous, and the centrosome preferentially localized near the nucleus. Finally, because MGE cells with an acute invalidation of N-cadherin presented centrosomal movements no longer coordinated with nuclear movements, we conclude that a pure substrate of cadherin promotes synchronous nuclear and centrosomal movements. Results moreover suggest that increased centrosomal motility does not impair the capacity of the MC to dock to the plasma membrane.

Materials and Methods

Animals

Pregnant Swiss mouse were purchased from Janvier Labs, and mouse embryos were produced in the animal facility of the laboratory by crossing wild type adults (Swiss, Janvier Labs). Experiments and animal care followed the European guidelines and were approved by the Ethical Committee Charles Darwin N°5 (E2CD5).

Cell Cultures

Cell Cultures for Live Cell Imaging and Immunostaining

Cultures were performed on glass coverslips previously treated with nitric acid 67%, ethanol 100% and then sterilized in the oven and fixed with paraffin at the bottom of perforated petri dishes which were used as a culture chamber for the video microscopy experiments. For immunostaining, cultures were performed on glass coverslips placed in 4-well boxes.

Co-cultures of MGE explants on dissociated cortical cells

Cortices from wild type E13.5 mouse embryos were dissociated mechanically and the cortical cells were spread as a monolayer onto glass coverslips coated with poly-lysine and laminin (PLL/LN) as explained in Bellion et al. (2005). Cortical cells were cultured for 2 to 3 h in Dulbecco's Modified

Eagle Medium/Nutrient Mixture F-12 (DMEM/F12) (1/1) supplemented with glucose, glutamax, penicillin/ streptomycin, 4-(2-hydroxyethyl)-1-piperazineethanesulfonic acid (HEPES) buffer, N2 and B27 before placing the explants of MGE. MGEs dissected from E13.5 green fluorescent protein (GFP)-expressing transgenic mouse embryos were divided into four to six explants and placed on the substrate of dissociated cortical cells. MGEs electroporated as explained in Baudoin et al. (2012) with a plasmid encoding the pericentrin-AKAP-450 centrosomal targeting (PACT) domain of pericentrin fused to the mKO1 fluorochrome (*pCAG-PACT-mKO1*) or with a plasmid encoding the LifeAct-RFP construct (*pCAG-LifeAct-RFP*, Ibidi) were cultured for 2–4 h for recovery before placing them in culture. To analyze centrosomal movements in cadherin invalidated MGE cells, MGE explants were co-electroporated with *pCAG-EGFP-N-cad(t)* and *pCAG-PACT-mKO1* plasmids as explained in Luccardini et al. (2013). Co-cultures were maintained in the culture medium described above for 24 h before time-lapse imaging.

Cultures of MGE explants on a protein substrate

Clean and sterile glass coverslips were coated with PLL/LN to prepare the laminin substrate. Coverslips were coated with the extracellular domain of N-cadherin fused to the human Fc receptor protein (Lambert et al., 2000) as explained in Luccardini et al. (2013) to prepare N-cadherin substrate. Briefly, coverslips were incubated overnight at 4°C with 4 μg/ml poly-L-lysine (Sigma) and 4 μg/ml goat anti-human Fc antibody (Jackson ImmunoResearch). Coverslips were then washed in borate buffer and incubated with 1 μg/cm^2 purified N-cad-hFc chimera protein for 3 h at 37°C. To prepare N-cadherin/laminin substrate, 4 μg/ml Laminin (Sigma) was added to the PLL and goat anti-human Fc antibody. GFP-expressing MGE explants dissected from E13.5 transgenic mouse embryos, electroporated or not with a plasmid encoding the PACT-mKO1 fusion protein, were placed on the protein substrate, and cultured 2–24 h before imaging.

Cultures for Electron Microscopy

Co-cultures of MGE explants on cortical axons

Co-cultures were performed on plastic coverslips coated with PLL/LN as explained in Baudoin et al. (2012). Because MGE cells cannot be identified by fluorescent markers in co-cultures destined to Electron Microscopy (EM) studies, they were cultured on cortical axons on which they were identified by their morphology. On this substrate, MGE cells exhibit the same migration cycle as on dissociated cortical cells (Bellion et al., 2005). Cortical explants dissected from E13.5 wild type mouse embryos were cultured for 3–5 days in DMEM/F12 (1/1) supplemented with glucose, glutamax, penicillin/streptomycin, HEPES buffer, N2 and B27. When long and numerous axons extended away from cortical explants and covered most of the surface surrounding explants, the MGE was then dissected from E12.5 wild type mouse embryos and cut equally into four to six explants. Explants were placed at the tip of corticofugal axons and cultured for 36–48 h, in order to observe the migration of numerous MGE cells on cortical axons. Co-cultures were then fixed in 1% paraformaldehyde, 1% glutaraldehyde in 0.12M PB/ 0.33 M sucrose at 4°C.

Cultures of MGE explants on a N-cadherin-Fc biomimetic substrate

Plastic coverslips (Thermanox) coated with the N-cadherin substrate were prepared as explained for glass coverslips (see above). The MGE dissected from E12.5 wild type mouse embryos were cut in half and deposited on a coverslip. After 24 h in culture in the DMEM/F12 culture medium (see above), cultures were fixed as described above in 1% paraformaldehyde, 1% glutaraldehyde in 0.12M PB/ 0.33 M sucrose at 4°C.

Electron Microscopy

Preparation of Ultra-Thin Sections

Cultures were post-fixed in 2% Osmium tetroxide (OsO_4) and contrasted with 1% uranyl acetate in maleate buffer. After dehydration in graded series of ethanol, cultures were transferred in araldite/ethanol (1/1) for 2 h and then overnight in 100% araldite. Small blocks with individual MGE cells migrating on either cortical axons or the N-cadherin substrate were isolated from the rest of the culture under a binocular microscope. These small regions were then embedded in a capsule of araldite with the plastic coverslip oriented parallel to the surface of the capsule. Ultra-thin sections (60 nm), parallel to the plastic coverslips, were collected on copper grids (Maxtaform Finder type H6, 200 mesh, Ted Pella Inc., Redding, CA, USA). Sections were contrasted with lead citrate solution.

Data Analysis

We selected several explants cultured on N-cadherin, which were surrounded by numerous migrating MGE cells (16 explants). An average of 6–11 grids were prepared with each culture. A total of 294 cells showing at least one centriole (30 grids, four independent cultures) were imaged, at minimum, at two different magnifications (×2000, ×20,000) with an ORIUS CCD camera (Gatan). In co-cultures performed on cortical axons, the density of MGE cells was strongly reduced compared to the density of MGE cells observed on the N-cadherin substrate. A total of 208 cells showing at least one centriole (98 grids, 10 independent cultures) were imaged and analyzed.

For each cell we measured the distance between the nuclear front and the centrosome, we characterized the plane of section of centriole(s) (transverse, longitudinal, oblique), and noted when centrioles were located within the leading process. The anchoring of the MC to the plasma membrane and the presence of ciliary structures (primary cilium, ciliary vesicle) at its distal end was also noted.

Time-lapse Recording

Time-lapse recording started 2–24 h after placement of explants on the laminin or N-cadherin substrate, and 24–36 h after placement of explants on the dissociated cortical cells. For time-lapse recording, the culture medium was replaced by a culture medium without phenol red and with an increased concentration of Hepes buffer (20 mM instead of 10 mM). Co-cultures and cultures were imaged on an inverted microscope (Leica CTR 4000) equipped with a spinning disk (Roper Scientific, Trenton, NJ, USA) and a QuantEM 512SC camera (Photometrics). Cells were recorded using an X63 immersion objective, every 3 min, for an average of 4–5 h. Acquisitions were controlled using Metamorph software (Roper Scientific, Trenton, NJ, USA).

Analyses of Recorded MGE Cells

Three independent culture experiments performed on each substrate of migration (dissociated cortical cells, laminin, N-cadherin, and N-cadherin/laminin) were analyzed in the present study. In experiments on cortical cells and N-cadherin, six to eight MGE cells exhibiting a correct expression pattern of PACT-mKO1 were selected for centrosomal and nuclear movement analysis in each experiment. In addition to its centrosome localization, the PACT construct was distributed throughout the cytoplasm and allowed for the identification of nuclear boundary. In experiments on laminin and N-cadherin/laminin, at least 15 cells were tracked in each experiment. Cell tracking was performed with either Metamorph or ImageJ (MTrackJ, NIH, USA).

Statistics

Statistical analyses were performed using XLSTAT software. Mean values for a parameter in two independent samples were compared using the Student *t*-test. Distributions into classes were compared by non-parametric statistical tests: the test of Mann-Whitney for two classes, and of Kolmogorov-Smirnov for five classes.

Immunostaining

Cultures were fixed with 4% paraformaldehyde in 0.12M phosphate buffer/0.33 M sucrose at 4°C. Cells were incubated for 2 h with a blocking solution containing 0.25% Triton, 10% normal goat serum, 2% bovine serum albumin (BSA) in phosphate buffer saline (PBS). The following primary antibodies were used: mouse anti-Arl13b (1:1000; UC Davis/NIH NeuroMab Facility), rat anti-Tubulin YL1/2 (1:2000; abcam). Appropriate Alexa Fluor dye-conjugated secondary antibody (1:500; Invitrogen) was used to detect primary antibodies. Bisbenzimide (1:5000) was used for fluorescent nuclear counterstaining. Culture were mounted in Mowiol-Dabco and observed using an upright fluorescent microscope at X100 magnification (DM6000; Leica).

Results

MGE cells contribute to 70% of cortical interneurons. We have previously shown that MGE cells exhibit the same migratory behavior in 3-dimensional organotypic cortical slices and on dissociated cortical cells (Bellion et al., 2005). When a piece of the MGE proliferative zone of a E12.5/E13.5 mouse embryo is placed on dissociated E13 cortical cells (see scheme in **Figure 1A1**), MGE cells exit the explant and migrate away with radially oriented trajectories. Cells present a polarized morphology with the nucleus facing the explant and the leading process extending at the opposite side (Bellion et al., 2005). After 24–36 h in culture, MGE cells distribute over a large area around their explant of origin (picture in **Figure 1A1**). In these co-cultures, MGE cells present a saltatory migration characterized by coordinated nuclear and centrosomal movements. The centrosome migrates first toward the cell front and then, the nucleus translocates toward the centrosome. During the nuclear resting phase, the centrosome can migrate far away from the nucleus in close association with the endoplasmic reticulum and Golgi apparatus (GA). We have recently shown that the MC of MGE cells can dock to the plasma membrane and organize a short primary cilium at the cell surface (Baudoin et al., 2012). About one third of MGE cells with the MC anchored to the plasma membrane have a primary cilium, making the MC a basal body. Plasma membrane anchoring could stabilize basal bodies and MCs, and thereby enhance the stabilization of MGE cell polarity.

We had previously shown that *N-cadherin* ablation and cadherin functional invalidation in MGE cells reduced cell motility and impaired cell polarization, identifying N-cadherin as an important cell-cell adhesion protein that controls the migration of cortical interneurons *in vivo* (Luccardini et al., 2013). Accordingly, MGE cells cultured on a biomimetic substrate of N-cad-Fc that consists of the extracellular domain of N-cadherin attached to a glass coverslips by the Fc receptor (Lambert et al., 2000) migrated actively. These observations confirmed that N-cadherin plays a unique role to control the migration of MGE cells as the extracellular domain of N-cadherin binds and activates N-cadherin receptors (Lambert et al., 2000). In particular, the motility of MGE cells was increased and the outgrowth of their leading process stimulated (Luccardini et al., 2013). Here, we first compared the motility and directionality of MGE cells cultured on a pure substrate of N-cadherin and on a pure substrate of laminin that binds integrin receptors and also controls cell polarity (Etienne-Manneville and Hall, 2003).

Migratory Behavior of MGE Cells on Pure Substrates of N-Cadherin or Laminin

As already reported (Luccardini et al., 2013), MGE cells migrate much faster on the biomimetic substrate of N-cadherin than on the "*in vivo*-like" substrate of cortical cells (**Figure 1**). However, frequent directional changes and polarity reversals prevented MGE cells cultured on a pure N-cadherin substrate from colonizing larger areas than MGE cells cultured on cortical cells (**Figures 1B,D**). On a pure laminin substrate, in contrast, MGE cells migrated for very short distances around their explant of origin. After 24 h in culture, migrated MGE cells aggregated to each other to form short chains in which cells presented small amplitude forwards and backwards gliding movements (**Figure 2A**). When N-cad-Fc was added to the laminin substrate, MGE cells distributed over a significantly larger area that nevertheless remained inferior to the area covered by MGE cells on the pure N-cadherin substrate (**Figure 1**). On the mixed laminin/N-cadherin substrate, MGE cells showed fast migration speed and their trajectories were straighter than on

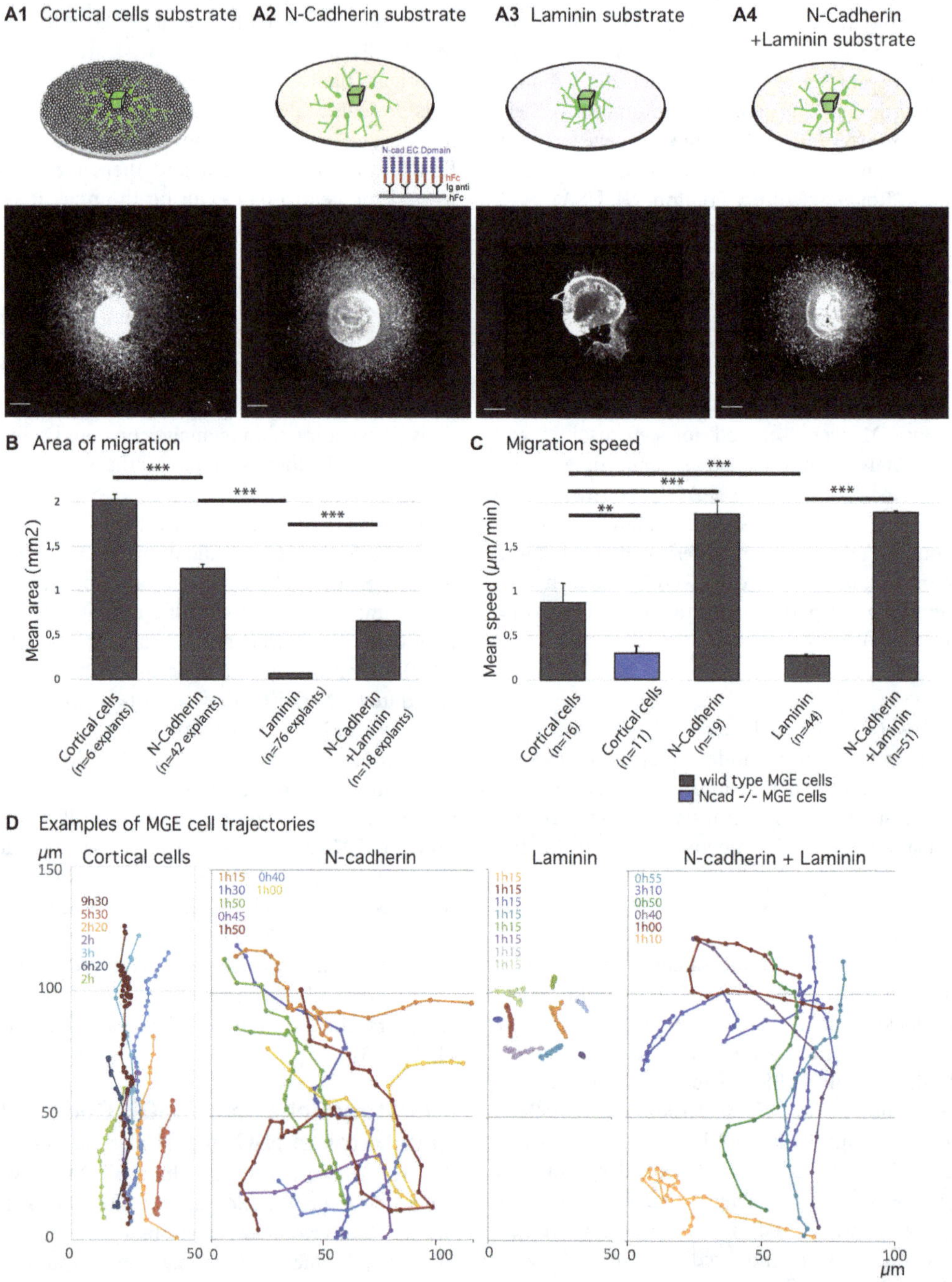

FIGURE 1 | Migratory behavior of medial ganglionic eminence (MGE) cells on various substrates of migration. (A1–B) Analysis of migration in fixed preparations. Schemes **(A1–A4)** illustrate co-culture and culture models compared in the present study. Co-culture of MGE explants on dissociated cortical cells **(A1)** mimics the *in vivo* situation. Biomimetic substrates are prepared on glass coverslips with the extracellular domain of N-cadherin fused to a human Fc fragment, N-cad-Fc (**A2**, see "Materials and Methods" Section), or with laminin **(A3)**, or with a mixture laminin/N-cad-Fc (**A4**, see "Materials and Methods" Section). Pictures below schemes illustrate the typical distribution of green fluorescent protein (GFP)-expressing MGE cells after 24 h of migration. Scale bars, 200 μm. Histogram in **(B)** gives the average area of migration covered by MGE cells around their explant of origin. The largest migration areas are observed on cortical cells **(A1)** and on N-cad-Fc substrate **(A3)**. Values significantly different ($^{**}p < 0.01$; $^{***}p < 0.001$). **(C,D)** Dynamic analysis of MGE cell migration using time-lapse videomicroscopy. Cells were imaged every 3 min for at least 30 min. Histogram **(C)** shows the mean instantaneous migration speed of the cell body of wild type (gray bars) and N-cadherin invalidated (blue) MGE cells on various substrates. Graphs in **(D)** are examples of cell trajectories at the front of the migration area (MGE explant up). Each cell track is shown in a specific color and the recording duration (hours, minutes) is indicated with the same color on the left upper corner. Dots indicate the position of the nucleus at each time point. MGE cells trajectories on dissociated cortical cells are rather straight and dots indicate the saltatory progression of the cell body.

(Continued)

FIGURE 1 | Continued
N-cad-Fc, alone or associated with laminin, strongly activates cell motility. On pure N-cadherin, MGE cells frequently turn or invert (green, yellow curves) their direction of migration. Cells movements on laminin are very slow. MGE cells are unbranched and form chains (see **Figure 2A**) in which cell bodies move alternatively forth and back. Trajectories are most often straight. On N-cadherin/laminin, trajectories are straighter than on N-cadherin (blue, orange curves).

N-cad-Fc (**Figure 1C**). On the N-cadherin/laminin substrate, neighboring MGE cells transiently migrated along each other and some of them exhibited polarity reversals (see yellow track in **Figure 1D**). As a consequence, the migration area of MGE cells was slightly but significantly reduced when compared to the migration area of MGE cells on a pure N-cadherin substrate (**Figure 1B**).

The morphologies of MGE cells and their spatial distribution strongly differed on the pure substrates of N-cadherin and of laminin (**Figures 2A,B**). Cells migrating on laminin exhibited bipolar shapes with short unbranched leading and trailing neurites whereas cells migrating on the pure N-cadherin substrate extended several long neurites at cell front and a thinner trailing process. On laminin, migrating MGE cells adhered to each other on their whole length. After 1 day in culture, they preferentially formed chains, with the exception of a few isolated cells. On N-cadherin, MGE cells moved on each other but never aggregated.

Cell dynamics and cell interactions appeared thus opposite on the pure substrates of N-cadherin and laminin. Cell motility was increased on the substrate of pure N-cadherin and decreased on the substrate of pure laminin. Cell-cell contacts were strengthened on laminin, and weakened on N-cadherin. Cell contacts moreover influenced MGE cell trajectories and the size of the area colonized by migrating MGE cells.

Primary Cilium Frequency in MGE Cells Migrating on N-Cadherin and on Laminin Substrates

MGE cells migrating on a pure N-cadherin substrate or on a pure laminin substrate, frequently reversed their direction of migration. We have proposed that the primary cilium protruding at the cell surface could help stabilizing the centrosome (Baudoin et al., 2012; Métin and Pedraza, 2014). We thus immunostained the primary cilium in MGE cells migrating on those pure protein substrates. Immunostaining revealed that a primary cilium was much less frequent on MGE cells migrating on a N-cadherin substrate than on MGE cells migrating on a laminin substrate (**Figure 2**). In contrast, the primary cilium was observed at similar frequencies on MGE cells migrating on the laminin substrate and on the "*in vivo*" like substrate of cortical cells (**Figures 2C,D**). This result shows that adhesion proteins distributed on the substrate of migration of MGE cells directly influenced the formation and/or the stabilization of their primary cilium, and that N-cadherin alone was unable to promote the assembly and/or the stabilization of the primary cilium. In contrast, we did not correlate the presence of a primary cilium with the capacity of migrating MGE cells to maintain a fixed polarity.

The primary cilium is assembled at the cell surface by the MC that docks to the plasma membrane. In order to determine whether the low frequency of primary cilia on MGE cells migrating on the pure N-cadherin substrate could result from a change in the subcellular positioning of the MC, we analyzed by EM the localization of the centrioles, especially the MC, in MGE cells migrating on the pure N-cadherin substrate. As a reference, the subcellular positioning of centrioles was analyzed in MGE cells migrating on the "*in vivo*-like" substrate of cortical axons (**Figure 3**).

Subcellular Localization of the Centrosome in MGE Cells Migrating on a N-Cadherin Substrate

Ultrathin sections were performed parallel to the surface of the coverslip in the plane of migration of MGE cells. Sections that comprised the cell body of MGE cells generally comprised a significant portion (up to 15 μm) of the neuritic processes extending from the cell body (**Figures 3A2,A2′**). A trailing process, much thinner than the leading process, was sometimes observed at the rear of the nucleus (black star in **Figure 3A2**). Depending on the phase of the migration cycle, the nuclear region, the cytoplasm and the leading process were either in continuity (**Figure 3A2**) or separated by constricted regions that identified the rostral swelling comprising the centrosome and the GA (**Figure 3A2**; Métin et al., 2008; Valiente and Marín, 2010). Our previous analyses (Bellion et al., 2005; Luccardini et al., 2013) showed that the GA was positioned at cell front in almost all MGE cells cultured on cortical axons.

MGE cells cultured on N-cad-Fc showed either a polarized morphology with a leading and a trailing process that differed in thickness and length (**Figure 3B2**) or a complex multipolar morphology (not illustrated). Multipolar MGE cells were few in our sample. The size of the cell body was increased on N-cadherin and a clear constriction between the nuclear compartment and the rostral cytoplasmic compartment was less frequently observed. The GA was most often located in the same compartment as the nucleus. Our previous studies showed that the GA was located at the rear of the nucleus in 30% of MGE cells cultured on N-cad-Fc (see histogram of Figure 1G in Luccardini et al., 2013).

We analyzed the centrosomal-nuclear distance in MGE cells (n = 213) cultured on N-cad-Fc and in MGE cells (n = 208) cultured on cortical axons as illustrated in **Figures 3C1–C3**. We defined 5 classes of distances between the centrosome and the nuclear edge facing the leading process, or the GA when the leading process was difficult to identify in ultrathin section (**Figure 3E**). In the present study, the nuclear edge facing the leading process or the GA was considered as the nuclear front in 100% of MGE cells migrating in cortical axons, and in only 70% of MGE cells cultured on N-cadherin. It was considered as the nuclear rear in the remaining 30% of MGE cells cultured on N-cadherin.

Surprisingly, the centrosome of MGE cells cultured on N-cad-Fc was less frequently located close to the nucleus (less than 2 μm away) as compared to the centrosome of MGE cells cultured on cortical cells (24% compared to 40%, **Figure 3F**). On N-cad-Fc, the centrosome was most often located at a

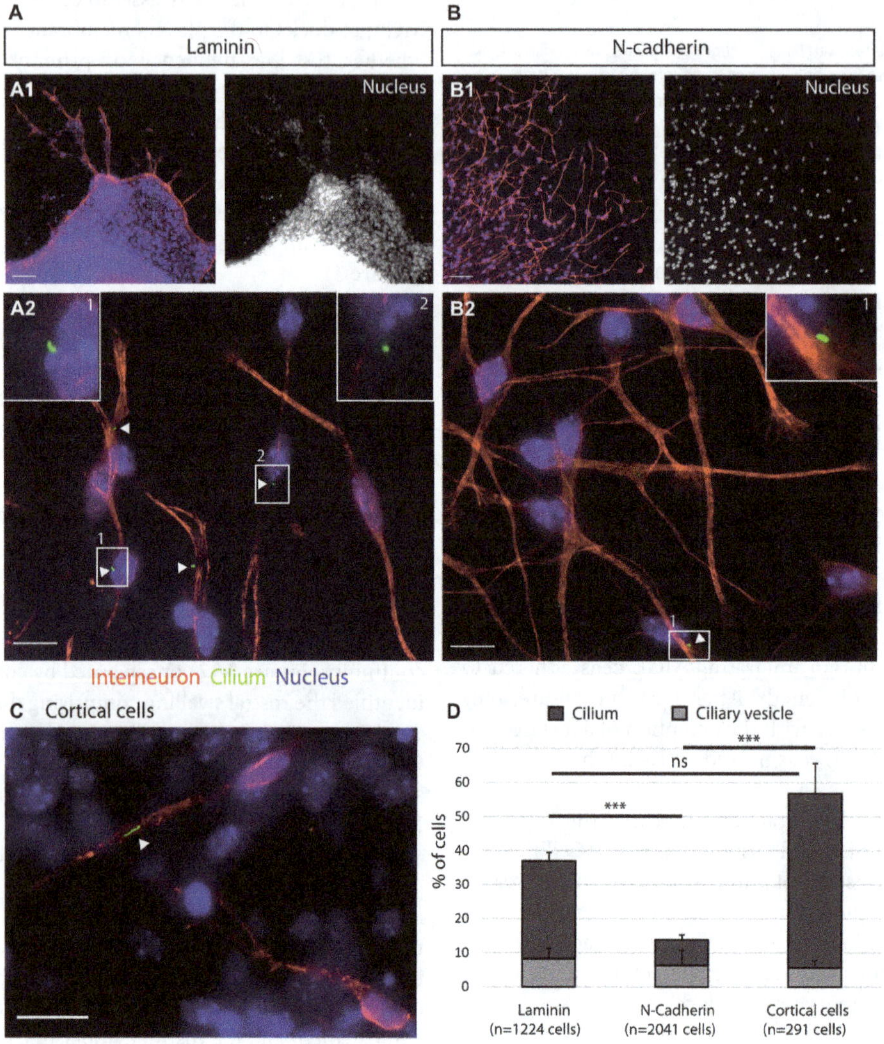

FIGURE 2 | Ciliogenesis in MGE cells depends on the substrate of migration. (A–C) Cells that migrated away from MGE explants on a glass coverslips coated with either laminin **(A)** or N-Cad-Fc **(B)** were immunostained for the ciliary protein Arl13b (green, white arrow heads) and for tyrosinated tubulin, a marker of dynamic microtubules (red). **A1** (resp. **B1**) are low magnification views of the cultures illustrated in **A2** (resp. **B2**). MGE cells migrating on cortical cells **(C)** were electroporated with LifeActRFP plasmid (red) and immunostained for the ciliary protein Arl13b (green, white arrow head). Arl13b antibodies label either small dots [diameter <0.5 μm, see enlarged insert 2 in panel **(A)**] or longer primary cilia [length > 0.5 μm, see enlarged inserts 1 in panels **(A,B)**]. Nuclei are labeled with DAPI (blue). Scale bars: 100 μm **(A1,B1)**, 10 μm **(A2,B2)**. **(D)** Percentage of ciliated MGE cells on laminin, N-cadherin and in co-cultures. Bars show the percentages of MGE exhibiting an Arl13b positive dot ("ciliary vesicle" in legend, light gray) and a primary cilium (Arl13b positive structure longer than 0.5 μm, dark gray). Error bars represent standard error of the mean (SEM). Mean values were compared using a *t*-test (***$p < 0.001$; ns, non significantly different).

distance between 2–5 μm from the nucleus, either at nuclear front or rear. Interestingly, in MGE cells cultured on cortical axons, the centrosome was able to escape the small perinuclear region and migrated into the leading process. Accordingly, the longest nuclear-centrosomal distances were observed in MGE cells cultured on cortical axons (mean value, 9.9 μm, table in **Figure 3G**) rather than in MGE cells cultured on N-cad-Fc (Table in **Figure 3G**, mean value 7.6 μm, significantly different by a *t*-test, $p = 0.0053$). These results show that the centrosome of MGE cells migrating on pure N-cadherin distributed in a perinuclear domain significantly larger than in MGE cells cultured on cortical axons. However, on N-cadherin, the cytoplasm rarely formed a rostral swelling. We then examined whether the distribution of the centrosome in a rather large cytoplasmic compartment surrounding the nucleus affected the frequency to which the MC docked to the plasma membrane.

Frequency of MC Docking to the Plasma Membrane in MGE Cells Migrating on N-Cadherin

The MC was detected in both MGE cells cultured on N-cad-Fc ($n = 92$) and MGE cells cultured on cortical axons ($n = 103$). In ultra-thin sections, the MC was sometimes accompanied by

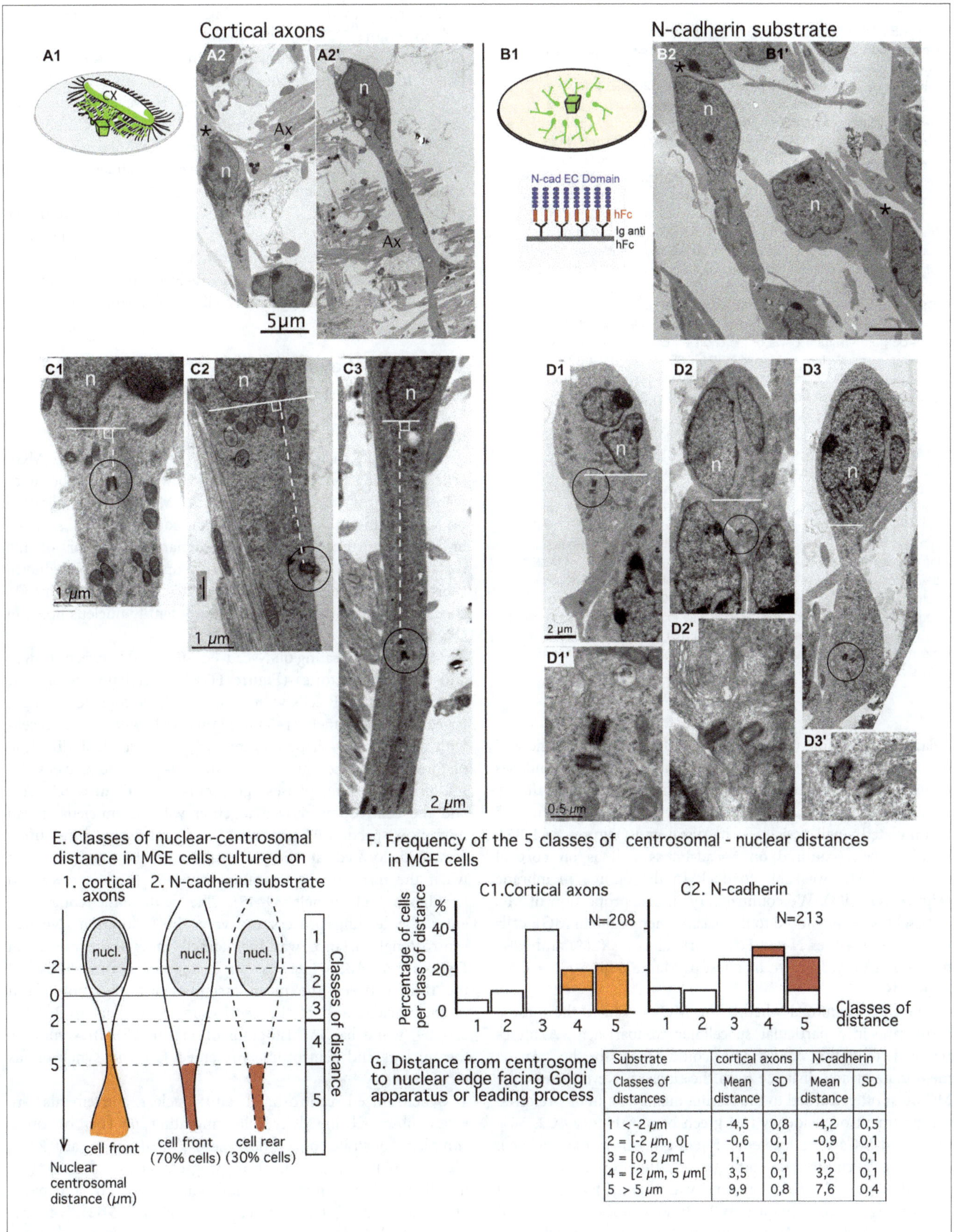

Substrate	cortical axons		N-cadherin	
Classes of distances	Mean distance	SD	Mean distance	SD
1 < -2 µm	-4,5	0,8	-4,2	0,5
2 = [-2 µm, 0[	-0,6	0,1	-0,9	0,1
3 = [0, 2 µm[	1,1	0,1	1,0	0,1
4 = [2 µm, 5 µm[	3,5	0,1	3,2	0,1
5 > 5 µm	9,9	0,8	7,6	0,4

FIGURE 3 | *Continued*

FIGURE 3 | Continued
Comparison of centrosomal position in MGE cells migrating on cortical axons vs. N-cadherin substrate using electron microscopy (EM) on ultrathin sections. (A1–B2) MGE cells were cultured on either cortical axons **(A2,A2′)** as schematized in (**A1**) or N-cad-Fc **(B2)** as schematized in **(B1)**. On these low magnification views of ultrathin sections, migrating MGE cells are polarized. Nuclei (n) are elongated on the polarization axis. A large process, likely the leading process, extends at one pole of the nucleus. No process **(A2′)** or a thin process resembling a trailing process (black stars in **A2**,**B2**) is observed at the opposite pole of the nucleus. Scale bars: 5 μm in **(A2,B2)**. **(C1–D3′)** Electron micrographs of MGE cells cultured on cortical axons **(C1–C3)** or on N-cad-Fc **(D1–D3′)** illustrate cells with different nucleus-centrioles distances: centrioles less than 2 μm in front of the nucleus **(C1,D1)**, more than 5 μm away from the nucleus **(C3,D3)** or between 2 and 5 μm **(C2,D2)**. The centriole-nuclear distance was measured as shown in panels **(C1–C3)** (white dotted line). **(D1′–D3′)** are enlarged views of the encircled centriole pair in panels **(D1–D3)**, respectively. Same scale in **(D1–D3)**, and in (**D1′–D3′**), respectively. **(E–G)** Quantitative analysis. Scheme E defines the five classes of nuclear centrosomal distances used in the present study. The nuclear membrane facing the Golgi apparatus (GA) or the leading process defines the origin of measurements (0). Distances measured away from the nucleus, on the polarity axis of the cell, are positive. Negative centrosomal-nuclear distances were subdivided into two classes (1 and 2), whereas positive centrosomal-nuclear distances were divided into three classes (3–5). In cultures on N-cad, MGE cells with the centrosome located at the nuclear rear (about 30% of MGE cells, see text) were not distinguishable from cells with the centrosome located at nuclear front. Histograms in F show the proportion of MGE cells in each class of nuclear-centrosomal distance in co-cultures on cortical axons **(C1)** and in cultures on N-cad **(C2)**. Orange and red bars identify cells in which the centriole was located in a process or in a cytoplasmic swelling, as illustrated in **(E)**. **(G)** Table indicates the mean nuclear-centrosomal distance and the standard deviation in each class of distance.

a daughter centriole (**Figures 4A4,B1,B4**). Most often, the MC was isolated and identified by the presence of lateral appendages and/or distal structures such as a large vesicle or a primary cilium (**Figures 4A1,A3,A4,B1,B2,B3**). In some cells, the MC accumulated small vesicles at its distal end (**Figures 4A1,B2**). In MGE cells cultured on N-cad-Fc as well as on cortical axons, the MC was able to dock to the plasma membrane (**Figures 4A2,B3**). We counted very similar proportion of MC or basal bodies anchored to the plasma membrane in MGE cells migrating on either N-cad-Fc or cortical axons (26% and 32%, not significantly different by a test of Mann-Whitney, $p = 0.67$, **Figure 4C**).

We then examined whether the MC docked to the plasma membrane in a particular subcellular compartment. Analyses revealed that the centrosome could dock to the plasma membrane at any distance from the nucleus. Nevertheless, the MC most often docked to the plasma membrane in its preferred compartment of residency (see green bars in **Figure 4C2**: 50% of docked MCs were located 2–5 μm away from the nucleus). In MGE cells cultured on cortical axons, the proportion of MCs docked to the plasma membrane was slightly biased toward the leading process (**Figure 4C1**: 30% of docked MCs, and 20% of undocked MCs, the difference is not significant by a Kolmogorov-Smirnov test).

According to the results in MGE cells immunostained for Arl13b (**Figure 2**), the proportion of MCs docked to the plasma membrane and associated with a primary cilium was two folds higher in MGE cells cultured on cortical axons (55%) than in MGE cells cultured on N-cad-Fc (27%). However, in this small sample, the difference is not significant by a Mann-Whitney test. It is noteworthy that MCs located into the cytoplasm associated with a large distal vesicle or small vesicles attached to distal appendages at the same frequency regardless of the substrate of migration (69 and 71% respectively, Table **D** in **Figure 4**). Therefore, the ability to assemble a primary cilium at the distal end of the MC was similar in both samples, showing that the interaction of MGE cells with a N-cad-Fc substrate of migration rather did not promote primary cilium elongation on the cell surface.

Dynamic Behavior of the Centrosome in MGE Cells Migrating on a N-Cadherin Substrate

Our EM analysis revealed that the MC of MGE cells migrating on a N-cad-Fc substrate docked to the plasma membrane at the same frequency as the MC of MGE cells migrating on cortical axons. However, the subcellular distribution of the centrosome in MGE cells migrating on a N-cadherin substrate and on cortical axons strongly differed. We thus analyzed the dynamic behavior of the centrosome in MGE cells cultured on a pure N-cadherin substrate. MGE cells were electroporated with a PACT-mKO1 construct to label the centrosome and identify nucleus position (**Figure 5**).

MGE cells migrating on N-cad-Fc alternated between straight and curved trajectories (**Figure 1D**) in correlation with their morphology. MGE cells with a bipolar shape followed straight trajectories (see panels 21–33 in **Figure 5A1**) whereas MGE cells with a multipolar shape continuously changed their direction of movements (see panels 3–15 and 39–51). The nucleus did not present resting phases (gray curves in **Figures 5A2,A3**) and the centrosome moved together with the nucleus (mean migration speed, 1.94 μm/min). The centrosome most often remained located at the same pole of the nucleus, even when the direction of migration reversed (pink arrow head in **Figure 5A1**, panels 39–45). The centrosome could also enter the leading process for very short duration. Nuclear centrosomal distance was maintained short (blue curves in **Figures 5A2,A3**, white bar in histogram **Figure 5D**) and the ratio between the mean instantaneous migration speed of the nucleus and of the centrosome was equal to 1 (1.05 ± 0.09, white bar in histogram of **Figure 5F**). In summary, the nucleus and centrosome presented fast and synchronous movements.

Synchronized centrosomal and nuclear movements are rarely observed in MGE cells migrating *in vivo* or on a complex substrate of cortical cells (Baudoin et al., 2012; **Figures 5B1,B2**). The nuclear progression is saltatory (see the distribution of nuclear positions in **Figure 1D**, and peaks of nuclear speed on gray curve in **Figure 5B2**), whereas centrosomal movements are progressive, with smaller peaks of migration speed and faster forward movements between

A,B. Cytoplasmic and cell surface location of mature centrioles (MC) and basal bodies in MGE cells cultured on cortical axons (A1-A4) or on N-cadherin substrate (B1-B4)

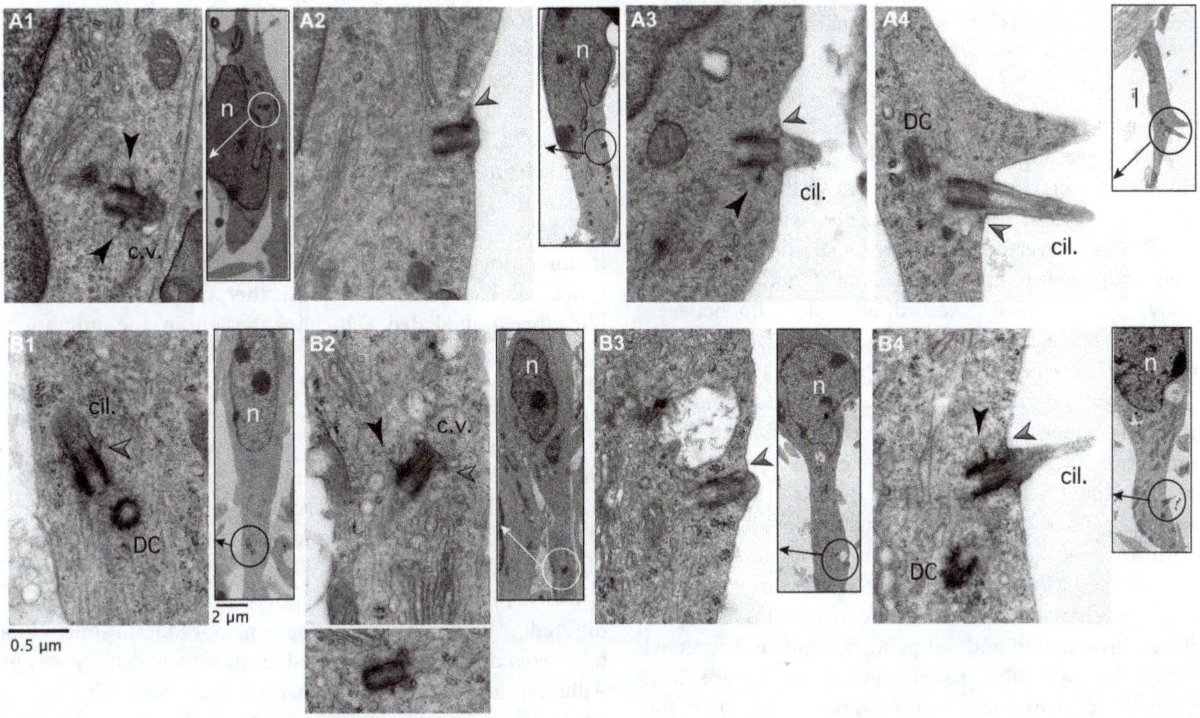

C. Influence of the distance to the nucleus on the docking of the MC to the plasma membrane

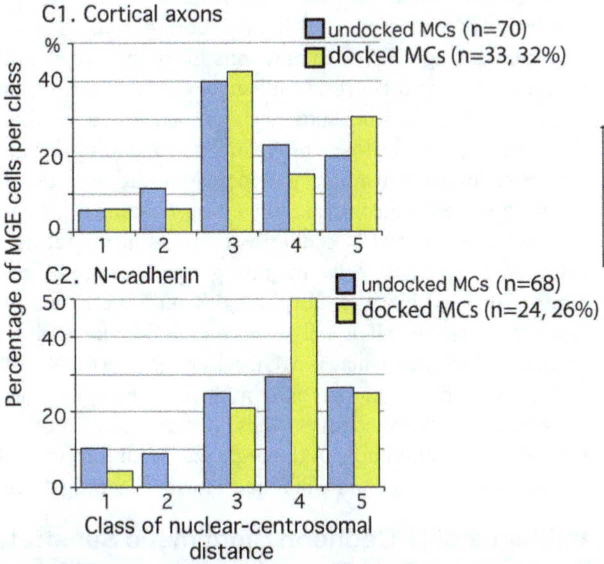

D. Frequency of ciliary structures (primary cilium, cil., or ciliary vesicle, c.v.) assocaited with cytoplasmic MC and plasma membrane anchored MC or basal bodies

Substrate

	cortical axons		N-cadherin	
Nber of MC	Total	with distal structure	Total	with distal structure
Pl. Memb.	20	12 cil. (60%)	15	4 cil. (27%)
cytopl.	28	20 c.v. (71%)	39	27 c.v. (69%)

FIGURE 4 | Mature centriole (MC) subcellular localization and ciliogenesis in MGE cells cultured on cortical axons or N-cadherin. (A1–B4) Panels show examples of MC with cytoplasmic localization **(A1,B1,B2)** or MC docked to the plasma membrane **(A2–A4,B3,B4)** in MGE cells cultured on cortical axons **(A1–A4)** and N-cad-Fc **(B1–B4)**. Inserts on the right side of panels are low magnification views of cells to localize the MC (circle). MC sectioned longitudinally show lateral appendages (black arrow heads) and/or distal appendages (gray arrow heads) which attach ciliary vesicles to the MC **(B1,B2)** or the MC to the plasma membrane **(A2–A4,B3,B4)**. The cilium is often attached to a basal body decorated with a long lateral appendage **(A3,B4)**. Same scale for all high magnification pictures and inserts (see **B1**). Cil., primary cilium; c.v., ciliary vesicle DC, daughter centriole; n, nucleus. **(C)** Histograms compare in MGEs cultured on either cortical axons or N-cad-Fc, the distribution of cytoplasmic MC (blue bars) and of MC docked to the plasma membrane (green bars) in the different classes of nuclear centrosomal

(*Continued*)

FIGURE 4 | Continued
distances (see **Figure 3E**). **(D)** Table gives the number of MC observed in the cytoplasm or docked to the plasma membrane, which exhibited a clear ciliary structure (primary cilium, cil.; ciliary vesicle, c.v.). Results confirm that primary cilia are less frequent on MGE cultured on N-cad-Fc than on cortical axons.

peaks (pink curve in **Figure 5B2**). The nuclear-centrosomal distance shows large amplitude variations, ranging from 0 to 20 μm (blue curve in **Figure 5B2**, and gray bar in histogram **Figure 5D**, significantly different from the white bar by a *t*-test, $p = 0.009$). Nevertheless, centrosomal movements are coordinated with nuclear movements even if both organelles do not move synchronously. Accordingly, the ratio between centrosomal and nuclear mean instantaneous migration speeds was close to 1 in the present sample (1.1 + 0.2, gray bar in histogram **Figure 5F**). To further understand the contribution of cadherin mediated cell-cell adhesion in those centrosomal and nuclear movements, we electroporated MGE cells with a dominant negative construct (pCAG-N-cad(t)) that sequesters endogenous catenins and interferes with signaling pathways downstream cadherin (Taniguchi et al., 2006). As previously reported (Luccardini et al., 2013), the migration speed of the nucleus was drastically reduced in MGE cells with cadherin invalidation and cell polarity frequently reversed (**Figures 5C1,C2**, and blue bar in histogram **Figure 5E**). Surprisingly, the centrosome remained more motile than the nucleus, moving from one nuclear pole to the other. Accordingly, the ratio between centrosomal and nuclear instantaneous migration speeds increased to 1.6 (±0.8), showing that cadherin invalidation in MGE cells partially disrupted the correlation between centrosomal and nuclear movements. This result suggests that cadherin activity promotes the synchronization of nuclear and centrosomal movements, which was indeed remarkably tight in MGE cells migrating on a pure N-cadherin substrate.

Discussion

In the embryonic brain, N-cadherin is present with other adhesive and guidance cues in the migratory pathway of MGE cells. Because we observed that N-cadherin was the most efficient protein substrate to promote the migration of MGE cells *in vitro*, we decided to further characterize the migratory behavior of MGE cells on this permissive substrate. We moreover compared the migration of MGE cells on a pure N-cadherin substrate with their migration on a pure laminin substrate. The migration speed of MGE cells was very slow on the pure laminin substrate and cells preferentially adhered to each other. On N-cadherin in contrast, contacts between MGE cells were minimal. Centrosomal movements were highly synchronized with nuclear movements. The MC remained able to dock to the plasma membrane but a primary cilium rarely formed. Therefore, cadherin signaling not only influences nuclear motility in migrating MGE cells, but moreover influences centrosomal movements and ciliogenesis.

Migratory Behavior of MGE Cells on a Pure Substrate of N-Cadherin or of Laminin

Two major types of cell adhesion regulate the cell migration: (1) cell-cell adhesion that is controlled, among other proteins, by classical cadherins that establish homophilic interactions; and (2) cell-extracellular matrix adhesion that is controlled, among others, by integrin receptors that link extra-cellular matrix (ECM) proteins as laminin or fibronectin to the actin cytoskeleton (Kawauchi, 2012). N-cadherin is expressed by MGE cells and by cells in their migratory pathway (Kadowaki et al., 2007). We previously showed that N-cadherin loss of function in migrating MGE cells altered cell motility and cell polarity (Luccardini et al., 2013). To further characterize the role of N-cadherin mediated cell-cell adhesion in the migration of cortical interneurons, we analyzed the migratory behavior of MGE cells on a biomimetic substrate of N-cadherin and on a pure laminin substrate that activates integrins, a class of cell surface receptors involved in neural migration and cell polarity (Lawson and Burridge, 2014). In contrast to laminin on which MGE cells moved very slowly, N-cadherin stimulated the outgrowth of leading processes and the motility of MGE cells. Additional differences distinguished MGE cells cultured on laminin or N-cadherin. First, reciprocal interactions between MGE cells differed. MGE cells migrating on N-cadherin only shortly interacted and never aggregated, even if their density was high. Adhesive interactions between MGE cells were thus minimal. On the laminin substrate in contrast, MGE cells exhibited long-lasting and tight reciprocal interactions that quickly led to the formation of chains or cell aggregates. On this latter substrate of migration, MGE cells not only interacted with the protein substrate, but moreover with neighboring cells. These tight and long-lasting cell-cell interactions likely involve N-cadherin receptors, among other receptors, suggesting that the response of MGE cells to the laminin substrate was perturbated by additional and uncontrolled cell-cell interactions. By adding laminin to the N-cadherin substrate, we increased the frequency and duration of cell-cell contacts, suggesting functional interactions between integrin and N-cadherin receptors in migrating MGE cells. Second, MGE cells migrating on N-cadherin and on laminin differed by their morphologies and trajectories. On the laminin substrate, MGE cells were mainly bipolar and showed straight trajectories, whereas MGE cells migrating on N-cadherin alternated between bipolar and multipolar morphologies and showed complex trajectories. These differences in morphology suggest major differences in the organization of the cytoskeleton on the two substrates and will require further investigations.

Influence of N-Cadherin Biomimetic Substrate on Centrosome Docking and on Primary Cilium Assembly

We have shown that the centrosome of GABAergic neurons born in the MGE of the basal telencephalon is a microtubule-organizing center that can moreover assemble a primary cilium at the distal end of the MC (Baudoin et al., 2012). An important function of the primary cilium is to anchor the centrosome to the plasma membrane (Pedersen et al., 2008; Reiter et al., 2012). In GABAergic neurons migrating a long distance from the basal

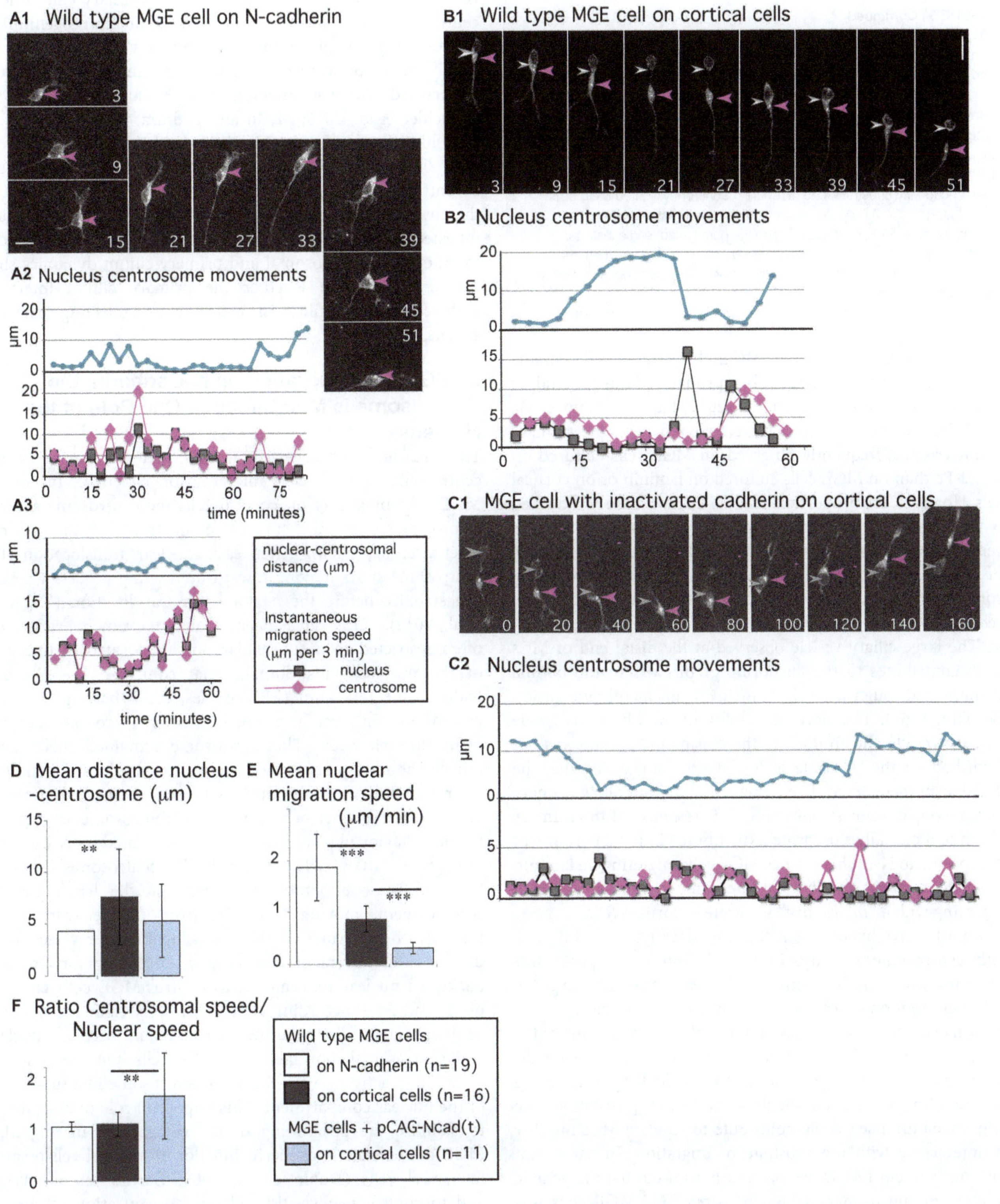

FIGURE 5 | Centrosomal movements in MGE cells migrating on a N-cadherin substrate and in MGE cells with cadherin invalidation. **(A1–C2)** Time-lapse sequences in **(A1,B1,C1)** illustrate the migratory behavior of MGE cells electroporated with a pericentrin expression vector that labels the centrosome (white dot, red arrow head) and the cytoplasm (gray labeling). Pericentrin expression is also used to track the nucleus (gray arrow head). Elapsed time is indicated in minutes in panels. Scale bars, 10 µm. Curves in **(A2,A3,B2,C2)**, represent the nuclear centrosomal distance (blue curve), the instantaneous migration speed of the nucleus (gray) and centrosome (pink) in migrating MGE cells. **(A1–A3)** Migration of wild type cells on a N-cad-Fc substrate. **(B1,B2)** Migration of a wild type cell on dissociated cortical cells.

(Continued)

FIGURE 5 | Continued
(C1,C2) Migration on dissociated cortical cells of a cell electroporated with the dominant negative construct N-cad(t). **(D–F)** Histograms show the mean value and standard deviation of the average nuclear centrosomal distance **(D)**, of the instantaneous migration speed of the nucleus **(E)**, and of the ratio between centrosomal and nuclear instantaneous migration speeds **(F)** in wild type MGE cells monitored on N-cad-Fc (white bars), on cortical cells (gray bars) and in cadherin invalidated MGE cells monitored on cortical cells (blue bars). The nuclear speed is maximal in wild type MGE cells migrating on the pure N-cadherin substrate, and minimal in cadherin invalidated MGE cells. $^{**}p < 0.01$; $^{***}p < 0.001$. Centrosomal and nuclear movements are synchronized in MGE cells migrating on the pure N-cadherin substrate; cadherin invalidation in MGE cells migrating on cortical cells disrupts the coordination between nuclear and centrosomal movements observed in wild type MGE cells.

telencephalon to the cortex, the MC is able to dock to the plasma membrane. It can associate with a primary cilium protruding at the cell surface (Baudoin et al., 2012; Higginbotham et al., 2012). In the cell samples that we analyzed here, the primary cilium was less frequently observed on MGE cells cultured on N-cad-Fc than on MGE cells cultured on laminin or on cortical cells. However, the proportion of MGE cells with the MC docked to the plasma membrane did not decrease when MGE cells were migrating on a pure substrate of N-cadherin. Moreover, the MC was able to dock on the cell surface at any distance from the nucleus. We observed ciliary vesicles at the same frequency in MGE cells cultured on cortical axons or on N-cad-Fc. The large ciliary vesicle observed at the distal end of MCs likely contributes to the anchoring of the MC to the plasma membrane through a mechanism involving membrane fusion (Sorokin, 1962). Therefore, the ability of the MC to assemble a ciliary vesicle and to dock to the plasma membrane was not perturbed on the substrate of N-cadherin, suggesting that the N-cadherin mediated cell-cell interaction did not allow primary cilium elongation or stabilization. This response of the primary cilium to a cell adhesion protein distributed in the environment was specific to N-cadherin since MGE cells migrating on laminin exhibited a primary cilium at the same frequency as MGE migrating with a "*in vivo like*" substrate of cortical cells.

An attractive hypothesis is that MC docking could interfere with centrosome motility. Our results do not support this hypothesis. Indeed, the centrosome moved twice faster in MGE cells cultured on N-cad-Fc than in MGE cells cultured on cortical cells, although it docked to the plasma membrane at the same frequency in both culture conditions. Even if our results argue against a role of plasma membrane docking to reducing MC motility, we cannot totally exclude this possibility. The primary cilium itself could contribute to regulate MCs motility by interacting with the substrate of migration. In agreement with our present results, we previously showed that the genetic ablation of the primary cilium in Kif3a KOs MGE cells was correlated to a slight increase in the motility of the centrosome (Baudoin et al., 2012).

Integrin receptors have been described on the primary cilium (McGlashan et al., 2006; Seeger-Nukpezah and Golemis, 2012). Adhesive interactions with the extracellular matrix could transiently stabilize the primary cilium and the basal body. Accordingly, the apical abscission of the primary cilium helps centrioles to move away from the basal lamina in progenitors of the cortical neuroepithelium (Das and Storey, 2014).

The role(s) of the primary cilium in cell migration is far from understood (Albrecht-Buehler, 1977; Katsumoto et al., 1994; Schneider et al., 2010; Métin and Pedraza, 2014). In adherent cells like fibroblasts or smooth muscle cells, the cilium has been shown to control cell directionality. The primary cilium of cortical interneurons concentrates receptors to factors in the environment that likely influence the migration of cortical interneurons (Higginbotham et al., 2012). The simultaneous monitoring of centrosomal and primary cilium dynamics shall permit to examine whether the primary cilium interferes with centriole motility in addition to collecting extrinsic signals.

In MGE Cells Migrating on N-Cadherin, the Centrosome is Maintained at One Pole of the Nucleus

The present study revealed an unexpected behavior of the centrosome in MGE cells migrating on N-cad-Fc. In control MGE cells migrating on cortical cells the centrosome showed a progressive forward migration in front of the nucleus (Métin et al., 2008). After each nuclear translocation, the centrosome starts moving toward the leading process where it can stabilize before the next nuclear translocation (Yanagida et al., 2012). On N-cad-Fc, centrosomal movements were most often restricted to a subcellular domain located at one pole of the nucleus. This domain, that contained the GA and endoplasmic reticulum (ER) vesicles, could be large and the centrosome only rarely escaped to enter a process emerging from the cell body. The centrosome remained there, even during the time period when the cell reversed its direction of migration and when the nucleus moved alternatively forward and backward. This behavior of the centrosome is opposite to the behavior observed in N-cadherin ablated or N-cadherin invalidated MGE cells, in which the centrosome exhibited fast and large amplitude movements in the whole nuclear compartment, moving from the front to the rear of the nucleus. N-cadherin KO MGE cells frequently reversed their direction of movement and showed alternating forward and backward nuclear movements, as control MGE cells cultured on N-cad-Fc (Luccardini et al., 2013). N-cadherin ablation or invalidation disrupted the coordination between nuclear and centrosomal movements in MGE cells. On the contrary, N-cadherin activation stabilized the centrosome in a sub-region of the nuclear compartment. This important role of N-cadherin to stabilize the positioning of the centrosome in migrating MGE cells recalls N-cadherin function to control cell polarity in neural cells (Dupin et al., 2009; Gärtner et al., 2012), and to control *in vivo*, the polarized organization of cortical progenitors in the proliferative neuroepithelium (Kadowaki et al., 2007). Accordingly, the expression level of N-cadherin has also been shown to control the polarity and migration speed of glial cells in a wound-healing test (Camand et al., 2012). In MGE cells migrating on N-cad-Fc, the nuclear and centrosomal movements were highly synchronized, which was not the case in MGE cells migrating on cortical cells. The regulatory mechanisms involved in this control remain to be explored.

In conclusion, we show here that N-cadherin-mediated cell-cell interactions are efficient signals for stimulating MGE cell motility, including centrosome motility. The negative correlation between centrosomal movements and primary cilium formation observed in MGE cells migrating on N-cadherin, remembers results in MGE cells with a genetic ablation of the primary cilium (Baudoin et al., 2012). In addition, our results show that N-cadherin mediated cell-cell interactions and integrin mediated ECM-cell interactions have distinct influences on the ciliogenesis in migrating MGE cells.

Acknowledgments

We thank René-Marc Mège for help with the biomimetic substrates, Melissa Martin for english corrections and all the members of the team for helpful discussions. This work was supported by Institut National de la Santé et de la Recherche Médicale (INSERM), Agence Nationale pour la Recherche (ANR Grant MRGENE), Fondation J. Lejeune and Fondation pour la Recherche sur le Cerveau. CL was supported by a grant from Neuropole Ile de France and by the Grant MRGENE from ANR. C. Métin's team is affiliated with the Paris School of Neuroscience and the Bio-Psy Laboratory of Excellence. We thank Institut du Fer à Moulin for Imaging Facility and Animal Facility.

References

Albrecht-Buehler, G. (1977). Phagokinetic tracks of 3T3 cells: parallels between the orientation of track segments and of cellular structures which contain actin or tubulin. *Cell* 12, 333–339. doi: 10.1016/0092-8674(77)90109-x

Anderson, S. A., Eisenstat, D. D., Shi, L., and Rubenstein, J. L. (1997). Interneuron migration from basal forebrain to neocortex: dependence on Dlx genes. *Science* 278, 474–476. doi: 10.1126/science.278.5337.474

Baudoin, J.-P., Viou, L., Launay, P.-S., Luccardini, C., Espeso Gil, S., Kiyasova, V., et al. (2012). Articletangentially migrating neurons assemble a primary cilium that promotes their reorientation to the cortical plate. *Neuron* 76, 1108–1122. doi: 10.1016/j.neuron.2012.10.027

Bellion, A., Baudoin, J.-P., Alvarez, C., Bornens, M., and Métin, C. (2005). Nucleokinesis in tangentially migrating neurons comprises two alternating phases: forward migration of the Golgi/centrosome associated with centrosome splitting and myosin contraction at the rear. *J. Neurosci.* 25, 5691–5699. doi: 10.1523/jneurosci.1030-05.2005

Butt, S. J. B., Fuccillo, M., Nery, S., Noctor, S., Kriegstein, A., Corbin, J. G., et al. (2005). The temporal and spatial origins of cortical interneurons predict their physiological subtype. *Neuron* 48, 591–604. doi: 10.1016/j.neuron.2005.09.034

Camand, E., Peglion, F., Osmani, N., Sanson, M., and Etienne-Manneville, S. (2012). N-cadherin expression level modulates integrin-mediated polarity and strongly impacts on the speed and directionality of glial cell migration. *J. Cell Sci.* 125, 844–857. doi: 10.1242/jcs.087668

Das, R. M., and Storey, K. G. (2014). Apical abscission alters cell polarity and dismantles the primary cilium during neurogenesis. *Science* 343, 200–204. doi: 10.1126/science.1247521

Dupin, I., Camand, E., and Etienne-Manneville, S. (2009). Classical cadherins control nucleus and centrosome position and cell polarity. *J. Cell Biol.* 185, 779–786. doi: 10.1083/jcb.200812034

Etienne-Manneville, S., and Hall, A. (2003). Cell polarity: par6, aPKC and cytoskeletal crosstalk. *Curr. Opin. Cell Biol.* 15, 67–72. doi: 10.1016/s0955-0674(02)00005-4

Flames, N., Pla, R., Gelman, D. M., Rubenstein, J. L. R., Puelles, L., and Marín, O. (2007). Delineation of multiple subpallial progenitor domains by the combinatorial expression of transcriptional codes. *J. Neurosci.* 27, 9682–9695. doi: 10.1523/jneurosci.2750-07.2007

Fogarty, M., Grist, M., Gelman, D., Marín, O., Pachnis, V., and Kessaris, N. (2007). Spatial genetic patterning of the embryonic neuroepithelium generates GABAergic interneuron diversity in the adult cortex. *J. Neurosci.* 27, 10935–10946. doi: 10.1523/jneurosci.1629-07.2007

Franco, S. J., Martinez-Garay, I., Gil-Sanz, C., Harkins-Perry, S. R., and Müller, U. (2011). Reelin regulates cadherin functionvia Dab1/Rap1 to control neuronal migration and lamination in the neocortex. *Neuron* 69, 482–497. doi: 10.1016/j.neuron.2011.01.003

Gärtner, A., Fornasiero, E. F., Munck, S., Vennekens, K. A. L., Seuntjens, E., Huttner, W. B., et al. (2012). N-cadherin specifies first asymmetry in developing neurons. *EMBO J.* 31, 1893–1903. doi: 10.1038/emboj.2012.41

Higginbotham, H., Eom, T.-Y., Mariani, L. E., Bachleda, A., Hirt, J., Gukassyan, V., et al. (2012). Arl13b in primary cilia regulates the migration and placement of interneurons in the developing cerebral cortex. *Dev. Cell* 23, 925–938. doi: 10.1016/j.devcel.2012.09.019

Higginbotham, H. R., and Gleeson, J. G. (2007). The centrosome in neuronal development. *Trends Neurosci.* 30, 276–283. doi: 10.1016/j.tins.2007.04.001

Jossin, Y., and Cooper, J. A. (2011). Reelin, Rap1 and N-cadherin orient the migration of multipolar neurons in the developing neocortex. *Nat. Neurosci.* 14, 697–703. doi: 10.1038/nn.2816

Kadowaki, M., Nakamura, S., Machon, O., Krauss, S., Radice, G. L., and Takeichi, M. (2007). N-cadherin mediates cortical organization in the mouse brain. *Dev. Biol.* 304, 22–33. doi: 10.1016/j.ydbio.2006.12.014

Katsumoto, T., Higaki, K., Ohno, K., and Onodera, K. (1994). The orientation of primary cilia during the wound response in 3Y1 cells. *Biol. Cell* 81, 17–21. doi: 10.1016/0248-4900(94)90050-7

Kawauchi, T. (2012). Cell adhesion and its endocytic regulation in cell migration during neural development and cancer metastasis. *Int. J. Mol. Sci.* 13, 4564–4590. doi: 10.3390/ijms13044564

Kawauchi, T., Sekine, K., Shikanai, M., Chihama, K., Tomita, K., Kubo, K.-I., et al. (2010). Rab GTPases-dependent endocytic pathways regulate neuronal migration and maturation through N-cadherin trafficking. *Neuron* 67, 588–602. doi: 10.1016/j.neuron.2010.07.007

Lambert, M., Padilla, F., and Mège, R. M. (2000). Immobilized dimers of N-cadherin-Fc chimera mimic cadherin-mediated cell contact formation: contribution of both outside-in and inside-out signals. *J. Cell Sci.* 113, 2207–2219. doi: 10.1159/000014630

Lawson, C. D., and Burridge, K. (2014). The on-off relationship of rho and rac during integrin-mediated adhesion and cell migration. *Small GTPases* 5:e27958. doi: 10.4161/sgtp.27958

Luccardini, C., Hennekinne, L., Viou, L., Yanagida, M., Murakami, F., Kessaris, N., et al. (2013). N-Cadherin sustains motility and polarity of future cortical interneurons during tangential migration. *J. Neurosci.* 33, 18149–18160. doi: 10.1523/JNEUROSCI.0593-13.2013

Marín, O., Valiente, M., Ge, X., and Tsai, L.-H. (2010). Guiding neuronal cell migrations. *Cold Spring Harb. Perspect. Biol.* 2:a001834. doi: 10.1101/cshperspect.a001834

McGlashan, S. R., Jensen, C. G., and Poole, C. A. (2006). Localization of extracellular matrix receptors on the chondrocyte primary cilium. *J. Histochem. Cytochem.* 54, 1005–1014. doi: 10.1369/jhc.5a6866.2006

Métin, C., and Pedraza, M. (2014). Cilia: traffic directors along the road of cortical development. *Neuroscientist* 20, 468–482. doi: 10.1177/1073858414543151

Métin, C., Vallee, R. B., Rakic, P., and Bhide, P. G. (2008). Modes and mishaps of neuronal migration in the mammalian brain. *J. Neurosci.* 28, 11746–11752. doi: 10.1523/JNEUROSCI.3860-08.2008

Miyoshi, G., Hjerling-Leffler, J., Karayannis, T., Sousa, V. H., Butt, S. J. B., Battiste, J., et al. (2010). Genetic fate mapping reveals that the caudal ganglionic eminence produces a large and diverse population of superficial cortical interneurons. *J. Neurosci.* 30, 1582–1594. doi: 10.1523/JNEUROSCI.4515-09.2010

Nery, S., Fishell, G., and Corbin, J. G. (2002). The caudal ganglionic eminence is a source of distinct cortical and subcortical cell populations. *Nat. Neurosci.* 5, 1279–1287. doi: 10.1038/nn971

Pedersen, L. B., Veland, I. R., Schrøder, J. M., and Christensen, S. T. (2008). Assembly of primary cilia. *Dev. Dyn.* 237, 1993–2006. doi: 10.1002/dvdy.21521

Reiter, J. F., Blacque, O. E., and Leroux, M. R. (2012). The base of the cilium: roles for transition fibres and the transition zone in ciliary formation, maintenance and compartmentalization. *EMBO Rep.* 13, 608–618. doi: 10.1038/embor.2012.73

Ridley, A. J., Schwartz, M. A., Burridge, K., Firtel, R. A., Ginsberg, M. H., Borisy, G., et al. (2003). Cell migration: integrating signals from front to back. *Science* 302, 1704–1709. doi: 10.1126/science.1092053

Schneider, L., Cammer, M., Lehman, J., Nielsen, S. K., Guerra, C. F., Veland, I. R., et al. (2010). Directional cell migration and chemotaxis in wound healing response to PDGF-AA are coordinated by the primary cilium in fibroblasts. *Cell. Physiol. Biochem.* 25, 279–292. doi: 10.1159/000276562

Seeger-Nukpezah, T., and Golemis, E. A. (2012). The extracellular matrix and ciliary signaling. *Curr. Opin. Cell Biol.* 24, 652–661. doi: 10.1016/j.ceb.2012.06.002

Solecki, D. J. (2012). Sticky situations: recent advances in control of cell adhesion during neuronal migration. *Curr. Opin. Neurobiol.* 22, 791–798. doi: 10.1016/j.conb.2012.04.010

Solecki, D. J., Model, L., Gaetz, J., Kapoor, T. M., and Hatten, M. E. (2004). Par6α signaling controls glial-guided neuronal migration. *Nat. Neurosci.* 7, 1195–1203. doi: 10.1038/nn1332

Sorokin, S. (1962). Centrioles and the formation of rudimentary cilia by fibroblasts and smooth muscle cells. *J. Cell Biol.* 15, 363–373. doi: 10.1083/jcb.15.2.363

Taniguchi, H., Kawauchi, D., Nishida, K., and Murakami, F. (2006). Classic cadherins regulate tangential migration of precerebellar neurons in the caudal hindbrain. *Development* 133, 1923–1931. doi: 10.1242/dev.02414

Ueda, M., Gräf, R., MacWilliams, H. K., Schliwa, M., and Euteneuer, U. (1997). Centrosome positioning and directionality of cell movements. *Proc. Natl. Acad. Sci. U S A* 94, 9674–9678. doi: 10.1073/pnas.94.18.9674

Valiente, M., and Marín, O. (2010). Neuronal migration mechanisms in development and disease. *Curr. Opin. Neurobiol.* 20, 68–78. doi: 10.1016/j.conb.2009.12.003

Wichterle, H., García-Verdugo, J. M., Herrera, D. G., and Alvarez-Buylla, A. (1999). Young neurons from medial ganglionic eminence disperse in adult and embryonic brain. *Nat. Neurosci.* 2, 461–466. doi: 10.1038/8131

Wonders, C. P., and Anderson, S. A. (2006). The origin and specification of cortical interneurons. *Nat. Rev. Neurosci.* 7, 687–696. doi: 10.1038/nrn1954

Yanagida, M., Miyoshi, R., Toyokuni, R., Zhu, Y., and Murakami, F. (2012). Dynamics of the leading process, nucleus and golgi apparatus of migrating cortical interneurons in living mouse embryos. *Proc. Natl. Acad. Sci. U S A* 109, 16737–16742. doi: 10.1073/pnas.1209166109

5

Neural Progenitor Cell Polarity and Cortical Development

Yoko Arai[1] *and Elena Taverna*[2]*

[1]Centre for Interdisciplinary Research in Biology (CIRB), Collège de France, CNRS UMR 7241/INSERM U1050, PSL Research University, Paris, France, [2]Department of Evolutionary Genetics, Max Planck Institute for Evolutionary Anthropology (MPG), Leipzig, Germany

***Correspondence:**
Elena Taverna
elena_taverna@eva.mpg.de

Neurons populating the cerebral cortex are generated during embryonic development from neural stem and progenitor cells in a process called neurogenesis. Neural stem and progenitor cells are classified into several classes based on the different location of mitosis (apical or basal) and polarity features (bipolar, monopolar and non-polar). The polarized architecture of stem cells is linked to the asymmetric localization of proteins, mRNAs and organelles, such as the centrosome and the Golgi apparatus (GA). Polarity affects stem cell function and allows stem cells to integrate environmental cues from distinct niches in the developing cerebral cortex. The crucial role of polarity in neural stem and progenitor cells is highlighted by the fact that impairment of cell polarity is linked to neurodevelopmental disorders such as Down syndrome, Fragile X syndrome, autism spectrum disorders (ASD) and schizophrenia.

Keywords: brain development, epithelial polarity, apical progenitors, basal progenitors, neural stem and progenitor cells, polarity, epithelial to mesenchymal transition (EMT), neurodevelopmental disorders

INTRODUCTION

The cerebral cortex is the center of higher cognitive functions. Neurons and glial cells populating the cerebral cortex arise sequentially during embryonic development from the division of neural stem and progenitor cells.

Polarity, that is the asymmetric spatial organization of cellular components and subcellular structures, is one of the main criteria used to classify and distinguish different types of stem and progenitor cells (Fietz and Huttner, 2011; Taverna et al., 2014). In actively dividing cells, such as neural stem cells, the polarity cues of the mother cells are used to generate different types of daughter cells: polarity is therefore instrumental in increasing cell type diversity (Fietz and Huttner, 2011). This is a crucial aspect in the central nervous system (CNS), particularly for cerebral cortex development and evolution, as enhanced cognitive functions in mammals are thought to arise from an increase in the diversity of cell types; in particular neural progenitor cell types in the developing cerebral cortex (Wilsch-Bräuninger et al., 2016; Arai and Pierani, 2014).

In this review article, we will focus on: (i) neural stem and progenitor cells and their polarity features; (ii) molecular mechanisms underlying neural stem and progenitor cell polarity; (iii) cell polarity and cell identity; and (iv) how the impairment of cellular polarity impacts cortical development.

NEUROGENESIS IN MAMMALS: CELL TYPES AND THEIR POLARITY FEATURES

Neural stem cells compared to neural progenitor cells differ with regards to their multipotency state: while neural stem cells are multipotent, neural progenitor cells are unipotent and fate restricted. They are classified based on several criteria, such as the location where they undergo mitosis, polarity features, and proliferation vs. differentiation potential (Taverna et al., 2014). Based on the location of their mitoses, neural stem and progenitor cells fall into two groups: apically-dividing and basally-dividing progenitor cells apical progenitors (APs) and basal progenitors (BPs), respectively (**Figure 1**; note that unless specified otherwise, the findings reported here refer to the developing dorsal telencephalon of rodents).

Apical Progenitors

The term apical stem and progenitor cells (APs) refer to cells undergoing mitosis at the apical surface of the ventricular zone (VZ; **Figure 1**). This category is comprised of cells which have a wide range of mitotic capacity and proliferation/differentiation potential. In the subsequent sections, we will describe the different AP subtypes in order from the most multipotent down to unipotent cells.

Neuroepithelial Cells

Before the onset of neurogenesis, the developing brain is formed mostly by neuroepithelial cells (NECs). They are highly polarized epithelial cells exhibiting apico-basal polarity (**Figure 1**). Their apical plasma membrane is integrated into the adherens junctional (AJ) belt and lines the lumen of the neural tube, which is filled with lipoprotein- and membrane particle-rich embryonic cerebrospinal fluid (Lehtinen et al., 2011). The AJs are cell junctions surrounding the cell, they are linked to the actin cytoskeleton and they separate the apical and the basal domain of NECs (for an historical perspective on AJs refer to Franke, 2009; and references therein; see also Farquhar and Palade, 1963; Takeichi, 1977; Stocker and Chenn, 2015). The basal plasma membrane of NECs spans the neuroepithelium and reaches the basal lamina, a rich source of extracellular molecules (Vaccarino et al., 1999a,b; Raballo et al., 2000; Götz and Huttner, 2005; Fietz et al., 2010). This highly dynamic and rich micro-environment provides a "stem cell niche" to the NECs during development (Lehtinen et al., 2011) that is crucial for the regulation of neurogenesis. NECs undergo interkinetic nuclear migration (INM), that is, they move their nuclei in the VZ in concert with the cell cycle: after completing mitosis at the ventricular surface, their nuclei undergo apical-to-basal migration during G1. After exiting from S-phase at the basal part of the VZ the nuclei undergo basal-to-apical migration, so that their successive mitosis will occur again at the ventricular surface (see Taverna and Huttner, 2010; Lee and Norden, 2013 and references therein). The NECs mitosis is confined to the ventricular surface, as the apical plasma membrane harbors the primary cilium that is nucleated by the centrosomes that also builds the mitotic spindle (see Taverna and Huttner, 2010; and references therein). NECs undergo proliferative divisions to expand the NEC pool. Ultimately, they develop into radial glial cells. Although it is not the main topics of this review article, it is important to mention that a proportion of NECs are embryonic neural stem cells from which adult neural stem cells originate (Furutachi et al., 2015). Using a strategy to follow the cell cycle progression of NECs, it has been shown that a subpopulation of NECs at early developmental stage gives rise to adult neural stem cells. This NECs subpopulation can be therefore considered as an embryonic neural stem cell (Furutachi et al., 2015). Embryonic neural stem cells slow down their cell-cycle speed allowing cells remain in a quiescence state. It still remains unclear how this embryonic neural stem cell population is determined during development and if adult neural stem cells can have also a radial glial origin.

Apical Radial Glial Cells

With the onset of neurogenesis, NECs differentiate into apical radial glial cells (aRGCs; Malatesta et al., 2003; Götz and Huttner, 2005). aRGCs are even more elongated than NECs. Their basolateral plasma membrane is divided in two sub-compartments: the apical and the basal process (**Figures 1**, **2**). The apical process is the portion of the basolateral plasma membrane residing in the VZ and it accommodates the nucleus during the different phases of INM. The basal process is the portion of the cell that traverses the sub-ventricular zone (SVZ) and the forming neuronal layers and reaches the basal lamina. Of note, as neurogenesis proceeds and neuronal layers are formed, the width of the cortical wall increases radially: therefore, the basal process elongates. The basal process functions as a guide for radial neuronal migration, allowing newborn excitatory cortical neurons to translocate from the place of birth to their final destination. In addition to providing a migratory scaffold for neurons in their journey to the cortical plate (CP), the basal process is a subcellular compartment involved in signaling and fate specification (Stenzel et al., 2014). Furthermore, live imaging has revealed that the basal process is a very dynamic entity, with the basal end changing from highly branched to club-like during cortical development (Yokota et al., 2010; **Figure 2**).

aRGCs have been extensively studied in the last decades and it is now clear that they contribute to neurogenesis mainly via the generation of a second type of neural progenitor cells: the BPs (Pontious et al., 2008; Kowalczyk et al., 2009). Interestingly, one of the main difference between apical and BPs is the absence of apical polarity cues in the latter.

Short Neural Precursors

Short neural precursors (SNPs, also known as apical intermediate progenitors) were first described in the mouse developing neocortex, where they exhibit several features in common with aRGCs, such as the bipolar morphology and the integration into the AJ belt (Gal et al., 2006; Tyler and Haydar, 2013). Unlike aRGCs, SNPs feature a basal process that does not traverse the neuronal layer, but it is confined to the VZ (**Figure 1**). A potentially similar cell type was reported to be present in the mouse ventral telencephalon, where aRGCs

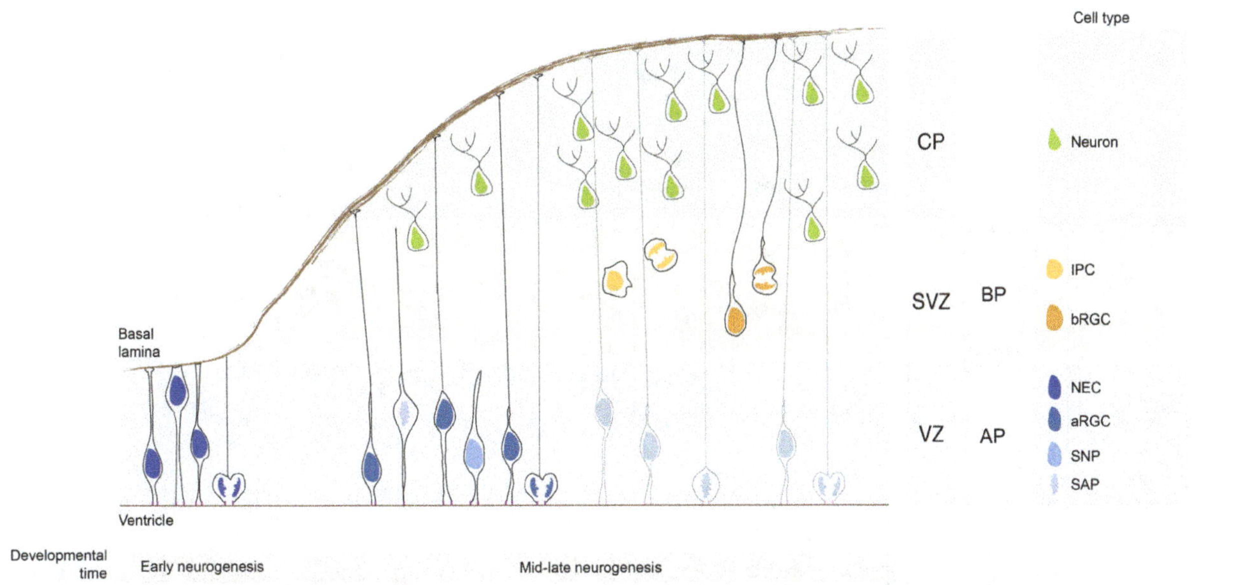

FIGURE 1 | Neural stem and progenitor cell types in the developing neocortex. During early neurogenesis, neuroepithelial cells (NECs) form the ventricular zone (VZ) and are responsible for the lateral expansion of the neocortex. During mid-late neurogenesis, apical progenitors (APs) divide and give rise to basal progenitors (BPs), which form a new proliferative zone, the subventricular zone (SVZ). The APs pool is mainly composed of apical radial glial cells (aRGCs) and a lower proportion of short neural precursors (SNPs) and sub-apical progenitors (SAPs). The BPs pool is composed by intermediate progenitor cells (IPCs) and basal radial glial cells (bRGCs). APs and BPs give rise to neurons that migrate basally and settle in the forming cortical plate (CP). The relative proportion of the different neural stem and progenitor cells changes greatly in species with different encephalyzation and gyrification. APs and BPs generate in a tightly controlled temporal order the pyramidal neurons populating the 6-layered neocortex (not depicted here for simplicity).

give rise to interneurons (Tan et al., 2016). As development proceed, the aRGCs in the ventral telencephalon grow radial glial fibers that no longer reach the basal lamina, but rather contact periventricular vessels (Tan et al., 2016). The vessel-anchored aRGCs undergo INM, divide apically (as SNPs do) and maintain the radial fiber throughout mitosis (unlike SNPs). Furthermore, a recent paper (Nowakowski et al., 2016) shows that in the human developing neocortex, during the mid-neurogenesis stage, aRGCs transform into "truncated" aRGCs, with a basal process that no longer reaches the basal lamina, but terminates in the depth of the cortical wall. Several interesting questions remain: are SNPs, vessel-anchored aRGCs in the mouse ventral telencephalon and truncated aRGCs in human related? Is the lack of basal attachment affecting the radial migration of the daughter cell after division? Is the daughter cell migrating for shorter distances?

Subapical Progenitors

Subapical progenitors (SAPs) were identified in the mouse ventral telencephalon and in the dorsal telencephalon of gyrencephalic species (Pilz et al., 2013). SAPs are anchored to the ventricle with an apical process. However, they undergo mitosis at a subapical location (Pilz et al., 2013; **Figure 1**). Most likely, in SAPs the centrosome is not docked at the apical plasma membrane and is therefore free to move basally to nucleate the mitotic spindle, as opposed to what happens in NECs where the centrosome is restricted to the apical side (see above).

Basal Progenitors

The term BPs indicates cells which undergo mitosis in the SVZ, the secondary germinal zone located basally compared to the VZ (**Figure 1**). BPs are generated by divisions of aRGCs and move basally via a process known as delamination. BPs are further divided into two classes: the intermediate progenitors (IPCs) and the basal radial glial cells (bRGCs).

Intermediate Progenitor Cells

IPCs represent the main class of BPs in rodents, as originally described independently by three different groups (Haubensak et al., 2004; Noctor et al., 2004; Miyata et al., 2004). IPCs are non-polar cells, as they lack both apical and basal polarity cues (**Figure 1**). The process of delamination of an IPC from the apical junctional belt very much resembles an epithelial-to-mesenchimal transition (EMT; Wilsch-Bräuninger et al., 2016), in which an epithelial cell gives rise to an unpolarized, highly motile cell (reviewed in Acloque et al., 2009; Itoh et al., 2013b). EMT is a process by which a polarized epithelial cell transforms into an unpolarized and highly motile mesenchymal cell. EMT occurs extensively during embryogenesis and it is crucial for gastrulation and neural crest formation. In pathological conditions, EMT is associated with in the initiation of metastasis and with cancer progression (Acloque et al., 2009; Itoh et al., 2013b; Wilsch-Bräuninger et al., 2016).

Basal Radial Glial Cells

Basal radial glial cells were first described in the developing neocortex of gyrencephalic species, namely in humans and

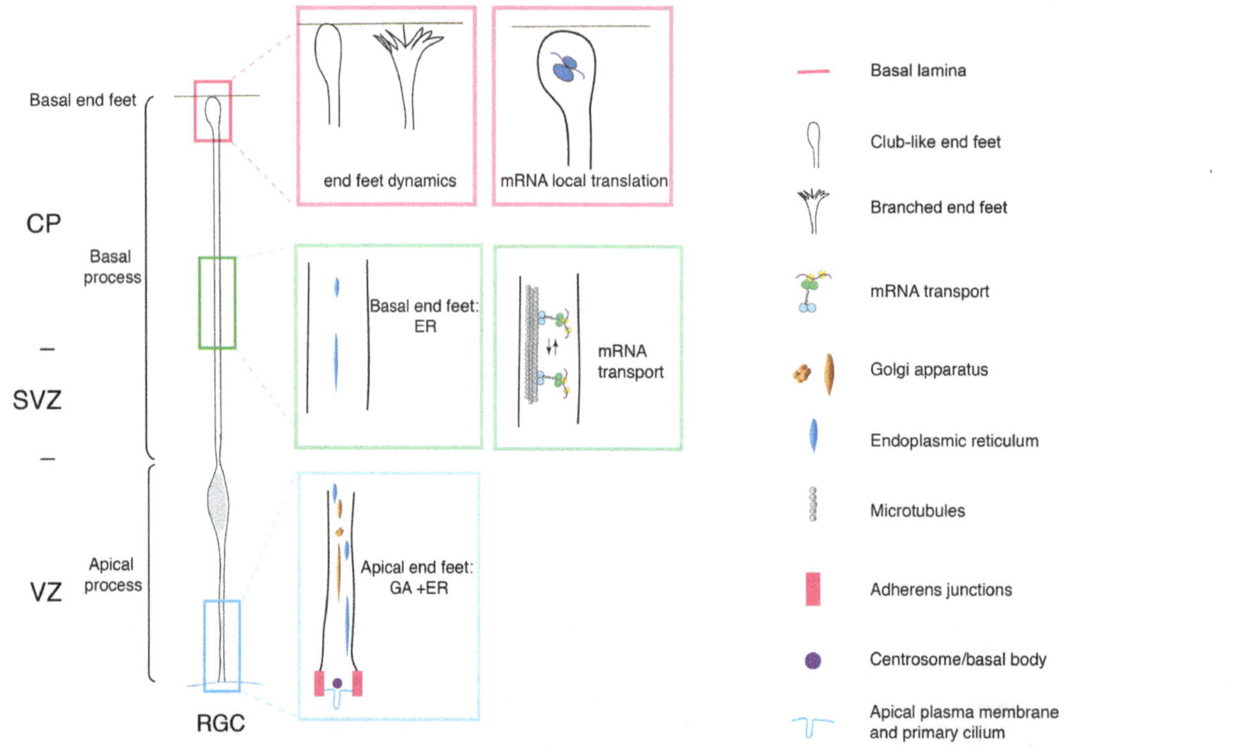

FIGURE 2 | Cell polarity and subcellular dynamics in apical radial glial cells. Apical radial glial cells (aRGCs) are highly polarized along their apico-basal axis. The adherens junctions maintain aRGC architecture and tissue integrity at the apical end feet. The basal process contacts the basal lamina with the basal end foot, where several mRNAs are transported and locally translated. The morphology of the basal end feet changes dynamically during neurogenesis. An organelle such as Golgi apparatus (GA) is distributed in the apical process exclusively. On the other hand, the endoplasmic reticulum (ER) is distributed globally in basal and apical processes. aRGC, apical radial glial cell; CP, cortical plate; SVZ, sub-ventricular zone and VZ, ventricular zone (the drawing is adapted from Taverna et al., 2016, licensed under a Creative Commons Attribution 4.0 International License).

ferrets, and were subsequently found, albeit at a much lower abundance, also in the lissencephalic developing rodent brain (Fietz et al., 2010; Hansen et al., 2010; Reillo et al., 2011; Wang et al., 2011; Reillo and Borrell, 2012; Sauerland et al., 2016). From an evolutionary perspective, the pool of bRGCs greatly expanded in humans and other gyrencephalic species, leading to the generation of two separate basal germinal zones: the inner and outer sub VZ (ISVZ and OSVZ, respectively; Smart et al., 2002). Recently, bRGCs have attracted great interest, as their abundance seems to correlate with the extent of brain expansion across species and with gyrification (Reillo et al., 2011; Kelava and Huttner, 2013). Several lines of evidence, including wide occurrence of bRGs in the marsupials and wallaby, suggest that bRGs might have been present in the ancestor of all mammals (Kelava et al., 2012; Sauerland et al., 2016). From a cell biological point of view, bRGCs are monopolar cells lacking an apical attachment (**Figure 1**). Interestingly, bRGCs still maintain an attachment to the basal lamina via a basal process (Hansen et al., 2010; Florio et al., 2015; Nowakowski et al., 2016). Functional manipulation has shown that the basal process is crucial for the maintenance of the proliferative capacity of bRGCs (Fietz et al., 2010). bRGCs appear to be a rather heterogeneous cell population, as shown by high resolution live imaging of the developing macaque neocortex (Betizeau et al., 2013). The heterogeneity was found to be both morphological and transcriptional. In particular, macaque bRGCs differ in term of presence vs. absence of apical-directed and basal-directed processes (Betizeau et al., 2013).

In summary, APs and BPs show striking differences in cell polarity. Evidences are accumulating that polarity influences the behavior of neural stem and progenitor cells during brain development.

MOLECULAR MECHANISMS OF NEURAL PROGENITOR CELL POLARITY

Key players of the maintenance of aRGCs polarity were found to be localized at the apical and basal end foot. The apical end foot of aRGCs is composed of the apical plasma membrane and the AJ belt (**Figure 2**). The apical plasma membrane represents a minor fraction of the total plasma membrane (1%–2%) and features the primary cilium that protrudes in the lumen of the ventricle and receives signals generated therein. The apical plasma membrane is delimited by the AJ, a subcellular structure that plays a crucial role in maintaining aRGCs architecture and function at the apical pole. At the cellular level, the AJ separates the apical and basolateral plasma membrane, while at the tissue level it maintains the integration of aRGCs in the neuroepithelium, securing tissue integrity. Consistent with this notion, perturbation of AJ components and polarity proteins localized at the apical end foot results in severe changes in APs morphology and function (Chenn and Walsh, 2002, 2003; Cappello et al., 2006, 2012; Katayama et al., 2011; Durak et al., 2016).

Among the polarity proteins regulating aRGCs function, Cdc42 represents a very interesting case, as it regulates the structure and function of aRGCs both at the apical and the basal pole. Indeed, the loss of function of Cdc42 results in the gradual loss of AJs and retraction of the apical processes, ultimately leading to an increase in the generation of IPCs and in turn premature neuronal differentiation (Cappello et al., 2006). Interestingly, the manipulation of Arp2/3 complex, a downstream effector of Cdc42, shows a phenotype similar to the Cdc42 mutant mouse, with altered aRGCs polarity, defective adhesion and an increased number of IPCs. Arp2/3 is an actin nucleator producing branched actin networks, suggesting a possible involvement of the actin cytoskeleton in maintaining aRGCs polarity. The actin cytoskeleton was found to be involved in the G1 apical-to-basal phase of INM in aRGCs and the pharmacological inhibition of actin contractility led to an increase in basal mitoses in the developing mouse neocortex (Schenk et al., 2009), suggesting a role for actin in maintaining a progenitor pool. The actin cytoskeleton is also crucial for vesicle trafficking, exocytosis and endocytosis. The formation of AJs requires the transport of cadherins and apical polarity proteins from trans-Golgi networks to the plasma membrane (Sheen et al., 2004). Furthermore, endocytosis may allow for the recycling of cadherins and the dynamic remodeling of the AJs in response to a change in aRGCs activity and function.

Cdc42 was found to be localized at the aRGCs basal pole, where it regulates the dynamics of the basal end feet (Yokota et al., 2010). As revealed by live imaging experiments, the basal end foot is a very dynamic structure, with small protrusions emanating from the basal process shaft, possibly engaging in cell-to-cell communication between aRGCs. The expression of the Cdc42 dominant negative results in morphological changes in the basal end feet, with a concomitant reduction in inter-radial glia interaction (Yokota et al., 2010). Of note, and consistent with the fact that Arp2/3 is a downstream effector of Cdc42, Arp2/3 was found to have an effect on the dynamics of the basal process. Upon conditional ablation of the Arp2/3 complex in aRGCs, the dynamics of basal process extension is altered and this ultimately results in an overall change in organization, orientation and length of the basal process (Wang et al., 2016).

CELL POLARITY AND SUBCELLULAR DYNAMICS

The extreme elongation of aRGCs and the division of the basolateral plasma membrane in apical and basal process pose very interesting questions. Is the subcellular organization different between the apical and the basal process? How do intracellular organelles, in particular the biosynthetic pathway, help build the apical and basal process? Using a panel of morphological approaches, it was recently shown that in aRGCs the Golgi apparatus (GA) is strongly polarized along the cell's apico-basal axis, and is confined to the apical process (Taverna et al., 2016; **Figure 2**). In contrast, the endoplasmic reticulum (ER) was found to be present in both the apical and the basal process. The confinement of the GA to the apical process of aRGCs impacts on the composition of the apical and basal process plasma membrane: the basal process plasma membrane was found to contain almost exclusively ER-derived glycans, whereas the apical process contains both ER- and Golgi-derived glycans. These observations prompted the authors to propose that the biosynthesis of the apical and basal process could rely on two different mechanisms: the delivery to the apical process plasma membrane is thought to largely occur via the canonical biosynthetic route (ER → GA–plasma membrane), whereas the delivery to the basal process plasma membrane has been proposed to occur via an unconventional route that bypasses the GA (ER → plasma membrane; Taverna et al., 2016; **Figure 2**).

What underlies the confinement of Golgi-derived glycans to the apical process? In neurons, the axon initial segment confines proteins and lipids to the axonal plasma membrane, thus contributing to maintain the identity of the axo-dendritic compartments (Rasband, 2010). One can speculate that a similar macromolecular complex could be involved in creating a boundary between the apical and the basal process, creating a diffusion barrier for membrane-bound and cytoplasmic molecules.

The enrichment of ER-derived glycans in the basal process plasma membrane may provide a specific environment for neuronal migration. Several questions remain to be answered. Do the particular glycans present in the membrane of the aRGCs have an influence on the behavior of the IPCs? Are ER-derived glycans influencing the migratory kinetics of neurons in their long journey along the basal process? Do early-born neurons, generated from less elongated aRGCs through IPCs, containing less ER-derived glycans than late-born neurons, generated from more elongated aRGCs? What is the glycan composition of the bRGC basal process?

Another important question is if any other organelle is asymmetrically distributed between apical and basal process. Interestingly, recent data has shown that mitochondria undergo extensive morphological changes in the developing neural tube of chick and mouse embryos. This study showed that mitochondria are thick and short in interphase APs, while they are thin and strongly connected in networks in neuronal cells (Mils et al., 2015).

Not only intracellular organelles but also *mRNAs* are distributed in a highly-polarized fashion along the apico-basal axis in aRGCs, a finding that opens an exciting avenue in the field of neural stem cell biology. In particular, it was first demonstrated that the *CyclinD2 mRNA* is highly enriched at the basal end foot (Tsunekawa et al., 2012), where it is locally translated into protein (Pilaz et al., 2016; **Figure 2**). This finding reveals that local translation can take place far away from the VZ, the germinal zone where the cell body and nucleus resides, even for proteins exerting their action in the nucleus, as is the case for CyclinD2. Possibly, the local translation of *CyclinD2* serves as a mechanism to strictly confine in space and time the function of CyclinD2 itself. Recently, FMRP were identified as the molecular motor responsible for *mRNA* transport to and localization at the basal end foot (Pilaz et al., 2016; Pilaz and Silver, 2017; **Figure 2**). The authors conducted an elegant and thorough characterization of the *mRNAs* localized at the basal end foot and showed that transcripts are locally translated (Pilaz et al., 2016). The local translation is somehow reminiscent of the local translation of *mRNA* in dendrites and axons (Bramham and Wells, 2007; Lin and Holt, 2008). In the case of neurons, transcripts can be translated on demand and in an activity-dependent manner. To push the parallel further, it would be extremely interesting to understand to which extent the transport and local translation of *mRNA* in the aRGCs basal end foot is regulated in a spatiotemporal manner by cell-to-cell interaction, either between neighbors aRGCs, or between aRGCs and the surrounding basal niche formed by meninges, basal lamina and Cajal-Retzius cells.

CELL BIOLOGICAL MECHANISMS OF APs TO BPs TRANSITION

Research in the last decade has focused on the fine cell biological mechanisms underlying APs-to-BPs fate transition and delamination (Acloque et al., 2009; Itoh et al., 2013b; Wilsch-Bräuninger et al., 2016), a process that very much resembles an epithelial-to-mesenchymal transition. Consistent with that parallel, the AJ components cadherins and catenins were found to have a role in the delamination of post-mitotic cell from aRGC and in the generation of bRGCs (Kadowaki et al., 2007; Stocker and Chenn, 2009, 2015; Itoh et al., 2013a; Martínez-Martínez et al., 2016). Conditional or focal reduction of N-Cadherin and αE-catenin, respectively, resulted in severe disruption in NECs structure and in turn affect cortical lamination (Kadowaki et al., 2007; Stocker and Chenn, 2009, 2015). Furthermore, a functional link between AJ complex and Wnt/β-catenin pro-proliferative signaling was observed in cortical progenitor cells (Hirabayashi et al., 2004; Stocker and Chenn, 2009).

One of the first detectable differences during fate transition and BP delamination is the change in the location of ciliogenesis. Cilia in APs are localized apically and they protrude in the ventricle from the apical plasma membrane, where they are tethered via the basal body (**Figure 2**). Elegant electron microscopy studies showed that in nascent BPs the cilium/basal body is located abventricularly, above the AJ belt (Wilsch-Bräuninger et al., 2012). The change in location of the cilium could favor cellular delamination either by favoring the "extrusion" of the apical plasma membrane from the AJ belt, or by increasing the endocytosis of the apical membrane components (though the two explanations are not mutually exclusive; Wilsch-Bräuninger et al., 2016). From a functional point of view, the relocation of the cilium could remove nascent BPs from the exposure to certain signals originating in the ventricle in favor of a signal originating in the VZ proper. An obvious question is if any other organelle undergoes reorganization upon fate transition. A good candidate in that respect is the GA, owing to the tight physical and functional link between the GA and the centrosome. Indeed, the GA in the aRGC's apical process was found to be neither perinuclear nor pericentrosomal. Interestingly, the GA was shown to become pericentrosomal in BPs upon delamination (Taverna et al., 2016). This data suggests that upon fate transition, the lack of polarity cues induces a reorganization at the centrosome-Golgi interface.

Another organelle involved in AP-to-BP fate transition is the ER. Recent findings show a role of the ER stress and unfolded protein response (UPR) in fate transition and neurogenesis (Laguesse et al., 2015). The authors focus on Elp3, a Elongator complex protein expressed in APs, where it maintains translational fidelity through the regulation of tRNA modification. Disruption of Elp3 decreases the speed of translation, promoting ER stress response and UPR upregulation. The knockout of Elp3 shows a progressive downregulation of UPR in APs and an amplification of IPCs leading to microcephaly (Laguesse et al., 2015). In a recent report, the authors also showed a role of Elp3 in the regulation of acetylation and membrane distribution of connexin-43 (Cx-43, Gja1; Laguesse et al., 2015). Cx-43 is a gap junction component expressed in APs where it plays a crucial role in cell-to-cell communication, INM and radial migration of neurons (Pearson et al., 2004; Sutor and Hagerty, 2005; Elias et al., 2007; Liu et al., 2010).

CELL POLARITY AND CELL FATE SPECIFICATION: RELEVANCE OF POLARITY FOR NEURAL STEM CELL FUNCTION

Cell polarity has important implications for neural stem cell fate for two main reasons: (i) the polarized organization allows progenitors to differentially respond to signals from the ventricle and/or from the basal pole; and (ii) the apical-basal polarity of aRGCs is the structural basis for their symmetric vs. asymmetric division, as defined by an equal vs. unequal distribution of cellular components to the daughter cells. Polarity is therefore instrumental in generating neural stem cell diversity.

Polarity and Differential Responses to Apical and Basal Niches

The organization of aRGCs along their apico-basal axis somehow mirrors the histological organization of the cortical wall. In that context, the basal and apical extensions of aRGCs could allow the aRGCs to sense, integrate and respond to different signals generated in different niches, either at the apical or at the basal pole. The apical plasma membrane delimits the ventricle, which is filled with cerebrospinal fluid, and contains different signaling molecules including morphogens (Lehtinen et al., 2011, 2013).

At the basal pole, the basal end feet are physically in contact with meninges, extracellular matrix and Cajal-Retzius cells which are sources for morphogens promoting proliferation and/or differentiation (Siegenthaler et al., 2009; Griveau et al., 2010). The basal end foot is therefore in a privileged position to sense and respond to basal extracellular signals. These signals could regulate local biological processes such as *mRNA* translation (Tsunekawa et al., 2012; Pilaz et al., 2016). It is interesting to note that due to their cellular organization, different neural stem cell subtypes have different level of access to signaling niches localized along the apico-basal axis of the cell and of the tissue. Since during development and evolution there is a progressive shift from apical to basal mitosis, it is tempting to speculate that this shift also represents a shift in signaling, with stem cells being regulated by basal and apical polarity cues during early development, and then being regulated mainly by basal polarity cues (Stenzel et al., 2014). This could also represent a way to restrict the expansion of the ventricular surface and favor the expansion of the basal part of the developing neocortex.

Polarity and Cell Division

The cell polarity of APs is the structural basis for symmetric vs. asymmetric division as it allows the equal vs. unequal distribution of cellular components to the daughter cells (Huttner and Kosodo, 2005). Several findings support the idea that the apical pole and subcellular structure therein are asymmetrically partitioned and influence cell fate. The apical plasma membrane constitutes a minor proportion of the total plasma membrane and can be either bisected or bypassed by the cleavage plane, resulting in only one daughter cell inheriting a portion of the apical plasma membrane (Kosodo et al., 2004). The cell inheriting the apical plasma membrane was reported to maintain proliferative potential (Kosodo et al., 2004). Not all the apical plasma membrane is partitioned based on the cleavage plane orientation: it was shown that the ciliary membrane, a specialized domain of the apical plasma membrane, is endocytosed at the onset of mitosis (Paridaen et al., 2013). The ciliary membrane preferentially associates with the mother centriole, is conserved throughout mitosis in association with one spindle pole and is asymmetrically inherited by one of the two daughter cells (Paridaen et al., 2013). The cell inheriting the ciliary membrane re-establishes the cilium faster and tend to maintain stem cell-like characteristics. These findings strongly suggest a role for the apical pole and subcellular structures therein in maintaining and influencing the choice between proliferation and differentiation.

It has also been shown that the basal process can be asymmetrically inherited by one of the two daughter cells, with the cell inheriting the basal process tending to maintain proliferative capacities (Konno et al., 2008; Shitamukai et al., 2011). How is the inheritance of the basal process linked to the choice between proliferation and differentiation? The inherited basal process could maintain aRGCs in a proliferative state thanks to the inheritance of the basal process-localized *mRNAs* and/or receptors for growth factors. Furthermore, data showed that both aRGCs and bRGCs are able to re-grow their basal process (Hansen et al., 2010; Shitamukai and Matsuzaki, 2012; Betizeau et al., 2013; Subramanian et al., 2017). What are the differences between an inherited vs. a regrown basal process? Is the re-growth of the basal process a mechanism to bypass the limitation imposed by the asymmetric inheritance of the basal process, so that both daughter cells are equally able to respond to extracellular signals? Is the re-grown basal process featuring different receptors compared to the inherited basal process? One might speculate that the newly delivered receptors in a re-grown basal process features different post-translational modifications and/or has a different desensitization status, allowing the two daughter cells to respond differentially to the same extracellular stimuli. Further research will be required to obtain a coherent picture on the interplay between polarity, asymmetric division and cell fate specification. It would also be extremely interesting to extend the pioneering work performed on aRGCs to other polarized progenitor cells, such as bRGCs, in order to understand to which extent similar cell biological principles are used in different cell types and how they act in generating neural stem cell diversity.

IMPAIRED CELL POLARITY AS A CAUSE OF NEURODEVELOPMENTAL DISORDERS

Neurodevelopmental defects comprise a substantial proportion of neuropsychiatric diseases and the general consensus is that they originate from early events in brain development (Feng et al., 2000; Bond et al., 2002; Chenn and Walsh, 2002; Tsai et al., 2005; Shu et al., 2006; Xie et al., 2007; Singh et al., 2010; Birnbaum et al., 2014). We here focus on neurodevelopmental disorders that are reported to be associated with polarity defects in neural stem and progenitor cells (Chenn and Walsh, 2003; Hirabayashi et al., 2004; Sheen et al., 2004; Mao et al., 2009; Katayama et al., 2011; Durak et al., 2015, 2016).

Down Syndrome

Down syndrome is the most common genetic cause of mental retardation. Patients diagnosed with Down syndrome showed an overall reduction of cerebrum gray matter volume (Weitzdoerfer et al., 2002) as well as a disorganized cortical lamination (Pinter et al., 2001). The reduction of Arp2/3 complex was reported in fetal Down syndrome brain and the conditional ablation of Arp2/3 complex in mice showed a reduction in neuronal number and highly disorganized cortical lamination (Wang et al., 2016). It would be important to understand to which extent the effects of Arp2/3 on the overall brain functions are due to the early effects of Arp2/3 on neural stem and progenitor cells, in particular on aRGCs (Tyler and Haydar, 2013).

Fragile X Syndrome and Autism Spectrum Disorders

Fragile-X syndrome (FXS) is the most common form of inherited intellectual disability and it is caused by mutations in *Fragile X Mental Retardation 1* (*FMR1*) gene. Loss-of-functions of FMR protein (FMRP) showed: (i) a switch from AP to BP fate, indicating the depletion of aRGCs pool (Saffary and Xie, 2011); (ii) defects in neuronal positioning due to the misregulation of

N-cadherin levels (La Fata et al., 2014); and (iii) early postnatal circuitry impairments possibly linked to abnormalities in the projection fibers (La Fata et al., 2014). Of interest, *FMR1* is also the most common single genetic cause of autism spectrum disorders (ASD; Hagerman et al., 2011; Bagni et al., 2012). In line with that, clinical crosstalk has been reported between FXS and ASD (Hagerman et al., 2011; Bagni et al., 2012). Considering the involvement of FMRP in *mRNA* transport in aRGCs (Pilaz et al., 2016; Pilaz and Silver, 2017), it would be interesting to understand if and how impaired *mRNA* transport in aRGCs contribute to the etiology of FXS and ASD (for an extensive discussion on the link between FXS, ASD, neural progenitors and cortical neurogenesis refer to Callan and Zarnescu, 2011; Packer, 2016; Marchetto et al., 2017 and references therein).

Ciliopathies

Ciliopathies are genetic disorders of ciliary structure or function. Joubert syndrome (JS) and related disorders are ciliopathies clinically characterized by ataxia, psychomotor delay and cognitive impairment (Cantagrel et al., 2008). The classical form of JS is caused by mutations in *Arl13b*, a cilia-specific small GTPase. *Arl13b* mutations lead to an inverted apico-basal polarity of aRGCs and impair the ability of primary cilia to convey extracellular signals such as insulin-like growth factor (Igf; Higginbotham et al., 2013). Igf is highly enriched in the CSF. It would be interesting to understand if the relocation of the primary cilium from the apical to the basolateral plasma membrane upon APs to BPs fate transition (Wilsch-Bräuninger et al., 2012) changes the degree of exposure to extracellular signals generated from the CSF.

Schizophrenia

Schizophrenia shares several common characteristics with ASD in term of behavioral, social and cognitive disturbances and also in term of genes implicated in the disease etiology (Carroll and Owen, 2009). *Disrupted In Schizophrenia* (*DISC1*) is a common susceptibility gene for those disorders and it is also associated with bipolar and mood disorders (Khanzada et al., 2017). Mutations in DISC1 gene lead to schizophrenic or depressive behavior (Clapcote et al., 2007; Mao et al., 2009; Dachtler et al., 2016). DISC1 is highly expressed in aRGCs during development and a knock-down of DISC1 showed a decreased proliferation of aRGCs and premature neurogenesis (Mao et al., 2009; De Rienzo et al., 2011; Ishizuka et al., 2011; Ye et al., 2017). The neuronal phenotypes observed are reminiscent of Cdc42 loss-of-functions (Yokota et al., 2010; Ishizuka et al., 2011). Consistent with that, DISC1 regulates aRGC proliferation through GSK3β, a downstream effector of Cdc42 (Clapcote et al., 2007; Ishizuka et al., 2011; Dachtler et al., 2016).

Taken together, these data suggest that alteration of aRGCs polarity can trigger neurodevelopmental and psychiatric disorders.

CONCLUDING REMARKS

In this review article, we discussed the polarity features of neural stem and progenitor cells in the developing cerebral cortex and their functional implications. Research in the last decades clearly showed that polarity affects neural stem and progenitor cells, including their architecture and shape, INM, proliferation vs. differentiation potential and asymmetric cell division. Nowadays concepts derived from work in mice are finally applied in an evolutionary perspective: one notable example is provided by aRGCs in humans, where their extreme elongation matches the massive growth of the cerebral cortex. In the future, it is likely that the functions of the basal process will receive increasing attention, both in aRGCs and bRGCs. Here are few questions that in our opinion deserve attention: which are the differences between a aRGC and a bRGC basal process? How is the growth of the basal process in a single RGC coordinated with the global tissue growth? Which is the role of intracellular traffic in the basal process elongation? How are the biological functions of the basal process (e.g., mRNA translation) affected by extracellular stimuli, and how are they coordinated with the rest of the cell? We are now witnessing a very exciting time, when thanks to several technological breakthroughs we can reasonably expect that several of these questions will be answered, leading to a better understanding of cerebral cortex development and evolution.

AUTHOR CONTRIBUTIONS

ET and YA wrote the manuscript.

ACKNOWLEDGMENTS

We thank Veronique Dubreuil, Nicola Maghelli, Jeanette Nardelli, Judith Paridaean and Jeremy Pulvers for their helpful comments and input on the manuscript.

REFERENCES

Acloque, H., Adams, M. S., Fishwick, K., Bronner-Fraser, M., and Nieto, M. A. (2009). Epithelial-mesenchymal transitions: the importance of changing cell state in development and disease. *J. Clin. Invest.* 119, 1438–1449. doi: 10.1172/jci38019

Arai, Y., and Pierani, A. (2014). Development and evolution of cortical fields. *Neurosci. Res.* 86, 66–76. doi: 10.1016/j.neures.2014.06.005

Bagni, C., Tassone, F., Neri, G., and Hagerman, R. (2012). Fragile X syndrome: causes, diagnosis, mechanisms, and therapeutics. *J. Clin. Invest.* 122, 4314–4322. doi: 10.1172/jci63141

Betizeau, M., Cortay, V., Patti, D., Pfister, S., Gautier, E., Bellemin-Ménard, A., et al. (2013). Precursor diversity and complexity of lineage relationships in the outer subventricular zone (OSVZ) of the primate. *Neuron* 80, 442–457. doi: 10.1016/j.neuron.2013.09.032

Birnbaum, R., Jaffe, A. E., Hyde, T. M., Kleinman, J. E., and Weinberger, D. R. (2014). Prenatal expression patterns of genes associated with neuropsychiatric disorders. *Am. J. Psychiatry* 171, 758–767. doi: 10.1176/appi.ajp.2014.13111452

Bond, J., Roberts, E., Mochida, G. H., Hampshire, D. J., Scott, S., Askham, J. M., et al. (2002). ASPM is a major determinant of cerebral cortical size. *Nat. Genet.* 32, 316–3120. doi: 10.1038/ng995

Bramham, C. R., and Wells, D. G. (2007). Dendritic mRNA: transport, translation and function. *Nat. Rev. Neurosci.* 8, 776–789. doi: 10.1038/nrn2150

Callan, M. A., and Zarnescu, D. C. (2011). Heads-up: new roles for the fragile X mental retardation protein in neural stem and progenitor cells. *Genesis* 49, 424–440. doi: 10.1002/dvg.20745

Cantagrel, V., Silhavy, J. L., Bielas, S. L., Swistun, D., Marsh, S. E., Marsh, S. E., et al. (2008). Mutations in the cilia gene ARL13B lead to the classical form of Joubert syndrome. *Am. J. Hum. Genet.* 83, 170–179. doi: 10.1016/j.ajhg.2008.06.023

Cappello, S., Attardo, A., Wu, X., Iwasato, T., Itohara, S., Wilsch-Bräuninger, M., et al. (2006). The Rho-GTPase cdc42 regulates neural progenitor fate at the apical surface. *Nat. Neurosci.* 9, 1099–1107. doi: 10.1038/nn1744

Cappello, S., Böhringer, C. R., Bergami, M., Conzelmann, K. K., Ghanem, A., Tomassy, G. S., et al. (2012). A radial glia-specific role of RhoA in double cortex formation. *Neuron* 73, 911–924. doi: 10.1016/j.neuron.2011.12.030

Carroll, L. S., and Owen, M. J. (2009). Genetic overlap between autism, schizophrenia and bipolar disorder. *Genome Med.* 1:102. doi: 10.1186/gm102

Chenn, A., and Walsh, C. A. (2002). Regulation of cerebral cortical size by control of cell cycle exit in neural precursors. *Science* 297, 365–369. doi: 10.1126/science.1074192

Chenn, A., and Walsh, C. A. (2003). Increased neuronal production, enlarged forebrains and cytoarchitectural distortions in β-catenin overexpressing transgenic mice. *Cereb. Cortex* 13, 599–606. doi: 10.1093/cercor/13.6.599

Clapcote, S. J., Lipina, T. V., Millar, J. K., Mackie, S., Christie, S., Ogawa, F., et al. (2007). Behavioral phenotypes of Discl missense mutations in mice. *Neuron* 54, 387–402. doi: 10.1016/j.neuron.2007.04.015

Dachtler, J., Elliott, C., Rodgers, R. J., Baillie, G. S., and Clapcote, S. J. (2016). Missense mutation in DISC1 C-terminal coiled-coil has GSK3β signaling and sex-dependent behavioral effects in mice. *Sci. Rep.* 6:18748. doi: 10.1038/srep18748

De Rienzo, G., Bishop, J. A., Mao, Y., Pan, L., Ma, T. P., Moens, C. B., et al. (2011). Discl regulates both β-catenin-mediated and noncanonical Wnt signaling during vertebrate embryogenesis. *FASEB J.* 25, 4184–4197. doi: 10.1096/fj.11-186239

Durak, O., de Anda, F. C., Singh, K. K., Leussis, M. P., Petryshen, T. L., Sklar, P., et al. (2015). Ankyrin-G regulates neurogenesis and Wnt signaling by altering the subcellular localization of β-catenin. *Mol. Psychiatry* 20, 388–397. doi: 10.1038/mp.2014.42

Durak, O., Gao, F., Kaeser-Woo, Y. J., Rueda, R., Martorell, A. J., Nott, A., et al. (2016). Chd8 mediates cortical neurogenesis via transcriptional regulation of cell cycle and Wnt signaling. *Nat. Neurosci.* 19, 1477–1488. doi: 10.1038/nn.4400

Elias, L. A., Wang, D. D., and Kriegstein, A. R. (2007). Gap junction adhesion is necessary for radial migration in the neocortex. *Nature* 448, 901–907. doi: 10.1038/nature06063

Farquhar, M. G., and Palade, G. E. (1963). Junctional complexes in various epithelia. *J. Cell Biol.* 17, 375–412. doi: 10.1083/jcb.17.2.375

Feng, Y., Olson, E. C., Stukenberg, P. T., Flanagan, L. A., Kirschner, M. W., and Walsh, C. A. (2000). LIS1 regulates CNS lamination by interacting with mNudE, a central component of the centrosome. *Neuron* 28, 665–679. doi: 10.1016/s0896-6273(00)00145-8

Fietz, S. A., and Huttner, W. B. (2011). Cortical progenitor expansion, self-renewal and neurogenesis—a polarized perspective. *Curr. Opin. Neurobiol.* 21, 23–35. doi: 10.1016/j.conb.2010.10.002

Fietz, S. A., Kelava, I., Vogt, J., Wilsch-Bräuninger, M., Stenzel, D., Fish, J. L., et al. (2010). OSVZ progenitors of human and ferret neocortex are epithelial-like and expand by integrin signaling. *Nat. Neurosci.* 13, 690–699. doi: 10.1038/nn.2553

Florio, M., Albert, M., Taverna, E., Namba, T., Brandl, H., Lewitus, E., et al. (2015). Human-specific gene ARHGAP11B promotes basal progenitor amplification and neocortex expansion. *Science* 347, 1465–1470. doi: 10.1126/science.aaa1975

Franke, W. W. (2009). Discovering the molecular components of intercellular junctions—a historical view. *Cold Spring Harb. Perspect. Biol.* 1:a003061. doi: 10.1101/cshperspect.a003061

Furutachi, S., Miya, H., Watanabe, T., Kawai, H., Yamasaki, N., Harada, Y., et al. (2015). Slowly dividing neural progenitors are an embryonic origin of adult neural stem cells. *Nat. Neurosci.* 18, 657–665. doi: 10.1038/nn.3989

Gal, J. S., Morozov, Y. M., Ayoub, A. E., Chatterjee, M., Rakic, P., and Haydar, T. F. (2006). Molecular and morphological heterogeneity of neural precursors in the mouse neocortical proliferative zones. *J. Neurosci.* 26, 1045–1056. doi: 10.1523/jneurosci.4499-05.2006

Götz, M., and Huttner, W. B. (2005). The cell biology of neurogenesis. *Nat. Rev. Mol. Cell Biol.* 6, 777–788. doi: 10.1038/nrm1739

Griveau, A., Borello, U., Causeret, F., Tissir, F., Boggetto, N., Karaz, S., et al. (2010). A novel role for Dbx1-derived Cajal-Retzius cells in early regionalization of the cerebral cortical neuroepithelium. *PLoS Biol.* 8:e1000440. doi: 10.1371/journal.pbio.1000440

Hagerman, R., Au, J., and Hagerman, P. (2011). FMR1 premutation and full mutation molecular mechanisms related to autism. *J. Neurodev. Disord.* 3, 211–224. doi: 10.1007/s11689-011-9084-5

Hansen, D. V., Lui, J. H., Parker, P. R., and Kriegstein, A. R. (2010). Neurogenic radial glia in the outer subventricular zone of human neocortex. *Nature* 464, 554–561. doi: 10.1038/nature08845

Haubensak, W., Attardo, A., Denk, W., and Huttner, W. B. (2004). Neurons arise in the basal neuroepithelium of the early mammalian telencephalon: a major site of neurogenesis. *Proc. Natl. Acad. Sci. U S A* 101, 3196–3201. doi: 10.1073/pnas.0308600100

Higginbotham, H., Guo, J., Yokota, Y., Umberger, N. L., Su, C. Y., Li, J., et al. (2013). Arl13b-regulated cilia activities are essential for polarized radial glial scaffold formation. *Nat. Neurosci.* 16, 1000–1007. doi: 10.1038/nn.3451

Hirabayashi, Y., Itoh, Y., Tabata, H., Nakajima, K., Akiyama, T., Masuyama, N., et al. (2004). The Wnt/β-catenin pathway directs neuronal differentiation of cortical neural precursor cells. *Development* 131, 2791–2801. doi: 10.1242/dev.01165

Huttner, W. B., and Kosodo, Y. (2005). Symmetric versus asymmetric cell division during neurogenesis in the developing vertebrate central nervous system. *Curr. Opin. Cell Biol.* 17, 648–657. doi: 10.1016/j.ceb.2005.10.005

Ishizuka, K., Kamiya, A., Oh, E. C., Kanki, H., Seshadri, S., Robinson, J. F., et al. (2011). DISC1-dependent switch from progenitor proliferation to migration in the developing cortex. *Nature* 473, 92–96. doi: 10.1038/nature09859

Itoh, Y., Moriyama, Y., Hasegawa, T., Endo, T. A., Toyoda, T., and Gotoh, Y. (2013a). Scratch regulates neuronal migration onset via an epithelial-mesenchymal transition-like mechanism. *Nat. Neurosci.* 16, 416–425. doi: 10.1038/nn.3336

Itoh, Y., Tyssowski, K., and Gotoh, Y. (2013b). Transcriptional coupling of neuronal fate commitment and the onset of migration. *Curr. Opin. Neurobiol.* 23, 957–964. doi: 10.1016/j.conb.2013.08.003

Kadowaki, M., Nakamura, S., Machon, O., Krauss, S., Radice, G. L., and Takeichi, M. (2007). N-cadherin mediates cortical organization in the mouse brain. *Dev. Biol.* 304, 22–33. doi: 10.1016/j.ydbio.2006.12.014

Katayama, K., Melendez, J., Baumann, J. M., Leslie, J. R., Chauhan, B. K., Nemkul, N., et al. (2011). Loss of RhoA in neural progenitor cells causes the disruption of adherens junctions and hyperproliferation. *Proc. Natl. Acad. Sci. U S A* 108, 7607–7612. doi: 10.1073/pnas.1101347108

Kelava, I., and Huttner, W. B. (2013). "Neural progenitors and evolution of mammalian neocortex," in *Stem Cells*, eds F. Calegari and C. Waskow (Enfield, NH: Science Publishers, Edenbridge Ltd., CRC Press/Taylor and Francis Group).

Kelava, I., Reillo, I., Murayama, A. Y., Kalinka, A. T., Stenzel, D., Tomancak, P., et al. (2012). Abundant occurrence of basal radial glia in the subventricular zone of embryonic neocortex of a lissencephalic primate, the common marmoset *Callithrix jacchus*. *Cereb. Cortex* 22, 469–481. doi: 10.1093/cercor/bhr301

Khanzada, N. S., Butler, M. G., and Manzardo, A. M. (2017). GeneAnalytics pathway analysis and genetic overlap among autism spectrum disorder, bipolar disorder and schizophrenia. *Int. J. Mol. Sci.* 18:E527. doi: 10.3390/ijms18030527

Konno, D., Shioi, G., Shitamukai, A., Mori, A., Kiyonari, H., Miyata, T., et al. (2008). Neuroepithelial progenitors undergo LGN-dependent planar divisions to maintain self-renewability during mammalian neurogenesis. *Nat. Cell Biol.* 10, 93–101. doi: 10.1038/ncb1673

Kosodo, Y., Röper, K., Haubensak, W., Marzesco, A.-M., Corbeil, D., and Huttner, W. B. (2004). Asymmetric distribution of the apical plasma membrane during neurogenic divisions of mammalian neuroepithelial cells. *EMBO J.* 23, 2314–2324. doi: 10.1038/sj.emboj.7600223

Kowalczyk, T., Pontious, A., Englund, C., Daza, R. A., Bedogni, F., Hodge, R., et al. (2009). Intermediate neuronal progenitors (basal progenitors) produce pyramidal-projection neurons for all layers of cerebral cortex. *Cereb. Cortex* 19, 2439–2450. doi: 10.1093/cercor/bhn260

La Fata, G., Gärtner, A., Domínguez-Iturza, N., Dresselaers, T., Dawitz, J., Poorthuis, R. B., et al. (2014). FMRP regulates multipolar to bipolar transition affecting neuronal migration and cortical circuitry. *Nat. Neurosci.* 17, 1693–1700. doi: 10.1038/nn.3870

Laguesse, S., Creppe, C., Nedialkova, D. D., Prévot, P. P., Borgs, L., Huysseune, S., et al. (2015). A dynamic unfolded protein response contributes to the control of cortical neurogenesis. *Dev. Cell* 35, 553–567. doi: 10.1016/j.devcel.2015.11.005

Lee, H. O., and Norden, C. (2013). Mechanisms controlling arrangements and movements of nuclei in pseudostratified epithelia. *Trends Cell Biol.* 23, 141–150. doi: 10.1016/j.tcb.2012.11.001

Lehtinen, M. K., Bjornsson, C. S., Dymecki, S. M., Gilbertson, R. J., Holtzman, D. M., and Monuki, E. S. (2013). The choroid plexus and cerebrospinal fluid: emerging roles in development, disease, and therapy. *J. Neurosci.* 33, 17553–17559. doi: 10.1523/JNEUROSCI.3258-13.2013

Lehtinen, M. K., Zappaterra, M. W., Chen, X., Yang, Y. J., Hill, A. D., Lun, A. D., et al. (2011). The cerebrospinal fluid provides a proliferative niche for neural progenitor cells. *Neuron* 69, 893–905. doi: 10.1016/j.neuron.2011.01.023

Lin, A. C., and Holt, C. E. (2008). Function and regulation of local axonal translation. *Curr. Opin. Neurobiol.* 18, 60–68. doi: 10.1016/j.conb.2008.05.004

Liu, X., Hashimoto-Torii, K., Torii, M., Ding, C., and Rakic, P. (2010). Gap junctions/hemichannels modulate interkinetic nuclear migration in the forebrain precursors. *J. Neurosci.* 30, 4197–4209. doi: 10.1523/JNEUROSCI.4187-09.2010

Malatesta, P., Hack, M. A., Hartfuss, E., Kettenmann, H., Klinkert, W., Kirchhoff, F., et al. (2003). Neuronal or glial progeny: regional differences in radial glia fate. *Neuron* 37, 751–764. doi: 10.1016/S0896-6273(03)00116-8

Mao, Y., Ge, X., Frank, C. L., Madison, J. M., Koehler, A. N., Doud, M. K., et al. (2009). Disrupted in schizophrenia 1 regulates neuronal progenitor proliferation via modulation of GSK3β/β-catenin signaling. *Cell* 136, 1017–1031. doi: 10.1016/j.cell.2008.12.044

Marchetto, M. C., Belinson, H., Tian, Y., Freitas, B. C., Fu, C., Vadodaria, K., et al. (2017). Altered proliferation and networks in neural cells derived from idiopathic autistic individuals. *Mol. Psychiatry* 22, 820–835. doi: 10.1038/mp.2016.95

Martínez-Martínez, M. Á., De Juan Romero, C., Fernández, V., Cárdenas, A., Götz, M., and Borrell, V. (2016). A restricted period for formation of outer subventricular zone defined by Cdh1 and Trnp1 levels. *Nat. Commun.* 7:11812. doi: 10.1038/ncomms11812

Mils, V., Bosch, S., Roy, J., Bel-Vialar, S., Belenguer, P., Pituello, F., et al. (2015). Mitochondrial reshaping accompanies neural differentiation in the developing spinal cord. *PLoS One* 10:e0128130. doi: 10.1371/journal.pone.0128130

Miyata, T., Kawaguchi, A., Saito, K., Kawano, M., Muto, T., and Ogawa, M. (2004). Asymmetric production of surface-dividing and non-surface-dividing cortical progenitor cells. *Development* 131, 3133–3145. doi: 10.1242/dev.01173

Noctor, S. C., Martínez-Cerdeño, V., Ivic, L., and Kriegstein, A. R. (2004). Cortical neurons arise in symmetric and asymmetric division zones and migrate through specific phases. *Nat. Neurosci.* 7, 136–144. doi: 10.1038/nn1172

Nowakowski, T. J., Pollen, A. A., Sandoval-Espinosa, C., and Kriegstein, A. R. (2016). Transformation of the radial glia scaffold demarcates two stages of human cerebral cortex development. *Neuron* 91, 1219–1227. doi: 10.1016/j.neuron.2016.09.005

Packer, A. (2016). Neocortical neurogenesis and the etiology of autism spectrum disorder. *Neurosci. Biobehav. Rev.* 64, 185–195. doi: 10.1016/j.neubiorev.2016.03.002

Paridaen, J. T., Wilsch-Bräuninger, M., and Huttner, W. B. (2013). Asymmetric inheritance of centrosome-associated primary cilium membrane directs ciliogenesis after cell division. *Cell* 155, 333–344. doi: 10.1016/j.cell.2013.08.060

Pearson, R. A., Catsicas, M., Becker, D. L., Bayley, P., Lüneborg, N. L., and Mobbs, P. (2004). Ca^{2+} signalling and gap junction coupling within and between pigment epithelium and neural retina in the developing chick. *Eur. J. Neurosci.* 19, 2435–2445. doi: 10.1111/j.0953-816x.2004.03338.x

Pilaz, L. J., Lennox, A. L., Rouanet, J. P., and Silver, D. L. (2016). Dynamic mRNA transport and local translation in radial glial progenitors of the developing brain. *Curr. Biol.* 26, 3383–3392. doi: 10.1016/j.cub.2016.10.040

Pilaz, L. J., and Silver, D. L. (2017). Moving messages in the developing brain-emerging roles for mRNA transport and local translation in neural stem cells. *FEBS Lett.* 591, 1526–1539. doi: 10.1002/1873-3468.12626

Pilz, G. A., Shitamukai, A., Reillo, I., Pacary, E., Schwausch, J., Stahl, R., et al. (2013). Amplification of progenitors in the mammalian telencephalon includes a new radial glial cell type. *Nat. Commun.* 4:2125. doi: 10.1038/ncomms3125

Pinter, J. D., Eliez, S., Schmitt, J. E., Capone, G. T., and Reiss, A. L. (2001). Neuroanatomy of Down's syndrome: a high-resolution MRI study. *Am. J. Psychiatry* 158, 1659–1665. doi: 10.1176/appi.ajp.158.10.1659

Pontious, A., Kowalczyk, T., Englund, C., and Hevner, R. F. (2008). Role of intermediate progenitor cells in cerebral cortex development. *Dev. Neurosci.* 30, 24–32. doi: 10.1159/000109848

Raballo, R., Rhee, J., Lyn-Cook, R., Leckman, J. F., Schwartz, M. L., and Vaccarino, F. M. (2000). Basic fibroblast growth factor (Fgf2) is necessary for cell proliferation and neurogenesis in the developing cerebral cortex. *J. Neurosci.* 20, 5012–5023.

Rasband, M. N. (2010). The axon initial segment and the maintenance of neuronal polarity. *Nat. Rev. Neurosci.* 11, 552–562. doi: 10.1038/nrn2852

Reillo, I., and Borrell, V. (2012). Germinal zones in the developing cerebral cortex of ferret: ontogeny, cell cycle kinetics, and diversity of progenitors. *Cereb. Cortex* 22, 2039–2054. doi: 10.1093/cercor/bhr284

Reillo, I., de Juan Romero, C., García-Cabezas, M. Á., and Borrell, V. (2011). A role for intermediate radial glia in the tangential expansion of the mammalian cerebral cortex. *Cereb. Cortex* 21, 1674–1694. doi: 10.1093/cercor/bhq238

Saffary, R., and Xie, Z. (2011). FMRP regulates the transition from radial glial cells to intermediate progenitor cells during neocortical development. *J. Neurosci.* 31, 1427–1439. doi: 10.1523/JNEUROSCI.4854-10.2011

Sauerland, C., Menzies, B. R., Glatzle, M., Seeger, J., Renfree, M. B., and Fietz, S. A. (2016). The basal radial glia occurs in marsupials and underlies the evolution of an expanded neocortex in therian mammals. *Cereb. Cortex* doi: 10.1093/cercor/bhw360 [Epub ahead of print].

Schenk, J., Wilsch-Bräuninger, M., Calegari, F., and Huttner, W. B. (2009). Myosin II is required for interkinetic nuclear migration of neural progenitors. *Proc. Natl. Acad. Sci. U S A* 106, 16487–16492. doi: 10.1073/pnas.0908928106

Sheen, V. L., Ganesh, V. S., Topcu, M., Sebire, G., Bodell, A., Hill, R. S., et al. (2004). Mutations in ARFGEF2 implicate vesicle trafficking in neural progenitor proliferation and migration in the human cerebral cortex. *Nat. Genet.* 36, 69–76. doi: 10.1038/ng1276

Shitamukai, A., Konno, D., and Matsuzaki, F. (2011). Oblique radial glial divisions in the developing mouse neocortex induce self-renewing progenitors outside the germinal zone that resemble primate outer subventricular zone progenitors. *J. Neurosci.* 31, 3683–3695. doi: 10.1523/JNEUROSCI.4773-10.2011

Shitamukai, A., and Matsuzaki, F. (2012). Control of asymmetric cell division of mammalian neural progenitors. *Dev. Growth Differ.* 54, 277–286. doi: 10.1111/j.1440-169x.2012.01345.x

Shu, T., Tseng, H. C., Sapir, T., Stern, P., Zhou, Y., Sanada, K., et al. (2006). Doublecortin-like kinase controls neurogenesis by regulating mitotic spindles and M phase progression. *Neuron* 49, 25–39. doi: 10.1016/j.neuron.2005.10.039

Siegenthaler, J. A., Ashique, A. M., Zarbalis, K., Patterson, K. P., Hecht, J. H., Kane, M. A., et al. (2009). Retinoic acid from the meninges regulates cortical neuron generation. *Cell* 139, 597–609. doi: 10.1016/j.cell.2009.10.004

Singh, K. K., Ge, X., Mao, Y., Drane, L., Meletis, K., Samuels, B. A., et al. (2010). Dixdc1 is a critical regulator of DISC1 and embryonic cortical development. *Neuron* 67, 33–48. doi: 10.1016/j.neuron.2010.06.002

Smart, I. H., Dehay, C., Giroud, P., Berland, M., and Kennedy, H. (2002). Unique morphological features of the proliferative zones and postmitotic compartments of the neural epithelium giving rise to striate and extrastriate cortex in the monkey. *Cereb. Cortex* 12, 37–53. doi: 10.1093/cercor/12.1.37

Stenzel, D., Wilsch-Bräuninger, M., Wong, F. K., Heuer, H., and Huttner, W. B. (2014). Integrin αvβ3 and thyroid hormones promote expansion of progenitors in embryonic neocortex. *Development* 141, 795–806. doi: 10.1242/dev.101907

Stocker, A. M., and Chenn, A. (2009). Focal reduction of αE-catenin causes premature differentiation and reduction of β-catenin signaling during cortical development. *Dev. Biol.* 328, 66–77. doi: 10.1016/j.ydbio.2009.01.010

Stocker, A. M., and Chenn, A. (2015). The role of adherens junctions in the developing neocortex. *Cell Adh. Migr.* 9, 167–174. doi: 10.1080/19336918.2015.1027478

Subramanian, L., Bershteyn, M., Paredes, M. F., and Kriegstein, A. R. (2017). Dynamic behaviour of human neuroepithelial cells in the developing forebrain. *Nat. Commun.* 8:14167. doi: 10.1038/ncomms14167

Sutor, B., and Hagerty, T. (2005). Involvement of gap junctions in the development of the neocortex. *Biochim. Biophys. Acta* 1719, 59–68. doi: 10.1016/j.bbamem.2005.09.005

Takeichi, M. (1977). Functional correlation between cell adhesive properties and some cell surface proteins. *J. Cell Biol.* 75, 464–474. doi: 10.1083/jcb.75.2.464

Tan, X., Liu, W. A., Zhang, X. J., Shi, W., Ren, S. Q., Li, Z., et al. (2016). Vascular influence on ventral telencephalic progenitors and neocortical interneuron production. *Dev. Cell* 36, 624–638. doi: 10.1016/j.devcel.2016.02.023

Taverna, E., Götz, M., and Huttner, W. B. (2014). The cell biology of neurogenesis: toward an understanding of the development and evolution of the neocortex. *Annu. Rev. Cell Dev. Biol.* 30, 465–502. doi: 10.1146/annurev-cellbio-101011-155801

Taverna, E., and Huttner, W. B. (2010). Neural progenitor nuclei IN Motion. *Neuron* 67, 906–914. doi: 10.1016/j.neuron.2010.08.027

Taverna, E., Mora-Bermúdez, F., Strzyz, P. J., Florio, M., Icha, J., Haffner, C., et al. (2016). Non-canonical features of the Golgi apparatus in bipolar epithelial neural stem cells. *Sci. Rep.* 6:21206. doi: 10.1038/srep21206

Tsai, J. W., Chen, Y., Kriegstein, A. R., and Vallee, R. B. (2005). LIS1 RNA interference blocks neural stem cell division, morphogenesis, and motility at multiple stages. *J. Cell Biol.* 170, 935–945. doi: 10.1083/jcb.200505166

Tsunekawa, Y., Britto, J. M., Takahashi, M., Polleux, F., Tan, S. S., and Osumi, N. (2012). Cyclin D2 in the basal process of neural progenitors is linked to non-equivalent cell fates. *EMBO J.* 31, 1879–1892. doi: 10.1038/emboj.2012.43

Tyler, W. A., and Haydar, T. F. (2013). Multiplex genetic fate mapping reveals a novel route of neocortical neurogenesis, which is altered in the Ts65Dn mouse model of Down syndrome. *J. Neurosci.* 33, 5106–5119. doi: 10.1523/JNEUROSCI.5380-12.2013

Vaccarino, F. M., Schwartz, M. L., Raballo, R., Nilsen, J., Rhee, J., Zhou, M., et al. (1999a). Changes in cerebral cortex size are governed by fibroblast growth factor during embryogenesis. *Nat. Neurosci.* 2, 246–253. doi: 10.1038/6350

Vaccarino, F. M., Schwartz, M. L., Raballo, R., Rhee, J., and Lyn-Cook, R. (1999b). Fibroblast growth factor signaling regulates growth and morphogenesis at multiple steps during brain development. *Curr. Top Dev. Biol.* 46, 179–200. doi: 10.1016/s0070-2153(08)60329-4

Wang, P. S., Chou, F. S., Ramachandran, S., Xia, S., Chen, H. Y., Guo, F., et al. (2016). Crucial roles of the Arp2/3 complex during mammalian corticogenesis. *Development* 143, 2741–2752. doi: 10.1242/dev.130542

Wang, X., Tsai, J. W., Lamonica, B., and Kriegstein, A. R. (2011). A new subtype of progenitor cell in the mouse embryonic neocortex. *Nat. Neurosci.* 14, 555–561. doi: 10.1038/nn.2807

Weitzdoerfer, R., Fountoulakis, M., and Lubec, G. (2002). Reduction of actin-related protein complex 2/3 in fetal Down syndrome brain. *Biochem. Biophys. Res. Commun.* 293, 836–841. doi: 10.1016/s0006-291x(02)00291-7

Wilsch-Bräuninger, M., Florio, M., and Huttner, W. B. (2016). Neocortex expansion in development and evolution—from cell biology to single genes. *Curr. Opin. Neurobiol.* 39, 122–132. doi: 10.1016/j.conb.2016.05.004

Wilsch-Bräuninger, M., Peters, J., Paridaen, J. T. M. L., and Huttner, W. B. (2012). Basolateral rather than apical primary cilia on neuroepithelial cells committed to delamination. *Development* 139, 95–105. doi: 10.1242/dev.069294

Xie, Z., Moy, L. Y., Sanada, K., Zhou, Y., Buchman, J. J., and Tsai, L. H. (2007). Cep120 and TACCs control interkinetic nuclear migration and the neural progenitor pool. *Neuron* 56, 79–93. doi: 10.1016/j.neuron.2007.08.026

Ye, F., Kang, E., Yu, C., Qian, X., Jacob, F., Yu, C., et al. (2017). DISC1 regulates neurogenesis via modulating kinetochore attachment of Ndel1/Nde1 during mitosis. *Neuron* doi: 10.1016/j.neuron.2017.10.010 [Epub ahead of print].

Yokota, Y., Eom, T. Y., Stanco, A., Kim, W. Y., Rao, S., Snider, W. D., et al. (2010). Cdc42 and Gsk3 modulate the dynamics of radial glial growth, inter-radial glial interactions and polarity in the developing cerebral cortex. *Development* 137, 4101–4110. doi: 10.1242/dev.048637

6

Cytoskeletal Proteins in Cortical Development and Disease: Actin Associated Proteins in Periventricular Heterotopia

*Gewei Lian and Volney L. Sheen **

Department of Neurology, Beth Israel Deaconess Medical Center and Harvard Medical School, Boston, MA, USA

***Correspondence:**
Volney L. Sheen, Department of Neurology, Beth Israel Deaconess Medical Center and Harvard Medical School, 3 Blackfan Circle, CLS-628H, Boston, MA 02115, USA
vsheen@bidmc.harvard.edu

The actin cytoskeleton regulates many important cellular processes in the brain, including cell division and proliferation, migration, and cytokinesis and differentiation. These developmental processes can be regulated through actin dependent vesicle and organelle movement, cell signaling, and the establishment and maintenance of cell junctions and cell shape. Many of these processes are mediated by extensive and intimate interactions of actin with cellular membranes and proteins. Disruption in the actin cytoskeleton in the brain gives rise to periventricular heterotopia (PH), a malformation of cortical development, characterized by abnormal neurons clustered deep in the brain along the lateral ventricles. This disorder can give rise to seizures, dyslexia and psychiatric disturbances. Anatomically, PH is characterized by a smaller brain (impaired proliferation), heterotopia (impaired initial migration) and disruption along the neuroependymal lining (impaired cell-cell adhesion). Genes causal for PH have also been implicated in actin-dependent processes. The current review provides mechanistic insight into actin cytoskeletal regulation of cortical development in the context of this malformation of cortical development.

Keywords: filamin, formin, RhoGTPases, actin cytoskeleton, proliferation, polarity, migration, periventricular heterotopia

Introduction

The cerebral cortex originates from an expansion of neural tube, which consists of a single-cell-layered, pseudostratified neuroepithelial cells (neural stem cells; Götz and Huttner, 2005). Neuroepithelial cells extend their processes from the apical side (ventricular zone) to the basal lamina, and undergo interkinetic nuclear migration along the apical-basal axis throughout the cell cycle. The nuclei locate to the basal lamina during G1 phase, staying at the basal lamina during S phase, and transition back to the apical side during G2 phase. Mitosis of most neural stem cells occurs at the apical surface, where adhesion proteins like N-cadherin and cytoskeleton-associated proteins form dense and dynamic adhesion structures. As neuroepithelial cells divide, neural cells adopt different cell fate specification—one proliferating neural stem cells and another differentiating neuronal cells by symmetric and asymmetric divisions (Cremisi et al., 2003). At an early stage of mouse corticogenesis, the neuroepithelial cells mainly adopt symmetric cell divisions to expand the neuroepithelial plane, thereby promoting enlargement the ventricle surface. As development progresses, the neuroepithelial cells begin to be progressively biased toward asymmetric division to generate one self-renewed progenitor and another differentiating intermediate progenitors (basal progenitors) or post-mitotic neurons. The post-mitotic neurons attach and migrate along radial glial scaffolds out of the expanding ventricular zone (germinal zone) creating a new overlying layer of cells called the preplate. The laminar position of neurons is characteristic of their birthdate, such that younger neuroblasts migrate past their older counterparts to form the more superficial layers of the cortex. Finally, once neurons reach their cortical destinations, they differentiate and adopt the complex dendritic and axonal connections that are characteristic of fully mature cortical neurons (Ohnuma and Harris, 2003). At later stages, neurogenesis declines and astroglial differentiation begins.

While different actin cytoskeletal mechanisms are often independently implicated in regulation of neural proliferation, migration and differentiation (Duong et al., 1994; Schaar and McConnell, 2005; Munro, 2006; Witte and Bradke, 2008; Solecki et al., 2009; Moon and Wynshaw-Boris, 2013), a primary role for the actin cytoskeleton in facilitating crosstalk between various cell membrane and intracellular molecules would suggest that shared actin dependent pathways could mediate these developmental processes. For example, cell fate specification of neural stem cells along the neuroependymal lining depends upon the actin cytoskeleton to direct cytokinesis and localization of cell fate determining proteins. This actin dependent process dictates whether progenitors produce daughter progeny capable of self-renewal or postmitotic neurons (Knoblich, 2008). Under a constant rate of cell cycle, the greater the number of progenitors that undergo self-renewal, the larger the number of neural progenitors generated, giving rise to more post-mitotic neurons and leading to bigger brain size. Conversely, increased differentiation will lead to a fewer neural progenitors over time, and ultimately fewer neurons and smaller brain size. In this respect, a shared actin cytoskeletal dependent pathway regulates both neural proliferation and differentiation, thereby maintaining a delicate tune of self-renewal vs. differentiation to direct formation of the cerebral cortex. Within this same framework, the same actin cytoskeletal pathways that regulate cell fate specification will also mediate neuronal migration, as intermediate progenitors and post-mitotic neurons will migrate toward the intermediate zone or cortical plate respectively, whereas progenitors remain restricted to the ventricular zone. In this review, we focus on a fundamental actin cytoskeletal pathway that singularly directs each of these developmental stages during corticogenesis.

Actin Cytoskeletal-Associated Proteins

The majority of actin cytoskeletal-associated proteins participate in the formation of actin filaments by regulating the dynamic processes of actin polymerization and de-polymerization. Actin polymerization occurs under the effect of actin-nucleating proteins, including Arp2/3 and formin proteins. The Arp2/3 complex nucleates G-actin in the lamellipodia to form short, branched actin filaments, whereas formins nucleate actin polymerization into long, unbranched filaments, which are important for both stress fiber formation and contractile ring assembly in mitosis (Bovellan et al., 2014; Fried et al., 2014; Khaitlina, 2014; Pan et al., 2014; Zhang et al., 2015). In addition, the actin polymerization state is also regulated by many small GTP-binding proteins like Rho GTPases, which cycle between active and inactive states through GTP to GDP exchange (Ciobanasu et al., 2013; Chen and Friml, 2014; Murali and Rajalingam, 2014). Actin polymerization coincides with a homeostatic de-polymerization of actin filaments through actin-severing molecules like cofilin and gelsolin, which bind and dissociate G-actin-GDP from actin filaments (Nag et al., 2013; Hild et al., 2014). Finally, the stability and contractile state of the actin cytoskeleton are regulated by many actin-crosslinking proteins, like filamins, actinin and myosin (Otey and Carpen, 2004; Ma and Adelstein, 2014; Modarres and Mofradt, 2014). Cooperative interaction between these various cytoskeletal-associated proteins can subserve multiple fundamental cell functions.

As F-actin-binding proteins, filamins are highly conserved and expressed in all eukaryotic cells. Filamins can crosslink actin filaments into orthogonal networks in the cellular cortical cytoplasm and participate in the anchoring of membrane proteins to the actin cytoskeleton (Gorlin et al., 1990). They also cross-link parallel stress fibers, thereby forming an aligned array in fibroblasts. Structurally, filamins are composed of a tandem calponin-homology (CH) actin-binding domain (ABD) at the N-terminus, 24 immunoglobulin-like repeat domains and a C-terminal dimerization domain. In vertebrates, filamins consist of three isoforms (FlnA, FlnB and FlnC) with molecular weights of ~280 kDa (Nakamura et al., 2011; Razinia et al., 2012). The *FLNA* gene is located on human chromosome X q28 and mouse chromosome X q37.89, encoding an approximate 2640-amino acid protein. FlnA is ubiquitously expressed in almost all the tissues, especially in developing brain. The *FLNB* gene resides on human chromosome 3 and mouse chromosome 14 and its encoded protein is predominantly expressed in bone, whereas FLNC is found in muscle tissue. Although FlnB and FlnC are expressed in the brain, they have not been clearly associated with neurological disorders (Sheen et al., 2002; Krakow et al., 2004; Okumura et al., 2013). FlnA, as a scaffolding protein, can interact with more than 45 proteins, including cell adhesion proteins (i.e., integrin) and cell cycle regulators. Recently, FlnA was found to be essential for formation of the E-cadherin-catenin adhesion complex (Feng et al., 2006; Ferland et al., 2009). FlnA also plays important roles in embryonic development by linking these important adhesion proteins and membrane receptors to the actin cytoskeleton. FlnA loss causes various tissue defects during embryonic development, including periventricular heterotopia (PH), skeletal malformation, disorders in vascular and cardiac development and intestinal defect (Fox et al., 1998; Sheen et al., 2001; Robertson et al., 2003). Missense mutations in *FLNA* gene, which are thought to lead to gain of function, are also associated with various human diseases, such as otopalatodigital syndrome, Melnick-Needles syndrome, thrombocytopenia, and intestinal pseudo-obstruction (Robertson et al., 2003). These roles for filamins in embryonic development are likely to be closely related to their functional mechanisms on diverse cellular processes in different types of cells, such as cell receptor signaling, endocytosis and exocytosis of membrane proteins through vesicle trafficking, and signaling transduction in the nucleus.

Formin(s) are members of a family of actin-nucleating, cytoskeletal-associated proteins, which stimulate actin nucleation at the barbed ends of actin to form linear filaments (Basu and Chang, 2007). The mammalian genome encodes more than 10 distinct formin proteins, such as mDia1-3, Daam1/2, and formin1/2. All the formin family of proteins includes two common domains, the formin homology 1 and 2 domains (FH1 and FH2). The FH1 domain contains a proline-rich sequence motif that can bind profilin and interact with certain proteins containing SRC Homology 3 (SH3) and WW domains. The WW domains are so named because of the presence of two conserved tryptophans (W) which are spaced 20–22 amino acids apart within the sequence (Bork and Sudol, 1994). Profilin-associated actin can be concentrated at the positive ends of actin filaments, and act as the major source of actin used for filament polymerization. The FH2 domain contains the actin-nucleating domain that can be associated with the fast-growing barbed end of actin filament and increase the actin polymerization rate by binding profilin/actin via its adjoining FH1 domains. The FH2 domain forms a ring-shaped dimer, which binds to the positive end of nascent actin filament and recruits two actin monomers for nucleation (Otomo et al., 2005). Flanking the FH1 and FH2 domains, the N-terminal GTPase-binding domain (GBD) and C-terminal autoregulatory domain (DAD) are also present in some subsets of formin proteins, and are important for formin activation (Gould et al., 2011). The binding of Rho GTPases to GBD is thought to open the DAD association with N-terminal autoinhibitory domain (DID), thereby changing the FH2 conformation and facilitating actin binding and polymerization. Except for the conserved FH2 domain, different subsets of formins display a distinct difference in other domain structures, which may endow formins with the capacity responding to varied sorts of cellular signals (Schönichen and Geyer, 2010). mDia 1-3 (Diaph1-3) genes are located in different genomic chromosomes, encode three 1100–1200 aa formin proteins carrying N-terminal GBD and DID domains, and C-terminal DAD domain. Loss of mDia proteins has been shown to disrupt apical adherens junctions, impact neuroepithelial polarity, and cause periventricular dysplasia in mouse and microcephaly in humans (Thumkeo et al., 2011). The *formin 1* (*Fmn1*) gene is located in mouse chromosome 2 and encodes a 1466-aa protein. It is predominantly expressed in the brain, kidney and developing limb buds, implying a potential role in development of various systems. The *formin 2* (*Fmn2*) gene is located on mouse chromosome 1 and encodes a 1578 aa protein. It is expressed in the central nervous system and developing mesenchyme, suggesting Fmn1 and Fmn2 may share some similar or common functions. Unlike the mDia proteins, it is not known whether Fmn1/2 contains GBD and DID domains. Collectively, expression of the formin genes in nervous system suggests that they may play diverse roles in neural cell adhesion, migration, proliferation and differentiation.

RhoGTPases are small GTP-binding proteins, the most commonly studied being RhoA, Rac and Cdc42 (Cook et al., 2014). They regulate many cell behaviors like polarity, adhesion, cell division and migration primarily by mediating actin cytoskeletal dynamics. Their regulation of actin polymerization is dependent on both Arp2/3- and formin1/2-nucleating processes. As master regulators of the cytoskeleton, RhoGTPases function between active and inactive states by exchanging GDP with GTP. The switch between activity states is modulated by three classes of regulatory proteins, referred to as guanine nucleotide exchange factors (RhoGEFs), GTPase activating proteins (RhoGAPs), and guanine nucleotide dissociation inhibitors (RhoGDIs). Although RhoA, Rac and Cdc42 all regulate actin remodeling and polymerization, they have distinctly different effects on actin reorganization through their respective downstream effectors. RhoA modulates actin polymerization, stress fiber assembly and focal adhesion formation through formins, Rock and myosin. Rac regulates actin filament polymerization through Arp2/3 and WAVE/WASP to produce lamellipodia and membrane ruffles at the leading edge. Cdc42 stimulates filament assembly and filopodia formation via WASP, Arp2/3 and formin. Collectively, RhoGTPases are expressed in neural cells during development of cerebral cortex, regulate downstream actin effectors (formins and Arps), and play pivotal roles in various neural cell developmental functions.

Periventricular Heterotopia is a malformation of cortical development, characterized by nodules of neurons ectopically located along the lateral ventricles. This disorder is thought to reflect impairments along several states of cortical development, including loss in neuroepithelial integrity, disrupted neural proliferation and cell fate specification, and impaired initial neural migration (Sheen, 2012). Mutations in the *FLNA* gene cause PH (Fox et al., 1998; Sheen et al., 2005). Filamins bind multiple cytoplasmic and cell surface receptors and molecules. Our work shows that filamins also bind formins and RhoGTPases, both of which have been implicated in some kinds of heterotopia formation (Thumkeo et al., 2011; Cappello, 2013). This trimeric complex provides a basic mechanism for modulation of broad actin cytoskeletal dependent processes, essential for cortical development and disease. Given the broad topic of cytoskeletal proteins in brain development, the current review focuses on filamin-associated proteins in corticogenesis, followed by their potential roles in causing PH.

The Actin Cytoskeleton and Neuroepithelial Integrity

The neuroepithelium forms tight cell -cell or -matrix adhesion junctions at the apical surface of the cortical ventricle. The actin cytoskeleton is also assembled into dense actin cables along the apical surface and anchored onto these adhesion sites through cytoskeletal-associated proteins, such as filamin, formin and catenins. The apical lining is enriched for cytoskeletal proteins and actin filaments play determinant roles on the stability of adhesion junctions, as well as the polarity and integrity of the neuroepithelium. FlnA has been found to be essential for formation of the E-cadherin-catenin adhesion complex and its loss causes aberrant adherens junctions in multiple tissues (Feng et al., 2006; Ferland et al., 2009). Furthermore, FlnA-deficient neural progenitors exhibit poor adhesion to extracellular matrix proteins such as laminin. MDia1 and mDia3 formin proteins are also both expressed in the developing brain, and mDia3 is especially concentrated at the apical surface of the neuroepithelium. Loss of mDia1 and mDia3 impairs neuroepithelial cell polarity with attenuated apical actin belts and impaired apical adherens junctions (Thumkeo et al., 2011). Similar to the above findings, β-catenin is a cytoskeleton-associated protein, linking cadherin(s) to actin filament. Mice with conditional loss of β-catenin show several abnormalities in the neuroepithelium, including loss of adherens junctions, and impairment of radial migration of neurons toward the superficial layers (Machon et al., 2003). Finally, RhoGTPases such as RhoA and Cdc42 are highly expressed in neuroepithelium and essential for assembly and stability of apical actin cables. Conditional loss of RhoA and Cdc42 in central nervous system impairs apical localization of cadherin, apical accumulation of actin filament and cell-cell junctions. Collectively, these observations raise the possibility of a fundamental filamin-RhoGTPase-formin pathway in maintaining the location and function of adhesions molecules such as cadherins, which are required to ensure neuroependymal integrity.

The Actin Cytoskeleton and Neural Progenitor Proliferation

Cytoskeletal-associated proteins may not regulate only the stability of cell-cell or cell-extracellular matrix adherens junctions, but also mediate cell proliferation by affecting cell cycle progression (Olson et al., 1995; Cappello et al., 2006; Woodhead et al., 2006; Katayama et al., 2011; Lian et al., 2012; Ercan-Sencicek et al., 2015). For example, actin regulates M (mitosis) phase progression, as the filaments are essential for cleavage furrow formation and completion of cytokinesis (Heng and Koh, 2010). Disruption of actin filaments by inhibitory agents such as latrunculin leads to cytokinesis failure due to a defect in the F-actin cable ring at the cleavage furrow (Lee and Song, 2007). FlnA shows strong expression in the cleavage furrow during mitosis. Additionally, functional loss of actin inhibits centrosome separation early in mitosis and leads to a delay in chromosome segregation late in mitosis (Rosenblatt et al., 2004; Cao et al., 2010). Finally, recent reports have suggested that the interaction of the cortical actin network with astral microtubules is crucial in establishing correct spindle orientation and in proper chromosome segregation in mammalian cells (Théry et al., 2005).

Prior to mitosis, G2-M phase entry requires remodeling of the actin cytoskeleton to change cell shape from an extended to a rounded morphology with cell retraction (Maddox and Burridge, 2003; Cao et al., 2010; Heng and Koh, 2010).This change in cell morphology initially requires activation of RhoA, which triggers a signaling cascade through formin and Rock to re-organize the actin cytoskeleton. Additionally, the cyclin dependent kinase 1 (Cdk1) promotes G2-M transition, and activated Cdk1 phosphorylates Rho GTPase activating protein (p190RhoGAP), down regulating p190RhoGAP hydrolysis of Rho-GTP and thereby promoting RhoA function (Maddox and Burridge, 2003). Our recent study shows that FlnA also regulates Cdk1 activity through Cdk1 phosphorylation and cyclin B degradation (Lian et al., 2012). Lastly, FlnA regulates RhoA activity through mediating p190RhoGAP accumulation in lipid rafts (Mammoto et al., 2007). Therefore, a potential signaling pathway underlying rearrangement of the actin filaments in G2-M phase involves a cascade beginning with FlnA, Cdk1, and p190RhoGAP, which then collectively mediate RhoA and formin/Rock function. This signaling pathway may also be crucial for cell cycle progression through M phase. Loss of FlnA impairs degradation of cyclin B1-related proteins, thereby delaying the onset and progression through mitosis (Lian et al., 2012). Furthermore, loss of FlnA increases the inhibitory phosphorylation of Cdk1 via its interaction with the kinase Wee1. In developing cerebral cortex, FlnA loss causes a decrease in proliferation rate of neural progenitors and a decline in neural progenitor pool size (Lian et al., 2012). This prolongation in cell cycle would relate to the impairment in actin filament rearrangement. Our understanding of the formin role in cell division is more limited, but insight can be gained from our understanding of formin function in other organ systems. Apart from a known interaction with filamins, Fmn1-deficient mice exhibit a reduction in digit number as well as the absence of a fibula due a defect in chondrocyte proliferation (Zhou et al., 2009). Fmn1 loss is linked to up-regulation of BMP and Msx1 but down-regulation of Fgf4 signals within the apical ectodermal ridge, which may influence mitosis. Finally, other RhoGTPase-related proteins also influence M phase progression. Both constitutively active and dominant negative Cdc42 inhibit cytokinesis (Drechsel et al., 1997), and loss of its downstream effector mDia3 causes chromosome misalignment during metaphase (Yasuda et al., 2004). Expression of dominant negative Rac1 retards adventricular nuclear migration, and promotes cytokinesis failures (Michaelson et al., 2008; Minobe et al., 2009).

The actin cytoskeleton mediates G1 phase progression after completion of mitosis. Disruption of actin polymerization by the cytochalasin D causes G1 phase arrest (Bohmer et al., 1996; Lian et al., 2012). The cytoskeletal-dependent effects on G1 progression is mediated through cyclin expression and cyclin-dependent kinase (Cdk) activation. More specifically, the actin cytoskeleton is required for anchorage-dependent expression of cyclin D1, activation of Cdk4/6, phosphorylation of the retinoblastoma protein and transition of G1 phase in non-transformed primary cells. In addition to this primary pathway, cytoskeletal-associated proteins regulate G1 phase progression through other secondary mechanisms. Inhibition of Cdc42, Rac1 and RhoA block G1 phase transition and serum-induced DNA synthesis (Olson et al., 1995; Leone et al., 2010). Active RhoA increases the expression of Skp2 protein, which promotes ubiquitinylation-dependent degradation of the Cdk inhibitor $p27^{kip1}$ (Mammoto et al., 2004). Conversely, RhoA inactivation results in higher levels of $p27^{kip1}$, thereby arresting cell cycle in G1 phase. RhoA inactivation or F-actin disruption are also shown to slow down the degradation of another Cdk inhibitor $p21^{Waf/Cip1}$ (Coleman et al., 2006). With respect to filamins, our prior study suggests that FlnA also regulates neural progenitor proliferation in G1 phase (Lian et al., 2012) and directs cadherin-catenin complex formation. β-catenin is known to mediate G1 phase progression and neural proliferation, and tethers cadherin to the actin cytoskeleton (Woodhead et al., 2006). Conditional deletion of β-catenin in developing mouse brain results in a dramatic defect in neural progenitor proliferation and severe brain malformation. In contrast, overexpression of a stabilized β-catenin causes a significant increase in neural progenitor number and massive expansion of the cerebral cortex (Chenn and Walsh, 2002). Similar to filamins, formins may play coordinative effects on cell proliferation through G1 phase. Our ongoing studies suggest that loss of filamin and formin can affect β-catenin translocation and cyclin D expression. Compared to loss of FlnB or Fmn1 alone, loss of both Fmn1 and FlnB in mice leads to a more severe reduction in body size, weight and growth plate length (Hu et al., 2014). These findings would suggest that these actin associated proteins can mediate cell proliferation in multiple organ systems.

From the discussion above, the filamin-formin-RhoGTPase pathway can potentially be implicated in several phases of the cell cycle through interactions with various cell cycle associated proteins. A prevailing role for these proteins in regulation of actin dependent vesicle trafficking would provide a common mechanism for the transport and degradation cell cycle and cell fate proteins, which oversee neural proliferation.

The Actin Cytoskeleton and Cell Polarity and Fate Specification

The neuroepithelium comprises a distinctive epithelial structure with apical-basal polarity. The actin cytoskeleton is selectively concentrated at the apical side along the ventricle of the developing cerebral cortex, forming a dense and dynamic filament belt to support tight adhesive junctions, cilium stability, and cell polarity, and to maintain a membrane barrier. Acting as regulators of cell shape and binding-partners for polarity proteins, the actin filament and its associated proteins are of key importance for regulating cell polarity (Ohno, 2001; Sawin, 2002; Etienne-Manneville, 2004; Witte and Bradke, 2008; Wang et al., 2009; Gonzalez-Billault et al., 2012). As an example, Rho-GTPases like RhoA, Cdc42 and Rac1 regulate actin cytoskeleton remodeling, focal adhesion formation and cell polarity (Etienne-Manneville, 2004; Iden and Collard, 2008; Gonzalez-Billault et al., 2012). Activated Cdc42 forms a stable hetero-tetrameric complex with polarizing proteins Par3, Par6, and atypical protein kinase C (PKCζ) and recruits these molecules to the leading edge to guide the reorientation of the microtubule and centrosome (Ohno, 2001; Etienne-Manneville, 2004). Cdc42-deficient neural progenitors exhibit multiple apical polarity-related defects including disorientation of cell division, aberrant location of the Par complex and adherens junctions, and severe impairments in the extension of nestin-positive radial fibers (Chen et al., 2006; Peng et al., 2013). Further, Cdc42 loss also causes PH and holoprosencephaly. As effectors of Rho-GTPases, formins and non-muscle myosin II have been shown to be indispensable for cell polarity (Habas et al., 2001; Ma et al., 2007). Depletion of the formin homologous protein Daam1 prevents Wnt/Fz activation of Rho and planar cell polarity during Xenopus gastrulation. Ablation of non-muscle myosin II-B in mice results in loss of neuroepithelial adhesion and severe hydrocephalus. Upstream of Rho GTPases, the association of FlnA with Wnt co-receptor Ror2 is required for Wnt5a-induced JNK activation, appropriate orientation of the microtubule organizing center and cell polarity (Nomachi et al., 2008). Further, loss of FlnA leads to a transition from bipolar neuron to multipolar neuron, suggesting a FlnA effect on neuronal polarity (Nagano et al., 2004). Given their physical interaction, filamins and RhoGTPases might regulate formin dependent polarized actin nucleation. Polarized actin provides a mechanism for establishment of neuroepithelial polarity.

Cytoskeletal proteins regulate cell proliferation not only by affecting cell cycle progression, but also through their control over cell fate specification (Chenn and Walsh, 2002; Taverna et al., 2014). During neuroepithelial cell fate specification, neural stem cells must undergo a decision process to undergo self-renewal or differentiate into intermediate progenitors or neurons. This process is dependent upon the asymmetric inheritance of cell fate determining proteins, which is regulated by polarized actin, actin dependent trafficking and degradation of cell fate proteins. In this respect cytoskeletal proteins could indirectly mediate cell fate. Cell fate determinants like Par3, aPKC, and numb as well as stem cell niche molecules like integrin and cadherin all directly or indirectly interact with the actin cytoskeleton, such that cell fate is influenced by cytoskeletal dynamics (Guo et al., 1996; Barros et al., 2003; Cappello et al., 2006; Woodhead et al., 2006). Furthermore, conditional deletion of Cdc42 at different stages of neurogenesis in mouse telencephalon results in an immediate increase in basal mitoses and altered differentiation of neural progenitors. In mesenchymal cells, loss of p190RhoGAP, which inactivates RhoA activity through GTP hydrolysis, causes a concomitant up-regulation of RhoA activity and increase in myogenic differentiation (but decrease in adipogenesis) (Sordella et al., 2003). In conditional RhoA-deleted embryos, RhoA-deficient neural progenitor cells exhibit accelerated proliferation and reduction in cell-cycle exit, indicating a change in cell fate specification (Katayama et al., 2011). Prior studies have shown that FlnA can bind to RhoA and integrin. Some of our initial observations suggest that loss of FlnA impairs cell cycle exit, in part through disruption of spindle orientation of neural progenitors during mitosis. Moreover, FlnA interactions with formins which nucleate actin in a polarized fashion would provide a basis for asymmetric delivery and localization of cell fate determining proteins.

The Actin Cytoskeleton and Neural Migration

Cell migration is a highly dynamic process involving cell adhesion, extension, protrusion of filopodia and lamellipodia at leading edge and formation of contractile structure at rear edge. All the events require the dynamic remodeling of actin cytoskeleton (Rottner and Stradal, 2011). A variety of literatures have reported that actin cytoskeleton and its associated proteins are essential for cell migration (Fox and Walsh, 1999; Ridley et al., 2003; Raftopoulou and Hall, 2004; Govek et al., 2005; Broussard et al., 2008). For instance, disruption of actin filaments with drug cytochalasin C in migrating cerebellar granule cells can completely block cell migration (Rivas and Hatten, 1995). Further, melanocytes lacking FLNA show defects in filopodia formation and abnormal surface blebbing, implying a necessary role for FLNA in promoting the assembly of the cortical actin network. Several types of FLNA-deficient cells like macrophages, melanocytes and Dictyostelium amoebae cells display profound defects in motility and chemotaxis (Cunningham et al., 1992; Cox et al., 1996). In contrast, re-expression of FLNA in the cells can rescue each of these phenotypes, further establishing the essential effects of FLNA on migration. FLNA also is concentrated at rear edge of migrating leukocytes, implying FLNA may execute some important functions on rear edge retraction via FLNA-crosslink-driven force (Ohta et al., 2006). Notably, recent studies using transgenetic FlnA-deficient mouse model result in some contradictory conclusions to FLNA effects on neural cell migration (Fox et al., 1998; Feng et al., 2006; Hart et al., 2006). FlnA loss does not affect *in vivo* migration of neural crest cells into neural-crest-derived tissues like endocardial cushion, and the membrane ruffling, locomotion and migration of *in vitro* cultured fibroblast cells also appear normal. However, BrdU pulse labeling in embryonic day 15 null FlnA brains shows that the migration of $BrdU^{+}$ cells into the cortical plate is slower than that of age matched wild type cells. Most $BrdU^{+}$ cells from null FlnA cerebral cortices migrate into intermediate zone, but not into the cortical plate, as seen in their wild type littermates by 3 days post-labeling (Zhang et al., 2013). Further, cultured neural progenitor cells from E13 FlnA-null cerebral cortex also show poor spreading on laminin-coated coverslips, implying impairment in cell adhesion on extracellular matrix (Zhang et al., 2013). Finally, FlnA regulates the stability and turnover of adhesion and migratory associated proteins such as paxillin (Zhang et al., 2012, 2013). These migratory defects may in part be related to FlnA interactions with Filip, which regulates the degradation of the actin binding protein and thereby influences neural migration and cell specification (Nagano et al., 2002, 2004). These findings would suggest that filamins may regulate neural motility but do not completely abolish the capacity of progenitors to migrate to their intended site. Thus, these cytoskeletal associated proteins may not form the primary mechanism required to allow cells to migrate, but rather mediate processes (i.e., trafficking of particular receptors/molecules) that influence the rate at which neural progenitors move.

RhoGTPases such as RhoA, Rac1 and Cdc42 regulate remodeling of actin cytoskeleton, thereby serving as key regulators for cell morphology and migration (Raftopoulou and Hall, 2004). Their effects on neural migration have been extensively studied. Basically, Cdc42 and Rac1 stimulate formation of filopodia and lamellipodia (Yang et al., 2012), to direct neurite outgrowth and promote neural cell migration (Chen et al., 2007), whereas RhoA promotes retraction of rear edge and nuclear translocation of neural cell but impairs neurite extension. Other small GTP-binding proteins such as Rnd2 and Rnd3 have also been implicated in neural migration, although their relationship with filamins and formins is not known (Heng et al., 2008; Azzarelli et al., 2014). As downstream effectors of Rho GTPases, formins play potential important roles in polymerization and remodeling of actin filament. For instance, mDia deficiency impairs tangential migration of cortical and olfactory inhibitory interneurons (Shinohara et al., 2012). mDia-deficient neuroblasts exhibit reduced separation of the centrosome from the nucleus, retard nuclear translocation and concomitantly impair F-actin movement and condensation at the cellular rear. In non-neural cells, mDia1 has been shown to regulate formation of stable actin filaments and turnover of focal adhesions. mDia1 deletion impairs focal contacts, and decreases lamellipodial thickness in migrating cells (Yamana et al., 2006). Other formins like Fmn1 and FLR also are shown to function in cellular migration (Zhou et al., 2009; Hu et al., 2014). Fmn1 protein is more similar in sequence to dishevelled-associated activator of morphogenesis-1 (Daam1). Mutations in mouse Fmn1 gene result in limb deformities and incompletely penetrant renal aplasia, and display altered cell protrusion at the leading edge, defective cell spreading, and less focal adhesions. Our recent findings show that formin(s) can physically interact with filamin(s) and they co-express in developing bone and brain tissues (Hu et al., 2014). Loss of both formin and filamin results in serve defects in cell proliferation and migration in developing mouse thoracic wall and brain, suggesting that filamin and formin play cooperative roles in cell proliferation and migration.

Cell migration is a complex and cooperative process with protrusion at cell leading edge and with concomitant retraction at rear edge. The molecular mechanisms underlying neural migration may include some signaling pathways from G protein-coupled receptors, tyrosine-kinase receptors, PI3K, MAPK and Rho GTPases and cytoskeletal reorganization (Witte and Bradke, 2008; Jurberg et al., 2014). Here, it needs to be underscored that these processes of signal transductions require directional and robust vesicle trafficking that cytoskeletal proteins regulate. For instance, directional vesicle trafficking from cell rear edge to leading edge may play crucial roles on cell migration. Thus in a manner similar to establishment of cell polarity by directing the localization of fate determining proteins, filamins, formins and RhoGTPases can coordinate similar processes during neural migration.

The functional roles of actin cytoskeletal genes in adhesion junctions and cell migration are also mutually interdependent. In the developing cerebral cortex, radial glial cells extend their end feet onto the apical lining of ventricle, where they form dense cell to cell/matrix connections via cell adhesion proteins like cadherins and integrins at the tips of the end feet. Newborn neuron or pre-neuron migrate out of ventricle along the radial glial fibers. Thus, loss of cytoskeletal-associated proteins causes destabilization of the interdependent adhesion complex (adhesion proteins and actin filament) and disconnection of radial glial at the apical lining. Impairment in the connection of radial glial end feet would interrupt migration along the radial glial tracks, thereby contributing to the neuronal migration defect. In addition, actin cytoskeletal and adhesion proteins are also enriched within the growth cone of migrating neuron. Loss of these proteins and/or disruption of their trafficking likely influence neuronal migration itself.

Finally, neural migration is dependent on the differentiation state of the precursor. For example, Rac1 is necessary for neural progenitor transition from G1 to S phase, at least in part by regulating cyclin D levels and retinoblastoma protein phosphorylation. Loss of Rac1 in progenitors impairs the migration of ventral GABAergic neurons into the cortical plate. Ablation of Rac1 from postmitotic progenitors does not result in similar defects (Vidaki et al., 2012).

Cytoskeletal-Associated Vesicle Trafficking: A Common Thread in Brain Development

Vesicle trafficking maintains the apical-basal polarity of neuroepithelium through directional vesicle transport and membrane protein sorting (transcytosis), thus underlying cell polarity, migration and asymmetric division (Rodriguez-Boulan et al., 2005). Vesicle trafficking includes endocytosis, exocytosis and endosomal recycling and sorting (Symons and Rusk, 2003). Endocytic trafficking is characterized by the internalization of plasma membrane and extracellular molecules via several distinct pathways: micropinocytosis, phagocytosis, and clathrin and caveolae-mediated endocytosis. This process is dependent on actin cytoskeletal-associated proteins like Rho GTPases (Ridley, 2006). For example, dominant-negative Cdc42 or Rac1 can block macropinocytosis, while constitutively active Cdc42 and Rac1 can restore the pinocytosis in immature dendritic cells (Garrett et al., 2000). Actin dynamics is also crucial for phagocytosis. Both Cdc42 and Rac participate in FcγR-mediated phagocytosis with Cdc42 directing pseudopod extension, and Rac functioning in pseudopod fusion and phagosome closure (Massol et al., 1998). During clathrin-mediated endocytosis, overexpression of constitutively active Rac1 and RhoA inhibits clathrin-mediated internalization of transferrin and EGF receptor in Hela cells (Lamaze et al., 1996), whereas RhoA can stimulate this process in polarized MDCK cells, suggesting that Rho GTPase function is dependent on cell polarity state (Leung et al., 1999). Caveolae are comprised of cholesterol-enriched internalized plasma membrane and are closely associated with actin filament. Integrins with caveolin have been shown to mediate RhoA activity in endothelial cells. Both RhoA and caveolin must co-localize and interact to mediate RhoA dependent actin remodeling (Nuno et al., 2009; Yang et al., 2011).

Formin and filamin proteins have been increasingly implicated in vesicle trafficking. MDia, together with myosin II, controls the initiation of E-cadherin endocytosis in the epithelium by regulating the lateral clustering of E-cadherin (Levayer et al., 2011). In oocytes, long-range transport of vesicles is regulated by Fmn2 through assembling an extensive actin network from the vesicles' surfaces to plasma membrane. The vesicles move directionally along these actin cables to reach the cell surface (Schuh, 2011). Recent work also reveals that filamin binds to the caveolae marker, caveolin, and is required for endocytic trafficking of caveolin (Muriel et al., 2011). The endocytic trafficking of caveolae towards a recycling endosome is impaired in FLNA-deficient HeLa and M2-melanoma cells.

Besides the effect on endocytic trafficking, actin cytoskeletal-associated proteins may also be involved in exocytosis. Actin-associated proteins (filamin, myosins and Cdc42) are present in the Golgi complex, and actin filament may function as tracks for the myosin-driven movement of vesicles. Expression of Cdc42 mutants slows the exit of the basolateral marker N-cadherin from the trans-Golgi network while also stimulating the exit of the apical marker neurotrophin receptor p75 (Musch et al., 2001). RhoGTPases associate with the Golgi apparatus in an ARF-dependent manner. The *ADP ribosylation factor guanine exchange factor 2* (*ARFGEF2* encodes for BIG2) is a guanine nucleotide-exchange factor for ARF1/3, which play an important role in vesicular trafficking from Golgi complex to plasma membrane. Inhibition of BIG2 disrupts membranous localization of adherens junction protein E-cadherin and beta-catenin by preventing their transport from the Golgi apparatus to the cell surface, leading to PH formation (Sheen et al., 2004; Zhang et al., 2012, 2013). Given that filamin can physically bind and interact with ARFGEF2 (Zhang et al., 2012), filamin and its associated proteins might orchestrate the vesicle exocytosis from Golgi to plasma membrane.

Genetics of Periventricular Heterotopia

Periventricular heterotopia is one of the most common malformation of cortical development and causes seizures, dyslexia, and psychiatric disturbances (Sheen, 2012). PH is characterized by bilateral ectopic neuronal nodules found along the lateral ventricles (Lu and Sheen, 2005). The nodules are caused by impaired migration from the ventricular zone and disruption in the integrity of the neuroependyma (Sheen, 2012). Mutations in the causative genes also cause microcephaly (meaning small brain) (Sheen et al., 2003, 2004).

The most common form of PH is inherited in an X-linked dominant fashion from mutations in the *FLNA* gene (Fox et al., 1998; Sheen et al., 2001, 2005). A second form of autosomal recessive PH with microcephaly (ARPHM) has been associated with mutations in the *ARFGEF2* gene. *ARFGEF2* encodes brefeldin-A inhibited guanine exchange factor-2 (BIG2) (Sheen et al., 2004). BIG2 is a protein kinase A anchoring protein (AKAP) which regulates Golgi-vesicle trafficking through its Sec7 domain. Recent work has identified cadherin receptor ligands in causing PH due to mutations in *FAT4* and *DCHS1* (Cappello et al., 2013).

Several mouse genes have been shown to cause PH formation and can be functionally linked. αSNAP is a SNARE-related protein, involved in vesicle fusion. Prior reports have shown that αSNAP mediates VE-cadherin localization through a β1-integrin-associated process (Andreeva et al., 2005). FlnA binds β1-integrin (Calderwood et al., 2001). Mekk4 binds and regulates FlnA (Chi et al., 2005), and therefore could indirectly regulate caveolin mediated endocytosis. The RhoGTPases bind FlnA and direct various aspects of intracellular actin dynamics, which are required for endosomal vesicle transport (Cappello et al., 2006; Katayama et al., 2011). Deficiency of the formin associated mDia disrupts integrity of neuroepithelium and causes periventricular dysplasia (Thumkeo et al., 2011). Similarly, Spred1 is a multidomain scaffolding protein that contains an ENA/VASP domain which modulates actin stress fiber remodeling, like filamins. Spred1 is also associated with specific endosomal vesicles (Phoenix and Temple, 2010). Finally, SCF-c-kit affects several downstream pathways including RAS/ERK and JAK/STAT pathways, both of which have been associated with Mekk4 and Spred1 activity (Rönnstrand, 2004; Soumiya et al., 2009).

Similar radiographic or anatomical findings of PH and potentially linked functions suggest that genes causal for PH might be involved in a common molecular pathway important in neural progenitor development. Prior studies have demonstrated a shared interaction between FlnA and Big2 in activating Arf to form vesicles at the cell membrane, and thereby regulate turnover/stability of cell adhesion molecules (Zhang et al., 2012, 2013).

Anatomical Phenotypes Associated with PH

Periventricular heterotopia refers to heterotopic neurons along the lateral ventricles which are caused by impaired motility/migration and disruption of the neuroependymal lining. For example, loss of FlnA results in fewer post mitotic cells reaching the cortical plate compared to wild type (WT) following BrdU incorporation. Cells remain in the intermediate and ventricular zones, consistent with a cell autonomous migratory defect (Zhang et al., 2013). Disruption in the neuroependymal lining has also been reported with FlnA inhibition (Adams et al., 2012). Loss of neuroependymal integrity is the primary cause of heterotopia formation.

While human and mouse genes associated with PH show brain heterotopia, they all also regulate neural proliferation. Human *ARFGEF2* mutations cause microcephaly. While microcephaly is not seen in females with *FLNA* mutations (likely due to mosaicism), males die at birth and have been reported to have thinner cortices, and loss of cortical convolutions consistent with underlying microcephaly (Guerrini et al., 2004). Human mutations in cadherin-associated DCHS1 and FAT4 alter progenitor proliferation (Cappello et al., 2013). FlnA null mice also have microcephaly (Lian et al., 2012). Disruption of Cdc42 and RhoA cause PH in mice and lead to changes in brain size and/or progenitor proliferation (Cappello et al., 2006; Katayama et al., 2011). Dysregulation of PH associated *Napa*, *Stem Cell Factor 1* (*SCF*) and *Spred1* genes also alter progenitor proliferation in mice (Chae et al., 2004; Ferland et al., 2009; Phoenix and Temple, 2010). Mekk4 loss causes PH and a smaller brain with increased cell death (Chi et al., 2005). Formins have been implicated in proliferation of mouse neuroepithelial cells (Thumkeo et al., 2011). Lastly, a nonsense mutation of the formin related DIAPH1 (human mDia1) in humans has been found to cause microcephaly (Ercan-Sencicek et al., 2015).

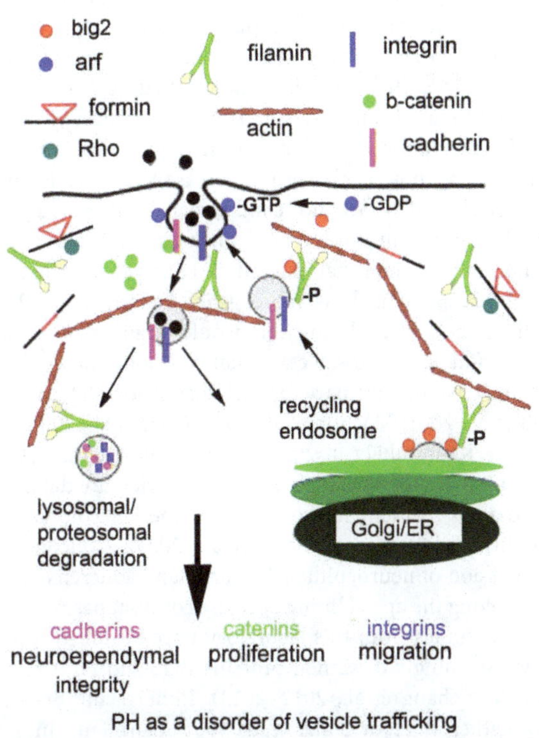

FIGURE 1 | Periventricular heterotopia as a disorder of vesicle trafficking. FlnA phosphorylation localizes Big2 to the cell membrane, thereby activating the Arfs. Arfs are required for vesicle formation. Fmn interactions with FlnA are hypothesized to alter endocytosis and Fmn2 regulates vesicle trafficking and ultimately lysosomal degradation. Disruption of these processes leads to loss of cell-cell adhesion, impairing neuroepithelial integrity. Loss of focal adhesion sites causes defects in neural migration and impaired degradation of cell cycle associated proteins causes a reduction in neural proliferation.

There are several reasons to believe that the heterotopia formation, disruption in neuroependyma integrity, and impairments in neural proliferation are integrally linked. First, from an anatomical basis, FlnA loss leads to a smaller brain through prolongation in cell progression through mitosis (M) phase (Lian et al., 2012). In cortical development, M phase occurs at the neuroepithelial lining suggesting a shared mechanism with PH formation (defects in adhesion/migration also occur at the neurependyma). Second, from a molecular standpoint, we have shown that Big2/FlnA regulate turnover of adhesion molecules (catenins and cadherins) at the neuroependyma (Zhang et al., 2013). These molecules have been show to regulate brain size and their associated molecules cause PH (Chenn and Walsh, 2002; Cappello et al., 2013). Lastly, a delay in differentiation would also lead to a delay in neural migration into the cortical plate.

Cellular and Molecular Mechanisms in PH

Periventricular heterotopia was initially thought to derive from a simple failure in neuronal migration given FLNA's regulation of the actin cytoskeleton (Fox et al., 1998). However, several observations indicate that PH formation may be more complex, derived from diverse processes associated with cytoskeletal dynamics. First, BrdU labeling shows that loss of FlnA in developing mouse brain results in slower migration of neurons, but no PH formation, implying that the impairment in neuronal migration may not be the primary reason for PH formation (Zhang et al., 2013). Second, conditional deletion of RhoA in developing brain causes severe PH formation, but loss of RhoA does not impair neuronal migration (Katayama et al., 2011; Cappello, 2013). Third, as more genes causative for PH are identified, their shared function would argue that adherens junctions and actin cytoskeletal dynamics along the ventricular lining may be the primary pivotal factor for PH formation (Brault et al., 2001; Machon et al., 2003; Chae et al., 2004; Sheen et al., 2004; Kadowaki et al., 2007; Ma et al., 2007; Thumkeo et al., 2011; Peng et al., 2013). Consistent with this view are the findings that the actin filament network around the heterotopia in the PH brains is disrupted (Ferland et al., 2009). Concomitantly, the expression of neuroepithelial polarity and adherens junction proteins along the apical lining decreases or disappears.

Recent studies from this laboratory have begun to reconcile how two seemingly dissimilar proteins Big2 and FlnA can give rise to PH (Zhang et al., 2012, 2013). Either acute or chronic loss of either Big2 or FlnA leads to impairments in neural migration during development of the cortex. Migratory neural cells show defects in filopodia extension and attachment onto extracellular matrix coated surfaces. Both proteins physically bind and interact within neural progenitors, and loss of protein expression of either FlnA or Big2 leads to compensatory upregulation of the other. As with many proteins that FlnA binds, Big2 localization is dependent on phosphorylation of the actin binding protein which redirects Big2 from the Golgi to the cell membrane. Relocalization to the membrane allows Big2 to activate Arf1. Arfs have been shown to reside at the cell surface with ARF1 and ARF3 mediating endocytosis (Dong et al., 2010; Kondo et al., 2012). The reciprocal regulation likely reflects a negative feedback, where loss of Big2 promotes phospho-FlnA expression to enhance redistribution of Big2 to the membrane. Conversely, loss of FlnA enhances Big2 expression to allow for Big2 delivery to the membrane. These studies begin to suggest an integral relationship between FlnA dependent actin dynamics and Big2 dependent regulation of vesicle formation and trafficking.

Periventricular Heterotopia as a Disorder of Vesicle Trafficking

Changes in Arf-dependent endocytosis have the potential to disrupt several cell developmental processes and provide a hypothetical model for PH formation (see the cartoon in **Figure 1**; Sheen, 2012). First, the primary anatomical defect leading to the PH phenotype (loss in neuroependymal integrity, impaired migration, and reduced proliferation) occurs within neural progenitors along the neuroepithelial lining. Genes implicated in PH (FlnA, Big2) regulate the stability, turnover and degradation of cell adhesion molecules (β-catenin, N-cadherin) and cell-ECM receptors (integrins, paxillin adaptor proteins). FlnA phosphorylation targets Big2 to the membrane, allowing for Arf-dependent activation and vesicle formation. Endocytosis occurs through a caveolin dependent mechanism leading to internalization of catenin/cadherin and integrins. Specificity for these molecules extends from their binding of filamins (Calderwood et al., 2001). Several associated PH genes (RhoA, αSNAP and Spredl) would be expected to participate in this process given their implied association with trafficking and/or endocytosis but their specific roles are not known. The downstream mechanisms that regulate endosomal and lysosomal/proteosomal processing in contributing to PH are also not known, although this review would point to a RhoA and Fmn dependent process.

In short, disruption of Big2 and FlnA (and presumably Fmn and RhoGTPases) would alter the stabilization, turnover and degradation of the cadherin, catenin and integrin proteins through impaired vesicle trafficking. Loss of cell adhesion (via altered cadherin) would disrupt the neuroependymal lining. Impaired cadherin stability would also alter catenin localization and function, thereby leading to impaired proliferation. Alteration of cell fate would be closely linked to proliferation and also effect neural migration. For example, slower progression through the cell cycle (as seen with loss of FlnA) causes delayed differentiation of neural progenitors at a given age (as seen with enhanced symmetric cell divisions from FlnA loss). This delayed differentiation would also lead to slower neural migration from the ventricular zone into the cortical plate. In this respect, many of the phenotypes seen with PH can be explained through changes in actin cytoskeletal regulation via FlnA-RhoA-Fmn2 (and Big2) within neural cells along the ventricular lining.

Conclusion

Actin cytoskeletal-associated proteins play a variety of diverse and key roles in cerebral cortex development. A basic mechanism for filamins, formins and RhoGTPases may extend from their regulation of dynamic vesicle trafficking, in directed neural progenitor development. Directional transport of actin cytoskeletal-associated vesicles toward apicolateral or basolateral membranes along the neuroepithelium may be crucial for establishing polarity and maintaining adherens junctions. Loss of this function appears to be the primary pathology underlying PH formation. Cytoskeletal-regulated vesicle trafficking may transmit extracellular signals into cytoplasm and nucleus, as well as mediate degradation of cell cycle associated proteins, thereby regulating cell cycle progression and proliferation. PH has been associated with microcephaly. Finally, directional vesicle trafficking, as well as regulation of turnover of proteins toward the leading edge of migratory neural cells, would be required for proper neuronal migration, and account for the impaired migration seen in this disorder.

Acknowledgments

This work was supported in part by the National Institutes of Health (1 R01 NS092062 01 to VLS).

References

Adams, M., Simms, R. J., Abdelhamed, Z., Dawe, H. R., Szymanska, K., Logan, C. V., et al. (2012). A meckelin-filamin A interaction mediates ciliogenesis. *Hum. Mol. Genet.* 21, 1272–1286. doi: 10.1093/hmg/ddr557

Andreeva, A. V., Kutuzov, M. A., Vaiskunaite, R., Profirovic, J., Meigs, T. E., Predescu, S., et al. (2005). G alpha12 interaction with alphaSNAP induces VE-cadherin localization at endothelial junctions and regulates barrier function. *J. Biol. Chem.* 280, 30376–30383. doi: 10.1074/jbc.m502844200

Azzarelli, R., Pacary, E., Garg, R., Garcez, P., van den Berg, D., Riou, P., et al. (2014). An antagonistic interaction between PlexinB2 and Rnd3 controls RhoA activity and cortical neuron migration. *Nat. Commun.* 5:3405. doi: 10.1038/ncomms4405

Barros, C. S., Phelps, C. B., and Brand, A. H. (2003). Drosophila nonmuscle myosin II promotes the asymmetric segregation of cell fate determinants by cortical exclusion rather than active transport. *Dev. Cell* 5, 829–840. doi: 10.1016/s1534-5807(03)00359-9

Basu, R., and Chang, F. (2007). Shaping the actin cytoskeleton using microtubule tips. *Curr. Opin. Cell Biol.* 19, 88–94. doi: 10.1016/j.ceb.2006.12.012

Bohmer, R. M., Scharf, E., and Assoian, R. K. (1996). Cytoskeletal integrity is required throughout the mitogen stimulation phase of the cell cycle and mediates the anchorage-dependent expression of cyclin D1. *Mol. Biol. Cell* 7, 101–111. doi: 10.1091/mbc.7.1.101

Bork, P., and Sudol, M. (1994). The WW domain: a signalling site in dystrophin? *Trends Biochem. Sci.* 19, 531–533. doi: 10.1016/0968-0004(94)90053-1

Bovellan, M., Romeo, Y., Biro, M., Boden, A., Chugh, P., Yonis, A., et al. (2014). Cellular control of cortical actin nucleation. *Curr. Biol.* 24, 1628–1635. doi: 10.1016/j.cub.2014.05.069

Brault, V., Moore, R., Kutsch, S., Ishibashi, M., Rowitch, D. H., McMahon, A. P., et al. (2001). Inactivation of the beta-catenin gene by Wnt1-Cre-mediated deletion results in dramatic brain malformation and failure of craniofacial development. *Development* 128, 1253–1264.

Broussard, J. A., Webb, D. J., and Kaverina, I. (2008). Asymmetric focal adhesion disassembly in motile cells. *Curr. Opin. Cell Biol.* 20, 85–90. doi: 10.1016/j.ceb.2007.10.009

Calderwood, D. A., Huttenlocher, A., Kiosses, W. B., Rose, D. M., Woodside, D. G., Schwartz, M. A., et al. (2001). Increased filamin binding to beta-integrin cytoplasmic domains inhibits cell migration. *Nat. Cell Biol.* 3, 1060–1068. doi: 10.1038/ncb1201-1060

Cao, J., Crest, J., Fasulo, B., and Sullivan, W. (2010). Cortical actin dynamics facilitate early-stage centrosome separation. *Curr. Biol.* 20, 770–776. doi: 10.1016/j.cub.2010.02.060

Cappello, S. (2013). Small Rho-GTPases and cortical malformations: fine-tuning the cytoskeleton stability. *Small GTPases* 4, 51–56. doi: 10.4161/sgtp.23093

Cappello, S., Attardo, A., Wu, X., Iwasato, T., Itohara, S., Wilsch-Brauninger, M., et al. (2006). The Rho-GTPase cdc42 regulates neural progenitor fate at the apical surface. *Nat. Neurosci.* 9, 1099–1107. doi: 10.1038/nn1744

Cappello, S., Gray, M. J., Badouel, C., Lange, S., Einsiedler, M., Srour, M., et al. (2013). Mutations in genes encoding the cadherin receptor-ligand pair DCHS1 and FAT4 disrupt cerebral cortical development. *Nat. Genet.* 45, 1300–1308. doi: 10.1038/ng.2765

Chae, T. H., Kim, S., Marz, K. E., Hanson, P. I., and Walsh, C. A. (2004). The hyh mutation uncovers roles for alpha Snap in apical protein localization and control of neural cell fate. *Nat. Genet.* 36, 264–270. doi: 10.1038/ng1302

Chen, X., and Friml, J. (2014). Rho-GTPase-regulated vesicle trafficking in plant cell polarity. *Biochem. Soc. Trans.* 42, 212–218. doi: 10.1042/BST20130269

Chen, L., Liao, G., Waclaw, R. R., Burns, K. A., Linquist, D., Campbell, K., et al. (2007). Rac1 controls the formation of midline commissures and the competency of tangential migration in ventral telencephalic neurons. *J. Neurosci.* 27, 3884–3893. doi: 10.1523/jneurosci.3509-06.2007

Chen, L., Liao, G., Yang, L., Campbell, K., Nakafuku, M., Kuan, C. Y., et al. (2006). Cdc42 deficiency causes Sonic hedgehog-independent holoprosencephaly. *Proc. Natl. Acad. Sci. U S A* 103, 16520–16525. doi: 10.1073/pnas.0603533103

Chenn, A., and Walsh, C. A. (2002). Regulation of cerebral cortical size by control of cell cycle exit in neural precursors. *Science* 297, 365–369. doi: 10.1126/science.1074192

Chi, H., Sarkisian, M. R., Rakic, P., and Flavell, R. A. (2005). Loss of mitogen-activated protein kinase kinase kinase 4 (MEKK4) results in enhanced apoptosis and defective neural tube development. *Proc. Natl. Acad. Sci. U S A* 102, 3846–3851. doi: 10.1073/pnas.0500026102

Ciobanasu, C., Faivre, B., and Le Clainche, C. (2013). Integrating actin dynamics, mechanotransduction and integrin activation: the multiple functions of actin binding proteins in focal adhesions. *Eur. J. Cell Biol.* 92, 339–348. doi: 10.1016/j.ejcb.2013.10.009

Coleman, M. L., Densham, R. M., Croft, D. R., and Olson, M. F. (2006). Stability of p21Waf1/Cip1 CDK inhibitor protein is responsive to RhoA-mediated regulation of the actin cytoskeleton. *Oncogene* 25, 2708–2716. doi: 10.1038/sj.onc.1209322

Cook, D. R., Rossman, K. L., and Der, C. J. (2014). Rho guanine nucleotide exchange factors: regulators of Rho GTPase activity in development and disease. *Oncogene* 33, 4021–4035. doi: 10.1038/onc.2013.362

Cox, D., Wessels, D., Soll, D. R., Hartwig, J., and Condeelis, J. (1996). Re-expression of ABP-120 rescues cytoskeletal, motility and phagocytosis defects of ABP-120- Dictyostelium mutants. *Mol. Biol. Cell* 7, 803–823. doi: 10.1091/mbc.7.5.803

Cremisi, F., Philpott, A., and Ohnuma, S. (2003). Cell cycle and cell fate interactions in neural development. *Curr. Opin. Neurobiol.* 13, 26–33. doi: 10.1016/s0959-4388(03)00005-9

Cunningham, C. C., Gorlin, J. B., Kwiatkowski, D. J., Hartwig, J. H., Janmey, P. A., Byers, H. R., et al. (1992). Actin-binding protein requirement for cortical stability and efficient locomotion. *Science* 255, 325–327. doi: 10.1126/science.1549777

Dong, C., Zhang, X., Zhou, F., Dou, H., Duvernay, M. T., Zhang, P., et al. (2010). ADP-ribosylation factors modulate the cell surface transport of G protein-coupled receptors. *J. Pharmacol. Exp. Ther.* 333, 174–183. doi: 10.1124/jpet.109.161489

Drechsel, D. N., Hyman, A. A., Hall, A., and Glotzer, M. (1997). A requirement for Rho and Cdc42 during cytokinesis in Xenopus embryos. *Curr. Biol.* 7, 12–23. doi: 10.1016/s0960-9822(06)00023-6

Duong, T., De Rosa, M. J., Poukens, V., Vinters, H. V., and Fisher, R. S. (1994). Neuronal cytoskeletal abnormalities in human cerebral cortical dysplasia. *Acta Neuropathol.* 87, 493–503. doi: 10.1007/bf00294176

Ercan-Sencicek, A. G., Jambi, S., Franjic, D., Nishimura, S., Li, M., El-Fishawy, P., et al. (2015). Homozygous loss of DIAPH1 is a novel cause of microcephaly in humans. *Eur. J. Hum. Genet.* 23, 165–172. doi: 10.1038/ejhg.2014.82

Etienne-Manneville, S. (2004). Cdc42–the centre of polarity. *J. Cell Sci.* 117(Pt. 8), 1291–1300. doi: 10.1242/jcs.01115

Feng, Y., Chen, M. H., Moskowitz, I. P., Mendonza, A. M., Vidali, L., Nakamura, F., et al. (2006). Filamin A (FLNA) is required for cell-cell contact in vascular development and cardiac morphogenesis. *Proc. Natl. Acad. Sci. U S A* 103, 19836–19841. doi: 10.1073/pnas.0609628104

Ferland, R. J., Batiz, L. F., Neal, J., Lian, G., Bundock, E., Lu, J., et al. (2009). Disruption of neural progenitors along the ventricular and subventricular zones in periventricular heterotopia. *Hum. Mol. Genet.* 18, 497–516. doi: 10.1093/hmg/ddn377

Fox, J. W., Lamperti, E. D., Ekioğlu, Y. Z., Hong, S. E., Feng, Y., Graham, D. A., et al. (1998). Mutations in filamin 1 prevent migration of cerebral cortical neurons in human periventricular heterotopia. *Neuron* 21, 1315–1325. doi: 10.1016/s0896-6273(00)80651-0

Fox, J. W., and Walsh, C. A. (1999). Periventricular heterotopia and the genetics of neuronal migration in the cerebral cortex. *Am. J. Hum. Genet.* 65, 19–24. doi: 10.1086/302474

Fried, S., Matalon, O., Noy, E., and Barda-Saad, M. (2014). WIP: more than a WASp-interacting protein. *J. Leukoc. Biol.* 96, 713–727. doi: 10.1189/jlb.2ru0314-162r

Garrett, W. S., Chen, L. M., Kroschewski, R., Ebersold, M., Turley, S., Trombetta, S., et al. (2000). Developmental control of endocytosis in dendritic cells by Cdc42. *Cell* 102, 325–334. doi: 10.1016/s0092-8674(00)00038-6

Gonzalez-Billault, C., Muñoz-Llancao, P., Henriquez, D. R., Wojnacki, J., Conde, C., and Caceres, A. (2012). The role of small GTPases in neuronal morphogenesis and polarity. *Cytoskeleton (Hoboken)* 69, 464–485. doi: 10.1002/cm.21034

Gorlin, J. B., Yamin, R., Egan, S., Stewart, M., Stossel, T. P., Kwiatkowski, D. J., et al. (1990). Human endothelial actin-binding protein (ABP-280, nonmuscle filamin): a molecular leaf spring. *J. Cell Biol.* 111, 1089–1105. doi: 10.1083/jcb.111.3.1089

Götz, M., and Huttner, W. B. (2005). The cell biology of neurogenesis. *Nat. Rev. Mol. Cell Biol.* 6, 777–788. doi: 10.1038/nrm1739

Gould, C. J., Maiti, S., Michelot, A., Graziano, B. R., Blanchoin, L., and Goode, B. L. (2011). The formin DAD domain plays dual roles in autoinhibition and actin nucleation. *Curr. Biol.* 21, 384–390. doi: 10.1016/j.cub.2011.01.047

Govek, E. E., Newey, S. E., and Van Aelst, L. (2005). The role of the Rho GTPases in neuronal development. *Genes Dev.* 19, 1–49. doi: 10.1101/gad.1256405

Guerrini, R., Mei, D., Sisodiya, S., Sicca, F., Harding, B., Takahashi, Y., et al. (2004). Germline and mosaic mutations of FLN1 in men with periventricular heterotopia. *Neurology* 63, 51–56. doi: 10.1212/01.wnl.0000132818.84827.4d

Guo, M., Jan, L. Y., and Jan, Y. N. (1996). Control of daughter cell fates during asymmetric division: interaction of Numb and Notch. *Neuron* 17, 27–41. doi: 10.1016/S0896-6273(00)80278-0

Habas, R., Kato, Y., and He, X. (2001). Wnt/Frizzled activation of Rho regulates vertebrate gastrulation and requires a novel Formin homology protein Daam1. *Cell* 107, 843–854. doi: 10.1016/s0092-8674(01)00614-6

Hart, A. W., Morgan, J. E., Schneider, J., West, K., McKie, L., Bhattacharya, S., et al. (2006). Cardiac malformations and midline skeletal defects in mice lacking filamin A. *Hum. Mol. Genet.* 15, 2457–2467. doi: 10.1093/hmg/ddl168

Heng, Y. W., and Koh, C. G. (2010). Actin cytoskeleton dynamics and the cell division cycle. *Int. J. Biochem. Cell Biol.* 42, 1622–1633. doi: 10.1016/j.biocel.2010.04.007

Heng, J. I., Nguyen, L., Castro, D. S., Zimmer, C., Wildner, H., Armant, O., et al. (2008). Neurogenin 2 controls cortical neuron migration through regulation of Rnd2. *Nature* 455, 114–118. doi: 10.1038/nature07198

Hild, G., Kalmár, L., Kardos, R., Nyitrai, M., and Bugyi, B. (2014). The other side of the coin: functional and structural versatility of ADF/cofilins. *Eur. J. Cell Biol.* 93, 238–251. doi: 10.1016/j.ejcb.2013.12.001

Hu, J., Lu, J., Lian, G., Ferland, R. J., Dettenhofer, M., and Sheen, V. L. (2014). Formin 1 and filamin B physically interact to coordinate chondrocyte proliferation and differentiation in the growth plate. *Hum. Mol. Genet.* 23, 4663–4673. doi: 10.1093/hmg/ddu186

Iden, S., and Collard, J. G. (2008). Crosstalk between small GTPases and polarity proteins in cell polarization. *Nat. Rev. Mol. Cell Biol.* 9, 846–859. doi: 10.1038/nrm2521

Jurberg, A. D., Aires, R., Nóvoa, A., Rowland, J. E., and Mallo, M. (2014). Compartment-dependent activities of Wnt3a/beta-catenin signaling during vertebrate axial extension. *Dev. Biol.* 394, 253–263. doi: 10.1016/j.ydbio.2014.08.012

Kadowaki, M., Nakamura, S., Machon, O., Krauss, S., Radice, G. L., and Takeichi, M. (2007). N-cadherin mediates cortical organization in the mouse brain. *Dev. Biol.* 304, 22–33. doi: 10.1016/j.ydbio.2006.12.014

Katayama, K., Melendez, J., Baumann, J. M., Leslie, J. R., Chauhan, B. K., Nemkul, N., et al. (2011). Loss of RhoA in neural progenitor cells causes the disruption of adherens junctions and hyperproliferation. *Proc. Natl. Acad. Sci. U S A* 108, 7607–7612. doi: 10.1073/pnas.1101347108

Khaitlina, S. Y. (2014). Intracellular transport based on actin polymerization. *Biochemistry (Mosc)* 79, 917–927. doi: 10.1134/s0006297914090089

Knoblich, J. A. (2008). Mechanisms of asymmetric stem cell division. *Cell* 132, 583–597. doi: 10.1016/j.cell.2008.02.007

Kondo, Y., Hanai, A., Nakai, W., Katoh, Y., Nakayama, K., and Shin, H. W. (2012). ARF1 and ARF3 are required for the integrity of recycling endosomes and the recycling pathway. *Cell Struct. Funct.* 37, 141–154. doi: 10.1247/csf.12015

Krakow, D., Robertson, S. P., King, L. M., Morgan, T., Sebald, E. T., Bertolotto, C., et al. (2004). Mutations in the gene encoding filamin B disrupt vertebral segmentation, joint formation and skeletogenesis. *Nat. Genet.* 36, 405–410. doi: 10.1038/ng1319

Lamaze, C., Chuang, T. H., Terlecky, L. J., Bokoch, G. M., and Schmid, S. L. (1996). Regulation of receptor-mediated endocytosis by Rho and Rac. *Nature* 382, 177–179. doi: 10.1038/382177a0

Lee, K., and Song, K. (2007). Actin dysfunction activates ERK1/2 and delays entry into mitosis in mammalian cells. *Cell Cycle* 6, 1487–1495. doi: 10.4161/cc.6.12.4303

Leone, D. P., Srinivasan, K., Brakebusch, C., and McConnell, S. K. (2010). The rho GTPase Rac1 is required for proliferation and survival of progenitors in the developing forebrain. *Dev. Neurobiol.* 70, 659–678. doi: 10.1002/dneu.20804

Leung, S. M., Rojas, R., Maples, C., Flynn, C., Ruiz, W. G., Jou, T. S., et al. (1999). Modulation of endocytic traffic in polarized Madin-Darby canine kidney cells by the small GTPase RhoA. *Mol. Biol. Cell* 10, 4369–4384. doi: 10.1091/mbc.10.12.4369

Levayer, R., Pelissier-Monier, A., and Lecuit, T. (2011). Spatial regulation of Dia and Myosin-II by RhoGEF2 controls initiation of E-cadherin endocytosis during epithelial morphogenesis. *Nat. Cell Biol.* 13, 529–540. doi: 10.1038/ncb2224

Lian, G., Lu, J., Hu, J., Zhang, J., Cross, S. H., Ferland, R. J., et al. (2012). Filamin a regulates neural progenitor proliferation and cortical size through Wee1-dependent Cdk1 phosphorylation. *J. Neurosci.* 32, 7672–7684. doi: 10.1523/JNEUROSCI.0894-12.2012

Lu, J., and Sheen, V. (2005). Periventricular heterotopia. *Epilepsy Behav.* 7, 143–149. doi: 10.1016/j.yebeh.2005.05.001

Ma, X., and Adelstein, R. S. (2014). The role of vertebrate nonmuscle Myosin II in development and human disease. *Bioarchitecture* 4, 88–102. doi: 10.4161/bioa.29766

Ma, X., Bao, J., and Adelstein, R. S. (2007). Loss of cell adhesion causes hydrocephalus in nonmuscle myosin II-B-ablated and mutated mice. *Mol. Biol. Cell* 18, 2305–2312. doi: 10.1091/mbc.e07-01-0073

Machon, O., van den Bout, C. J., Backman, M., Kemler, R., and Krauss, S. (2003). Role of beta-catenin in the developing cortical and hippocampal neuroepithelium. *Neuroscience* 122, 129–143. doi: 10.1016/s0306-4522(03)00519-0

Maddox, A. S., and Burridge, K. (2003). RhoA is required for cortical retraction and rigidity during mitotic cell rounding. *J. Cell Biol.* 160, 255–265. doi: 10.1083/jcb.200207130

Mammoto, A., Huang, S., and Ingber, D. E. (2007). Filamin links cell shape and cytoskeletal structure to Rho regulation by controlling accumulation of p190RhoGAP in lipid rafts. *J. Cell Sci.* 120(Pt. 3), 456–467. doi: 10.1242/jcs.03353

Mammoto, A., Huang, S., Moore, K., Oh, P., and Ingber, D. E. (2004). Role of RhoA, mDia and ROCK in cell shape-dependent control of the Skp2–p27kip1 pathway and the G1/S transition. *J. Biol. Chem.* 279, 26323–26330. doi: 10.1074/jbc.m402725200

Massol, P., Montcourrier, P., Guillemot, J. C., and Chavrier, P. (1998). Fc receptor-mediated phagocytosis requires CDC42 and Rac1. *EMBO J.* 17, 6219–6229. doi: 10.1093/emboj/17.21.6219

Michaelson, D., Abidi, W., Guardavaccaro, D., Zhou, M., Ahearn, I., Pagano, M., et al. (2008). Rac1 accumulates in the nucleus during the G2 phase of the cell cycle and promotes cell division. *J. Cell Biol.* 181, 485–496. doi: 10.1083/jcb.200801047

Minobe, S., Sakakibara, A., Ohdachi, T., Kanda, R., Kimura, M., Nakatani, S., et al. (2009). Rac is involved in the interkinetic nuclear migration of cortical progenitor cells. *Neurosci. Res.* 63, 294–301. doi: 10.1016/j.neures.2009.01.006

Modarres, H. P., and Mofradt, M. R. (2014). Filamin: a structural and functional biomolecule with important roles in cell biology, signaling and mechanics. *Mol. Cell Biomech.* 11, 39–65. doi: 10.3970/mcb.2014.011.039

Moon, H. M., and Wynshaw-Boris, A. (2013). Cytoskeleton in action: lissencephaly, a neuronal migration disorder. *Wiley Interdiscip. Rev. Dev. Biol.* 2, 229–245. doi: 10.1002/wdev.67

Munro, E. M. (2006). PAR proteins and the cytoskeleton: a marriage of equals. *Curr. Opin. Cell Biol.* 18, 86–94. doi: 10.1016/j.ceb.2005.12.007

Murali, A., and Rajalingam, K. (2014). Small Rho GTPases in the control of cell shape and mobility. *Cell Mol. Life Sci.* 71, 1703–1721. doi: 10.1007/s00018-013-1519-6

Muriel, O., Echarri, A., Hellriegel, C., Pavón, D. M., Beccari, L., and Del Pozo, M. A. (2011). Phosphorylated filamin A regulates actin-linked caveolae dynamics. *J. Cell Sci.* 124(Pt. 16), 2763–2776. doi: 10.1242/jcs.080804

Musch, A., Cohen, D., Kreitzer, G., and Rodriguez-Boulan, E. (2001). cdc42 regulates the exit of apical and basolateral proteins from the trans-Golgi network. *EMBO J.* 20, 2171–2179. doi: 10.1093/emboj/20.9.2171

Nag, S., Larsson, M., Robinson, R. C., and Burtnick, L. D. (2013). Gelsolin: the tail of a molecular gymnast. *Cytoskeleton (Hoboken)* 70, 360–384. doi: 10.1002/cm.21117

Nagano, T., Morikubo, S., and Sato, M. (2004). Filamin A and FILIP (Filamin A-Interacting Protein) regulate cell polarity and motility in neocortical subventricular and intermediate zones during radial migration. *J. Neurosci.* 24, 9648–9657. doi: 10.1523/jneurosci.2363-04.2004

Nagano, T., Yoneda, T., Hatanaka, Y., Kubota, C., Murakami, F., and Sato, M. (2002). Filamin A-interacting protein (FILIP) regulates cortical cell migration out of the ventricular zone. *Nat. Cell Biol.* 4, 495–501. doi: 10.1038/ncb808

Nakamura, F., Stossel, T. P., and Hartwig, J. H. (2011). The filamins: organizers of cell structure and function. *Cell Adh. Migr.* 5, 160–169. doi: 10.4161/cam.5.2.14401

Nomachi, A., Nishita, M., Inaba, D., Enomoto, M., Hamasaki, M., and Minami, Y. (2008). Receptor tyrosine kinase Ror2 mediates Wnt5a-induced polarized cell migration by activating c-Jun N-terminal kinase via actin-binding protein filamin A. *J. Biol. Chem.* 283, 27973–27981. doi: 10.1074/jbc.M802325200

Nuno, D. W., Harrod, J. S., and Lamping, K. G. (2009). Sex-dependent differences in Rho activation contribute to contractile dysfunction in type 2 diabetic mice. *Am. J. Physiol. Heart Circ. Physiol.* 297, H1469–H1477. doi: 10.1152/ajpheart.00407.2009

Ohno, S. (2001). Intercellular junctions and cellular polarity: the PAR-aPKC complex, a conserved core cassette playing fundamental roles in cell polarity. *Curr. Opin. Cell Biol.* 13, 641–648. doi: 10.1016/s0955-0674(00)00264-7

Ohnuma, S., and Harris, W. A. (2003). Neurogenesis and the cell cycle. *Neuron* 40, 199–208. doi: 10.1016/S0896-6273(03)00632-9

Ohta, Y., Hartwig, J. H., and Stossel, T. P. (2006). FilGAP, a Rho- and ROCK-regulated GAP for Rac binds filamin A to control actin remodelling. *Nat. Cell Biol.* 8, 803–814. doi: 10.1038/ncb1437

Okumura, A., Hayashi, M., Shimojima, K., Ikeno, M., Uchida, T., Takanashi, J., et al. (2013). Whole-exome sequencing of a unique brain malformation with periventricular heterotopia, cingulate polymicrogyria and midbrain tectal hyperplasia. *Neuropathology* 33, 553–560. doi: 10.1111/neup.12007

Olson, M. F., Ashworth, A., and Hall, A. (1995). An essential role for Rho, Rac and Cdc42 GTPases in cell cycle progression through G1. *Science* 269, 1270–1272. doi: 10.1126/science.7652575

Otey, C. A., and Carpen, O. (2004). Alpha-actinin revisited: a fresh look at an old player. *Cell Motil. Cytoskeleton.* 58, 104–111. doi: 10.1002/cm.20007

Otomo, T., Otomo, C., Tomchick, D. R., Machius, M., and Rosen, M. K. (2005). Structural basis of Rho GTPase-mediated activation of the formin mDia1. *Mol. Cell* 18, 273–281. doi: 10.1016/j.molcel.2005.04.002

Pan, J., Lordier, L., Meyran, D., Rameau, P., Lecluse, Y., Kitchen-Goosen, S., et al. (2014). The formin DIAPH1 (mDia1) regulates megakaryocyte proplatelet formation by remodeling the actin and microtubule cytoskeletons. *Blood* 124, 3967–3977. doi: 10.1182/blood-2013-12-544924

Peng, X., Lin, Q., Liu, Y., Jin, Y., Druso, J. E., Antonyak, M. A., et al. (2013). Inactivation of Cdc42 in embryonic brain results in hydrocephalus with ependymal cell defects in mice. *Protein Cell* 4, 231–242. doi: 10.1007/s13238-012-2098-2

Phoenix, T. N., and Temple, S. (2010). Spred1, a negative regulator of Ras-MAPK-ERK, is enriched in CNS germinal zones, dampens NSC proliferation and maintains ventricular zone structure. *Genes Dev.* 24, 45–56. doi: 10.1101/gad.1839510

Raftopoulou, M., and Hall, A. (2004). Cell migration: Rho GTPases lead the way. *Dev. Biol.* 265, 23–32. doi: 10.1016/j.ydbio.2003.06.003

Razinia, Z., Mäkelä, T., Ylänne, J., and Calderwood, D. A. (2012). Filamins in mechanosensing and signaling. *Annu. Rev. Biophys.* 41, 227–246. doi: 10.1146/annurev-biophys-050511-102252

Ridley, A. J. (2006). Rho GTPases and actin dynamics in membrane protrusions and vesicle trafficking. *Trends Cell Biol.* 16, 522–529. doi: 10.1016/j.tcb.2006.08.006

Ridley, A. J., Schwartz, M. A., Burridge, K., Firtel, R. A., Ginsberg, M. H., Borisy, G., et al. (2003). Cell migration: integrating signals from front to back. *Science* 302, 1704–1709. doi: 10.1126/science.1092053

Rivas, R. J., and Hatten, M. E. (1995). Motility and cytoskeletal organization of migrating cerebellar granule neurons. *J. Neurosci.* 15, 981–989.

Robertson, S. P., Twigg, S. R., Sutherland-Smith, A. J., Biancalana, V., Gorlin, R. J., Horn, D., et al. (2003). Localized mutations in the gene encoding the cytoskeletal protein filamin A cause diverse malformations in humans. *Nat. Genet.* 33, 487–491. doi: 10.1038/ng1119

Rodriguez-Boulan, E., Kreitzer, G., and Müsch, A. (2005). Organization of vesicular trafficking in epithelia. *Nat. Rev. Mol. Cell Biol.* 6, 233–247. doi: 10.1038/nrm1593

Rönnstrand, L. (2004). Signal transduction via the stem cell factor receptor/c-Kit. *Cell. Mol. Life Sci.* 61, 2535–2548. doi: 10.1007/s00018-004-4189-6

Rosenblatt, J., Cramer, L. P., Baum, B., and McGee, K. M. (2004). Myosin II-dependent cortical movement is required for centrosome separation and positioning during mitotic spindle assembly. *Cell* 117, 361–372. doi: 10.1016/s0092-8674(04)00341-1

Rottner, K., and Stradal, T. E. (2011). Actin dynamics and turnover in cell motility. *Curr. Opin. Cell Biol.* 23, 569–578. doi: 10.1016/j.ceb.2011.07.003

Sawin, K. E. (2002). Cell polarity: following formin function. *Curr. Biol.* 12, R6–R8. doi: 10.1016/s0960-9822(01)00637-6

Schaar, B. T., and McConnell, S. K. (2005). Cytoskeletal coordination during neuronal migration. *Proc. Natl. Acad. Sci. U S A* 102, 13652–13657. doi: 10.1073/pnas.0506008102

Schönichen, A., and Geyer, M. (2010). Fifteen formins for an actin filament: a molecular view on the regulation of human formins. *Biochim. Biophys. Acta* 1803, 152–163. doi: 10.1016/j.bbamcr.2010.01.014

Schuh, M. (2011). An actin-dependent mechanism for long-range vesicle transport. *Nat. Cell Biol.* 13, 1431–1436. doi: 10.1038/ncb2353

Sheen, V. L. (2012). Periventricular Heterotopia: shuttling of proteins through vesicles and actin in cortical development and disease. *Scientifica (Cairo)* 2012:480129. doi: 10.6064/2012/480129

Sheen, V. L., Dixon, P. H., Fox, J. W., Hong, S. E., Kinton, L., Sisodiya, S. M., et al. (2001). Mutations in the X-linked filamin 1 gene cause periventricular nodular heterotopia in males as well as in females. *Hum. Mol. Genet.* 10, 1775–1783. doi: 10.1093/hmg/10.17.1775

Sheen, V. L., Feng, Y., Graham, D., Takafuta, T., Shapiro, S. S., and Walsh, C. A. (2002). Filamin A and Filamin B are co-expressed within neurons during periods of neuronal migration and can physically interact. *Hum. Mol. Genet.* 11, 2845–2854. doi: 10.1093/hmg/11.23.2845

Sheen, V. L., Ganesh, V. S., Topcu, M., Sebire, G., Bodell, A., Hill, R. S., et al. (2004). Mutations in ARFGEF2 implicate vesicle trafficking in neural progenitor proliferation and migration in the human cerebral cortex. *Nat. Genet.* 36, 69–76. doi: 10.1038/ng1276

Sheen, V. L., Jansen, A., Chen, M. H., Parrini, E., Morgan, T., Ravenscroft, R., et al. (2005). Filamin a mutations cause periventricular heterotopia with Ehlers-Danlos syndrome. *Neurology* 64, 254–262. doi: 10.1212/01.wnl.0000149512.79621.df

Sheen, V. L., Topçu, M., Berkovic, S., Yalnizoglu, D., Blatt, I., Bodell, A., et al. (2003). Autosomal recessive form of periventricular heterotopia. *Neurology* 60, 1108–1112. doi: 10.1212/01.wnl.0000055898.00349.02

Shinohara, R., Thumkeo, D., Kamijo, H., Kaneko, N., Sawamoto, K., Watanabe, K., et al. (2012). A role for mDia, a Rho-regulated actin nucleator, in tangential migration of interneuron precursors. *Nat. Neurosci.* 15, 373–380, S1–S2. doi: 10.1038/nn.3020

Solecki, D. J., Trivedi, N., Govek, E. E., Kerekes, R. A., Gleason, S. S., and Hatten, M. E. (2009). Myosin II motors and F-actin dynamics drive the coordinated movement of the centrosome and soma during CNS glial-guided neuronal migration. *Neuron* 63, 63–80. doi: 10.1016/j.neuron.2009.05.028

Sordella, R., Jiang, W., Chen, G. C., Curto, M., and Settleman, J. (2003). Modulation of Rho GTPase signaling regulates a switch between adipogenesis and myogenesis. *Cell* 113, 147–158. doi: 10.1016/s0092-8674(03)00271-x

Soumiya, H., Fukumitsu, H., and Furukawa, S. (2009). Stem cell factor induces heterotopic accumulation of cells (heterotopia) in the mouse cerebral cortex. *Biomed. Res.* 30, 121–128. doi: 10.2220/biomedres.30.121

Symons, M., and Rusk, N. (2003). Control of vesicular trafficking by Rho GTPases. *Curr. Biol.* 13, R409–R418. doi: 10.1016/S0960-9822(03)00324-5

Taverna, E., Götz, M., and Huttner, W. B. (2014). The cell biology of neurogenesis: toward an understanding of the development and evolution of the neocortex. *Annu. Rev. Cell Dev. Biol.* 30, 465–502. doi: 10.1146/annurev-cellbio-101011-155801

Théry, M., Racine, V., Pépin, A., Piel, M., Chen, Y., Sibarita, J. B., et al. (2005). The extracellular matrix guides the orientation of the cell division axis. *Nat. Cell Biol.* 7, 947–953. doi: 10.1038/ncb1307

Thumkeo, D., Shinohara, R., Watanabe, K., Takebayashi, H., Toyoda, Y., Tohyama, K., et al. (2011). Deficiency of mDia, an actin nucleator, disrupts integrity of neuroepithelium and causes periventricular dysplasia. *PLoS One* 6:e25465. doi: 10.1371/journal.pone.0025465

Vidaki, M., Tivodar, S., Doulgeraki, K., Tybulewicz, V., Kessaris, N., Pachnis, V., et al. (2012). Rac1-dependent cell cycle exit of MGE precursors and GABAergic interneuron migration to the cortex. *Cereb. Cortex* 22, 680–692. doi: 10.1093/cercor/bhr145

Wang, Z., Sandiford, S., Wu, C., and Li, S. S. (2009). Numb regulates cell-cell adhesion and polarity in response to tyrosine kinase signalling. *EMBO J.* 28, 2360–2373. doi: 10.1038/emboj.2009.190

Witte, H., and Bradke, F. (2008). The role of the cytoskeleton during neuronal polarization. *Curr. Opin. Neurobiol.* 18, 479–487. doi: 10.1016/j.conb.2008.09.019

Woodhead, G. J., Mutch, C. A., Olson, E. C., and Chenn, A. (2006). Cell-autonomous beta-catenin signaling regulates cortical precursor proliferation. *J. Neurosci.* 26, 12620–12630. doi: 10.1523/jneurosci.3180-06.2006

Yamana, N., Arakawa, Y., Nishino, T., Kurokawa, K., Tanji, M., Itoh, R. E., et al. (2006). The Rho-mDia1 pathway regulates cell polarity and focal adhesion turnover in migrating cells through mobilizing Apc and c-Src. *Mol. Cell Biol.* 26, 6844–6858. doi: 10.1128/mcb.00283-06

Yang, B., Radel, C., Hughes, D., Kelemen, S., and Rizzo, V. (2011). p190 RhoGTPase-activating protein links the beta1 integrin/caveolin-1 mechanosignaling complex to RhoA and actin remodeling. *Arterioscler. Thromb. Vasc. Biol.* 31, 376–383. doi: 10.1161/ATVBAHA.110.217794

Yang, T., Sun, Y., Zhang, F., Zhu, Y., Shi, L., Li, H., et al. (2012). POSH localizes activated Rac1 to control the formation of cytoplasmic dilation of the leading process and neuronal migration. *Cell Rep.* 2, 640–651. doi: 10.1016/j.celrep.2012.08.007

Yasuda, S., Oceguera-Yanez, F., Kato, T., Okamoto, M., Yonemura, S., Terada, Y., et al. (2004). Cdc42 and mDia3 regulate microtubule attachment to kinetochores. *Nature* 428, 767–771. doi: 10.1038/nature02452

Zhang, J., Neal, J., Lian, G., Hu, J., Lu, J., and Sheen, V. (2013). Filamin A regulates neuronal migration through brefeldin A-inhibited guanine exchange factor 2-dependent Arf1 activation. *J. Neurosci.* 33, 15735–15746. doi: 10.1523/JNEUROSCI.1939-13.2013

Zhang, J., Neal, J., Lian, G., Shi, B., Ferland, R. J., and Sheen, V. (2012). Brefeldin A-inhibited guanine exchange factor 2 regulates filamin A phosphorylation and neuronal migration. *J. Neurosci.* 32, 12619–12629. doi: 10.1523/JNEUROSCI.1063-12.2012

Zhang, Y., Wang, F., Niu, Y., Liu, H. L., Rui, R., Cui, X. S., et al. (2015). Formin mDia1, a downstream molecule of FMNL1, regulates Profilin1 for actin assembly and spindle organization during mouse oocyte meiosis. *Biochim. Biophys. Acta* 1853, 317–327. doi: 10.1016/j.bbamcr.2014.11.005

Zhou, F., Leder, P., Zuniga, A., and Dettenhofer, M. (2009). Formin1 disruption confers oligodactylism and alters Bmp signaling. *Hum. Mol. Genet.* 18, 2472–2482. doi: 10.1093/hmg/ddp185

7

Resurgent Sodium Current in Neurons of the Cerebral Cortex

Giulia Quattrocolo, Keagan Dunville and Maximiliano José Nigro**

Center for Neural Computation, Egil and Pauline Braathen and Fred Kavli Center for Cortical Microcircuits, Kavli Institute for Systems Neuroscience, Norwegian University of Science and Technology, Trondheim, Norway

***Correspondence:**
Giulia Quattrocolo
Giulia.quattrocolo@ntnu.no
Maximiliano José Nigro
Maximiliano.j.nigro@ntnu.no

In the late '90, Dr. Indira Raman, at the time a postdoctoral fellow with Dr. Bruce Bean, at Harvard University, identified a new type of sodium current, flowing through the channels that reopens when the membrane is repolarized. This current, called "resurgent Sodium current," was originally identified in cerebellar Purkinje neurons and has now been confirmed in around 20 different neuronal types. Since moving to Northwestern University in 1999 to establish her own research group, Dr. Raman has dedicated great efforts in identifying the mechanisms supporting the resurgent Sodium current and how its biophysical properties shape the firing of the different cell types. Her work has impacted greatly the field of cellular neurophysiology, from basic research to translation neuroscience. In fact, alterations in the resurgent sodium currents have been observed in several neuropathologies, from Huntington's disease to epilepsy. In this Perspective we will focus on the current knowledge on the expression and function of the resurgent Sodium current in neurons of the cerebral cortex and hippocampus. We will also briefly highlight the role of Dr. Raman's as teacher and mentor, not only for her pupils, but for the whole scientific community.

Keywords: resurgent sodium current, cortical neurons, hippocampus, sodium channels, neurophysiology

INTRODUCTION

Neuronal voltage-gated Sodium channels (VGSCs) are responsible for the large and transient inward current (I_{NaT}) underlying the upstroke of the action potential (AP) (Hodgkin and Huxley, 1952a). After opening, VGSCs quickly inactivate and require strong membrane hyperpolarization to become available (Hodgkin and Huxley, 1952b). Many neurons express subthreshold non-inactivating Sodium currents: a persistent sodium current (I_{NaP}) flowing through non-inactivated VGSCs, and resurgent Sodium current (I_{NaR}) that activates upon membrane repolarization (Stafstrom et al., 1982; Crill, 1996; Raman and Bean, 1997). Subthreshold sodium currents can powerfully shape spike after-potentials and repetitive firing (Raman and Bean, 1997; Khaliq et al., 2003; Yamada-Hanff and Bean, 2013). I_{NaR} has first been described in isolated cerebellar Purkinje neurons, where it contributes to the generation of complex spikes and repetitive spontaneous firing (Raman and Bean, 1997; Khaliq et al., 2003). I_{NaR} has been identified in many different cell-types throughout the brain, with conserved biophysical properties (Lewis and Raman, 2014). Thanks to the elegant work of Dr. Raman and collaborators, I_{NaR}, together with I_{NaT}, is the best characterized component of the Sodium current. Indeed, Dr. Raman's original description highlighted the role of I_{NaR} in bursting in Purkinje neurons and developed a model for its generation hypothesizing the existence of a blocking particle that enters the pore at open states and is released upon repolarization (Raman and Bean, 1997, 2001). Later, Dr. Raman led her laboratory on a quest to decipher the structural and molecular mechanisms of I_{NaR}, discovering the interaction of alpha and beta subunits of VGSCs underlying open channel block and the identity of the blocking particle (Grieco et al., 2005; Aman and Raman, 2007, 2010; Aman et al., 2009; Bant and Raman, 2010; Lewis and Raman, 2011, 2013). Following its description in Purkinje cells, the discovery of I_{NaR} in other cell-types has propelled research on the molecular underpinnings and physiological role of I_{NaR} in the brainstem, basal ganglia and peripheral sensory neurons (Do and Bean, 2003; Cummins et al., 2005; Enomoto et al., 2006; Barbosa et al., 2015), as well as its involvement in disorders such as pain, long QT syndrome and epilepsy (Jarecki et al., 2010; Hargus et al., 2011). In this review we want to focus on I_{NaR} in neurons of the cerebral cortex, where the work of Dr. Raman inspired our own first steps in the field of neurophysiology. The authors started their journey in neuroscience by studying the expression of I_{NaR} in cortical neurons and were deeply inspired by the solidity and elegance of the experimental work of Dr. Raman. One of us (GQ) had the chance to attend Dr. Raman's "Great experiments in Cellular Neurophysiology" course at Northwestern University, experiencing her outstanding teaching.

EXPRESSION OF I_{NaR} IN CORTICAL AND HIPPOCAMPAL NEURONS

Soon after Raman and Bean (1997) first described it in cerebellar Purkinje cells, the I_{NaR} has been identified in several cell types of the cerebellum, brainstem, basal ganglia, and dorsal root ganglia (Lewis and Raman, 2014). Raman and Bean (1997) also described the absence of I_{NaR} in acutely isolated pyramidal neurons of the CA3 region. In the cerebral cortex, I_{NaR} was first reported in layer II of the rat perirhinal cortex (Castelli et al., 2007a). This first report was followed shortly by an examination of the expression of I_{NaR} across the hippocampus and parahippocampal region (Castelli et al., 2007b). In the perirhinal and entorhinal cortices 75–100% of excitatory neurons express I_{NaR} depending on layer localization. In these regions the resurgent conductance amounts to 1.5–3% of the conductance of the transient component. As opposed to other types of neurons, the channels responsible for the I_{NaR} in cortical neurons are enriched in the axon initial segment. Indeed, application of TTx to the axon initial segment of perirhinal neurons abolished I_{NaR} to a larger extent than when applied to the soma/proximal apical dendrite (Castelli et al., 2007a). Moreover, patch clamp recordings from acutely isolated cortical neurons rarely show I_{NaR} (Castelli et al., 2007a). In the parahippocampal region, I_{NaR} is expressed most prominently by layer II excitatory neurons of the medial entorhinal cortex (MEC) (Castelli et al., 2007b). In MEC layer II, I_{NaR} was found in all recorded neurons, with an amplitude representing 3.6% that of I_{NaT}, the second largest among neurons of the cerebral cortex (Castelli et al., 2007b; Nigro et al., 2012). MEC layer II neurons express all three components of the Sodium current: I_{NaT}, I_{NaP}, and I_{NaR}. The developmental expression of the I_{NaR} in MEC layer II follows a trajectory that is independent from that of the other components, increasing steadily in amplitude from postnatal day (P) 5 to P10 (Nigro et al., 2012). In parallel, the percent of neurons expressing I_{NaR} also increases in the same developmental window (Nigro et al., 2012).

In the hippocampus I_{NaR} is expressed in subpopulations of excitatory neurons in the dentate gyrus (60%), ventral CA1 (40%), and the majority of subicular neurons (Castelli et al., 2007b; Barker et al., 2017). Interestingly, I_{NaR} does not seem to be expressed by pyramidal neurons of the dorsal hippocampus or in CA3 pyramidal neurons recorded from brain slices (Castelli et al., 2007b). Future studies correlating I_{NaR} expression to transcriptomic cell types might shed light on the molecular identity of neurons expressing I_{NaR} and the molecular mechanisms underlying its expression in the cortex (see below).

CONTRIBUTION OF I_{NaR} TO FIRING PROPERTIES OF CORTICAL NEURONS

Several neuron types expressing I_{NaR} show spontaneous firing with relatively high firing rates and bursting, e.g., Purkinje cells, subthalamic neurons, neurons of the cerebellar nuclei (Lewis and Raman, 2014). I_{NaR} endows these cell-types with the ability to produce repetitive spiking spontaneously (i.e., in absence of synaptic activity) at high frequencies by preventing fast inactivation through open channel block (Raman and Bean, 2001; Khaliq et al., 2003). At depolarized membrane potentials, the open channel block competes with fast inactivation, and during repolarization, the transition from open channel block to open states allows Sodium ions to flow and initiate a new cycle of spiking (Raman and Bean, 2001). Excitatory neurons of the cerebral cortex do not produce spontaneous repetitive firing, nor they reach high firing frequency, but fire trains of action potentials with different degrees of adaptation. I_{NaR} has been shown to contribute to repetitive firing in layer II pyramidal neurons of the rat perirhinal cortex (Castelli et al., 2007a). These neurons produce repetitive firing up to 30 Hz upon depolarizing current injection, a firing frequency much lower than other I_{NaR} expressing neurons outside the cerebral cortex. However, even at those firing frequencies I_{NaR} contributes to most of the Sodium current during the interspike interval promoting depolarization and repetitive firing (Castelli et al., 2007a).

By injecting AP waveforms (recorded in current clamp) in voltage clamp experiments, Raman and Bean (1997) demonstrated that I_{NaR} provides a major contribution to the generation of complex spikes in Purkinje neurons. Inspired by these original experiments, Alessi et al. (2016) tested the contribution of different ionic conductances to the generation of the depolarizing afterpotential (DAP) in MEC layer II stellate cells. The authors described two mechanisms generating DAPs in these cells acting at different membrane voltages. At hyperpolarized holding potentials T-type Calcium channels provide most of the depolarization following the fast afterhyperpolarization (fAHP). However, at holding voltages closer to the resting potential, subthreshold Sodium currents (I_{NaP} and I_{NaR}) are the major contributors to the DAP (Alessi et al., 2016). During spatial navigation, MEC layer II stellate cells show a spatially modulated firing pattern characterized by regularly spaced firing fields arranged in a hexagonal matrix, as described for grid cells (Fyhn et al., 2004; Hafting et al., 2005; Domnisoru et al., 2013; Schmidt-Hieber and Hausser, 2013;

Rowland et al., 2018). MEC stellate cells with grid firing patterns also show a higher probability of generating bursts of APs during navigation (Latuske et al., 2015; Bant et al., 2020). Interestingly, bursting probability and amplitude of I_{NaR} show a gradient along the dorso-ventral axis of the MEC that correlates with the gradient in spacing and field size of grid cells along the same axis (Bant et al., 2020). The authors observed that using bursts increased the performance of decoding the animal's position during navigation as compared to isolated spikes. The higher information content of burst points to a cellular mechanism to maximize signal-to-noise ratio in dorsal MEC grid cells (Bant et al., 2020). We would like to highlight that these interesting results were obtained by Dr. Jason Bant, a previous student of Dr. Raman, teaming up with Dr. Lisa Giocomo, who pioneered the study of the topographic organization of biophysical properties in MEC.

MOLECULAR MECHANISM OF I_{NaR} IN CORTICAL NEURONS

Patch clamp experiments from Purkinje neurons obtained from Nav1.6 (*Scn8a*) null mice showed that this subunit contributes to most of the I_{NaR} in these neurons (Raman et al., 1997). However, the alpha subunit on its own cannot generate I_{NaR}. Indeed Nav1.6 is also expressed in CA3 neurons that do not express I_{NaR} (Raman and Bean, 1997). The mechanism generating I_{NaR} involves a blocking particle that interacts with the alpha subunit (Raman and Bean, 2001). In a series of elegant experiments, Grieco et al. (2005) demonstrated that the blocking particle consists of the beta subunit Navβ4 (Grieco et al., 2005). Knockdown expression of the Navβ4 in cerebellar granule cells and peripheral sensory neurons strongly reduced I_{NaR}, further highlighting the role of this beta subunit in generating I_{NaR} (Bant and Raman, 2010; Barbosa et al., 2015). In cortical neurons, Nav1.6 is expressed at high levels in the axon initial segment correlating with the subcellular expression of I_{NaR} in these neurons (Castelli et al., 2007a; Royeck et al., 2008; Buffington and Rasband, 2013). On the other hand, most of the cortical cells in which I_{NaR} has been observed express Navβ4 at very low levels (Buffington and Rasband, 2013) or completely lack *scn4b* expression (Yu et al., 2003; Lewis and Raman, 2014; **Table 1**). *In situ* hybridization (ISH) data from the Allen Brain Institute suggest a low level of expression in a subpopulation of layer II stellate cells in the dorsal MEC, which correlates with the dorso-ventral gradient of I_{NaR} in these neurons (Lein et al., 2007; Bant et al., 2020). In the hippocampus, *scn4b* is expressed in the dorsal CA1, where I_{NaR} is not expressed (Castelli et al., 2007b). The absence of I_{NaR} in CA1 pyramidal neurons might be explained by a slicing artifact by which the axon initial segment of CA1 neurons was lost. However, the recordings in CA1 were performed from coronal slices that preserve cellular integrity (Dougherty et al., 2012). Additionally, *scn4b* expression might not be sufficient for I_{NaR} expression in all cell types. A recent single cell transcriptomic analysis of the whole cortex and hippocampus by the Allen Brain Institute (Yao et al., 2021) showed that expression of *scn4b* is restricted to a handful of layer V neurons, none of whom are known to express I_{NaR}. The discrepancy between ISH and single cell transcriptomic in MEC might be due to the sparseness of *scn4b* expressing neurons in this region (**Figure 1**). Additionally, this discrepancy may arise because of sample processing differences between ISH and single cell transcriptomics. In ISH, the tissue remains intact and preserves cytosolic compartments, like distal neuronal processes, that are otherwise destroyed in tissue homogenization for single cell RNA processing. Alternatively, single cell RNA sequencing intrinsically yields low rates of capture (Zheng et al., 2017) and read efficiency which must be accounted for computationally (Galfrè et al., 2021). Tissue homogenization is similar between bulk and single cell RNA sequencing and differences in technique should yield similar results. Bulk transcriptomic analysis comparing the dorsal and ventral MEC from adult mice in Ramsden et al. (2015), however, demonstrates that *scn4b* is significantly upregulated in the dorsal MEC at P60 (**Figure 1B**). Moreover, it is expressed at a level which drives distance-based clustering separation between the dorsal and ventral MEC (Ramsden et al., 2015). This discrepancy in the single cell dataset may not be related to weakness in gene detection or homogenization methods. Instead, gene expression differences in the dorsal-ventral axis in the adult single cell dataset may not have been considered and thus cells in ventral layer II may mask *scnb4* expression in dorsal layer II. Interestingly, a subgroup of pyramidal tract (PT) projecting layer V neurons showed a significant expression of *scn4b*, suggesting the possible expression of I_{NaR} in this type of cells. The expression of *scn4b* in layer V cortical neurons shows a gradient along the rostrocaudal axis of the telencephalon. Strong *scn4b* expression in layer V is evident in motor areas, sensory cortices, anterior cingulate and retrosplenial cortex. *Scn4b* seems to be absent in association areas, including the insula, parahippocampal area and medial prefrontal areas (**Figures 1C–G**). Future electrophysiological experiments might corroborate the presence of I_{NaR} in these cortical neurons. The molecular nature of the blocking particle in cortical neurons also remains enigmatic, particularly in the perirhinal cortex, ventral CA1 and dentate gyrus. Current approaches to characterize the transcriptomic and electrophysiological profile of neurons will shed light on the molecular underpinnings of I_{NaR} in cortical neurons (Cadwell et al., 2016).

I_{NaR} IN EPILEPSY

The contribution of I_{NaR} to repetitive spiking, DAP and burst generation suggests that it might play a role in disorders where neuronal excitability is altered, such as epilepsy. This component of the Sodium current is expressed in cortical areas that are strongly affected in temporal lobe epilepsy (TLE), such as MEC, perirhinal cortex, hippocampus and subiculum. I_{NaR} expressing MEC layer II neurons are spared in temporal lobe epilepsy, but they show an increased excitability (Bear et al., 1996). The increased excitability is in part due to a reorganization of the synaptic network (Kuman et al., 2007), however intrinsic mechanisms are also at play. Indeed, in the absence of synaptic inputs, layer II MEC neurons show a higher firing rate in response to current injection in a rat model of TLE (Hargus et al., 2011). These changes in intrinsic excitability correlate

TABLE 1 | Cell-types where I_{NaR} expression and/or *scn4b* has been investigated.

Cell type	I_{NaR} expression	*scn4b* expression by ISH	References
CA3 pyramidal neuron	No	No	Raman and Bean, 1997; Yu et al., 2003 Allen Institute
Dorsal CA1 pyramidal neuron	No	Low	Yu et al., 2003 Allen Institute Castelli et al., 2007b
Ventral CA1 pyramidal neuron	35% of tested neurons	No	Yu et al., 2003 Allen Institute Castelli et al., 2007b
Dentate granule cells	60% of tested neurons	No	Yu et al., 2003 Allen Institute Castelli et al., 2007b
Subiculular pyramidal neurons	Most tested neurons	Yes	Allen Institute Barker et al., 2017
MEC LII stellate cells	Yes	Low in dorsal MEC (not detectable with single cell transcriptomics)	Allen Institute Castelli et al., 2007b
MEC LII pyramidal cells	Yes	Possibly in dorsal MEC	Allen Institute Castelli et al., 2007b
MEC LIII pyramidal cells	80% of tested neurons	No	Allen Institute Castelli et al., 2007b
MEC LV pyramidal neurons	70% of tested neurons	No	Allen Institute Castelli et al., 2007b
Perirhinal LII pyramidal neurons	90% of tested neurons	No	Allen Institute Castelli et al., 2007b
Perirhinal LV pyramidal neurons	80% of tested neurons	No	Allen Institute Castelli et al., 2007b
Neocortical LV pyramidal neurons	Unknown	Yes (detectable also with single cell transcriptomics)	Yu et al., 2003 Allen Institute

with an increased amplitude of all components of the Sodium current (Hargus et al., 2011). The molecular underpinnings of the increased excitability reside in an increased expression of the Nav1.6 subunit. Indeed, pharmacological blockade of Nav1.6 channels with 4,9-anidro-tetrodotoxin rescued the excitability of TLE MEC layer II neurons to levels like control neurons (Hargus et al., 2013). Moreover, similar alterations in intrinsic excitability and Sodium currents are recapitulated in mice carrying a mutated Nav1.6 isoform (Ottolini et al., 2017; Pan and Cummins, 2020). An increased excitability and augmented I_{NaR} and I_{NaP} have recently been described in human excitatory cortical neurons differentiated from pluripotent stem-cells obtained from patients affected by early infantile epileptic encephalopathy type 13 (*Scn8a*-related epilepsy) (Tidball et al., 2020).

DISCUSSION

In the current perspective we aimed at reviewing the state-of-the-art of the research on the I_{NaR} in neurons of the cerebral cortex. The expression of I_{NaR} has been reported in nine cortical cell-types, and we propose its expression in a population of layer V PT neurons based on their expression of Navβ4. The contribution of I_{NaR} to the firing behavior of cortical neurons has been well demonstrated in the perirhinal and entorhinal cortices. In these areas, I_{NaR} supports repetitive firing, DAPs and bursting. Bursting in LII MEC neurons has been proposed to maximize signal-to-noise ratio in grid cells and might represent a cellular mechanism for a reliable transmission of spatial information to the hippocampus (Bant et al., 2020).

The molecular mechanisms underlying I_{NaR} in cortical neurons are yet to be described. The molecular identity of the blocking particle in many cortical cell types remains unknown and future studies describing the correlation of trascriptomics and electrophysiology will allow to uncover potential candidates. These studies will also provide molecular targets for pharmacological treatments of epileptic encephalopaties involving I_{NaR}.

With this perspective, we wished to emphasize the pivotal influence of Dr. Raman's work on the mechanism of open-channel block, molecular identity of the blocking particle, and physiological role of I_{NaR} in cerebellar Purkinje neurons. Her findings sparked the quest for I_{NaR} in the cerebral cortex and provided the foundations for our current understanding of the role of I_{NaR} in the firing properties of cortical neurons.

In addition to her scientific contribution, Dr. Raman has also always been interested in forging new generations of scientists. Anyone who had the privilege of attending a class or a lecture given by Dr. Raman knows it will not be boring. Her scientific knowledge will engage you and her ability to introduce interesting anecdotes on the "behind the scenes" will enchant you. Her outstanding teaching abilities have been recognized by multiple awards received at Northwestern University, but her drive to good mentoring and good science has not stopped in Chicago. Dr. Raman has contributed to a series of feature articles titled "Living science" published in eLIFE from 2015 to 2019 (Raman, 2015a,b, 2016, 2017, 2019). In addition, her piece on good mentoring (Raman, 2014) faithfully describes the challenges faced by both the trainee and the advisor.

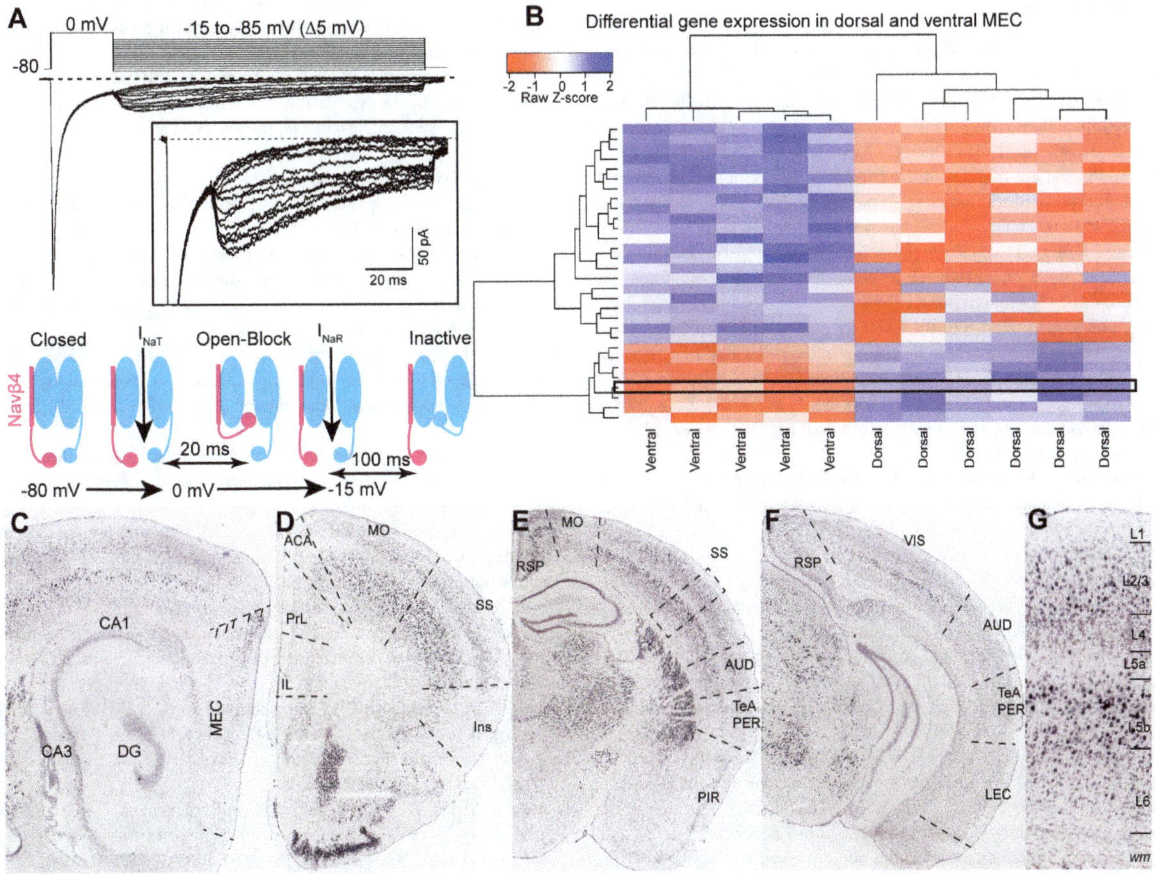

FIGURE 1 | (A) Representative voltage-clamp recording of sodium currents in a layer II neuron in MEC. Sodium currents were evoked by the voltage steps shown in the upper panel. A 20 ms step to 0 mV evoked INaT and was followed by a family of repolarizing steps from −15 to −85 mV to elicit INaR. Insert shows an expanded view of the INaR. The schematic in the lower panel shows the sequence of events generating INaR in sodium channels associated with a Navβ4 subunit.
(B) Differentially expressed gene analysis of data from Ramsden et al. (2015). Gene expression driven separation between ventral and dorsal medial entorhinal cortex from P60 mice. *Scn4b* is highlighted by a black rectangle and appears as one of 8 genes significantly enriched in the dorsal adult MEC. Heatmap displays 34 genes significantly up or downregulated in either ventral or dorsal MEC samples (p-val. < 0.05, $\log_2$FC threshold ± 1.5, Benjamini-Hochberg corrected; hierarchical clustering performed by pairwise-Spearman correlation matrix). **(C–G)** ISH experiments from the Allen Institute showing the expression of *scn4b* across the cerebral cortex. **(C)** *Scn4b* is expressed in the dorsal MEC. **(D–F)** Expression of *scn4b* in the isocortex decreases from rostral **(C)** to caudal **(F)** regions. **(G)** Magnification of the somatosensory (SS) area highlighted by a dotted box in **(C)**. CA, Cornu Ammonis; DG, dentate gyrus; MEC, medial entorhinal cortex; IL, infralimbic; PrL, prelimbic; ACA, anterior cingulate area; MO, motor area; SS, somatosensory area; Ins, insula; AUD, auditory area; TeA, temporal association area; PER, perirhinal cortex; PIR, piriform cortex; RSP, retrosplenial area; VIS, visual area; LEC, lateral entorhinal cortex. Image credit: For **(A)**: adapted from Nigro et al. (2012) with permission from Elsevier. For **(C–G)** Allen Institute. 2004 Allen Institute for Brain Science. Allen Mouse Brain Atlas. Available from: https://mouse.brain-map.org/.

Dr. Raman contribution to science and her effort to make the scientific world a better place for young trainees and women has left a mark on the authors as well as, we are sure, on all the people that had trained with her and have known her.

AUTHOR CONTRIBUTIONS

GQ and MN conceived the study and analyzed the data. KD analyzed the data. All authors wrote the manuscript.

FUNDING

This study has been supported by the Centre of Excellence scheme of the Research Council of Norway—Centre for Neural Computation (Grant No. 223262), and the Kavli Foundation. This project has received funding from the European Union's Horizon 2020 Research and Innovation Programme under the Marie Skłodowska-Curie Grant Nos. 885955 to MN and 839988 to GQ.

REFERENCES

Alessi, C., Raspanti, A., and Magistretti, J. (2016). Two distinct types of depolarizing afterpotentials are differentially expressed in stellate and pyramidal-like neurons of entorhinal-cortex layer II. *Hippocampus* 26, 380–404. doi: 10.1002/hipo.22529

Aman, T. K., Grieco-Calub, T. M., Chen, C., Ruscon, R., Slat, E. A., Isom, L. L., et al. (2009). Regulation of persistent Na current by interactions between beta subunits of voltage-gated Na channels. *J. Neurosci.* 29, 2027–2042. doi: 10.1523/JNEUROSCI.4531-08.2009

Aman, T. K., and Raman, I. M. (2007). Subunit dependence of Na channel slow inactivation and open channel block in cerebellar neurons. *Biophys. J.* 92, 1938–1951. doi: 10.1529/biophysj.106.093500

Aman, T. K., and Raman, I. M. (2010). Inwardly permeating Na ions generate the voltage dependence of resurgent Na current in cerebellar Purkinje neurons. *J. Neurosci.* 30, 5629–5634. doi: 10.1523/JNEUROSCI.0376-10.2010

Bant, J. S., Hardcastle, K., Ocko, S. A., and Giocomo, L. M. (2020). Topography in the bursting dynamics of entorhinal neurons. *Cell Rep.* 30, 2349.e7–2359.e7. doi: 10.1016/j.celrep.2020.01.057

Bant, J. S., and Raman, I. M. (2010). Control of transient, resurgent, and persistent current by open-channel block by Na channel beta4 in cultured cerebellar granule neurons. *Proc. Natl. Acad. Sci. U.S.A.* 107, 12357–12362. doi: 10.1073/pnas.1005633107

Barbosa, C., Tan, Z.-Y., Wang, R., Xie, W., Strong, J. A., Patel, R. R., et al. (2015). Navβ4 regulates fast resurgent sodium currents and excitability in sensory neurons. *Mol. Pain* 11:60. doi: 10.1186/s12990-015-0063-9

Barker, B. S., Nigam, A., Ottolini, M., Gaykema, R. P., Hargus, N. J., and Patel, M. K. (2017). Pro-excitatory alterations in sodium channel activity facilitate subiculum neuron hyperexcitability in temporal lobe epilepsy. *Neurobiol. Dis.* 108, 183–194. doi: 10.1016/j.nbd.2017.08.018

Bear, J., Fountain, N. B., and Lothman, E. W. (1996). Responses of the superficial entorhinal cortex in vitro in slices from naive and chronically epileptic rats. *J. Neurophysiol.* 76, 2928–2940. doi: 10.1152/jn.1996.76.5.2928

Buffington, S. A., and Rasband, M. N. (2013). Na+ channel-dependent recruitment of Navβ4 to axon initial segments and nodes of Ranvier. *J. Neurosci.* 33, 6191–6202. doi: 10.1523/JNEUROSCI.4051-12.2013

Cadwell, C. R., Palasantza, A., Jiang, X., Berens, P., Deng, Q., Yilmaz, M., et al. (2016). Electrophysiological, transcriptomic and morphologic profiling of single neurons using Patch-seq. *Nat. Biotechnol.* 34, 199–203. doi: 10.1038/nbt.3445

Castelli, L., Biella, G., Toselli, M., and Magistretti, J. (2007a). Resurgent Na+ current in pyramidal neurones of rat perirhinal cortex: axonal location of channels and contribution to depolarizing drive during repetitive firing. *J. Physiol.* 582(Pt 3), 1179–1193. doi: 10.1113/jphysiol.2007.135350

Castelli, L., Nigro, M. J., and Magistretti, J. (2007b). Analysis of resurgent sodium-current expression in rat parahippocampal cortices and hippocampal formation. *Brain Res.* 1163, 44–55. doi: 10.1016/j.brainres.2007.05.065

Crill, W. E. (1996). Persistent sodium current in mammalian central neurons. *Annu. Rev. Physiol.* 58, 349–362. doi: 10.1146/annurev.ph.58.030196.002025

Cummins, T. R., Dib-Hajj, S. D., Herzog, R. I., and Waxman, S. G. (2005). $Na_V1.6$ channels generate resurgent sodium currents in spinal sensory neurons. *FEBS Lett.* 579, 2166–2170. doi: 10.1016/j.febslet.2005.03.009

Do, M. T., and Bean, B. P. (2003). Subthreshold sodium currents and pacemaking of subthalamic neurons: modulation by slow inactivation. *Neuron* 39, 109–120. doi: 10.1016/s0896-6273(03)00360-X

Domnisoru, C., Kinkhabwala, A. A., and Tank, D. W. (2013). Membrane potential dynamics of grid cells. *Nature* 495, 199–204. doi: 10.1038/nature11973

Dougherty, K. A., Islam, T., and Johnston, D. (2012). Intrinsic excitability of CA1 pyramidal neurons from the rat dorsal and ventral hippocampus. *J. Physiol.* 590, 5707–5722. doi: 10.1113/jphysiol.2012.242693

Enomoto, A., Han, J. M., Hsiao, C. F., Wu, N., and Chandler, S. H. (2006). Participation of sodium currents in burst generation and control of membrane excitability in mesencephalic trigeminal neurons. *J. Neurosci.* 26, 3412–3422. doi: 10.1523/JNEUROSCI.5274-05.2006

Fyhn, M., Molden, S., Witter, M. P., Moser, E. I., and Moser, M. B. (2004). Spatial representation in the entorhinal cortex. *Science* 305, 1258–1264. doi: 10.1126/science.1099901

Galfrè, S. G., Morandin, F., Pietrosanto, M., Cremisi, F., and Helmer-Citterich, M. (2021). COTAN: scRNA-seq data analysis based on gene co-expression. *NAR Genom. Bioinform.* 3, 1–11.

Grieco, T. M., Malhotra, J. D., Chen, C., Isom, L. L., and Raman, I. M. (2005). Open-channel block by the cytoplasmic tail of sodium channel beta4 as a mechanism for resurgent sodium current. *Neuron* 45, 233–244. doi: 10.1016/j.neuron.2004.12.035

Hafting, T., Fyhn, M., Molden, S., Moser, M. B., and Moser, E. I (2005). Microstructure of a spatial map in the entorhinal cortex. *Nature* 436, 801–806. doi: 10.1038/nature03721

Hargus, N. J., Merrick, E. C., Nigam, A., Kalmar, C. L., Baheti, A. R., Bertam, E. H., et al. (2011). Temporal lobe epilepsy induces intrinsic alterations in Na channel gating in layer II medial entorhinal cortex neurons. *Neurobiol. Dis.* 41, 361–376. doi: 10.1016/j.nbd.2010.10.004

Hargus, N. J., Nigam, A., Bertram, E. H., and Patel, M. K. (2013). Evidence for a role of Nav1.6 in facilitating increases in neuronal hyperexcitability during epileptogenesis. *J. Neurophysiol.* 110, 1144–1157. doi: 10.1152/jn.00383.2013

Hodgkin, A. L., and Huxley, A. F. (1952a). A quantitative description of membrane current and its application to conduction and excitation in nerve. *J. Physiol.* 117, 500–544. doi: 10.1113/jphysiol.1952.sp004764

Hodgkin, A. L., and Huxley, A. F. (1952b). The components of membrane conductance in the giant axon of Loligo. *J. Physiol.* 116, 449–472. doi: 10.1113/jphysiol.1952.sp004718

Jarecki, B. W., Piekarz, A. D., Jackson, J. O., and Cummins, T. R. (2010). Human voltage-gated sodium channel mutations that cause inherited neuronal and muscle channelopathies increase resurgent sodium currents. *J. Clin. Invest.* 120, 369–378. doi: 10.1172/JCI40801

Khaliq, Z. M., Gouwens, N. W., and Raman, I. M. (2003). The contribution of resurgent sodium current to high-frequency firing in Purkinje neurons: an experimental and modeling study. *J. Neurosci.* 23, 4899–4912. doi: 10.1523/JNEUROSCI.23-12-04899.2003

Kuman, S. S., Jin, X., Buckmaster, P. S., and Huguenard, J. R. (2007). Recurrent circuits in layer II of medial entorhinal cortex in a model of temporal lobe epilepsy. *J. Neurosci.* 27, 1239–1246. doi: 10.1523/JNEUROSCI.3182-06.2007

Latuske, P., Toader, O., and Allen, K. (2015). Interspike intervals reveal functionally distinct cell populations in the medial entorhinal cortex. *J. Neurosci.* 35, 10963–10976.

Lein, E. S., Hawrylycz, M. J., Ao, N., Ayres, M., Bensinger, A., Bernard, A., et al. (2007). Genome-wide atlas of gene expression in the adult mouse brain. *Nature* 445, 168–176. doi: 10.1038/nature05453

Lewis, A. H., and Raman, I. M. (2011). Cross-species conservation of open channel block by Na channel beta4 peptides reveals structural features required for resurgent sodium current. *J. Neurosci.* 31, 11527–11536. doi: 10.1523/JNEUROSCI.1428-11.2011

Lewis, A. H., and Raman, I. M. (2013). Interactions among DIV voltage-sensor movement, fast inactivation, and resurgent Na current induced by the Navbeta4 open channel-blocking peptide. *J. Gen. Physiol.* 142, 191–206. doi: 10.1085/jgp.201310984

Lewis, A. H., and Raman, I. M. (2014). Resurgent current of voltage-gated Na(+) channels. *J. Physiol.* 592, 4825–4838. doi: 10.1113/jphysiol.2014.277582

Nigro, M. J., Quattrocolo, G., and Magistretti, J. (2012). Distinct developmental patterns in the expression of transient, persistent, and resurgent Na+ currents in entorhinal cortex layer-II neurons. *Brain Res.* 1463, 30–41. doi: 10.1016/j.brainres.2012.04.049

Ottolini, M., Barker, B. S., Gaykema, R. P., Meisler, M. H., and Patel, M. K. (2017). Aberrant sodium channel currents and hyperexcitability of medial entorhinal cortex neurons in a mouse model of SCN8A encephalopathy. *J. Neurosci.* 37, 7643–7655. doi: 10.1523/JNEUROSCI.2709-16.2017

Pan, Y., and Cummins, T. R. (2020). Distinct functional alterations in SCN8A epilepsy mutant channels. *J. Physiol.* 598, 381–401.

Raman, I. M. (2014). How to be a graduate advisee. *Neuron* 81, 9–11. doi: 10.1016/j.neuron.2013.12.030

Raman, I. M. (2015a). Teaching for the future. *eLife* 4:e05846. doi: 10.7554/eLife.05846

Raman, I. M. (2015b). Triaging Shakespeare. *eLife* 4:e07157. doi: 10.7554/eLife.07157

Raman, I. M. (2016). The truth is in the distribution. *eLife* 5:e21723. doi: 10.7554/eLife.21723

Raman, I. M. (2017). The humanity of science. *eLife* 6:e27982. doi: 10.7554/eLife.27982

Raman, I. M. (2019). Power analysis. *eLife* 8:e52232. doi: 10.7554/eLife.52232

Raman, I. M., and Bean, B. P. (1997). Resurgent sodium current and action potential formation in dissociated cerebellar Purkinje neurons. *J. Neurosci.* 17, 4517–4526. doi: 10.1523/JNEUROSCI.17-12-04517.1997

Raman, I. M., and Bean, B. P. (2001). Inactivation and recovery of sodium currents in cerebellar Purkinje neurons: evidence for two mechanisms. *Biophys. J.* 80, 729–737. doi: 10.1016/S0006-3495(01)76052-3

Raman, I. M., Sprunger, L. K., Meisler, M. H., and Bean, B. P. (1997). Altered subthreshold sodium currents and disrupted firing patterns in Purkinje neurons of Scn8a mutant mice. *Neuron* 19, 881–891. doi: 10.1016/s0896-6273(00)80969-1

Ramsden, H. L., Sürmeli, G., McDonagh, S. G., and Nolan, M. F. (2015). Laminar, and dorsoventral molecular organization of the medial entorhinal cortex revealed by large-scale anatomical analysis of gene expression. *PLoS Comput. Biol.* 11:e1004032. doi: 10.1371/journal.pcbi.1004032

Rowland, D. C., Obenhaus, H. A., Skytøen, E. R., Zhang, Q., Kentros, C. G., Moser, E. I., et al. (2018). Functional properties of stellate cells in medial entorhinal cortex layer II. *eLife* 7:e36664. doi: 10.7554/eLife.36664

Royeck, M., Horstmann, M. T., Remy, S., Reitze, M., Yaari, Y., and Beck, H. (2008). Role of axonal NaV1.6 sodium channels in action potential initiation of CA1 pyramidal neurons. *J. Neurophysiol.* 100, 2361–2380. doi: 10.1152/jn.90332.2008

Schmidt-Hieber, C., and Hausser, M. (2013). Cellular mechanisms of spatial navigation in the medial entorhinal cortex. *Nat. Neurosci.* 16, 325–331. doi: 10.1038/nn.3340

Stafstrom, C. E., Schwindt, P. C., and Crill, W. E. (1982). Negative slope conductance due to a persistent subthreshold sodium current in cat neocortical neurons in vitro. *Brain Res.* 236, 221–226.

Tidball, A. M., Lopez-Santiago, L. F., Yuan, Y., Glenn, T. W., Margolis, J. L., Walker, J. C., et al. (2020). Variant-specific changes in persistent or resurgent sodium current in SCN8A-related epilepsy patient-derived neurons. *Brain* 143, 3025–3040. doi: 10.1093/brain/awaa247

Yamada-Hanff, J., and Bean, B. P. (2013). Persistent sodium current drives conditional pacemaking in CA1 pyramidal neurons under muscarinic stimulation. *J. Neurosci.* 33, 15011–15021. doi: 10.1523/JNEUROSCI.0577-13.2013

Yao, Z., van Velthoven, C. T. J., Nguyen, T. N., Goldy, J., Sedeno-Cortes, A. E., Baftizadeh, F., et al. (2021). A taxonomy of transcriptomic cell types across the isocortex and hippocampal formation. *Cell* 184, 3222.e6–3241.e6. doi: 10.1016/j.cell.2021.04.021

Yu, F. H., Westenbroek, R. E., Silos-Santiago, I., McCormick, K. A., Lawson, D., Ge, P., et al. (2003). Sodium channel beta4, a new disulfide-linked auxiliary subunit with similarity to beta2. *J. Neurosci.* 23, 7577–7585. doi: 10.1523/JNEUROSCI.23-20-07577.2003

Zheng, G. X., Terry, J. M., Belgrader, P., Ryvkin, P., Bent, Z. W., Wilson, R., et al. (2017). Massively parallel digital transcriptional profiling of single cells. *Nat. Commun.* 8:14049.

8

Impact of Prenatal Environmental Stress on Cortical Development

Seiji Ishii [1] ***and Kazue Hashimoto-Torii*** [1, 2, 3*]

[1] Center for Neuroscience Research, Children's National Medical Center, Children's Research Institute, Washington, DC, USA, [2] Department of Pediatrics, Pharmacology and Physiology, School of Medicine and Health Sciences, The George Washington University, Washington, DC, USA, [3] Department of Neurobiology, School of Medicine, Kavli Institute for Neuroscience, Yale University, New Haven, CT, USA

***Correspondence:**
*Kazue Hashimoto-Torii,
Center for Neuroscience Research,
Children's Research Institute,
Children's National Medical Center,
and Department of Pediatrics,
Pharmacology and Physiology, The
George Washington University School
of Medicine and Health Sciences, 111
Michigan Avenue N.W., M7633,
Washington, DC, 20010-2970, USA
KHTorii@childrensnational.org*

Prenatal exposure of the developing brain to various types of environmental stress increases susceptibility to neuropsychiatric disorders such as autism, attention deficit hyperactivity disorder and schizophrenia. Given that even subtle perturbations by prenatal environmental stress in the cerebral cortex impair the cognitive and memory functions, this review focuses on underlying molecular mechanisms of pathological cortical development. We especially highlight recent works that utilized animal exposure models, human specimens or/and induced Pluripotent Stem (iPS) cells to demonstrate: (1) molecular mechanisms shared by various types of environmental stressors, (2) the mechanisms by which the affected extracortical tissues indirectly impact the cortical development and function, and (3) interaction between prenatal environmental stress and the genetic predisposition of neuropsychiatric disorders. Finally, we discuss current challenges for achieving a comprehensive understanding of the role of environmentally disturbed molecular expressions in cortical maldevelopment, knowledge of which may eventually facilitate discovery of interventions for prenatal environment-linked neuropsychiatric disorders.

Keywords: cortical development, prenatal environmental stress, alcohol, autism, schizophrenia, maternal immune activation, gene-environment interaction, iPS cells

Introduction

The development of the cerebral cortex consists of very intricate multifaceted steps including proliferation/differentiation of neural progenitor cells, neuronal migration and maturation (Whitford et al., 2002; Kriegstein and Noctor, 2004; Kriegstein et al., 2006; Ayala et al., 2007; Barnes and Polleux, 2009; Rakic, 2009; Rakic et al., 2009; Evsyukova et al., 2013; Lewis et al., 2013), and it can be impaired by exposure to environmental stress (Ben-Ari, 2008; Deverman and Patterson, 2009; Thompson et al., 2009). Even subtle disturbances in the development of the cerebral cortex impair cognitive and memory functions (Berger-Sweeney and Hohmann, 1997; Arnsten, 2009). Accordingly, ever increasing attention is being paid to understanding the underlying non-genomic alterations thought to govern impairment.

Alcohol is known as one of the most prevalent prenatal environmental stress, and prenatal alcohol exposure-linked impairments are categorized under the term "Fetal Alcohol Spectrum

---

Abbreviations: iPS cells, induced Pluripotent Stem cells; FASD, fetal alcohol spectrum disorder; HSP(s), Heat Shock Protein(s); HSF1, Heat Shock Factor 1; MIA, maternal immune activation; IL-6, interleukin-6; DISC1, disrupted-in-schizophrenia-1.

Disorder (FASD)." FASD patients show higher rates of co-morbidity with various types of neuropsychiatric problems, such as attention deficit hyperactivity disorder (ADHD) and epilepsy (Mattson and Riley, 1998). Histological analysis using postmortem tissues from FASD patients documented various anomalies in the brain, including heterotopias, microcephaly, hydrocephaly, and agenesis of the corpus callosum (Clarren and Smith, 1978; Roebuck et al., 1998; Muralidharan et al., 2013). Many of these morphological phenotypes, as well as behavioral phenotypes of human patients, have been reproduced by non-human primate, rodent and other vertebrate models of fetal alcohol exposure, and therefore, these animal models have been used for understanding etiology of FASD and other health problems linked to prenatal alcohol exposure (Miller and Nowakowski, 1991; Kelly et al., 2009; Wilson and Cudd, 2011; Patten et al., 2014). Furthermore, these animal studies found that fetal alcohol exposure particularly affects the development of the cerebral cortex, in multiple cellular events including proliferation, differentiation, apoptosis, migration, synaptogenesis and dendritogenesis, depending on the regimens and timing of exposure (Lindsley et al., 2006; Thompson et al., 2009; Miranda, 2012).

Similarly, clinical and epidemiological studies identified a variety of environmental stressors, exposure to which increases the risk of neuropsychiatric diseases (Schmitt et al., 2014). Importantly, rodent and non-human primate models of prenatal exposure to those environmental factors, including hypoxia (Golan et al., 2009; Howell and Pillai, 2014), drugs such as cocaine (Gressens et al., 1992; Cabrera-Vera et al., 2000; Stanwood et al., 2001; Lidow and Song, 2001a,b; Crandall et al., 2004; Thompson et al., 2009), and heavy metals such as methylmercury (Kakita et al., 2001; Hashimoto-Torii et al., 2014), have shown that these factors cause similar structural anomalies in the cortex as well as similar abnormal behaviors (Thompson et al., 2009). These findings imply that different environmental challenges provide common impacts on cortical development, thereby resulting in similar endophenotypes.

Here, we review recent publications that found molecular mechanisms underlying pathological cortical development elicited by exposure to prenatal environmental stress and discuss how various types of prenatal environmental stress similarly affect cortical development and increase the risk of neuropsychiatric disorders.

Early Response Genes That Protect or Disturb Cortical Development under the Conditions of Exposure to Environmental Stress

Based on recent findings using prokaryotes, genes that respond (either by increase or decrease of expression) to environmental stress can be classified mainly into two groups (Mitchell et al., 2009; Levine et al., 2013; Young et al., 2013). The first group consists of genes that exhibit altered expression immediately upon exposure to multiple types of environmental insult. The second group consists of genes that exhibit altered expression profiles only upon exposure to specific types of environmental stress and are generally altered gradually post exposure. Thus, orchestrated changes in the activities of these two types of genes are likely to occur in developing cortices. The following section focuses on the first group of genes that immediately respond to environmental stress and may lead to common endophenotypes (Gluckman and Hanson, 2004), discussing how these genes change the molecular landscape of cortical development and contribute to the pathogenesis elicited by prenatal environmental stress.

Stress Responsive Signaling

The cellular stress activates multiple signaling pathways that are well-positioned to help restore homeostasis upon sudden environmental changes, or, in the long run, enforce a new gene expression program so cells can tolerate the new environment. These signaling pathways and genes include molecular chaperone encoding genes, genes involved in the unfolded protein response, Mitogen-Activated Protein Kinase (MAPK) and Growth Arrest and DNA Damage 45 (GADD45) signaling pathways (Yang et al., 2009). The Heat Shock Protein (HSP) pathway is a major molecular chaperone signaling pathway, the activation of which has been identified as one of immediate molecular responses to various types of environmental stress, including alcohol, heat, heavy metals and viral infection (Nollen and Morimoto, 2002; Hashimoto-Torii et al., 2011, 2014).

Our recent study using knockout mice of *Heat shock factor 1* (*Hsf1*), a canonical transcription factor that controls transcription of *Hsp* genes revealed that activation of this signaling is required to reduce the risk of cortical malformation, such as heterotopias and small size of the cortex, upon prenatal exposure to various types of environmental stress, thereby reducing susceptibility to epilepsy (Hashimoto-Torii et al., 2014). Histological analysis immediately after prenatal stress exposure revealed that the increase of these cortical malformations in *Hsf1* knockout mice is due to the increase of cell death and suspension of cell cycling, suggesting *Hsf1*'s roles in cellular protection against environmental stress. Interestingly, the canonical downstream targets of *Hsf1*, *Hsps* mediate proapoptotic effects of *Hsf1* but not the effects on cell cycling (**Figure 1**). El Fatimy et al. (2014) showed that, many cortical genes that are critically involved in the control of cell cycling/proliferation and the neuronal migration are under the control of *Hsf1* and the family gene *Hsf2*. Thus, the activation of HSF1 immediately alters expressions of various types of genes to protect the embryonic cortex from environmental stress.

Another example of a stress responsive transcriptional factor that protects the fetal brain from prenatal environmental stress is Nuclear Factor Erythroid 2-Related Factor 2 (Nfe2l2/Nrf2). The transcriptional activity is increased in response to such as alcohol (Narasimhan et al., 2011), kainate induced excitotoxic damage (Rojo et al., 2008a) and hydrogen peroxide induced oxidative stress (Rojo et al., 2008b). The target genes include multiple genes that encode antioxidant proteins (Dong et al., 2008; Muramatsu et al., 2013). Prenatal exposure to methamphetamine (speed) plus *Nrf2* loss of function lead to reduced motor activity, smaller body weight etc. in the offspring (Ramkissoon and Wells, 2013).

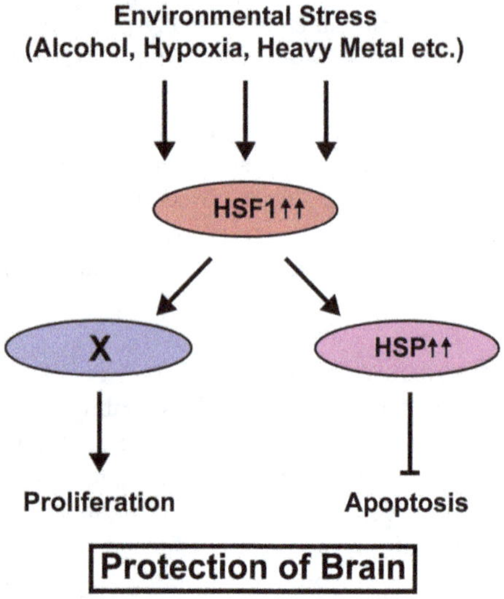

FIGURE 1 | HSF1-mediated protection of neural progenitor cells from various types of environmental stress. Upon exposure to environmental stress, HSF1 is activated and HSPs transcribed by HSF1 inhibit cell death. HSF1 also keeps cell cycling/proliferation under stress exposure. The downstream player X is still unknown.

Interestingly, the gender dependent differences were observed in the severity of the phenotypes.

These lines of evidence suggest that multiple cellular mechanisms provoked by the stress response genes act to ensure fetal cortical tolerance to environmental stress, and thus decrease the prevalence and severity of ensuing neuropsychiatric diseases (Hashimoto-Torii et al., 2014).

MicroRNAs

Post-transcriptional controls have been demonstrated to be critically involved in the control of normal cortical development (Grabowski, 2011; DeBoer et al., 2013; Yano et al., 2015). MicroRNAs (miRNAs) are non-coding RNAs that are involved in post-transcriptional regulation of the expression of a wide variety of genes (Ambros, 2004). Because of their nature as short RNAs for post-transcriptional regulation of genes, they are likely to change the molecular landscape of the cell immediately and temporally in response to environmental challenges (Leung and Sharp, 2010).

In a comprehensive miRNA profiling study using a neurosphere model of alcohol exposure, Miranda and his colleagues found a reduction in expressions of *miR-21*, *miR-335*, *miR-9*, and *miR-153* 24 h after exposure (Sathyan et al., 2007).

MiR-9 knockout mouse displays smaller brain size (Shibata et al., 2011). The analysis of those embryonic brains suggested that impaired proliferation and differentiation of neural progenitor cells in stage dependent manner may lead to the smaller brain. Consistent with this *in vivo* observation, *miR-9* knockdown inhibited the proliferation and promoted the migration of the neural progenitor cells *in vitro* (Delaloy et al., 2010). The control of these biological events by *miR-9* may be mediated by controlling expression levels of the downstream targets such as *Forkhead box G1* (*Foxg1/Bf1*) (Shibata et al., 2008, 2011), *embryonic lethal, abnormal vision, Drosophila like 2* (*Elavl2/HuB*) (Sathyan et al., 2007), *Fibroblast growth factor receptor 1* (*Fgfr1*) (Pappalardo-Carter et al., 2013), *Forkhead box P2* (*Foxp2*) (Pappalardo-Carter et al., 2013), *Stathmin 1* (*Stmn1*) (Delaloy et al., 2010), *Nuclear receptor subfamily 2, group E, member 1* (*Nr2e1/Tlx*) (Zhao et al., 2009; Shibata et al., 2011), *Inhibitor of DNA binding 4* (*Id4*) (Shibata et al., 2008), *Paired box 6* (*Pax6*) (Shibata et al., 2011), *Meis homeobox 2* (*Meis2*) (Shibata et al., 2011), *GS homeobox 2* (*Gsh2*) (Shibata et al., 2011), *Islet1* (*Isl1*) (Shibata et al., 2011), *RE1-silencing transcription factor* (*Rest*) (Packer et al., 2008), and *Actin-like 6A* (*Actl6a/BAF53a*) (Yoo et al., 2009). Thus, reduced expression of *miR-9* by alcohol exposure is also likely to inhibit those events by the similar mechanism. The miR-153 and miR-21 also similarly control the cellular proliferation (Zhong et al., 2012; Wu et al., 2013).

Reduction of *miR-9* expression and the target gene expressions in the zebrafish whole-embryo (Tal et al., 2012) and the embryonic forebrain (Pappalardo-Carter et al., 2013) exposed to alcohol also supports this hypothesis. However, in the conditions of exposure to different contexts of maternal stress induced by such as restraint of the body and forced swimming, expression of *miR-9* was increased in the brain of offspring (Zucchi et al., 2013). Similarly, the expression of *miR-21* has also been reported to be increased in the different ambience, such as in the mouse brain exposed to ionizing radiation (Shi et al., 2012a), in the endothelial cells under the exposure to shear stress (Weber et al., 2010), and in the embryonic fibroblasts exposed to arsenite (Ling et al., 2012). The expression of *miR-153* is also upregulated by hydrogen peroxidase induced oxidative stress (Narasimhan et al., 2014) and nicotine exposure (Tsai et al., 2014). These lines of evidence indicate that the microRNAs are susceptible to the environmental changes and that the overall changes of various types of microRNAs may determine the phenotypes specific to types/regimens of the environmental stress exposure. The fact that miR-335 knockdown reverses the effects of miR-21 knockdown in the cell proliferation and death also supports this possibility (Sathyan et al., 2007).

Maternal, Placental, and Extracortical Tissues Exhibit Indirect Effects as a Result of Environmental Stress

Beside direct molecular changes within embryonic cortical cells, evidences exist that indirect impacts of environmental stress from maternal, placental, and other extracortical tissues exert a critical influence on cortical development (Velasquez et al., 2013).

Maternal infection is well defined by epidemiological studies as a risk factor for neurodevelopmental disorders such as autism and schizophrenia (Hagberg et al., 2012; Depino, 2013; Meldrum et al., 2013). Mouse offspring that have been exposed to maternal infection display abnormalities reminiscent of the behavioral, histological, and molecular characteristics of autism (Patterson, 2011), while fetal brain infection does not cause these abnormalities (Meldrum et al., 2013). Mouse offspring exposed to maternal immune activation (MIA), which is elicited by poly-riboinosinic-polyribocytidylic acid or lipopolysaccharide, also reproduce the behavioral and histological abnormalities of autism (Meyer et al., 2006; Smith et al., 2007; Hsiao et al., 2012; Carpentier et al., 2013), suggesting that activation of maternal immune system triggered by infection is critical for manifestation of deficits. These early findings have proven MIA model useful in the investigation of the molecular mechanisms at play in unraveling maternal effects on the pathophysiology of autism.

Smith et al. (2007) demonstrated that a proinflammatory cytokine interleukin-6 (IL-6) supplied from the maternal tissues might mediate the MIA effects on the fetal cortex. A single maternal injection of IL-6 in the middle of corticogenesis causes deficits in prepulse inhibition and lateral inhibition in the offspring (Smith et al., 2007), both of which are linked to autism and schizophrenia (Solomon et al., 1981; Wynn et al., 2004; Bertone et al., 2005; Perry et al., 2007). They also demonstrated that inhibition of IL-6 by application of the antibody or using the knockout dam, significantly ameliorated such as cognitive and exploratory deficits in mouse offspring exposed to MIA (Smith et al., 2007). The gene expression profiles were also reversed by inhibition of IL-6 in the cortices of the MIA offspring. These results provided evidence that IL-6 may owe the indirect effects of MIA on fetal cortical development.

Indirect effects of MIA on cortical development may also involve the effects from gastrointestinal tissues of offspring. Autism is often associated with gastrointestinal barrier defects (Buie et al., 2010; Coury et al., 2012), and rodent MIA models reproduce these defects (Hsiao et al., 2013). Hsiao and colleagues made an interesting observation that probiotic treatment of gastrointestinal barrier defects improved behavioral abnormalities such as anxiety-like behavior, decreased prepulse inhibition, and deficits in ultrasonic vocal communication in the MIA offspring. Their study also suggested the possibility that gastrointestinal barrier deficit-induced increase of serum metabolites such as 4-ethylphenylsulfate, indolepyruvate, glycolate, imidazole propionate, and N-acetylserine, may contribute to behavior abnormality in the MIA offspring (Hsiao et al., 2013). Of these, the most dramatically affected metabolite, 4-ethylphenylsulfate, has been known as a uremic toxin, and the administration of this metabolite induces anxiety-like behavior in the mouse (Hsiao et al., 2013). As a recent study suggested the link between the uremic toxin and the depression in the chronic kidney disease (Hsu et al., 2013), the 4-ethylphenylsulfate in serum may be the common factor that affects the brain function in various pathophysiological conditions.

Serotonin derived from placenta may also indirectly affect embryonic brain development. Recent studies demonstrated that the placenta is the major source of serotonin at early embryonic stage, while the dorsal raphe nuclei in the hindbrain take over from late embryonic stage to adulthood (Bonnin et al., 2011). Abnormal serotonin levels in the brain have been linked to autism (Chugani et al., 1999; Whitaker-Azmitia, 2001; Gaspar et al., 2003), and the role of serotonin in the normal development of thalamocortical projections also has been reported (Bonnin et al., 2007). In addition, it has been demonstrated that prenatal intake of selective serotonin reuptake inhibitors increases the risk of cognitive impairment in mouse progeny (Smit-Rigter et al., 2012; Kinast et al., 2013). Importantly, serotonin level is lower in the cortices of the offspring exposed to environmental stress such as maternal infection (Fatemi et al., 2008; Wang et al., 2009) and cocaine (Cabrera-Vera et al., 2000). Therefore, environmental stressors may indirectly affect the cortical development as a result of disruption in the synthesis/release of serotonin in/from the placenta (Velasquez et al., 2013).

Interaction between a Susceptible Genotype and Environmental Risk Factors

Genome wide association studies have shown a polygenic component contributes to the risk of schizophrenia and autism (Purcell et al., 2014). Similarly, many epidemiological studies as well as the aforementioned results from studies of animal exposure models have shown these disorders also include a "polyepigenetic" component that is influenced by various types of environmental stress (Weinberger, 1987; Caspi and Moffitt, 2006; Ben-Ari, 2008; van Os et al., 2010; Bregant et al., 2013). However, just how the polyepigenetic component increases the risk of disease manifestation by interacting with polygenic component is largely unknown.

One relatively new approach to help answering this question is the use of induced Pluripotent Stem (iPS) cells taken from subjects diagnosed with polygenic diseases such as schizophrenia or autism. iPS cells are not only becoming useful tools to obtain functional human cortical neurons (Mariani et al., 2012; Shi et al., 2012b; Espuny-Camacho et al., 2013; Lancaster et al., 2013) for understanding the pathogenesis of disease, but are also being utilized for drug screening (Han et al., 2011). To examine potential interactions between genetic predisposition and the environmental risk factors, we recently used iPS cells derived from schizophrenia patients, and exposed the differentiated neural progenitor cells to environmental stress including alcohol, methylmercury and hydrogen peroxide. Single cell RNA detection revealed augmented cell-to-cell variable activation of HSF1-HSP signaling in the schizophrenia patients' neural progenitor cells, individual cell lines of which carry different genetic risks for schizophrenia (**Figure 2**). This finding suggests that variable responses of HSF1-HSP signaling among a population of neural progenitor cells exposed to environmental

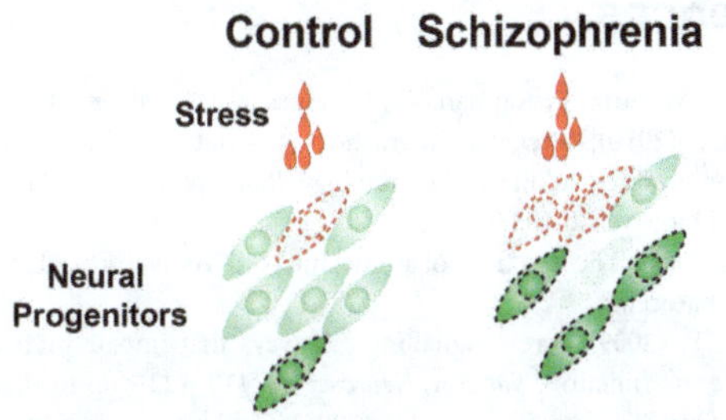

FIGURE 2 | Cell-to-cell variability of HSF1 activation in response to environmental challenges is increased in schizophrenia neural progenitor cells. The number of cells that are in the levels of excess or very little activation of HSF1 was increased in the schizophrenia cells (Hashimoto-Torii et al., 2014; Brennand et al., 2015). These outlier cells may be at the risk of manifesting pathophysiological features (indicated by the cells surrounded by broken lines).

stress is predetermined by genetic predisposition and may increase the risk of the onset of schizophrenia as well as other neuropsychiatric diseases (Hashimoto-Torii et al., 2014; Brennand et al., 2015).

Using *Disrupted-in-schizophrenia-1* gene (*Disc1*) mutant mice combined with MIA, *in vivo* evidence for the interaction of gene and prenatal environment in the pathogenesis of schizophrenia and depression was also provided. The *Disc1* is one of the risk genes for psychiatric disorders such as schizophrenia and mood disorders (St Clair et al., 1990; Millar et al., 2000). The transgenic mice expressing the dominant negative form of *Disc1* that was found in the patient (Millar et al., 2000), displayed hyperactivity and impaired social interaction (Pletnikov et al., 2008). When this transgenic mouse was subjected to MIA, neurobehavioral phenotypes such as anxiety, depression-like behavior, and a decrease in social interaction and an increase in aggressiveness were unraveled (Abazyan et al., 2010). Two other *Disc1* mutant mouse lines with point mutations at Q31L and L100P, which show schizophrenia and depression related phenotypes, respectively (Clapcote et al., 2007), were also subjected to MIA. MIA exposure augmented the impairment in prepulse inhibition, lateral inhibition, spatial object recognition, and social motivation of those *Disc1* mutant mice (Lipina et al., 2013). Importantly, the production of IL-6 was concomitantly increased by the combination of *Disc1* mutations and the MIA in the fetal mouse brains (Lipina et al., 2013). Thus, these mouse models that combine *Disc1* mutation and MIA will become powerful models for understanding the molecular mechanisms underlying interactions between the gene and prenatal environmental factors that increase the risk of the psychiatric diseases.

Outlook

As outlined in this review, research on polyepigenetic mechanisms associated with many types of environmental stress that disturb cortical development and on potential prophylactic or preventative interventions of these disturbances are just beginning to emerge. To further facilitate this type of research, patient-derived iPS cells will become one of several powerful tools. Although there are a number of limitations in their use, easy application of environmental stress and the potential for high throughput analysis substantiate their usefulness. Challenges include: (1) limited availability of iPS cell lines that are fully characterized; (2) lack of validated differentiation protocols for specific types of neurons; and (3) lack of validated *in vivo* approaches (e.g., efficient transplantation methods to animal models, etc.) that allow observation of the iPS cells during cortical development.

A type of the environmental stress can lead to various phenotypes in the cerebral cortex, however, this variability cannot be explained exclusively by different regimens of exposure. Recent studies have revealed potential factors that may affect the resultant phenotypes, including gender (Mooney and Varlinskaya, 2011; Ramkissoon and Wells, 2013) and probabilistic molecular responses of individual cells to the environmental stress (Hashimoto-Torii et al., 2014) (**Figure 2**) etc. Thus, the next important questions will be: (1) if such molecular differences of individual cells elicited by environmental stress are sustained for long periods of time and ultimately result in altered cortical function, and (2) which molecules mediate the gender specific effects of prenatal environmental stress.

Another recent interesting observation that needs to be addressed at the molecular level is the transgenerational effects of prenatal exposure to environmental stress, as reported in the cases of alcohol (Govorko et al., 2012). This observation opens up a whole new field of research that might eventually lead to an understanding of why FASD and other environment-linked disorders show familial and geographical linkages.

Acknowledgments

We thank Miki Masuda, Drs. Alexander I. Son, and Masaaki Torii for their comments on the manuscript. We also thank NIH/NIAAA R00AA1838705, CTSI-CN, NARSAD/Scott-Gentle Foundation and ABMRF for their respective support.

References

Abazyan, B., Nomura, J., Kannan, G., Ishizuka, K., Tamashiro, K. L., Nucifora, F., et al. (2010). Prenatal interaction of mutant DISC1 and immune activation produces adult psychopathology. *Biol. Psychiatry* 68, 1172–1181. doi: 10.1016/j.biopsych.2010.09.022

Ambros, V. (2004). The functions of animal microRNAs. *Nature* 431, 350–355. doi: 10.1038/nature02871

Arnsten, A. F. (2009). Stress signalling pathways that impair prefrontal cortex structure and function. *Nat. Rev. Neurosci.* 10, 410–422. doi: 10.1038/nrn2648

Ayala, R., Shu, T., and Tsai, L. H. (2007). Trekking across the brain: the journey of neuronal migration. *Cell* 128, 29–43. doi: 10.1016/j.cell.2006.12.021

Barnes, A. P., and Polleux, F. (2009). Establishment of axon-dendrite polarity in developing neurons. *Annu. Rev. Neurosci.* 32, 347–381. doi: 10.1146/annurev.neuro.31.060407.125536

Ben-Ari, Y. (2008). Neuro-archaeology: pre-symptomatic architecture and signature of neurological disorders. *Trends Neurosci.* 31, 626–636. doi: 10.1016/j.tins.2008.09.002

Berger-Sweeney, J., and Hohmann, C. F. (1997). Behavioral consequences of abnormal cortical development: insights into developmental disabilities. *Behav. Brain Res.* 86, 121–142. doi: 10.1016/S0166-4328(96)02251-6

Bertone, A., Mottron, L., Jelenic, P., and Faubert, J. (2005). Enhanced and diminished visuo-spatial information processing in autism depends on stimulus complexity. *Brain* 128, 2430–2441. doi: 10.1093/brain/awh561

Bonnin, A., Goeden, N., Chen, K., Wilson, M. L., King, J., Shih, J. C., et al. (2011). A transient placental source of serotonin for the fetal forebrain. *Nature* 472, 347–350. doi: 10.1038/nature09972

Bonnin, A., Torii, M., Wang, L., Rakic, P., and Levitt, P. (2007). Serotonin modulates the response of embryonic thalamocortical axons to netrin-1. *Nat. Neurosci.* 10, 588–597. doi: 10.1038/nn1896

Bregant, T., Rados, M., Vasung, L., Derganc, M., Evans, A. C., Neubauer, D., et al. (2013). Region-specific reduction in brain volume in young adults with perinatal hypoxic-ischaemic encephalopathy. *Eur. J. Paediatr. Neurol.* 17, 608–614. doi: 10.1016/j.ejpn.2013.05.005

Brennand, K., Savas, J. N., Kim, Y., Tran, N., Simone, A., Hashimoto-Torii, K., et al. (2015). Phenotypic differences in hiPSC NPCs derived from patients with schizophrenia. *Mol. Psychiatry* 20, 361–368. doi: 10.1038/mp.2014.22

Buie, T., Campbell, D. B., Fuchs, G. J. III, Furuta, G. T., Levy, J., Vandewater, J., et al. (2010). Evaluation, diagnosis, and treatment of gastrointestinal disorders in individuals with ASDs: a consensus report. *Pediatrics* 125(Suppl. 1), S1–S18. doi: 10.1542/peds.2009-1878c

Cabrera-Vera, T. M., Garcia, F., Pinto, W., and Battaglia, G. (2000). Neurochemical changes in brain serotonin neurons in immature and adult offspring prenatally exposed to cocaine. *Brain Res.* 870, 1–9. doi: 10.1016/S0006-8993(00)02382-9

Carpentier, P. A., Haditsch, U., Braun, A. E., Cantu, A. V., Moon, H. M., Price, R. O., et al. (2013). Stereotypical alterations in cortical patterning are associated with maternal illness-induced placental dysfunction. *J. Neurosci.* 33, 16874–16888. doi: 10.1523/JNEUROSCI.4654-12.2013

Caspi, A., and Moffitt, T. E. (2006). Gene-environment interactions in psychiatry: joining forces with neuroscience. *Nat. Rev. Neurosci.* 7, 583–590. doi: 10.1038/nrn1925

Chugani, D. C., Muzik, O., Behen, M., Rothermel, R., Janisse, J. J., Lee, J., et al. (1999). Developmental changes in brain serotonin synthesis capacity in autistic and nonautistic children. *Ann. Neurol.* 45, 287–295.

Clapcote, S. J., Lipina, T. V., Millar, J. K., Mackie, S., Christie, S., Ogawa, F., et al. (2007). Behavioral phenotypes of Disc1 missense mutations in mice. *Neuron* 54, 387–402. doi: 10.1016/j.neuron.2007.04.015

Clarren, S. K., and Smith, D. W. (1978). The fetal alcohol syndrome. *N. Engl. J. Med.* 298, 1063–1067. doi: 10.1056/NEJM197805112981906

Coury, D. L., Ashwood, P., Fasano, A., Fuchs, G., Geraghty, M., Kaul, A., et al. (2012). Gastrointestinal conditions in children with autism spectrum disorder: developing a research agenda. *Pediatrics* 130(Suppl. 2), S160–S168. doi: 10.1542/peds.2012-0900n

Crandall, J. E., Hackett, H. E., Tobet, S. A., Kosofsky, B. E., and Bhide, P. G. (2004). Cocaine exposure decreases GABA neuron migration from the ganglionic eminence to the cerebral cortex in embryonic mice. *Cereb. Cortex* 14, 665–675. doi: 10.1093/cercor/bhh027

DeBoer, E. M., Kraushar, M. L., Hart, R. P., and Rasin, M. R. (2013). Post-transcriptional regulatory elements and spatiotemporal specification of neocortical stem cells and projection neurons. *Neuroscience* 248, 499–528. doi: 10.1016/j.neuroscience.2013.05.042

Delaloy, C., Liu, L., Lee, J. A., Su, H., Shen, F., Yang, G. Y., et al. (2010). MicroRNA-9 coordinates proliferation and migration of human embryonic stem cell-derived neural progenitors. *Cell Stem Cell* 6, 323–335. doi: 10.1016/j.stem.2010.02.015

Depino, A. M. (2013). Peripheral and central inflammation in autism spectrum disorders. *Mol. Cell. Neurosci.* 53, 69–76. doi: 10.1016/j.mcn.2012.10.003

Deverman, B. E., and Patterson, P. H. (2009). Cytokines and CNS development. *Neuron* 64, 61–78. doi: 10.1016/j.neuron.2009.09.002

Dong, J., Sulik, K. K., and Chen, S. Y. (2008). Nrf2-mediated transcriptional induction of antioxidant response in mouse embryos exposed to ethanol *in vivo*: implications for the prevention of fetal alcohol spectrum disorders. *Antioxid. Redox Signal.* 10, 2023–2033. doi: 10.1089/ars.2007.2019

El Fatimy, R., Miozzo, F., Le Mouel, A., Abane, R., Schwendimann, L., Saberan-Djoneidi, D., et al. (2014). Heat shock factor 2 is a stress-responsive mediator of neuronal migration defects in models of fetal alcohol syndrome. *EMBO Mol. Med.* 6, 1043–1061. doi: 10.15252/emmm.201303311

Espuny-Camacho, I., Michelsen, K. A., Gall, D., Linaro, D., Hasche, A., Bonnefont, J., et al. (2013). Pyramidal neurons derived from human pluripotent stem cells integrate efficiently into mouse brain circuits *in vivo*. *Neuron* 77, 440–456. doi: 10.1016/j.neuron.2012.12.011

Evsyukova, I., Plestant, C., and Anton, E. S. (2013). Integrative mechanisms of oriented neuronal migration in the developing brain. *Annu. Rev. Cell Dev. Biol.* 29, 299–353. doi: 10.1146/annurev-cellbio-101512-122400

Fatemi, S. H., Reutiman, T. J., Folsom, T. D., Huang, H., Oishi, K., Mori, S., et al. (2008). Maternal infection leads to abnormal gene regulation and brain atrophy in mouse offspring: implications for genesis of neurodevelopmental disorders. *Schizophr. Res.* 99, 56–70. doi: 10.1016/j.schres.2007.11.018

Gaspar, P., Cases, O., and Maroteaux, L. (2003). The developmental role of serotonin: news from mouse molecular genetics. *Nat. Rev. Neurosci.* 4, 1002–1012. doi: 10.1038/nrn1256

Gluckman, P. D., and Hanson, M. A. (2004). Living with the past: evolution, development, and patterns of disease. *Science* 305, 1733–1736. doi: 10.1126/science.1095292

Golan, M. H., Mane, R., Molczadzki, G., Zuckerman, M., Kaplan-Louson, V., Huleihel, M., et al. (2009). Impaired migration signaling in the hippocampus following prenatal hypoxia. *Neuropharmacology* 57, 511–522. doi: 10.1016/j.neuropharm.2009.07.028

Govorko, D., Bekdash, R. A., Zhang, C., and Sarkar, D. K. (2012). Male germline transmits fetal alcohol adverse effect on hypothalamic proopiomelanocortin gene across generations. *Biol. Psychiatry* 72, 378–388. doi: 10.1016/j.biopsych.2012.04.006

Grabowski, P. (2011). Alternative splicing takes shape during neuronal development. *Curr. Opin. Genet. Dev.* 21, 388–394. doi: 10.1016/j.gde.2011.03.005

Gressens, P., Kosofsky, B. E., and Evrard, P. (1992). Cocaine-induced disturbances of corticogenesis in the developing murine brain. *Neurosci. Lett.* 140, 113–116. doi: 10.1016/0304-3940(92)90694-3

Hagberg, H., Gressens, P., and Mallard, C. (2012). Inflammation during fetal and neonatal life: implications for neurologic and neuropsychiatric disease in children and adults. *Ann. Neurol.* 71, 444–457. doi: 10.1002/ana.22620

Han, S. S., Williams, L. A., and Eggan, K. C. (2011). Constructing and deconstructing stem cell models of neurological disease. *Neuron* 70, 626–644. doi: 10.1016/j.neuron.2011.05.003

Hashimoto-Torii, K., Kawasawa, Y. I., Kuhn, A., and Rakic, P. (2011). Combined transcriptome analysis of fetal human and mouse cerebral cortex exposed to alcohol. *Proc. Natl. Acad. Sci. U.S.A.* 108, 4212–4217. doi: 10.1073/pnas.1100903108

Hashimoto-Torii, K., Torii, M., Fujimoto, M., Nakai, A., El Fatimy, R., Mezger, V., et al. (2014). Roles of heat shock factor 1 in neuronal response to fetal environmental risks and its relevance to brain disorders. *Neuron* 82, 560–572. doi: 10.1016/j.neuron.2014.03.002

Howell, K. R., and Pillai, A. (2014). Effects of prenatal hypoxia on schizophrenia-related phenotypes in heterozygous reeler mice: a gene x environment interaction study. *Eur. Neuropsychopharmacol.* 24, 1324–1336. doi: 10.1016/j.euroneuro.2014.05.011

Hsiao, E. Y., McBride, S. W., Chow, J., Mazmanian, S. K., and Patterson, P. H. (2012). Modeling an autism risk factor in mice leads to permanent immune dysregulation. *Proc. Natl. Acad. Sci. U.S.A.* 109, 12776–12781. doi: 10.1073/pnas.1202556109

Hsiao, E. Y., McBride, S. W., Hsien, S., Sharon, G., Hyde, E. R., McCue, T., et al. (2013). Microbiota modulate behavioral and physiological abnormalities associated with neurodevelopmental disorders. *Cell* 155, 1451–1463. doi: 10.1016/j.cell.2013.11.024

Hsu, H. J., Yen, C. H., Chen, C. K., Wu, I. W., Lee, C. C., Sun, C. Y., et al. (2013). Association between uremic toxins and depression in patients with chronic kidney disease undergoing maintenance hemodialysis. *Gen. Hosp. Psychiatry* 35, 23–27. doi: 10.1016/j.genhosppsych.2012.08.009

Kakita, A., Wakabayashi, K., Su, M., Piao, Y. S., and Takahashi, H. (2001). Experimentally induced leptomeningeal glioneuronal heterotopia and underlying cortical dysplasia of the lateral limbic area in rats treated transplacentally with methylmercury. *J. Neuropathol. Exp. Neurol.* 60, 768–777.

Kelly, S. J., Goodlett, C. R., and Hannigan, J. H. (2009). Animal models of fetal alcohol spectrum disorders: impact of the social environment. *Dev. Disabil. Res. Rev.* 15, 200–208. doi: 10.1002/ddrr.69

Kinast, K., Peeters, D., Kolk, S. M., Schubert, D., and Homberg, J. R. (2013). Genetic and pharmacological manipulations of the serotonergic system in early life: neurodevelopmental underpinnings of autism-related behavior. *Front. Cell. Neurosci.* 7:72. doi: 10.3389/fncel.2013.00072

Kriegstein, A. R., and Noctor, S. C. (2004).Patterns of neuronal migration in the embryonic cortex. *Trends Neurosci.* 27, 392–399. doi: 10.1016/j.tins.2004.05.001

Kriegstein, A., Noctor, S., and Martinez-Cerdeno, V. (2006). Patterns of neural stem and progenitor cell division may underlie evolutionary cortical expansion. *Nat. Rev. Neurosci.* 7, 883–890. doi: 10.1038/nrn2008

Lancaster, M. A., Renner, M., Martin, C. A., Wenzel, D., Bicknell, L. S., Hurles, M. E., et al. (2013). Cerebral organoids model human brain development and microcephaly. *Nature* 501, 373–379. doi: 10.1038/nature12517

Leung, A. K., and Sharp, P. A. (2010). MicroRNA functions in stress responses. *Mol. Cell* 40, 205–215. doi: 10.1016/j.molcel.2010.09.027

Levine, J. H., Lin, Y., and Elowitz, M. B. (2013). Functional roles of pulsing in genetic circuits. *Science* 342, 1193–1200. doi: 10.1126/science.1239999

Lewis, T. L. Jr., Courchet, J., and Polleux, F. (2013). Cell biology in neuroscience: cellular and molecular mechanisms underlying axon formation, growth, and branching. *J. Cell Biol.* 202, 837–848. doi: 10.1083/jcb.201305098

Lidow, M. S., and Song, Z. M. (2001a). Effect of cocaine on cell proliferation in the cerebral wall of monkey fetuses. *Cereb. Cortex* 11, 545–551. doi: 10.1093/cercor/11.6.545

Lidow, M. S., and Song, Z. M. (2001b). Primates exposed to cocaine *in utero* display reduced density and number of cerebral cortical neurons. *J. Comp. Neurol.* 435, 263–275. doi: 10.1002/cne.1028

Lindsley, T. A., Miller, M. W., Littner, Y., and Bearer, C. F. (2006). Signaling pathways regulating cell motility: a role in ethanol teratogenicity? *Alcohol. Clin. Exp. Res.* 30, 1445–1450. doi: 10.1111/j.1530-0277.2006.00173.x

Ling, M., Li, Y., Xu, Y., Pang, Y., Shen, L., Jiang, R., et al. (2012). Regulation of miRNA-21 by reactive oxygen species-activated ERK/NF-kappaB in arsenite-induced cell transformation. *Free Radic. Biol. Med.* 52, 1508–1518. doi: 10.1016/j.freeradbiomed.2012.02.020

Lipina, T. V., Zai, C., Hlousek, D., Roder, J. C., and Wong, A. H. (2013). Maternal immune activation during gestation interacts with Disc1 point mutation to exacerbate schizophrenia-related behaviors in mice. *J. Neurosci.* 33, 7654–7666. doi: 10.1523/JNEUROSCI.0091-13.2013

Mariani, J., Simonini, M. V., Palejev, D., Tomasini, L., Coppola, G., Szekely, A. M., et al. (2012). Modeling human cortical development *in vitro* using induced pluripotent stem cells. *Proc. Natl. Acad. Sci. U.S.A.* 109, 12770–12775. doi: 10.1073/pnas.1202944109

Mattson, S. N., and Riley, E. P. (1998). A review of the neurobehavioral deficits in children with fetal alcohol syndrome or prenatal exposure to alcohol. *Alcohol. Clin. Exp. Res.* 22, 279–294. doi: 10.1111/j.1530-0277.1998.tb03651.x

Meldrum, S. J., Strunk, T., Currie, A., Prescott, S. L., Simmer, K., and Whitehouse, A. J. (2013). Autism spectrum disorder in children born preterm-role of exposure to perinatal inflammation. *Front. Neurosci.* 7:123. doi: 10.3389/fnins.2013.00123

Meyer, U., Nyffeler, M., Engler, A., Urwyler, A., Schedlowski, M., Knuesel, I., et al. (2006). The time of prenatal immune challenge determines the specificity of inflammation-mediated brain and behavioral pathology. *J. Neurosci.* 26, 4752–4762. doi: 10.1523/JNEUROSCI.0099-06.2006

Millar, J. K., Wilson-Annan, J. C., Anderson, S., Christie, S., Taylor, M. S., Semple, C. A., et al. (2000). Disruption of two novel genes by a translocation co-segregating with schizophrenia. *Hum. Mol. Genet.* 9, 1415–1423. doi: 10.1093/hmg/9.9.1415

Miller, M. W., and Nowakowski, R. S. (1991). Effect of prenatal exposure to ethanol on the cell cycle kinetics and growth fraction in the proliferative zones of fetal rat cerebral cortex. *Alcohol. Clin. Exp. Res.* 15, 229–232. doi: 10.1111/j.1530-0277.1991.tb01861.x

Miranda, R. C. (2012). MicroRNAs and fetal brain development: implications for ethanol teratology during the second trimester period of neurogenesis. *Front. Genet.* 3:77. doi: 10.3389/fgene.2012.00077

Mitchell, A., Romano, G. H., Groisman, B., Yona, A., Dekel, E., Kupiec, M., et al. (2009). Adaptive prediction of environmental changes by microorganisms. *Nature* 460, 220–224. doi: 10.1038/nature08112

Mooney, S. M., and Varlinskaya, E. I. (2011). Acute prenatal exposure to ethanol and social behavior: effects of age, sex, and timing of exposure. *Behav. Brain Res.* 216, 358–364. doi: 10.1016/j.bbr.2010.08.014

Muralidharan, P., Sarmah, S., Zhou, F. C., and Marrs, J. A. (2013). Fetal Alcohol spectrum disorder (FASD) associated neural defects: complex mechanisms and potential therapeutic targets. *Brain Sci.* 3, 964–991. doi: 10.3390/brainsci3020964

Muramatsu, H., Katsuoka, F., Toide, K., Shimizu, Y., Furusako, S., and Yamamoto, M. (2013). Nrf2 deficiency leads to behavioral, neurochemical and transcriptional changes in mice. *Genes Cells* 18, 899–908. doi: 10.1111/gtc.12083

Narasimhan, M., Mahimainathan, L., Rathinam, M. L., Riar, A. K., and Henderson, G. I. (2011). Overexpression of Nrf2 protects cerebral cortical neurons from ethanol-induced apoptotic death. *Mol. Pharmacol.* 80, 988–999. doi: 10.1124/mol.111.073262

Narasimhan, M., Riar, A. K., Rathinam, M. L., Vedpathak, D., Henderson, G., and Mahimainathan, L. (2014). Hydrogen peroxide responsive miR153 targets Nrf2/ARE cytoprotection in paraquat induced dopaminergic neurotoxicity. *Toxicol. Lett.* 228, 179–191. doi: 10.1016/j.toxlet.2014.05.020

Nollen, E. A., and Morimoto, R. I. (2002). Chaperoning signaling pathways: molecular chaperones as stress-sensing 'heat shock' proteins. *J. Cell Sci.* 115, 2809–2816.

Packer, A. N., Xing, Y., Harper, S. Q., Jones, L., and Davidson, B. L. (2008). The bifunctional microRNA miR-9/miR-9* regulates REST and CoREST and is downregulated in Huntington's disease. *J. Neurosci.* 28, 14341–14346. doi: 10.1523/JNEUROSCI.2390-08.2008

Pappalardo-Carter, D. L., Balaraman, S., Sathyan, P., Carter, E. S., Chen, W. J., and Miranda, R. C. (2013). Suppression and epigenetic regulation of MiR-9 contributes to ethanol teratology: evidence from zebrafish and murine fetal neural stem cell models. *Alcohol. Clin. Exp. Res.* 37, 1657–1667. doi: 10.1111/acer.12139

Patten, A. R., Fontaine, C. J., and Christie, B. R. (2014). A comparison of the different animal models of fetal alcohol spectrum disorders and their use in studying complex behaviors. *Front. Pediatr.* 2:93. doi: 10.3389/fped.2014.00093

Patterson, P. H. (2011). Modeling autistic features in animals. *Pediatr. Res.* 69, 34R–40R. doi: 10.1203/PDR.0b013e318212b80f

Perry, W., Minassian, A., Lopez, B., Maron, L., and Lincoln, A. (2007). Sensorimotor gating deficits in adults with autism. *Biol. Psychiatry* 61, 482–486. doi: 10.1016/j.biopsych.2005.09.025

Pletnikov, M. V., Ayhan, Y., Nikolskaia, O., Xu, Y., Ovanesov, M. V., Huang, H., et al. (2008). Inducible expression of mutant human DISC1 in mice is associated with brain and behavioral abnormalities reminiscent of schizophrenia. *Mol. Psychiatry* 13, 173–186. doi: 10.1038/sj.mp.4002079

Purcell, S. M., Moran, J. L., Fromer, M., Ruderfer, D., Solovieff, N., Roussos, P., et al. (2014). A polygenic burden of rare disruptive mutations in schizophrenia. *Nature* 506, 185–190. doi: 10.1038/nature12975

Rakic, P. (2009). Evolution of the neocortex: a perspective from developmental biology. *Nat. Rev. Neurosci.* 10, 724–735. doi: 10.1038/nrn2719

Rakic, P., Ayoub, A. E., Breunig, J. J., and Dominguez, M. H. (2009). Dominguez, decision by division: making cortical maps. *Trends Neurosci.* 32, 291–301. doi: 10.1016/j.tins.2009.01.007

Ramkissoon, A., and Wells, P. G. (2013). Developmental role of nuclear factor E2-related factor 2 in mitigating methamphetamine fetal toxicity and postnatal neurodevelopmental deficits. *Free Radic. Biol. Med.* 65, 620–631. doi: 10.1016/j.freeradbiomed.2013.07.043

Roebuck, T. M., Mattson, S. N., and Riley, E. P. (1998). A review of the neuroanatomical findings in children with fetal alcohol syndrome or prenatal exposure to alcohol. *Alcohol. Clin. Exp. Res.* 22, 339–344. doi: 10.1111/j.1530-0277.1998.tb03658.x

Rojo, A. I., Rada, P., Egea, J., Rosa, A. O., Lopez, M. G., and Cuadrado, A. (2008a). Functional interference between glycogen synthase kinase-3 beta and the transcription factor Nrf2 in protection against kainate-induced hippocampal cell death. *Mol. Cell. Neurosci.* 39, 125–132. doi: 10.1016/j.mcn.2008.06.007

Rojo, A. I., Sagarra, M. R., and Cuadrado, A. (2008b). GSK-3beta down-regulates the transcription factor Nrf2 after oxidant damage: relevance to exposure of neuronal cells to oxidative stress. *J. Neurochem.* 105, 192–202. doi: 10.1111/j.1471-4159.2007.05124.x

Sathyan, P., Golden, H. B., and Miranda, R. C. (2007). Competing interactions between micro-RNAs determine neural progenitor survival and proliferation after ethanol exposure: evidence from an *ex vivo* model of the fetal cerebral cortical neuroepithelium. *J. Neurosci.* 27, 8546–8557. doi: 10.1523/JNEUROSCI.1269-07.2007

Schmitt, A., Malchow, B., Hasan, A., and Falkai, P. (2014). The impact of environmental factors in severe psychiatric disorders. *Front. Neurosci.* 8:19. doi: 10.3389/fnins.2014.00019

Shi, Y., Kirwan, P., Smith, J., Robinson, H. P., and Livesey, F. J. (2012b). Human cerebral cortex development from pluripotent stem cells to functional excitatory synapses. *Nat. Neurosci.* 15, 477–486, S1. doi: 10.1038/nn.3041

Shi, Y., Zhang, X., Tang, X., Wang, P., Wang, H., and Wang, Y. (2012a). MiR-21 is continually elevated long-term in the brain after exposure to ionizing radiation. *Radiat. Res.* 177, 124–128. doi: 10.1667/RR2764.1

Shibata, M., Kurokawa, D., Nakao, H., Ohmura, T., and Aizawa, S. (2008). MicroRNA-9 modulates Cajal-Retzius cell differentiation by suppressing Foxg1 expression in mouse medial pallium. *J. Neurosci.* 28, 10415–10421. doi: 10.1523/JNEUROSCI.3219-08.2008

Shibata, M., Nakao, H., Kiyonari, H., Abe, T., and Aizawa, S. (2011). MicroRNA-9 regulates neurogenesis in mouse telencephalon by targeting multiple transcription factors. *J. Neurosci.* 31, 3407–3422. doi: 10.1523/JNEUROSCI.5085-10.2011

Smith, S. E., Li, J., Garbett, K., Mirnics, K., and Patterson, P. H. (2007). Maternal immune activation alters fetal brain development through interleukin-6. *J. Neurosci.* 27, 10695–10702. doi: 10.1523/JNEUROSCI.2178-07.2007

Smit-Rigter, L. A., Noorlander, C. W., von Oerthel, L., Chameau, P., Smidt, M. P., and van Hooft J. A. (2012). Prenatal fluoxetine exposure induces life-long serotonin 5-HT(3). receptor-dependent cortical abnormalities and anxiety-like behaviour. *Neuropharmacology* 62, 865–870. doi: 10.1016/j.neuropharm.2011.09.015

Solomon, P. R., Crider, A., Winkelman, J. W., Turi, A., Kamer, R. M., and Kaplan, L. J. (1981). Disrupted latent inhibition in the rat with chronic amphetamine or haloperidol-induced supersensitivity: relationship to schizophrenic attention disorder. *Biol. Psychiatry* 16, 519–537.

St Clair, D., Blackwood, D., Muir, W., Carothers, A., Walker, M., Spowart, G., et al. (1990). Association within a family of a balanced autosomal translocation with major mental illness. *Lancet* 336, 13–16. doi: 10.1016/0140-6736(90)91520-K

Stanwood, G. D., Washington, R. A., and Levitt, P. (2001). Identification of a sensitive period of prenatal cocaine exposure that alters the development of the anterior cingulate cortex. *Cereb. Cortex* 11, 430–440. doi: 10.1093/cercor/11.5.430

Tal, T. L., Franzosa, J. A., Tilton, S. C., Philbrick, K. A., Iwaniec, U. T., Turner, R. T., et al. (2012). MicroRNAs control neurobehavioral development and function in zebrafish. *FASEB J.* 26, 1452–1461. doi: 10.1096/fj.11-194464

Thompson, B. L., Levitt, P., and Stanwood, G. D. (2009). Stanwood, Prenatal exposure to drugs: effects on brain development and implications for policy and education. *Nat. Rev. Neurosci.* 10, 303–312. doi: 10.1038/nrn2598

Tsai, P. C., Bake, S., Balaraman, S., Rawlings, J., Holgate, R. R., Dubois, D., et al. (2014). MiR-153 targets the nuclear factor-1 family and protects against teratogenic effects of ethanol exposure in fetal neural stem cells. *Biol. Open* 3, 741–758. doi: 10.1242/bio.20147765

van Os, J., Kenis, G., and Rutten, B. P. (2010). The environment and schizophrenia. *Nature* 468, 203–212. doi: 10.1038/nature09563

Velasquez, J. C., Goeden, N., and Bonnin, A. (2013). Placental serotonin: implications for the developmental effects of SSRIs and maternal depression. *Front. Cell. Neurosci.* 7:47. doi: 10.3389/fncel.2013.00047

Wang, S., Yan, J. Y., Lo, Y. K., Carvey, P. M., and Ling, Z. (2009). Dopaminergic and serotoninergic deficiencies in young adult rats prenatally exposed to the bacterial lipopolysaccharide. *Brain Res.* 1265, 196–204. doi: 10.1016/j.brainres.2009.02.022

Weber, M., Baker, M. B., Moore, J. P., and Searles, C. D. (2010). MiR-21 is induced in endothelial cells by shear stress and modulates apoptosis and eNOS activity. *Biochem. Biophys. Res. Commun.* 393, 643–648. doi: 10.1016/j.bbrc.2010.02.045

Weinberger, D. R. (1987). Implications of normal brain development for the pathogenesis of schizophrenia. *Arch. Gen. Psychiatry* 44, 660–669. doi: 10.1001/archpsyc.1987.01800190080012

Whitaker-Azmitia, P. M. (2001). Serotonin and brain development: role in human developmental diseases. *Brain Res. Bull.* 56, 479–485. doi: 10.1016/S0361-9230(01)00615-3

Whitford, K. L., Dijkhuizen, P., Polleux, F., and Ghosh, A. (2002). Molecular control of cortical dendrite development. *Annu. Rev. Neurosci.* 25, 127–149. doi: 10.1146/annurev.neuro.25.112701.142932

Wilson, S. E., and Cudd, T. A. (2011). Focus on: the use of animal models for the study of fetal alcohol spectrum disorders. *Alcohol Res. Health* 34, 92–98.

Wu, Z., He, B., He, J., and Mao, X. (2013). Upregulation of miR-153 promotes cell proliferation via downregulation of the PTEN tumor suppressor gene in human prostate cancer. *Prostate* 73, 596–604. doi: 10.1002/pros.22600

Wynn, J. K., Dawson, M. E., Schell, A. M., McGee, M., Salveson, D., and Green, M. F. (2004). Prepulse facilitation and prepulse inhibition in schizophrenia patients and their unaffected siblings. *Biol. Psychiatry* 55, 518–523. doi: 10.1016/j.biopsych.2003.10.018

Yang, Z., Song, L., and Huang, C. (2009). Gadd45 proteins as critical signal transducers linking NF-kappaB to MAPK cascades. *Curr. Cancer Drug Targets* 9, 915–930. doi: 10.2174/156800909790192383

Yano, M., Ohtsuka, T., and Okano, H. (2015). RNA-binding protein research with transcriptome-wide technologies in neural development. *Cell Tissue Res.* 359, 135–144. doi: 10.1007/s00441-014-1923-8

Yoo, A. S., Staahl, B. T., Chen, L., and Crabtree, G. R. (2009). MicroRNA-mediated switching of chromatin-remodelling complexes in neural development. *Nature* 460, 642–646. doi: 10.1038/nature08139

Young, J. W., Locke, J. C., and Elowitz, M. B. (2013). Rate of environmental change determines stress response specificity. *Proc. Natl. Acad. Sci. U.S.A.* 110, 4140–4145. doi: 10.1073/pnas.1213060110

Zhao, C., Sun, G., Li, S., and Shi, Y. (2009). A feedback regulatory loop involving microRNA-9 and nuclear receptor TLX in neural stem cell fate determination. *Nat. Struct. Mol. Biol.* 16, 365–371. doi: 10.1038/nsmb.1576

Zhong, Z., Dong, Z., Yang, L., and Gong, Z. (2012). miR-21 induces cell cycle at S phase and modulates cell proliferation by down-regulating hMSH2 in lung cancer. *J. Cancer Res. Clin. Oncol.* 138, 1781–1788. doi: 10.1007/s00432-012-1287-y

Zucchi, F. C., Yao, Y., Ward, I. D., Ilnytskyy, Y., Olson, D. M., Benzies, K., et al. (2013). Maternal stress induces epigenetic signatures of psychiatric and neurological diseases in the offspring. *PLoS ONE* 8:e56967. doi: 10.1371/journal.pone.0056967

9

Cell Polarity in Cerebral Cortex Development—Cellular Architecture Shaped by Biochemical Networks

Andi H. Hansen†, Christian Duellberg†, Christine Mieck†, Martin Loose and Simon Hippenmeyer**

Institute of Science and Technology Austria, Klosterneuburg, Austria

***Correspondence:**
Martin Loose
martin.loose@ist.ac.at
Simon Hippenmeyer
simon.hippenmeyer@ist.ac.at

†These authors have contributed equally to this work.

The human cerebral cortex is the seat of our cognitive abilities and composed of an extraordinary number of neurons, organized in six distinct layers. The establishment of specific morphological and physiological features in individual neurons needs to be regulated with high precision. Impairments in the sequential developmental programs instructing corticogenesis lead to alterations in the cortical cytoarchitecture which is thought to represent the major underlying cause for several neurological disorders including neurodevelopmental and psychiatric diseases. In this review article we discuss the role of cell polarity at sequential stages during cortex development. We first provide an overview of morphological cell polarity features in cortical neural stem cells and newly-born postmitotic neurons. We then synthesize a conceptual molecular and biochemical framework how cell polarity is established at the cellular level through a break in symmetry in nascent cortical projection neurons. Lastly we provide a perspective how the molecular mechanisms applying to single cells could be probed and integrated in an *in vivo* and tissue-wide context.

Keywords: cerebral cortex, polarity, neurogenesis, neuronal migration, axon, dendrite, break in symmetry, GTPases

ESTABLISHMENT OF CELLULAR POLARITY IN SEQUENTIAL STAGES OF CORTICAL DEVELOPMENT

Neural Stem Cell Polarity

The mammalian cerebral cortex emerges from the neuroectoderm. At the end of neurulation and neural tube closure, occurring from embryonic day (E) 7 to E9 in mice, the early neuroepithelium is composed of neuroepithelial stem cells (NESCs) from which all subsequent neural progenitor cells and their neuron lineages derive (**Figure 1**). NESCs are highly polarized and their nuclei exhibit interkinetic nuclear migration whereby they translocate from the ventricular (apical) side to the more basal side in concert with the cell cycle (Lee and Norden, 2013). NESC polarity correlates with the asymmetric distribution of cell fate determinants which are thought to control the fine balance between symmetric and asymmetric progenitor divisions (Shitamukai and Matsuzaki, 2012). Such balance is critical for the generation of the correct number of radial glia progenitor cells (RGPCs), which are not only lineally related to NESCs but exhibit even more polarized cellular morphology with an extended basal process (Taverna et al., 2014). In the initial stages of neurogenesis, NESCs arrange the mitotic spindle in parallel (division plane perpendicular) to the ventricular zone (VZ) and divide mostly symmetrically, thereby expanding the progenitor pool (Postiglione and Hippenmeyer, 2014; Taverna et al., 2014). The disruption of the mitotic spindle, anchored to the lateral walls of NESCs, results in the precocious generation of neurons and apoptosis (Yingling et al., 2008). Thus the correct cellular polarization of the earliest neural progenitor cells in the developing cerebral cortex is absolutely essential for the correct lineage progression and eventual neuron production. While it has been well established that components of the planar cell polarity signaling pathway play critical roles in establishing and maintaining progenitor polarity (Knoblich, 2008; Homem et al., 2015), the signaling cues and molecular mechanisms that instruct polarization and the break of symmetry in NESCs are not well understood *in vivo*.

Radial glia progenitors (RGPs) have been demonstrated to be the major neural progenitors in the developing cortex responsible for producing the vast majority of cortical excitatory neurons (Malatesta et al., 2000; Noctor et al., 2001; Anthony et al., 2004; Lui et al., 2011; Franco and Muller, 2013; Borrell and Götz, 2014; Taverna et al., 2014). The RGP division patterns and dynamics determine the number of neurons in the mature cortex. RGP cell division during mitosis occurs at the surface of the embryonic VZ and can be either symmetric or asymmetric, which is defined by the fate of the two daughter cells (Lui et al., 2011; Gao et al., 2014; Taverna et al., 2014; Homem et al., 2015). The extrinsic and intracellular signaling cues that instruct the mode of cell division are not well understood. The directional segregation of cell fate determinants such as Notch, components of the planar cell polarity signaling module, or entire centrosomes (i.e., duplicated centrioles) in dividing neural stem cells indicates however that polarized secretion and/or trafficking is a key mechanism (Wang et al., 2009; Lui et al., 2011; Paridaen et al., 2013; Taverna et al., 2014). Symmetric RGP divisions generate two RGPs to amplify the progenitor pool or two postmitotic neurons. In contrast, asymmetric divisions produce a renewing RGP and a neuron or an intermediate progenitor (IP). IPs can further divide symmetrically in the subventricular zone (SVZ) to produce neurons (Noctor et al., 2004; Kowalczyk et al., 2009). Interestingly, IPs adopt a multipolar morphology (Noctor et al., 2004; Kowalczyk et al., 2009) and it is currently not known whether the transition from bipolar (RGP) to multipolar (IP) state could correlate with, or even be instructive, for the neurogenic potential in dividing IPs. RGPs may also produce other types of transient amplifying progenitors, such as short neural precursors (SNPs; Stancik et al., 2010) and outer SVZ radial glial progenitors (oRGs aka basal RGs or bRGs; Fietz et al., 2010; Hansen et al., 2010; Shitamukai et al., 2011; Wang X. et al., 2011; Kelava et al., 2012; Betizeau et al., 2013; Florio et al., 2015; Johnson et al., 2015; Pollen et al., 2015). Although oRGs like RGPs are bipolar, they have been shown to adopt different morphological states and thus likely exhibit distinct cellular polarity since they lack apical attachment at the ventricle. Distinct oRG morphologies may reflect distinct competence states with respect to the number and types of neurons which are generated (Betizeau et al., 2013). Although the above studies provide a framework of stem cell polarity and lineage progression at the cellular level (**Figure 1**), the underlying molecular and biochemical mechanisms of progenitor cell polarization are still poorly defined.

Polarity in Nascent Postmitotic Neurons—Implications for Neuronal Migration

The basal processes of RGPs serve as a scaffold for nascent cortical neurons, which migrate from the VZ/SVZ through the intermediate zone (IZ), in order to reach the cortical plate (CP; Rakic, 1972; Evsyukova et al., 2013). Cortical layering occurs in an "inside-out" fashion whereby earlier born neurons populate deep layers and later born neurons occupy progressively upper layers (Angevine and Sidman, 1961; Rakic, 1974). Newly-born cortical neurons migrate, in a step-wise fashion coupled with changes in cell polarity, from the VZ/SVZ through IZ zone in order to reach the CP where they position themselves at their final location (**Figure 1**; Rakic, 1972; Nadarajah and Parnavelas, 2002; Noctor et al., 2004; Tsai et al., 2005; Marín et al., 2010; Hippenmeyer, 2014). Timelapse and videomicroscopy approaches (Tabata and Nakajima, 2008; Noctor, 2011; Tsai and Vallee, 2011) with the goal to trace the migration paths of individual cortical projection neurons have impressively revealed that: (1) radially migrating neurons proceed though several distinct migratory phases; (2) change their morphology and polarize along the way; and (3) adjust their mode of migration while transiting through the different zones along the radial migratory path (Nadarajah et al., 2001; Tabata and Nakajima, 2003; Noctor et al., 2004; Tsai et al., 2005; Sekine et al., 2011; **Figure 1**). From these observations through live-imaging, it is evident that nascent migrating neurons undergo a series of morphological changes including the depolarization and repolarization within the SVZ/IZ. The molecular mechanisms controlling these morphological transitions are poorly defined but if they are perturbed or delayed, the development of the cortical cytoarchitecture may be compromised. This is in particular relevant in humans that suffer from e.g., Lissencephaly (a severe cortical malformation disorder) where the loss of *LIS1* activity results in a defect to repolarize migrating neurons which in turn accumulate in ectopic positions instead of properly migrating into the developing CP (Tsai et al., 2005; Wynshaw-Boris et al., 2010). LIS1 is only one of many molecules which are involved in more than one cellular polarization process. As such LIS1 plays a role in neural progenitor polarization and in the establishment of polarity in postmitotic neurons. It will thus be important to precisely dissect the sequential and/or distinct functions of proteins orchestrating cellular polarity during development.

Establishment of Axon and Dendrite Compartments in Cortical Projection Neurons

After nascent cortical projection neurons, exhibiting bipolar (BP) morphology, have delaminated from the neuroepithelium at the ventricular surface they move radially away to the SVZ. Within

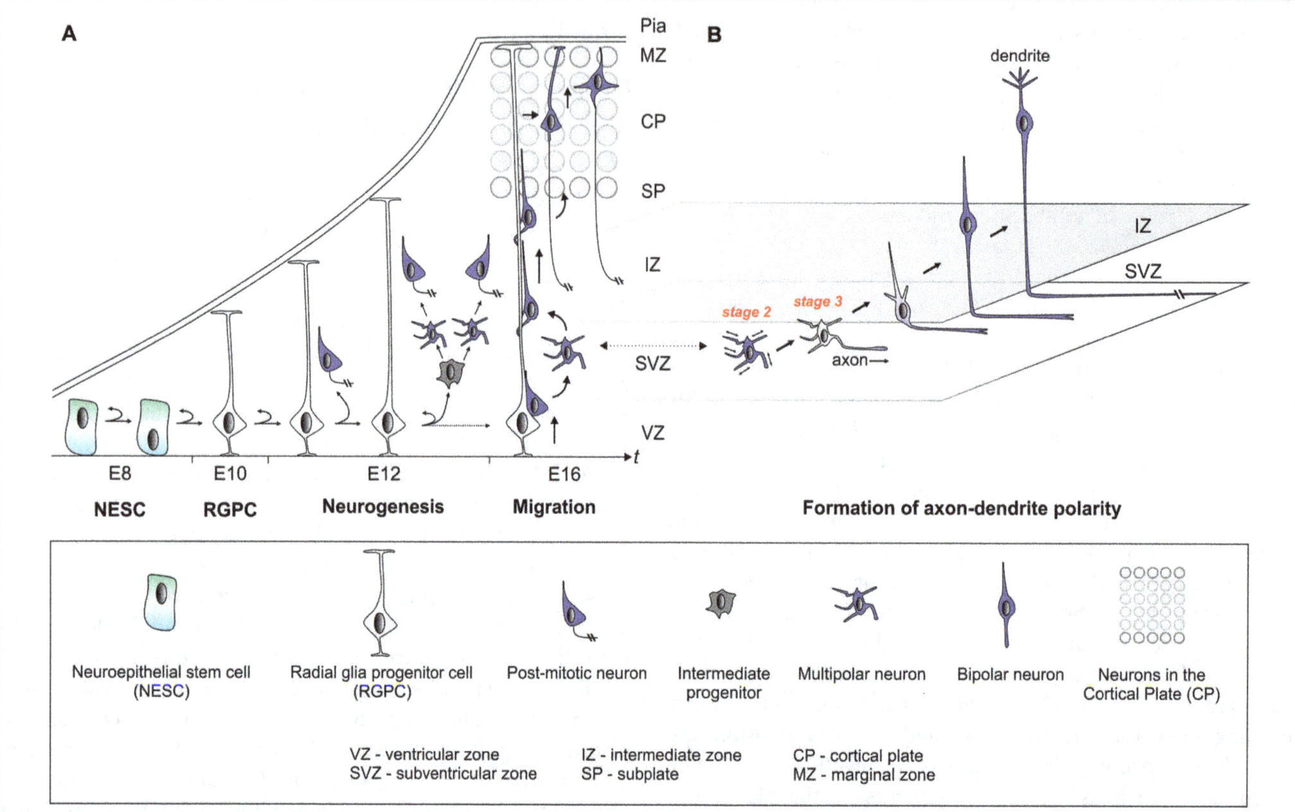

FIGURE 1 | Establishment of cell polarity in cerebral cortex development. **(A)** The early neuroepithelium is composed of highly polarized neuroepithelial stem cells (NESCs, apical-basal polarity is indicated). NESCs give rise to radial glia progenitor stem cells (RGPCs) which exhibit even more polarized cellular morphology with an extended basal process. During neurogenesis symmetric radial glia progenitor (RGP) divisions may generate two RGPs but asymmetric divisions produce a renewing RGP and a neuron or an intermediate progenitor (IP). IPs further divide symmetrically in the subventricular zone (SVZ) to produce neurons. The basal processes of RGPs serve as a scaffold for nascent post-mitotic neurons, which migrate in a step-wise fashion coupled with changes in cell polarity, from the ventricular zone (VZ)/SVZ through the intermediate zone (IZ) in order to reach the cortical plate (CP). After nascent cortical projection neurons have delaminated from the neuroepithelium at the ventricular surface they move radially away to the SVZ exhibiting bipolar (BP) morphology. Within the SVZ/IZ, neurons "sojourn" for about 24 h or longer and most adopt a multipolar (MP) morphology, extending and retracting processes in all directions. At one point fundamental cellular polarization events take place that predetermine the future axon of the neuron before the neuron again adopts a bipolar morphology and starts locomoting along the radial glial fiber through the IZ. Once reaching the subplate (SP), neurons enter the CP and migrate towards the marginal zone (MZ) where they detach from the radial glial fiber. Finally, neurons settle in their appropriate position in the CP and the leading process will eventually become the dendrite. **(B)** This panel depicts the migrating neuron from panel **(A)** in higher detail with the leading and trailing processes which eventually become the dendrite and axon, respectively.

the SVZ neurons "sojourn" for about 24 h or longer and most adopt a multipolar (MP) morphology, extending and retracting processes in all directions (Tabata and Nakajima, 2003; Noctor et al., 2004). While this stage is critical for the progression of the sequential migration program it is also essential for establishing the cellular compartments that later transform into axonal and dendritic processes. During this phase, multipolar (MP) neurons tend to migrate tangentially in an apparent random fashion (Noctor et al., 2004; Jossin and Cooper, 2011). At one point however, fundamental cellular polarization events take place that predetermine the future axon of the neuron (Barnes and Polleux, 2009) before the neuron again adopts a bipolar morphology (**Figure 1**). In the remainder of this review we synthesize a framework of neuronal polarization based upon *in vitro* biochemical, cell culture and genetic loss of function experiments *in vivo*. We reflect upon the relative contribution of extrinsic cues and cell-intrinsic molecular and biochemical signaling modules that dictate the break in symmetry and control polarization of cortical projection neurons.

EXTRACELLULAR CUES CONTROLLING PROJECTION NEURON POLARITY IN CORTEX DEVELOPMENT

Developing cortical neurons can break symmetry in the absence of external cues suggesting that the role of the extracellular signals in the *in vivo* context is solely to activate/trigger an intrinsic symmetry-breaking pathway. The intrinsic signaling pathways on the other hand are dependent on the internal biochemical state of the cell (**Figures 2, 3** and see below for detailed discussion). Albeit cell intrinsic mechanisms have received much more attention than extracellular regulatory cues it is clear that in the developing cortex, cell-to-cell interactions,

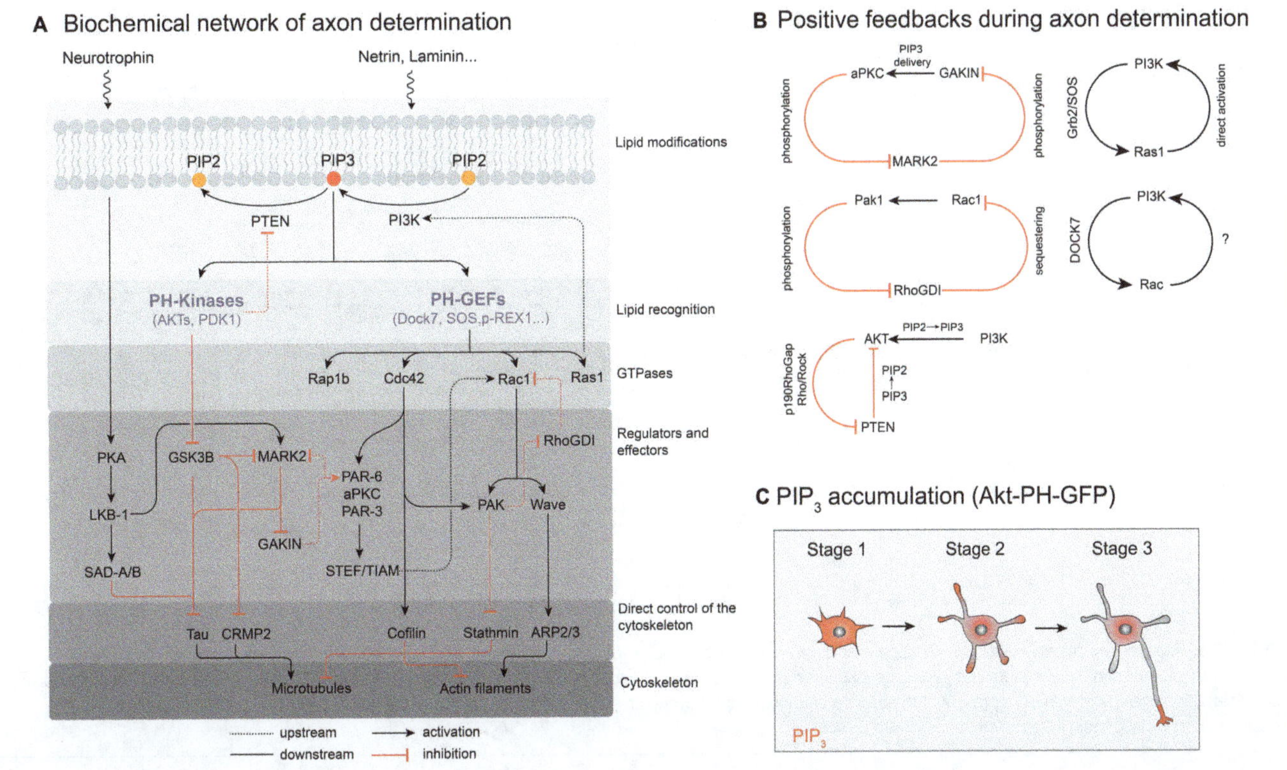

FIGURE 2 | Molecular signaling pathways controlling neuronal polarization. **(A)** A simplified illustration of the biochemical network of axon determination. Only interactions localized to the nascent axon are shown. **(B)** Positive feedback loops in the process of axon determination. **(C)** Probing PIP_3 localization and accumulation in polarizing neurons with Akt-pleckstrin-homology (PH)-GFP as a probe for PIP_3.

the local microenvironment and long-range signaling constitute essential factors for the establishment of projection neuron polarity *in vivo*.

Cell-Cell Interactions

Nascent projection neurons are embedded in a heterogeneous environment and cell-cell interactions are likely to play an important role in neuronal polarization (Jossin, 2011; Gartner et al., 2015; Namba et al., 2015). It has been suggested that the radial glial scaffold, on which neurons perform locomotion in the IZ, could be involved in the MP-to-BP transition. Experiments inhibiting the cell-adhesion molecule N-cadherin have shown that newly-born neurons expressing a dominant-negative form of N-cadherin establish abnormal leading processes (Gartner et al., 2012, 2015). These experiments have also indicated that radial glial-neuron interactions mediated by N-cadherin play an essential role in the initial radial alignment of nascent neurons and thus possibly (albeit in an indirect manner) in the subsequent MP-to-BP transition. Interestingly, polarized N-cadherin localization has been shown to occur in a single neurite during MP-to-BP transition and thus likely represents one of the earliest consequences of the symmetry-break (Gartner et al., 2012). In such context, it has been proposed that the interaction of multipolar cells and RGPs mediated by N-cadherin leads to the establishment of axon-dendrite polarity through polarized distribution of active RhoA in the neurite contacting the RGC and active Rac1 on the opposite side where the axon is formed (Xu et al., 2015). Physical interactions between pioneering axons from earlier generated neurons and the dynamic neurites from newly born neurons have been shown to contribute to polarization in MP neurons (Namba et al., 2014, 2015). These interactions involve the cell adhesion molecule transient axonal glycoprotein 1 (TAG-1). The highest expression of TAG-1 has been observed in the lower IZ (Namba et al., 2014), exactly where nascent neurons switch from MP-to-BP morphology. Current models propose that TAG-1 is expressed in both MP cells and pioneering axons and thus could mediate homophilic cell-cell contacts. Indeed, shRNA-mediated knockdown of TAG-1 results in the disruption of the MP-to-BP transition and axon specification. The underlying mechanism of TAG-1 action in polarization may involve: (1) an increase in physical tension in the immature neurite leading to axon induction and formation; and (2) contact-mediated activation of signaling molecules that instruct axon specification (Namba et al., 2015). Interestingly, N-cadherin is mainly expressed in the upper IZ (Xu et al., 2015) but TAG-1 in the lower IZ (Namba et al., 2014). Thus N-cadherin and TAG-1 could act as two separate polarity inducing cues which might work complementary in axon-dendrite formation as proposed by the Kaibuchi laboratory (Xu et al., 2015). Whether the induction of cellular polarization within these

C. elegans embryo: Protein	Neurons: Protein	Localization pattern	Expression ↑ No. of axons	Expression ↓ No. of axons	Comment	References
PKC-3	aPKC-λ	A	+	0	Both PKC-3 isoforms can bind to PAR-3 and compete for PAR-3 binding. The neurite localized PKM-ζ disrupts the aPKC-PAR-3 complex and prevents neuron specification. Conversely, aPKC-λ-PAR-3-PAR-6 facilitates axonogenesis. In C. elegans there is one expressed aPKC that builds dynamic complexes with cdc42, PAR-6 and PAR-3. The stoichiometry and lifetime of this complexes is still poorly understood.	*Parker et al., 2013
	PKM-ζ	B	0	+		
PAR-3	PAR-3	A	+	0	Nematode and mammalian PAR-3 is able to oligomerize and form a complex with aPKC and PAR-6. PAR-3 oligomerization is crucial for membrane-attachment and stabilizes microtubules in mammalian neurons.	*Parker et al., 2013; *Nishimura et al., 2005; *Shi et al., 2003; *Chen et al., 2013; Feng et al., 2007
PAR-6	PAR-6	A	+	0	PAR-6 binds to PAR-3 via its PDZ domain. Both, PAR-6 and PAR-3 are able to bind PKC-3. The complex of PAR-6/PAR-3/PKC-3 is crucial for axon formation in C. elegans and in neurons.	*Shi et al., 2003
cdc42	cdc42	C	+	0	Cdc42 is recruiting the PAR-6-aPKC complex to the membrane in the C. elegans zygote and in neurons. Cdc42 has been shown to enhance aPKC's kinase activity in epithelial cells and astrocytes.	*DaSilva et al., 2005; *Garvalov et al., 2007; *Schwamborn and Puschel, 2004; Etienne-Manneville and Hall, 2001, Yamanaka et al., 2001
PAR-1	MARK2	A	0	+	PAR-1 is phosphorylated by aPKC in both systems. In C. elegans this reaction detaches PAR-1 from the membrane, which is still to be confirmed for neuronal PAR-1.	Wu et al., 2011; *Chen et al., 2006
	SAD-A/-B	C			The double knockout of SAD-A and -B neurons have multiple processes of similar length that stain for markers of dendrites and axons.	*Kishi et al., 2005; Moravcevic et al., 2010
PAR-2	-		.		PAR-2 recruits PAR-1 to the cell membrane in C.elegans, in neurons PAR-1 binds the cell membrane via its KA1 domain.	Motegi et al., 2011; Moravcevic et al., 2010
LGL-1	LGL-1	A	+	0	LGL forms a complex with PAR-6 and aPKC. LGL activates the small GTPase Rab10 and promotes axonal membrane trafficking.	*Wang et al., 2011; Plant et al., 2003
PAR-4	LKB1	A	+	0	Neuronal LKB1 is phosphorylated by PKA which leads to downstream activation of kinases like MARK and SAD.	*Shelly et al., 2007; *Lizcano et al., 2004; *Barnes et al., 2007; *Kishi et al., 2005
PAR-5	14-3-3	C			14-3-3 proteins are recruited to phosphorylated serines and threonines. PAR-5 releases PAR-3 from the membrane. In C.elegans PAR-5 is required for mutual exclusion of the anterior and posterior PAR domains.	Morton et al., 2002

Localization (C. elegans embryo): anterior posterior

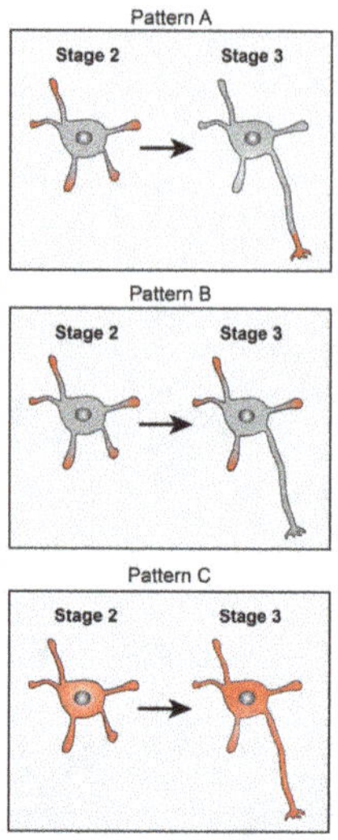

FIGURE 3 | Table of key polarity proteins in *C. elegans* and their neuronal homologs. The localization of the nematode proteins is illustrated according to their anterior or posterior domain affiliation. In neurons the respective localization is classified according to the indicated patterns (A–C). A supernumerary axon phenotype is indicated by a plus sign, while 0 represents the absence of an axon upon overexpression or downregulation of the respective polarity protein. References describing neuronal protein systems are marked with an asterisk.

two distinct zones correlates with a certain neuron type (e.g., derived from either RGCs or IPs) remains to be determined.

Secreted Factors

Reelin

Newly born cortical projection neurons migrate from the VZ to the CP in order to reach their final target area (Marín et al., 2010; Hippenmeyer, 2014). A key regulatory module controlling neuronal migration includes the Reelin pathway (Honda et al., 2011). The function of Reelin in neuronal migration has been studied extensively for decades and several hypotheses concerning the mechanism of Reelin action have been put forward (Honda et al., 2011). However, it has also become clear recently that Reelin fulfills an important role in the polarization of nascent projection neurons (Jossin and Cooper, 2011; Jossin, 2011). Reelin is mainly expressed by Cajal-Retzius cells in the marginal one (MZ) in the developing cortex (Ogawa et al., 1995). The Reelin protein primarily binds to its two cognate receptors, very low density lipoprotein receptor (VLDLR) and apolipoprotein E receptor 2 (ApoER2/LRP8; D'Arcangelo et al., 1999), which are mainly expressed in RGPs and nascent migrating neurons (Perez-Garcia et al., 2004). Binding of Reelin to its receptors triggers the activation of a Src family kinase (SFK) called Fyn which in turn phosphorylates the adaptor protein disabled-1 (DAB1; Howell et al., 1997, 1999). Phosphorylated DAB1 functions as a hub for several downstream intracellular signals and has been shown to activate the effectors CRK, C3G and PI3K which in turn regulate the activity of Limk1, Akt and Rap1 to eventually modulate the dynamic cytoskeleton (Honda et al., 2011; Sekine et al., 2014). Thus the Reelin-DAB1 pathway translates extracellular cues into cytoskeletal changes in migrating neurons (Frotscher, 2010; Forster et al., 2010). How Reelin might regulate dynamic polarization events in nascent cortical projection neurons is less well understood. Interestingly however, it has been shown that while VLDLR is mainly localized on the leading processes of migrating neurons in the MZ, ApoER2 is primarily localized to neuronal processes and the cell membranes of multipolar neurons in the SVZ and lower IZ. In addition to strong expression of Reelin in the MZ, it was also demonstrated that Reelin is also expressed in the IZ at early developmental stages (Hirota et al., 2015). *Ex vivo* experiments where exogenous Reelin was added to cultured brain slices have shown an effect on the morphology and dynamic behavior of nascent neurons in the IZ (Britto et al., 2014). Thus, based on the expression pattern of Reelin and its cognate receptors it is conceivable that Reelin could play a prominent role during the polarization process of nascent cortical projection neurons. Indeed, Jossin and Cooper propose a three step model (Jossin and Cooper, 2011) how Reelin controls the radial orientation of multipolar neurons in SVZ/IZ. First, multipolar neurons migrate tangentially in a stochastic manner in the SVZ/IZ until they encounter Reelin which leads to the activation of the small GTPase RAP1, likely via pDAB1-CRK/CRKL-C3G signaling (Ballif et al., 2004; Voss et al., 2008). Next, active RAP1 triggers an increase of the surface level of N-Cadherin in multipolar neurons. These increased cell surface levels of N-Cadherin could then allow the multipolar neurons to sample local microenvironmental cues which then could initiate the break in symmetry and induce polarization. The cortical projection neurons then progressively exit the multipolar stage and adopt a bipolar morphology (Jossin, 2011; Jossin and Cooper, 2011). Altogether, the above data and model indicates that Reelin acts as a critical cue for the directional movement of nascent migrating cortical projection neurons and could serve as a critical extracellular cue for modulating polarization of nascent migrating cortical projection neurons. It will be intriguing to decipher the precise intracellular and biochemical signaling pathways controlling RAP1-dependent N-Cadherin trafficking and how N-Cadherin-dependent signaling triggers the break in symmetry.

Neurotrophins

Brain derived neurotrophic factor (BDNF) and neurotrophin-3 (NT-3) are highly expressed in the developing brain and have been shown to stimulate axon specification and elongation (Morfini et al., 1994; Nakamuta et al., 2011). Both, BDNF and NT-3 as extracellular regulators of neuronal polarity are of special interest since they act in an autocrine and/or paracrine manner in cell-culture (Nakamuta et al., 2011). This feature indicates that neurons are able to produce extracellular stimuli (in form of secreted neurotrophins) that activate the intrinsic machinery for axon-dendrite specification in a cell-autonomous and non-cell-autonomous manner. BDNF and NT-3 bind to tropomyosin related kinases receptors (TRK), TRK-B and TRK-C respectively (Chao, 2003). Upon TRK receptor binding, the small GTPase Ras and PI3K are activated. This leads to the production of phosphatidylinositol (3,4,5)-trisphosphate (PIP_3) and the activation of its downstream signaling pathways (Reichardt, 2006). Neurotrophin signaling through TRK receptors also leads to increased levels of inositol triphosphate (IP3)-induced calcium release which in turn activates the calmodulin-dependent protein kinase kinase (CaMKK) and calmodulin-dependent protein kinase I (CamKI; Nakamuta et al., 2011). The activation of CaMKK and CamKI triggers the phosphorylation of microtubule affinity regulating kinase 2 (MARK2). This leads to the phosphorylation of downstream microtubule associated proteins (MAPs) MAP2/4, Tau and DCX which reduces microtubule stability (Drewes et al., 1997; Schaar et al., 2004; Nakamuta et al., 2011). Interestingly, acute knockdown of MARK2 has been shown to stall MP-to-BP transition in the IZ in mice (Sapir et al., 2008). Thus, proper regulation of MARK2 appears to be essential for neuronal polarization *in vivo*.

BDNF signaling via TrkB has been demonstrated in culture experiments to lead to the activation of LKB1 (liver kinase b1 in mammals and PAR-4 in *C. elegans* (**Figures 2, 3**; Shelly et al., 2007). Loss of function of LKB1 either by genetic knockout or knockdown by shRNA in nascent cortical projection neurons results in striking phenotypes: axon specification is completely abolished while the dendrite appears to still be specified (Barnes et al., 2007; Shelly et al., 2007). In contrast, overexpression of LKB1 in neural progenitors and postmitotic neurons lead to formation of multiple axons. In a biochemical pathway downstream of BDNF/TrkB, LKB1 is phosphorylated by protein kinase A (PKA) or ribosomal S6 kinase (p90RSK) at Serine 431 (Collins et al., 2000; Sapkota et al., 2001). Phosphorylated LKB1 leads to downstream activation of MARK2 (Shelly et al., 2007) and the SAD kinases which in turn phosphorylate Tau-1 (Kishi et al., 2005; Barnes et al., 2007). Remarkably, SAD-A/B double knockout precisely mimic the LKB1 loss of function phenotype with complete absence of the axon (Kishi et al., 2005). In summary, the above studies established a model whereby BDNF signaling via TrkB results in the activation of LKB1 which is translated into an intracellular symmetry break in multipolar cortical projection neurons while sojourning in the SVZ/IZ. Phosphorylated LKB1 localizes into the nascent axon and is required for axon extension and development. It will be interesting to determine the extent of specificity and functional redundancy of individual downstream components along the BDNF/TrkB-LKB1-SAD-A/B signaling module while executing the break in symmetry.

Semaphorins

Semaphorins consist of a large family of membrane bound or secreted proteins (Nakamura et al., 2000). The secreted semaphorin, Sema3A have been shown to act as a chemotactic factor for migrating cortical projection neurons (Polleux et al., 2000; Chen et al., 2008). Sema3A expression is highest near the pial surface in the developing cortex and the Sema3A expression domain establishes a descending gradient across the emerging cortical layers (Polleux et al., 2000; Chen et al., 2008). Sema3A binds its co-receptors Plexin and Neuropilin (Negishi et al., 2005) and it has been suggested that Sema3A may actively control the process of symmetry breaking and cellular polarization. Sema3A activates a number of downstream cascades resulting in the tuning of relative levels of cGMP and cyclic adenosine 3′,5′-monophosphate (cAMP) which negatively affects axon formation by downregulation of PKA-dependent phosphorylation of LKB1 (Shelly et al., 2011). Interestingly, exposure of undifferentiated neurites to local sources of Sema3A in hippocampal neuron cell culture leads to the suppression of axon-formation but promotion of dendrite formation in culture conditions (Shelly et al., 2011). Strikingly, *in vivo* knockdown of the Sema3A receptor neuropilin-1 in rat embryonic cortical progenitors results in severe polarization defects. Furthermore, Sema4D inactivates Ras (Oinuma et al., 2004) while it activates RhoA (Swiercz et al., 2002) which prevents axon formation and/or outgrowth via reduced actin dynamics and actin contraction. Thus, Sema3A acting via the neuropilin-1 receptor and semaphorins in general are critically involved in the symmetry break and polarization of nascent projection neurons in the developing cortex (Shelly et al., 2011).

TGF-β

The transforming growth factor β (TGF-β) has been reported to play an important role in the polarization of nascent cortical projection neurons in the developing cerebral cortex (Yi et al., 2010). Upon binding of one of the three TGF-β ligands (TGF-β1-3) to the type II TGF-β receptor (TβR2), this receptor is recruited to the type I TGF-β receptor (TβR1) to form a complex which triggers the phosphorylation of the two receptors by the serine/threonine kinase domain (Shi and Massagué, 2003). The TβR2-TβR1 receptor complex has been shown to phosphorylate Par-6 which in turn regulates Cdc42/Rac1 activity by recruiting the ubiquitin ligase Smurf1 which promotes proteasomal degradation of the RhoA GTPase. This results in reduced activity of RhoA in the nascent axon thereby stimulating its outgrowth (Gonzalez-Billault et al., 2012). Thus, RhoA activity can be precisely regulated in response to TGF-β signaling thereby controlling the dynamics of the local actin organization which is essential for axon specification and thus cellular polarization (Yi et al., 2010). Interestingly, TGF-β2-3 is highly expressed near the VZ/SVZ. Thus nascent developing neurons could be exposed to a gradient which delivers a uniform stimuli for axon specification (Yi et al., 2010). However, the majority of MP neurons extend their axons tangentially (Hatanaka and Yamauchi, 2013) rather than towards the ventricular side. It is thus conceivable that TGF-β might only act as a stimulus for axon specification rather than an axon guidance cue (Yi et al., 2010). Bone morphogenic protein (BMP), also a member of the TGF-β superfamily appears to play important functions in the MP-to-BP transition as well. BMPs are known to signal via the intracellular downstream mediator SMAD which leads to the suppression of collapsin response mediator protein 2 (CRMP2), a transcription factor known to promote microtubule assembly (Shi and Massagué, 2003; Sun et al., 2010). Strikingly, upon suppression of CRMP2 or overexpression of dominant negative forms of CRMP2 multipolar cells accumulate in the SVZ/IZ in the developing cortex. While these findings suggest that a BMP-SMAD signaling pathway, via CRMP2, regulates the polarization of cortical projection neurons the precise molecular and biochemical mechanisms remain to be determined (Sun et al., 2010). Altogether, different members of the TFG-β superfamily play important roles in multipolar cortical neurons and direct neuronal polarization through distinct signaling pathways.

INTRINSIC BIOCHEMICAL NETWORKS THAT MEDIATE NEURONAL POLARITY

While the above sections illustrated the role of extracellular cues for triggering and/or execution of neuronal polarization, the intrinsic molecular mechanisms involved in symmetry breaking will be discussed in the sections below with a focus on *in vitro* and cell culture experiments. Isolated neurons in cell culture form one axon and several dendrites. External chemical or physical cues of instructive or antagonistic nature that determine axon formation have been identified (Lamoureux et al., 2002; Gomez et al., 2007; Shelly et al., 2011). However, cultured neuronal cells are able to polarize even in the absence of any external cue (Dotti et al., 1988) suggesting that cells have intrinsic ability to break symmetry, which is solely activated externally. What are the functional cell-intrinsic networks that underlie cell polarization and determine the biochemical state of the cell? Based on Turing's idea of a reaction-diffusion mechanism to explain how spatial order during embryogenesis may arise (Turing, 1990), Gierer and Meinhardt developed a conceptual framework for pattern formation, which is based on the local activation in the form of self-enhancing feedback, which amplifies and reinforces spatially asymmetric distributions of molecules, coupled to long-range inhibitory processes (Meinhardt and Gierer, 2000). While this concept was originally developed to explain spatial patterning during morphogenesis, it also provides a framework to understand cell polarity. Accordingly, cell polarization is seen as a self-organized process (Wennekamp et al., 2013), which involves local symmetry breaking, signal amplification and long-range inhibition (Wang, 2009; Chau et al., 2012).

Previous work was able to identify many molecular players involved in the processes that allow a neuron to choose the one neurite to become an axon (Barnes and Polleux, 2009). While cell polarization can theoretically arise from a single molecular species that features a positive feedback (Altschuler et al., 2008), symmetry breaking in neurons likely reflects interactions among multiple, partially redundant pathways with crosstalk among them (Namba et al., 2015). This network can be subdivided into several, partially overlapping modules, each of which comprises a subset of molecular players that encode for specific cellular functions. To a rough approximation, the output of one module can serve as the input for a module downstream. Here, we want to illustrate how these functional modules orchestrate neuronal polarization and how they are embedded in a more complex biochemical network giving rise to axon specification. Importantly, individual modules are often evolutionarily conserved among species and pathways that regulate cell polarization in seemingly distinct tissues and contexts are remarkably similar. Accordingly we can to some degree take advantage of known cell polarization concepts in yeast, *C. elegans* and migrating cells (Iden and Collard, 2008), with the goal to anticipate a better understanding of the molecular processes that underlie axon specification.

PIP/PI$_3$K Module

Molecules involved in the initial symmetry breaking event are commonly localized to the plasma membrane, where not only integral membrane proteins receive extracellular signals, but where also peripherally binding membrane proteins bind reversibly to the membrane (Cho and Stahelin, 2005). This restricts the diffusion of these proteins, increases the efficiency of protein-protein interactions and/or modulates their catalytic activity (Vaz et al., 1984; Leonard and Hurley, 2011; Ebner et al., 2017). As a result, the membrane can be interpreted as a computational platform where transient protein clusters integrate, interpret and amplify incoming biochemical signals (Groves and Kuriyan, 2010).

One component of membrane-based signaling pathways that was found to be essential for the establishment of intracellular organization include phosphoinositides (PIPs). Even though they represent only about 1% of membrane phospholipids (Di Paolo and De Camilli, 2006), the associated signaling pathways control cell growth, division, survival and differentiation, and allow to generate highly polarized neuronal morphologies such as growth cones and synapses (Sasaki et al., 2007). Cells use a precisely defined spatiotemporal distribution of PIPs to control the activity of intracellular signaling pathways. For cell polarity, it is the asymmetry of phosphatidylinositol-3,4,5-phosphate ($PI(3,4,5)P_3$ = PIP_3) at the plasma membrane that is used to establish a polarity axis in the cell. The intramembranous PIP_3 concentration is controlled by activation of the phosphoinositide-3-kinase (PI3K; Whitman et al., 1985) as well as phosphatases such as phosphatase and tensin homolog (PTEN; Lee et al., 1999) that directly antagonize PI3K by dephosphorylating PIP_3 to $PI(4,5)P_2$ (PIP_2) (Carracedo and Pandolfi, 2008). Overexpression of PTEN or inhibition of the PI3K were both found to abolish cell polarization and axon specification (Shi et al., 2003; Jiang et al., 2005). In contrast, reduction of PTEN expression results in neurons with multiple axons (Jiang et al., 2005). Together, these results demonstrate that the activities of these enzymes need to be tightly balanced to produce one and only one axon.

Since polarization is a dynamic spatiotemporal process, not only the total amount of phosphoinositides but also their distribution in space and time needs to be precisely regulated. In cells, the intracellular distribution of PIP_3 can be visualized using a fluorescent reporter protein that specifically binds to PIP_3; e.g., GFP fused to the Pleckstrin-homology (PH) domain of the serine/threonine kinase Akt (Gray et al., 1999). This probe visualized PIP_3 accumulation at the tip of a neurite contributing to neuronal polarity and axon specification (Ménager et al., 2004). In contrast, EGFP-PLCd1-PH, which binds to PI(4, 5)P2 or IP3 showed a homogeneous distribution in cultured neuronal cells (Ménager et al., 2004).

The localized accumulation of PIP_3 likely represents the first spatial landmark that establishes the polarity axes of the cell. *In vivo*, activity of PI3K and PIP_3 production is most likely regulated by asymmetric distribution of extracellular factors (Namba et al., 2015), still, neurons polarize in cell culture without obvious asymmetries in their environment (Dotti et al., 1988). This suggest that starting from a homogeneous distribution of signaling molecules, dedicated biochemical circuits are able to amplify small fluctuations of signaling lipids in the plasma membrane. These interactions eventually break the symmetry of the cell and control cell morphogenesis (Wennekamp et al., 2013). The biochemical network underlying phosphoinositide polarity was studied in detail in other model systems. For example, *Dictyostelium discoideum* cells (Malchow et al., 1973), leukocytes and neutrophils (Trepat et al., 2012) polarize in response to a gradient of the chemoattractant cAMP or a variety of chemokines respectively by establishing domains of different phosphoinositides: PIP_3 at the leading edge of the cell and PIP_2 at its tail (Petrie et al., 2009). Importantly, and similar to neurons, the ability to break symmetry is independent from directional sensing, as cells that are placed in a uniform distribution of chemoattractant are still able to polarize (Petrie et al., 2009). Again, this illustrates the intrinsic ability of biochemical networks to polarize the cell in the absence of exogenous spatial signals (Wedlich-Soldner and Li, 2003). While phosphoinositide signaling was found to spatially organize the actin cytoskeleton, the initial symmetry breaking event itself does not depend on actin filaments. Fluorescently-labeled PH_{Akt} and PTEN, which acted as probes for PIP_3 and PIP_2 respectively, were found to self-organize into traveling waves in *Dictyostelium discoideum* cells even in the presence of the actin polymerization inhibitor latrunculin A (Gerisch et al., 2012). Importantly, this finding indicates that the ability to break symmetry in the membrane is established upstream and independent of the cytoskeleton. Instead, a PIP_3-dependent negative regulation of PTEN recruitment to the membrane was suggested to allow PIP_3 to accumulate. In addition, PTEN localization and activity has been found to be dependent on the small GTPase RhoA, which was found to restrict PTEN to the rear of chemotaxing leukocytes (Li et al., 2005) and *Dictyostelium* cells. Arai et al. (2010) further suggest a Ras-dependent positive feedback of PI3K activity to stabilize the polarized state of the cell. In addition, negative regulation of PTEN activity downstream of the PIP_3 activated AKT kinase has been reported, which constitutes a parallel mechanism to maintain and stabilize polarity (Papakonstanti et al., 2007).

While phosphoinositides are the most important lipid species for cellular signaling there are also other lipid species involved in neuronal polarization: plasma membrane ganglioside sialidase (PMGS), which controls the ganglioside content in the plasma membrane of neurons was also found to show an asymmetric distribution of its activity: it is enriched in one of the stage 2 neurites and facilitates axon outgrowth by enhancing Rac and PI3K activity (Da Silva et al., 2005). Thus, the asymmetric distribution of two different kinds of lipid species appears to control the polarity of the cell.

GEFs and Small GTPases

Which biochemical circuits underlie signal amplification in neurons? By now, the identity of several PI3K-dependent GTPases involved in neuronal polarization is known, such as H-Ras (Yoshimura et al., 2006b), Cdc42 (Garvalov et al., 2007) or Rap1B (Schwamborn and Püschel, 2004; Nakamura et al., 2013). Similar to PI3K (Shi et al., 2003) their overexpression results in supernumerary axons (see **Figure 3**), while their knock down prevents axon formation (Schwamborn and Püschel, 2004; Yoshimura et al., 2006b; Garvalov et al., 2007; Nakamura et al., 2013), however, these proteins do not interact with PIP_3 themselves. Instead, the phosphorylation state of phosphoinositides in the plasma membrane is recognized by soluble guanine nucleotide exchange factors (GEFs) that contain PIP3 binding domains, such as GEFs of the Dbl and DOCK180 families (Rossman et al., 2005; Laurin and Côté, 2014). These protein families in turn activate GTPases while recruiting them to the membrane (Cherfils and Zeghouf, 2013). Though a systematic characterization of GEFs that directly interact with PIP_3 and control cell polarization is not complete yet, candidate proteins include SOS and RasGFR, both members of the Dbl family of GEFs that contain a canonical DH-PH domain structure (Zheng, 2001). The PH (Pleckstrin homology) domain binds to phosphoinositides and thereby controls localization and the DH (Dbl homology) domain is responsible for catalyzing nucleotide exchange (Zheng, 2001). Dock7, a Dock180 related protein that catalyzes the nucleotide exchange of Racl (Watabe-Uchida et al., 2006), was found to specifically bind PIP_3 via its DHR-1 domain (Kobayashi et al., 2001; Cote et al., 2005). Importantly, Dock7 is enriched in one of the stage 2 neurites—potentially the designated axon—supposedly controlling polarization and morphogenesis of the neuron (Watabe-Uchida et al., 2006). Controlled by these regulators, small GTPases can show phosphoinositide dependent activity patterns and a characteristic spatial distribution in the cell. However, direct evidence that GEF enrichment is a direct consequence of elevated PIP_3 levels in a stage 2 neurite is largely missing. Accordingly, the spatial distribution of GEFs could also depend on another PIP_3 binding protein which is recruited to and initiates a nascent axon.

As a result of their activation, GTP-bound GTPases engage in specific protein-protein interactions. By recruiting so-called effector proteins to the plasma membrane small GTPases determining the spatiotemporal activation pattern of other protein systems in the cell (Cherfils and Zeghouf, 2013). Effector proteins can be categorized in two classes: first, they can control cell morphology by directly acting on regulators of the actin or microtubule cytoskeleton, namely by increasing actin dynamicity and microtubule stabilization in the axon while stabilizing actin filaments in dendrites (Neukirchen and Bradke, 2011). For example, activation of Racl leads to a stabilization of axon microtubules via the stathmin pathway (Watabe-Uchida et al., 2006) while triggering actin remodeling (Hall et al., 2001; Gonzalez-Billault et al., 2012). In contrast, active RhoA promotes actin stabilization and contraction in dendrites as revealed by fluorescent activity sensors (Gonzalez-Billault et al., 2012). Second, effector proteins can be involved in the regulation of other small GTPases (DerMardirossian et al., 2004) or constituents of supramolecular complexes with various functions (Joberty et al., 2000; Lin et al., 2000). For example, they can act as coincidence detector for multiple binding partners (Carlton and Cullen, 2005) or signal to additional levels of regulation. For example, a common theme for the activation of small GTPases is that they comprise positive feedback loops. These self-amplifying circuits may not only lead to a local enrichment of GTPases on the membrane, but can also lead to collective, switch-like activation of proteins (Mizuno-Yamasaki et al., 2012). Accordingly, these kind of interactions can give rise to nonlinear signaling circuits with emergent properties, which can be crucial for breaking the symmetry and spatially organizing the cell (Yoshimura et al., 2006a).

The importance of positive feedback regulation for the symmetry breaking is probably best characterized in single-cell organisms such as yeast (Johnson et al., 2011). Despite the much lower complexity of this model organism, the general architecture of the biochemical network leading to cell polarization is most probably similar. In yeast, Cdc42 is the main spatial organizer of the cell as it regulates asymmetric cell division. Active, GTP-bound Cdc42 binds to the plasma membrane via its prenylated C-terminus, while GDP-bound Cdc42 is kept soluble in the cytoplasm via its interaction with its Guanosine nucleotide dissociation inhibitor (GDI) Rdil. Cdc42-GTP is thought to form a locally confined protein cluster on the membrane by a local amplification of spontaneous asymmetries. The positive feedback is thought to arise from an effector-GEF complex, where the activated GTPase recruits an effector protein that in turn interacts with its activator. In yeast, a small, transient patch of Cdc42-GTP would recruit the scaffolding protein Bem-1 to the membrane, which interacts with the Cdc42 GEF Cdc24. Bem-1 not only binds to Cdc24 but also boosts its GEF activity. Thus Bem-1 efficiently catalyzes proximal Cdc42-GDP to exchange their nucleotide to Cdc42-GTP which again is able to recruit more Bem-1-Cdc24 complex (Nern and Arkowitz, 1998; Gulli et al., 2000; Johnson et al., 2011). Effector-GEF interactions have been found to be involved for the regulation of many different small GTPases (Mizuno-Yamasaki et al., 2012) and might be generally required for collective, switch-like activation of GTPases. These kind of decisive signaling reactions are of crucial importance for the cell, as they not only lead to cell polarization, but also regulate other fundamental processes such as membrane trafficking and the dynamic properties of the actin and microtubule cytoskeletons, thereby controlling the morphogenesis of the cell.

While the role of many proteins involved in neuronal polarity has been studied in neuronal cell culture, the function of Cdc42 has also been studied *in vivo* (Garvalov et al., 2007). Only about 30% of neurons derived from Cdc42 null mice were able to form a Tau-1 positive axon and the activity levels of the actin regulator cofilin were disturbed. However, when axon formation in Cdc42 null cells was initiated by cytochalasin, axons formed even if the drug was washed away. This indicates that Cdc42 is needed for the initial steps of axon specification but is dispensable for axon outgrowth (Garvalov et al., 2007).

The PAR System

During cell polarization, the asymmetric distribution of phosphoinositides provides an initial signal to a number of protein systems that together control cell morphogenesis. One of those protein systems is the PAR system, which is recruited downstream of activated Cdc42 (Etienne-Manneville and Hall, 2001; Yamanaka et al., 2001; Nishimura et al., 2005). The PAR system is a set of highly conserved proteins that organize cell polarity in all metazoan cells. In neurons, it was found that the PAR system is required for axon dendrite polarity (Shi et al., 2003; Chen et al., 2006), migration (Sapir et al., 2008) and dendrite development (Terabayashi et al., 2007). However, a complete mechanistic characterization of how these proteins regulate axon formation is missing.

The PAR system is probably best studied in the nematode *Caenorhabditis elegans*, where it controls the first division. In a single cell embryo, the PAR proteins self-organize into two non-overlapping domains (anterior and posterior domain) to govern asymmetric spindle positioning and ultimately the generation of daughter cells with different fate (Kemphues et al., 1988; Gönczy and Rose, 2005). The PAR proteins have been categorized in anterior PARs (aPARs; PAR-3, PAR-6, PKC-3, cdc42) and posterior PARs (pPARs; PAR-2, PAR-1, LGL-1), all of which are peripheral membrane proteins. Their mutual exclusion is thought to arise from cross-phosphorylation by the two kinases PKC-3 and PAR-1, which leads to membrane detachment, controls oligomerization state and hence their diffusivity (Feng et al., 2007; Hoege and Hyman, 2013; Arata et al., 2016). PKC-3 can phosphorylate all posterior PARs (Hao et al., 2006; Hoege et al., 2010), in return, PAR-1 phosphorylates PAR-3 (Guo and Kemphues, 1995; Benton and St Johnston, 2003; Motegi et al., 2011). A network of regulatory biochemical interactions between aPARs and pPARs is thought to finely tune the activity of these kinases, leading to two dynamically stable cellular domains that govern a plethora of downstream events (Goehring, 2014).

Apart from PAR-2, the PAR system is conserved among most multicellular organisms and defines polarity via mutual exclusion in different contexts such as anterior-posterior polarity in *Drosophila* oocytes and apical-basal polarity in epithelial tissues (Morton et al., 2002; Goldstein and Macara, 2007; Thompson, 2013). The overall importance of the PAR system for axon dendrite polarity was firmly established in dissociated hippocampal cell culture system and enrichment of anterior PARs at the tip of the outgrowing axon has been observed (Shi et al., 2003). Subsequent knock down or overexpression studies of several PAR members showed that genetic manipulation of the PAR system either results in no or supernumerary axons (**Figure 3**). If mutual exclusion among aPARs and pPARs is a universal feature of the PAR system one would expect the posterior PAR-1 homolog MARK2 to be absent from the tip of the axon. Surprisingly, fluorescence sensors to measure MARK2 activity in the developing axon of cortical neurons showed highest kinase activity in the growing axon tip (Moravcevic et al., 2010; Timm et al., 2011). This indicates that both active PAR-1 kinases and aPARs are co-localizing at tip of the outgrowing axon and mutual exclusion of the "opposing" PAR complexes is not a requirement for axon dendrite polarity establishment. On a functional level, antagonism between MARK2 and the aPAR complex has been suggested (Chen et al., 2006). Analog to the *C. elegans* system, aPKC phosphorylates MARK2, which results in membrane detachment and most likely in reduced activity. Overexpression of MARK2 in hippocampal neurons prevented axon formation while knock down caused multiple axons (Chen et al., 2006; Wu et al., 2011). The opposite was seen for aPKC overexpression, which resulted in multiple axons (**Figure 3**; Parker et al., 2013). The overexpression phenotype of MARK2 was rescued by simultaneous overexpression of aPARs. No rescue was observed with a non phosphorylatable MARK2, indicating that direct inhibition of MARK2 by aPKC is responsible for the observed rescue. In a simple view, this could mean that MARK2 is a negative regulator of axon formation which is specifically inhibited by axon enriched aPARs via aPKC phosphorylation. However, *in vivo* knock out of the other PAR-1 homologs (SAD-kinases) also inhibited axon formation (see also above), indicating that a fine balance between these activities is needed (Kishi et al., 2005). Both, MARK2 and SAD kinases have to be activated by LKB1/PAR-4 (Lizcano et al., 2004; Shelly and Poo, 2011), which itself is downstream of cAMP/PKA signaling (Shelly et al., 2007). Thus, the PAR system not only translates PIP_3 dependent signaling into altered cytoskeleton dynamics but also integrates the input of heterotrimeric G protein receptor ligands. Interestingly and in contrast to *C. elegans*, LKB1/PAR-4 is enriched in the axon (Shelly et al., 2007) while it is homogenously distributed in the *C. elegans* zygote (Goehring, 2014). Knockdown of LGL-1 prevents axon formation but the precise role of LGL-1 in axon development is still poorly understood (Plant et al., 2003; Wang T. et al., 2011).

Another fundamental difference between the neuronal and nematode PAR system is their dependence on a previous symmetry breaking event. In *C. elegans*, the sperm entry marks a single symmetry breaking event that starts actomyosin based flows and facilitates PAR domain establishment whereas no asymmetries of PIP_3 have been reported. The PAR system in neurons is clearly downstream of regulators that directly control or are controlled by PIP_3, such as PI3K or ATK/GSK3b, Cdc42 and Rap1B (Insolera et al., 2011), whereas initial polarity formation in *C. elegans* does not depend on these PIP_3 controlled proteins (Schlesinger et al., 1999; Insolera et al., 2011). A possible explanation for this difference could be that neurons have to screen their environment during development (open systems) to remain a certain degree of plasticity while communication with the extracellular space is less important in the early stages of worm development. Thus, the PAR system is integrated into a more complex signaling network in neurons while it constitutes a rather autonomous polarity system in *C. elegans*. Since many PAR system intrinsic reactions (like phosphorylation events) seem to be conserved, it is still not clear how these reactions have to occur in space and time in neurons for faithful axon dendrite polarity establishment. Super resolution microscopy and higher temporal resolution of simultaneous activity monitoring of PARs and PIP_3 may be required to solve the question of how PARs fulfil their functions during neuronal development.

Closing the Loop

So far, we have only considered biochemical reactions downstream of an initial asymmetry of PIP_3. For robust symmetry breaking, a self-enforcing loop is required, which would give rise to a local accumulation of PIP_3 despite its rapid diffusion in the plasma membrane and the proteins in the cytoplasm. One possible functional network could originate from PIP_3 and at the same time further increase its local concentration on the membrane. Therefore, the described functional modules need to talk to each other and eventually feed back to the activity of PI3K.

The molecular players involved for this regulatory network could for example be GTPases or their GEFs and effector proteins, which would not only translate local PIP_3 enrichment into altered cytoskeleton dynamics and transport, but themselves further enhance the activity of PI3K. For example, Ras-GTP (Sasaki et al., 2004) and Rac1-GTP (Srinivasan et al., 2003) in combination with actin polymerization (Peyrollier et al., 2000; Wang et al., 2002) or via additional players like the Par6/Par3 aPKC complex where found to activate PI3K

(Motegi et al., 2011; Laurin and Côté, 2014). Indeed, these proteins were all found to be required for axon formation (Shi et al., 2003; Yoshimura et al., 2006b; Tahirovic et al., 2010). H-Ras is a direct activator of PI3K and is also activated downstream of PI3K (Rodriguez-Viciana et al., 1994; Yang et al., 2012). Interestingly, this feedback loop results in H-Ras translocation via vesicle based transport into the future axon, which depletes H-RAS from the other neurites, presumably leading to reduced PI3K activity in other neurites and subsequently to inhibition of their outgrowth (Fivaz et al., 2008). While the idea of this amplifying circuit is at least partially based on experimentally verified protein-protein interactions, the emergent properties of this network have not been tested yet. For example, the role of PTEN localization and activity for phosphoinositide polarization in neurons is not yet clear (Kreis et al., 2014) and there might be functional networks that involve either less or a different set of molecular players. Furthermore, the connectivity of those circuits could even change with time, different extracellular inputs or in different subcellular locations.

Another layer of regulation can also be performed on the level of GDP dissociation inhibitors (GDIs), whose main function is to maintain their target, lipid-modified GTPases in an inactive, soluble state (Cherfils and Zeghouf, 2013). There is evidence that the affinity of RhoGDIs for different GTPases can be modulated by phosphorylation. For example, the kinase PAK1 is an effector protein of Rac1 that was found to phosphorylate RhoGDIs (DerMardirossian et al., 2004). Phosphorylation of these GDIs can enhance the dissociation of Rac1 from the GDI complex, thereby increasing the rate of Rac1 activation. As this leads to further stimulation of PAK1 activity such interaction may give rise to another positive feedback and symmetry breaking in neurons (**Figure 2B**).

Finally, and in addition to molecular processes that depend on locally confined phosphorylation and dephosphorylation of PIPs, PIP_3 can also accumulate in the outgrowing axon with the help of directed microtubule-based transport. For example, the plus-end directed kinesin-like motor Gakin transports PIP_3-containing vesicles through the interaction with the adaptor protein α-centaurin (Horiguchi et al., 2006). MARK2, a homolog of PAR-1, inhibits this transport by phosphorylating Gakin thereby preventing the development of axons (Yoshimura et al., 2010). MARK2 itself is deactivated by the PIP_3-regulated kinase aPKC (Chen et al., 2006; Ivey et al., 2014). Thus a high local PIP_3 concentration could inhibit MARK2 in the axon shaft, further enhancing directed transport of PIP_3-containing vesicles to the growth cone. Accordingly, this could result in a self-perpetuating feedback loop supporting axon outgrowth (Yoshimura et al., 2010).

Collectively, these feedback loops stabilize polarity that can arise from short-lived local concentration fluctuations of external signals, temporal fluctuations in the output signal strength of receptors (Ladbury and Arold, 2012) or subtle heterogeneities on a coverslip. These small differences then lead to high and persistent activity of modulators that favor actin dynamicity and microtubule stability in the designated axon. Studies using drugs that either stabilized microtubules (Witte et al., 2008) or destabilized actin filaments (Bradke and Dotti, 1999) are sufficient to induce the formation of multiple axons, consistent with the view that the effects of the above mentioned circuits are transmitted via selective modulation of the cytoskeleton. In particular, these are the MARK2/SAD target and microtubule stabilizing tau proteins, microtubule destabilizers such as stathmin, actin dynamics modulators cofilin and WAVE and/ or inactivation of regulators that prevent axon outgrowth such as the RhoA/Rock module. This ultimately gives rise to a permanent molecular difference between axon and dendrites that will later on be manifested in a functional/electrophysiological difference of the two compartments, axon and dendrites. How this compartmentalization is maintained is not well understood and probably also relies on long range inhibitory signals, but future research will be needed to entangle the exact communications of these compartments during neuronal development.

CONCLUSION AND PERSPECTIVES

The phenomenon of neuronal polarization has been extensively studied in the last decades. Many of the analyses used the elegant cell culture system developed by Dotti et al. (1988). Thus the current model of neuronal polarization is to a large extent based on single hippocampal cells in an isolated system. Still, these extensive *in vitro* biochemical and cell biological analyses have provided a solid understanding of the general principles of cell polarization. A key question however remains: what are the cell-intrinsic biophysical and molecular mechanisms that induce the initial break in symmetry in cortical progenitor cells and developing cortical projection neurons *in vivo*? In order to address this question it will be essential to establish tools that allow the visualization and/or manipulation of the precise localization of molecular markers at high resolution in an *in situ* tissue context. The CRISPR-Cas9-dependent SLENDR method promises a high-throughput platform to visualize the endogenous localization of candidate proteins at high micro- to nanometer resolution (Mikuni et al., 2016). Given that a number of "polarity signaling systems" seem quite sensitive to perturbation and not particularly resilient, the precise determination of "polarity gene" function at distinct stages in development represents a current challenge in the field. In order to probe the function of genes encoding regulators of neuronal polarity *in vivo*, the genetic mosaic analysis with double markers (MADM) technology (Zong et al., 2005; Hippenmeyer et al., 2010; Hippenmeyer, 2013) offers an experimental opportunity. By exploiting MADM, one can induce sparse genetic mosaics with wild-type and mutant cells labeled in two distinct colors at high resolution. In combination with live-imaging such an experimental MADM paradigm enables: (1) the dissection of the cell-autonomous gene function; and (2) determination of the relative contribution of non-cell-autonomous effects *in situ* at the global tissue level (Beattie et al., 2017). Altogether, the experimental platforms above promise a robust approach to determine the so far unknown functions of regulators implicated in the polarization process of progenitor cells and nascent cortical projection neurons. A key open question in a functional context is: what is the level of redundancy and specificity in extracellular cues and intracellular amplification mechanisms? Interestingly, the process of MP-to-BP transition appears to involve not only dynamic cytoskeletal-associated processes but also regulation at the transcriptional level (Hippenmeyer, 2014; Ohtaka-Maruyama and Okado, 2015). It will be important to analyze transcriptional responses at high temporal resolution and evaluate the influence on the general biochemical cell state. In future experiments it will be also important to establish biochemical and biophysical methods and assays that should allow the precise analysis of the break in symmetry at high molecular and/or structural resolution. In a broader context it will be important to address the question whether cell-type diversity may imply the necessity for adaptation in the mechanisms controlling polarization? In other words, how conserved is the process of symmetry break and polarization in distinct classes of neurons with different morphologies? The future analysis of the core signaling modules controlling cell polarity in a variety of brain areas and at high cellular and molecular resolution promises great conceptual advance.

AUTHOR CONTRIBUTIONS

AHH, CD, CM, ML and SH contributed equally to the writing of the initial draft. All authors revised the manuscript.

ACKNOWLEDGMENTS

This work was supported by IST Austria institutional funds; the European Union (FP7-CIG618444 to SH) and a program grant from the Human Frontiers Science Program (RGP0053/2014 to SH). CD was supported by a postdoctoral ISTFELLOW fellowship and CM was a postdoctoral fellow of the FWF Herta Firnberg programme.

REFERENCES

Altschuler, S. J., Angenent, S. B., Wang, Y., and Wu, L. F. (2008). On the spontaneous emergence of cell polarity. *Nature* 454, 886–889. doi: 10.1038/nature07119

Angevine, J. B. Jr., and Sidman, R. L. (1961). Autoradiographic study of cell migration during histogenesis of cerebral cortex in the mouse. *Nature* 192, 766–768. doi: 10.1038/192766b0

Anthony, T. E., Klein, C., Fishell, G., and Heintz, N. (2004). Radial glia serve as neuronal progenitors in all regions of the central nervous system. *Neuron* 41, 881–890. doi: 10.1016/s0896-6273(04)00140-0

Arai, Y., Shibata, T., Matsuoka, S., Sato, M. J., Yanagida, T., and Ueda, M. (2010). Self-organization of the phosphatidylinositol lipids signaling system for random cell migration. *Proc. Natl. Acad. Sci. U S A* 107, 12399–12404. doi: 10.1073/pnas.0908278107

Arata, Y., Hiroshima, M., Pack, C. G., Ramanujam, R., Motegi, F., Nakazato, K., et al. (2016). Cortical polarity of the RING protein PAR-2 is maintained by exchange rate kinetics at the cortical-cytoplasmic boundary. *Cell rep.* 17:316. doi: 10.1016/j.celrep.2016.09.044

Ballif, B. A., Arnaud, L., Arthur, W. T., Guris, D., Imamoto, A., and Cooper, J. A. (2004). Activation of a Dab1/CrkL/C3G/Rap1 pathway in Reelin-stimulated neurons. *Curr. Biol.* 14, 606–610. doi: 10.1016/j.cub.2004.03.038

Barnes, A. P., Lilley, B. N., Pan, Y. A., Plummer, L. J., Powell, A. W., Raines, A. N., et al. (2007). LKB1 and SAD kinases define a pathway required for the polarization of cortical neurons. *Cell* 129, 549–563. doi: 10.1016/j.cell.2007.03.025

Barnes, A. P., and Polleux, F. (2009). Establishment of axon-dendrite polarity in developing neurons. *Annu. Rev. Neurosci.* 32, 347–381. doi: 10.1146/annurev.neuro.31.060407.125536

Beattie, R., Postiglione, M. P., Burnett, L. E., Laukoter, S., Streicher, C., Pauler, F. M., et al. (2017). Mosaic analysis with double markers reveals distinct sequential functions of lgl1 in neural stem cells. *Neuron* 94, 517.e3–533.e3. doi: 10.1016/j.neuron.2017.04.012

Benton, R., and St Johnston, D. (2003). *Drosophila* PAR-1 and 14-3-3 inhibit Bazooka/PAR-3 to establish complementary cortical domains in polarized cells. *Cell* 115, 691–704. doi: 10.1016/s0092-8674(03)00938-3

Betizeau, M., Cortay, V., Patti, D., Pfister, S., Gautier, E., Bellemin-Ménard, A., et al. (2013). Precursor diversity and complexity of lineage relationships in the outer subventricular zone of the primate. *Neuron* 80, 442–457. doi: 10.1016/j.neuron.2013.09.032

Borrell, V., and Götz, M. (2014). Role of radial glial cells in cerebral cortex folding. *Curr. Opin. Neurobiol.* 27, 39–46. doi: 10.1016/j.conb.2014.02.007

Bradke, F., and Dotti, C. G. (1999). The role of local actin instability in axon formation. *Science* 283, 1931–1934. doi: 10.1126/science.283.5409.1931

Britto, J. M., Tait, K. J., Lee, E. P., Gamble, R. S., Hattori, M., and Tan, S. S. (2014). Exogenous Reelin modifies the migratory behavior of neurons depending on cortical location. *Cereb. Cortex* 24, 2835–2847. doi: 10.1093/cercor/bht123

Carlton, J. G., and Cullen, P. J. (2005). Coincidence detection in phosphoinositide signaling. *Trends Cell Biol.* 15, 540–547. doi: 10.1016/j.tcb.2005.08.005

Carracedo, A., and Pandolfi, P. P. (2008). The PTEN-PI3K pathway: of feedbacks and cross-talks. *Oncogene* 27, 5527–5541. doi: 10.1038/onc.2008.247

Chao, M. V. (2003). Neurotrophins and their receptors: a convergence point for many signalling pathways. *Nat. Rev. Neurosci.* 4, 299–309. doi: 10.1038/nrn1078

Chau, A. H., Walter, J. M., Gerardin, J., Tang, C., and Lim, W. A. (2012). Designing synthetic regulatory networks capable of self-organizing cell polarization. *Cell* 151, 320–332. doi: 10.1016/j.cell.2012.08.040

Chen, S., Chen, J., Shi, H., Wei, M., Castaneda-Castellanos, D. R., Bultje, R. S., et al. (2013). Regulation of microtubule stability and organization by mammalian Par3 in specifying neuronal polarity. *Dev. Cell* 24, 26–40. doi: 10.1016/j.devcel.2012.11.014

Chen, G., Sima, J., Jin, M., Wang, K. Y., Xue, X. J., Zheng, W., et al. (2008). Semaphorin-3A guides radial migration of cortical neurons during development. *Nat. Neurosci.* 11, 36–44. doi: 10.1038/nn2018

Chen, Y. M., Wang, Q. J., Hu, H. S., Yu, P. C., Zhu, J., Drewes, G., et al. (2006). Microtubule affinity-regulating kinase 2 functions downstream of the PAR-3/PAR-6/atypical PKC complex in regulating hippocampal neuronal polarity. *Proc. Natl. Acad. Sci. U S A* 103, 8534–8539. doi: 10.1073/pnas.0509955103

Cherfils, J., and Zeghouf, M. (2013). Regulation of small GTPases by GEFs, GAPs and GDIs. *Physiol. Rev.* 93, 269–309. doi: 10.1152/physrev.00003.2012

Cho, W., and Stahelin, R. V. (2005). Membrane-protein interactions in cell signaling and membrane trafficking. *Annu. Rev. Biophys. Biomol. Struct.* 34, 119–151. doi: 10.1146/annurev.biophys.33.110502.133337

Collins, S. P., Reoma, J. L., Gamm, D. M., and Uhler, M. D. (2000). LKB1, a novel serine/threonine protein kinase and potential tumour suppressor, is phosphorylated by cAMP-dependent protein kinase (PKA) and prenylated *in vivo*. *Biochem. J.* 345, 673–680. doi: 10.1042/0264-6021:3450673

Cote, J. F., Motoyama, A. B., Bush, J. A., and Vuori, K. (2005). A novel and evolutionarily conserved PtdIns(3,4,5)P3-binding domain is necessary for DOCK180 signalling. *Nat. Cell Biol.* 7, 797–807. doi: 10.1038/ncb1280

D'Arcangelo, G., Homayouni, R., Keshvara, L., Rice, D. S., Sheldon, M., and Curran, T. (1999). Reelin is a ligand for lipoprotein receptors. *Neuron* 24, 471–479. doi: 10.1016/s0896-6273(00)80860-0

Da Silva, J. S., Hasegawa, T., Miyagi, T., Dotti, C. G., and Abad-Rodriguez, J. (2005). Asymmetric membrane ganglioside sialidase activity specifies axonal fate. *Nat. Neurosci.* 8, 606–615. doi: 10.1038/nn1442

DerMardirossian, C., Schnelzer, A., and Bokoch, G. M. (2004). Phosphorylation of RhoGDI by Pak1 mediates dissociation of Rac GTPase. *Mol. Cell* 15, 117–127. doi: 10.1016/j.molcel.2004.05.019

Di Paolo, G., and De Camilli, P. (2006). Phosphoinositides in cell regulation and membrane dynamics. *Nature* 443, 651–657. doi: 10.1038/nature05185

Dotti, C. G., Sullivan, C. A., and Banker, G. A. (1988). The establishment of polarity by hippocampal neurons in culture. *J. Neurosci.* 8, 1454–1468.

Drewes, G., Ebneth, A., Preuss, U., Mandelkow, E. M., and Mandelkow, E. (1997). MARK, a novel family of protein kinases that phosphorylate microtubule-associated proteins and trigger microtubule disruption. *Cell* 89, 297–308. doi: 10.1016/s0092-8674(00)80208-1

Ebner, M., Lucic, I., Leonard, T. A., and Yudushkin, I. (2017). PI(3,4,5)P3 engagement restricts Akt activity to cellular membranes. *Mol. Cell* 65, 416.e6–431.e6. doi: 10.1016/j.molcel.2016.12.028

Etienne-Manneville, S., and Hall, A. (2001). Integrin-mediated activation of Cdc42 controls cell polarity in migrating astrocytes through PKCζ. *Cell* 106, 489–498. doi: 10.1016/s0092-8674(01)00471-8

Evsyukova, I., Plestant, C., and Anton, E. S. (2013). Integrative mechanisms of oriented neuronal migration in the developing brain. *Annu. Rev. Cell Dev. Biol.* 29, 299–353. doi: 10.1146/annurev-cellbio-101512-122400

Feng, W., Wu, H., Chan, L. N., and Zhang, M. (2007). The Par-3 NTD adopts a PB1-like structure required for Par-3 oligomerization and membrane localization. *EMBO J.* 26, 2786–2796. doi: 10.2210/pdb2ns5/pdb

Fietz, S. A., Kelava, I., Vogt, J., Wilsch-Brauninger, M., Stenzel, D., Fish, J. L., et al. (2010). OSVZ progenitors of human and ferret neocortex are epithelial-like and expand by integrin signaling. *Nat. Neurosci.* 13, 690–699. doi: 10.1038/nn.2553

Fivaz, M., Bandara, S., Inoue, T., and Meyer, T. (2008). Robust neuronal symmetry breaking by Ras-triggered local positive feedback. *Curr. Biol.* 18, 44–50. doi: 10.1016/j.cub.2007.11.051

Florio, M., Albert, M., Taverna, E., Namba, T., Brandl, H., Lewitus, E., et al. (2015). Human-specific gene *ARHGAP11B* promotes basal progenitor amplification and neocortex expansion. *Science* 347, 1465–1470. doi: 10.1126/science.aaa1975

Forster, E., Bock, H. H., Herz, J., Chai, X., Frotscher, M., and Zhao, S. (2010). Emerging topics in Reelin function. *Eur. J. Neurosci.* 31, 1511–1518. doi: 10.1111/j.1460-9568.2010.07222.x

Franco, S. J., and Muller, U. (2013). Shaping our minds: stem and progenitor cell diversity in the mammalian neocortex. *Neuron* 77, 19–34. doi: 10.1016/j.neuron.2012.12.022

Frotscher, M. (2010). Role for Reelin in stabilizing cortical architecture. *Trends Neurosci.* 33, 407–414. doi: 10.1016/j.tins.2010.06.001

Gao, P., Postiglione, M. P., Krieger, T. G., Hernandez, L., Wang, C., Han, Z., et al. (2014). Deterministic progenitor behavior and unitary production of neurons in the neocortex. *Cell* 159, 775–788. doi: 10.1016/j.cell.2014.10.027

Gartner, A., Fornasiero, E. F., and Dotti, C. G. (2015). Cadherins as regulators of neuronal polarity. *Cell Adh. Migr.* 9, 175–182. doi: 10.4161/19336918.2014.983808

Gartner, A., Fornasiero, E. F., Munck, S., Vennekens, K., Seuntjens, E., Huttner, W. B., et al. (2012). N-cadherin specifies first asymmetry in developing neurons. *EMBO J.* 31, 1893–1903. doi: 10.1038/emboj.2012.41

Garvalov, B. K., Flynn, K. C., Neukirchen, D., Meyn, L., Teusch, N., Wu, X., et al. (2007). Cdc42 regulates cofilin during the establishment of neuronal polarity. *J. Neurosci.* 27, 13117–13129. doi: 10.1523/jneurosci.3322-07.2007

Gerisch, G., Schroth-Diez, B., Muller-Taubenberger, A., and Ecke, M. (2012). PIP3 waves and PTEN dynamics in the emergence of cell polarity. *Biophys. J.* 103, 1170–1178. doi: 10.1016/j.bpj.2012.08.004

Goehring, N. W. (2014). PAR polarity: from complexity to design principles. *Exp. Cell Res.* 328, 258–266. doi: 10.1016/j.yexcr.2014.08.009

Goldstein, B., and Macara, I. G. (2007). The PAR proteins: fundamental players in animal cell polarization. *Dev. Cell* 13, 609–622. doi: 10.1016/j.devcel.2007.10.007

Gomez, N., Chen, S., and Schmidt, C. E. (2007). Polarization of hippocampal neurons with competitive surface stimuli: contact guidance cues are preferred over chemical ligands. *J. R. Soc. Interface* 4, 223–233. doi: 10.1098/rsif.2006.0171

Gönczy, P., and Rose, L. S. (2005). "Asymmetric cell division and axis formation in the embryo," in *WormBook*, ed. The *C. elegans* Research Community, 1–20. doi: 10.1895/wormbook.1.30.1

Gonzalez-Billault, C., Muñoz-Llancao, P., Henriquez, D. R., Wojnacki, J., Conde, C., and Caceres, A. (2012). The role of small GTPases in neuronal morphogenesis and polarity. *Cytoskeleton* 69, 464–485. doi: 10.1002/cm.21034

Gray, A., Van Der Kaay, J., and Downes, C. P. (1999). The pleckstrin homology domains of protein kinase B and GRP1 (general receptor for phosphoinositides-1) are sensitive and selective probes for the cellular detection of phosphatidylinositol 3,4-bisphosphate and/or phosphatidylinositol 3,4,5-trisphosphate *in vivo*. *Biochem. J.* 344, 929–936. doi: 10.1042/0264-6021:3440929

Groves, J. T., and Kuriyan, J. (2010). Molecular mechanisms in signal transduction at the membrane. *Nat. Struct. Mol. Biol.* 17, 659–665. doi: 10.1038/nsmb.1844

Gulli, M. P., Jaquenoud, M., Shimada, Y., Niederhauser, G., Wiget, P., and Peter, M. (2000). Phosphorylation of the Cdc42 exchange factor Cdc24 by the PAK-like kinase Cla4 may regulate polarized growth in yeast. *Mol. Cell* 6, 1155–1167. doi: 10.1016/s1097-2765(00)00113-1

Guo, S., and Kemphues, K. J. (1995). par-1, a gene required for establishing polarity in *C. elegans* embryos, encodes a putative Ser/Thr kinase that is asymmetrically distributed. *Cell* 81, 611–620. doi: 10.1016/0092-8674(95)90082-9

Hall, C., Brown, M., Jacobs, T., Ferrari, G., Cann, N., Teo, M., et al. (2001). Collapsin response mediator protein switches RhoA and Rac1 morphology in N1E-115 neuroblastoma cells and is regulated by Rho kinase. *J. Biol. Chem.* 276, 43482–43486. doi: 10.1074/jbc.c100455200

Hansen, D. V., Lui, J. H., Parker, P. R., and Kriegstein, A. R. (2010). Neurogenic radial glia in the outer subventricular zone of human neocortex. *Nature* 464, 554–561. doi: 10.1038/nature08845

Hao, Y., Boyd, L., and Seydoux, G. (2006). Stabilization of cell polarity by the *C. elegans* RING protein PAR-2. *Dev. Cell* 10, 199–208. doi: 10.1016/j.devcel.2005.12.015

Hatanaka, Y., and Yamauchi, K. (2013). Excitatory cortical neurons with multipolar shape establish neuronal polarity by forming a tangentially oriented axon in the intermediate zone. *Cereb. Cortex* 23, 105–113. doi: 10.1093/cercor/bhr383

Hippenmeyer, S. (2013). Dissection of gene function at clonal level using mosaic analysis with double markers. *Front. Biol.* 8, 557–568. doi: 10.1007/s11515-013-1279-6

Hippenmeyer, S. (2014). Molecular pathways controlling the sequential steps of cortical projection neuron migration. *Adv. Exp. Med. Biol.* 800, 1–24. doi: 10.1007/978-94-007-7687-6_1

Hippenmeyer, S., Youn, Y. H., Moon, H. M., Miyamichi, K., Zong, H., Wynshaw-Boris, A., et al. (2010). Genetic mosaic dissection of Lis1 and Ndel1 in neuronal migration. *Neuron* 68, 695–709. doi: 10.1016/j.neuron.2010.09.027

Hirota, Y., Kubo, K., Katayama, K., Honda, T., Fujino, T., Yamamoto, T. T., et al. (2015). Reelin receptors ApoER2 and VLDLR are expressed in distinct spatiotemporal patterns in developing mouse cerebral cortex. *J. Comp. Neurol.* 523, 463–478. doi: 10.1002/cne.23691

Hoege, C., Constantinescu, A. T., Schwager, A., Goehring, N. W., Kumar, P., and Hyman, A. A. (2010). LGL can partition the cortex of one-cell *Caenorhabditis elegans* embryos into two domains. *Curr. Biol.* 20, 1296–1303. doi: 10.1016/j.cub.2010.05.061

Hoege, C., and Hyman, A. A. (2013). Principles of PAR polarity in *Caenorhabditis elegans* embryos. *Nat. Rev. Mol. Cell Biol.* 14, 315–322. doi: 10.1038/nrm3558

Homem, C. C., Repic, M., and Knoblich, J. A. (2015). Proliferation control in neural stem and progenitor cells. *Nat. Rev. Neurosci.* 16, 647–659. doi: 10.1038/nrn4021

Honda, T., Kobayashi, K., Mikoshiba, K., and Nakajima, K. (2011). Regulation of cortical neuron migration by the Reelin signaling pathway. *Neurochem. Res.* 36, 1270–1279. doi: 10.1007/s11064-011-0407-4

Horiguchi, K., Hanada, T., Fukui, Y., and Chishti, A. H. (2006). Transport of PIP3 by GAKIN, a kinesin-3 family protein, regulates neuronal cell polarity. *J. Cell Biol.* 174, 425–436. doi: 10.1083/jcb.200604031

Howell, B. W., Hawkes, R., Soriano, P., and Cooper, J. A. (1997). Neuronal position in the developing brain is regulated by mouse disabled-1. *Nature* 389, 733–737. doi: 10.1038/39607

Howell, B. W., Herrick, T. M., and Cooper, J. A. (1999). Reelin-induced tyrosine [corrected] phosphorylation of disabled 1 during neuronal positioning. *Genes Dev.* 13, 643–648. doi: 10.1101/gad.13.6.643

Iden, S., and Collard, J. G. (2008). Crosstalk between small GTPases and polarity proteins in cell polarization. *Nat. Rev. Mol. Cell Biol.* 9, 846–859. doi: 10.1038/nrm2521

Insolera, R., Chen, S., and Shi, S. H. (2011). Par proteins and neuronal polarity. *Dev. Neurobiol.* 71, 483–494. doi: 10.1002/dneu.20867

Ivey, R. A., Sajan, M. P., and Farese, R. V. (2014). Requirements for pseudosubstrate arginine residues during autoinhibition and phosphatidylinositol 3,4,5-$(PO_4)_3$-dependent activation of atypical PKC. *J. Biol. Chem.* 289, 25021–25030. doi: 10.1074/jbc.M114.565671

Jiang, H., Guo, W., Liang, X., and Rao, Y. (2005). Both the establishment and the maintenance of neuronal polarity require active mechanisms: critical roles of GSK-3beta and its upstream regulators. *Cell* 120, 123–135. doi: 10.1016/s0092-8674(04)01258-9

Joberty, G., Petersen, C., Gao, L., and Macara, I. G. (2000). The cell-polarity protein Par6 links Par3 and atypical protein kinase C to Cdc42. *Nat. Cell Biol.* 2, 531–539. doi: 10.1038/35019573

Johnson, J. M., Jin, M., and Lew, D. J. (2011). Symmetry breaking and the establishment of cell polarity in budding yeast. *Curr. Opin. Genet. Dev.* 21, 740–746. doi: 10.1016/j.gde.2011.09.007

Johnson, M. B., Wang, P. P., Atabay, K. D., Murphy, E. A., Doan, R. N., Hecht, J. L., et al. (2015). Single-cell analysis reveals transcriptional heterogeneity of neural progenitors in human cortex. *Nat. Neurosci.* 18, 637–646. doi: 10.1038/nn.3980

Jossin, Y. (2011). Polarization of migrating cortical neurons by Rap1 and N-cadherin: revisiting the model for the reelin signaling pathway. *Small GTPases* 2, 322–328. doi: 10.4161/sgtp.18283

Jossin, Y., and Cooper, J. A. (2011). Reelin, Rap1 and N-cadherin orient the migration of multipolar neurons in the developing neocortex. *Nat. Neurosci.* 14, 697–703. doi: 10.1038/nn.2816

Kelava, I., Reillo, I., Murayama, A. Y., Kalinka, A. T., Stenzel, D., Tomancak, P., et al. (2012). Abundant occurrence of basal radial glia in the subventricular zone of embryonic neocortex of a lissencephalic primate, the common marmoset Callithrix jacchus. *Cereb. Cortex* 22, 469–481. doi: 10.1093/cercor/bhr301

Kemphues, K. J., Priess, J. R., Morton, D. G., and Cheng, N. S. (1988). Identification of genes required for cytoplasmic localization in early *C. elegans* embryos. *Cell* 52, 311–320. doi: 10.1016/s0092-8674(88)80024-2

Kishi, M., Pan, Y. A., Crump, J. G., and Sanes, J. R. (2005). Mammalian SAD kinases are required for neuronal polarization. *Science* 307, 929–932. doi: 10.1126/science.1107403

Knoblich, J. A. (2008). Mechanisms of asymmetric stem cell division. *Cell* 132, 583–597. doi: 10.1016/j.cell.2008.02.007

Kobayashi, S., Shirai, T., Kiyokawa, E., Mochizuki, N., Matsuda, M., and Fukui, Y. (2001). Membrane recruitment of DOCK180 by binding to PtdIns(3,4,5)P3. *Biochem. J.* 354, 73–78. doi: 10.1042/0264-6021:3540073

Kowalczyk, T., Pontious, A., Englund, C., Daza, R. A., Bedogni, F., Hodge, R., et al. (2009). Intermediate neuronal progenitors (basal progenitors) produce pyramidal-projection neurons for all layers of cerebral cortex. *Cereb. Cortex* 19, 2439–2450. doi: 10.1093/cercor/bhn260

Kreis, P., Leondaritis, G., Lieberam, I., and Eickholt, B. J. (2014). Subcellular targeting and dynamic regulation of PTEN: implications for neuronal cells and neurological disorders. *Front. Mol. Neurosci.* 7:23. doi: 10.3389/fnmol.2014.00023

Ladbury, J. E., and Arold, S. T. (2012). Noise in cellular signaling pathways: causes and effects. *Trends Biochem. Sci.* 37, 173–178. doi: 10.1016/j.tibs.2012.01.001

Lamoureux, P., Ruthel, G., Buxbaum, R. E., and Heidemann, S. R. (2002). Mechanical tension can specify axonal fate in hippocampal neurons. *J. Cell Biol.* 159, 499–508. doi: 10.1083/jcb.200207174

Laurin, M., and Côté, J.-F. (2014). Insights into the biological functions of Dock family guanine nucleotide exchange factors. *Genes Dev.* 28, 533–547. doi: 10.1101/gad.236349.113

Lee, H. O., and Norden, C. (2013). Mechanisms controlling arrangements and movements of nuclei in pseudostratified epithelia. *Trends Cell Biol.* 23, 141–150. doi: 10.1016/j.tcb.2012.11.001

Lee, J. O., Yang, H., Georgescu, M. M., Di Cristofano, A., Maehama, T., Shi, Y., et al. (1999). Crystal structure of the PTEN tumor suppressor: implications for its phosphoinositide phosphatase activity and membrane association. *Cell* 99, 323–334.

Leonard, T. A., and Hurley, J. H. (2011). Regulation of protein kinases by lipids. *Curr. Opin. Struct. Biol.* 21, 785–791. doi: 10.1016/j.sbi.2011.07.006

Li, Z., Dong, X., Wang, Z., Liu, W., Deng, N., Ding, Y., et al. (2005). Regulation of PTEN by Rho small GTPases. *Nat. Cell Biol.* 7, 399–404. doi: 10.1038/ncb1236

Lin, D., Edwards, A. S., Fawcett, J. P., Mbamalu, G., Scott, J. D., and Pawson, T. (2000). A mammalian PAR-3-PAR-6 complex implicated in Cdc42/Rac1 and aPKC signalling and cell polarity. *Nat. Cell Biol.* 2, 540–547. doi: 10.1038/35019582

Lizcano, J. M., Göransson, O., Toth, R., Deak, M., Morrice, N. A., Boudeau, J., et al. (2004). LKB1 is a master kinase that activates 13 kinases of the AMPK subfamily, including MARK/PAR-1. *EMBO J.* 23, 833–843. doi: 10.1038/sj.emboj.7600110

Lui, J. H., Hansen, D. V., and Kriegstein, A. R. (2011). Development and evolution of the human neocortex. *Cell* 146, 18–36. doi: 10.1016/j.cell.2011.06.030

Malatesta, P., Hartfuss, E., and Götz, M. (2000). Isolation of radial glial cells by fluorescent-activated cell sorting reveals a neuronal lineage. *Development* 127, 5253–5263.

Malchow, D., Fuchila, J., and Jastorff, B. (1973). Correlation of substrate specificity of cAMP-phosphodiesterase in Dictyostelium discoideum with chemotactic activity of cAMP-analogues. *FEBS Lett.* 34, 5–9. doi: 10.1016/0014-5793(73)80690-8

Marín, O., Valiente, M., Ge, X., and Tsai, L.-H. (2010). Guiding neuronal cell migrations. *Cold Spring Harb. Perspect. Biol.* 2:a001834. doi: 10.1101/cshperspect.a001834

Meinhardt, H., and Gierer, A. (2000). Pattern formation by local self-activation and lateral inhibition. *Bioessays* 22, 753–760. doi: 10.1002/1521-1878(200008)22:8<753::AID-BIES9>3.0.CO;2-Z

Ménager, C., Arimura, N., Fukata, Y., and Kaibuchi, K. (2004). PIP_3 is involved in neuronal polarization and axon formation. *J. Neurochem.* 89, 109–118. doi: 10.1046/j.1471-4159.2004.02302.x

Mikuni, T., Nishiyama, J., Sun, Y., Kamasawa, N., and Yasuda, R. (2016). High-throughput, high-resolution mapping of protein localization in mammalian brain by *in vivo* genome editing. *Cell* 165, 1803–1817. doi: 10.1016/j.cell.2016.04.044

Mizuno-Yamasaki, E., Rivera-Molina, F., and Novick, P. (2012). GTPase networks in membrane traffic. *Annu. Rev. Biochem.* 81, 637–659. doi: 10.1146/annurev-biochem-052810-093700

Moravcevic, K., Mendrola, J. M., Schmitz, K. R., Wang, Y. H., Slochower, D., Janmey, P. A., et al. (2010). Kinase associated-1 domains drive MARK/PAR1 kinases to membrane targets by binding acidic phospholipids. *Cell* 143, 966–977. doi: 10.1016/j.cell.2010.11.028

Morfini, G., DiTella, M. C., Feiguin, F., Carri, N., and Cáeres, A. (1994). Neurotrophin-3 enhances neurite outgrowth in cultured hippocampal pyramidal neurons. *J. Neurosci. Res.* 39, 219–232. doi: 10.1002/jnr.490390212

Morton, D. G., Shakes, D. C., Nugent, S., Dichoso, D., Wang, W., Golden, A., et al. (2002). The *Caenorhabditis elegans* par-5 gene encodes a 14-3-3 protein required for cellular asymmetry in the early embryo. *Dev. Biol.* 241, 47–58. doi: 10.1006/dbio.2001.0489

Motegi, F., Zonies, S., Hao, Y., Cuenca, A. A., Griffin, E., and Seydoux, G. (2011). Microtubules induce self-organization of polarized PAR domains in *C. elegans* zygotes. *Nat. Cell Biol.* 13, 1361–1367. doi: 10.1038/ncb2354

Nadarajah, B., Brunstrom, J. E., Grutzendler, J., Wong, R. O., and Pearlman, A. L. (2001). Two modes of radial migration in early development of the cerebral cortex. *Nat. Neurosci.* 4, 143–150. doi: 10.1038/83967

Nadarajah, B., and Parnavelas, J. G. (2002). Modes of neuronal migration in the developing cerebral cortex. *Nat. Rev. Neurosci.* 3, 423–432. doi: 10.1038/nrn845

Nakamura, F., Kalb, R. G., and Strittmatter, S. M. (2000). Molecular basis of semaphorin-mediated axon guidance. *J. Neurobiol.* 44, 219–229. doi: 10.1002/1097-4695(200008)44:2<219::AID-NEU11>3.0.CO;2-W

Nakamura, T., Yasuda, S., Nagai, H., Koinuma, S., Morishita, S., Goto, A., et al. (2013). Longest neurite-specific activation of Rap1B in hippocampal neurons contributes to polarity formation through RalA and Nore1A in addition to PI3-kinase. *Genes Cells* 18, 1020–1031. doi: 10.1111/gtc.12097

Nakamuta, S., Funahashi, Y., Namba, T., Arimura, N., Picciotto, M. R., Tokumitsu, H., et al. (2011). Local application of neurotrophins specifies axons through inositol 1,4,5-trisphosphate, calcium, and Ca^{2+}/calmodulin-dependent protein kinases. *Sci. Signal.* 4:ra76. doi: 10.1126/scisignal.2002011

Namba, T., Funahashi, Y., Nakamuta, S., Xu, C., Takano, T., and Kaibuchi, K. (2015). Extracellular and intracellular signaling for neuronal polarity. *Physiol. Rev.* 95, 995–1024. doi: 10.1152/physrev.00025.2014

Namba, T., Kibe, Y., Funahashi, Y., Nakamuta, S., Takano, T., Ueno, T., et al. (2014). Pioneering axons regulate neuronal polarization in the developing cerebral cortex. *Neuron* 81, 814–829. doi: 10.1016/j.neuron.2013.12.015

Negishi, M., Oinuma, I., and Katoh, H. (2005). Plexins: axon guidance and signal transduction. *Cell. Mol. Life Sci.* 62, 1363–1371. doi: 10.1007/s00018-005-5018-2

Nern, A., and Arkowitz, R. A. (1998). A GTP-exchange factor required for cell orientation. *Nature* 391, 195–198. doi: 10.1038/34458

Neukirchen, D., and Bradke, F. (2011). Neuronal polarization and the cytoskeleton. *Semin. Cell Dev. Biol.* 22, 825–833. doi: 10.1016/j.semcdb.2011.08.007

Nishimura, T., Yamaguchi, T., Kato, K., Yoshizawa, M., Nabeshima, Y., Ohno, S., et al. (2005). PAR-6-PAR-3 mediates Cdc42-induced Rac activation through the Rac GEFs STEF/Tiam1. *Nat. Cell Biol.* 7, 270–277. doi: 10.1038/ncb1227

Noctor, S. C. (2011). Time-lapse imaging of fluorescently labeled live cells in the embryonic mammalian forebrain. *Cold Spring Harb. Protoc.* 2011, 1350–1361. doi: 10.1101/pdb.prot066605

Noctor, S. C., Flint, A. C., Weissman, T. A., Dammerman, R. S., and Kriegstein, A. R. (2001). Neurons derived from radial glial cells establish radial units in neocortex. *Nature* 409, 714–720. doi: 10.1038/35055553

Noctor, S. C., Martínez-Cerdeño, V., Ivic, L., and Kriegstein, A. R. (2004). Cortical neurons arise in symmetric and asymmetric division zones and migrate through specific phases. *Nat. Neurosci.* 7, 136–144. doi: 10.1038/nn1172

Ogawa, M., Miyata, T., Nakajima, K., Yagyu, K., Seike, M., Ikenaka, K., et al. (1995). The reeler gene-associated antigen on Cajal-Retzius neurons is a crucial molecule for laminar organization of cortical neurons. *Neuron* 14, 899–912. doi: 10.1016/0896-6273(95)90329-1

Ohtaka-Maruyama, C., and Okado, H. (2015). Molecular pathways underlying projection neuron production and migration during cerebral cortical development. *Front. Neurosci.* 9:447. doi: 10.3389/fnins.2015.00447

Oinuma, I., Ishikawa, Y., Katoh, H., and Negishi, M. (2004). The Semaphorin 4D receptor Plexin-B1 is a GTPase activating protein for R-Ras. *Science* 305, 862–865. doi: 10.1126/science.1097545

Papakonstanti, E. A., Ridley, A. J., and Vanhaesebroeck, B. (2007). The p110delta isoform of PI 3-kinase negatively controls RhoA and PTEN. *EMBO J.* 26, 3050–3061. doi: 10.1038/sj.emboj.7601763

Paridaen, J. T., Wilsch-Bräuninger, M., and Huttner, W. B. (2013). Asymmetric inheritance of centrosome-associated primary cilium membrane directs ciliogenesis after cell division. *Cell* 155, 333–344. doi: 10.1016/j.cell.2013.08.060

Parker, S. S., Mandell, E. K., Hapak, S. M., Maskaykina, I. Y., Kusne, Y., Kim, J. Y., et al. (2013). Competing molecular interactions of aPKC isoforms regulate neuronal polarity. *Proc. Natl. Acad. Sci. U S A* 110, 14450–14455. doi: 10.1073/pnas.1301588110

Perez-Garcia, C. G., Tissir, F., Goffinet, A. M., and Meyer, G. (2004). Reelin receptors in developing laminated brain structures of mouse and human. *Eur. J. Neurosci.* 20, 2827–2832. doi: 10.1111/j.1460-9568.2004.03733.x

Petrie, R. J., Doyle, A. D., and Yamada, K. M. (2009). Random versus directionally persistent cell migration. *Nat. Rev. Mol. Cell Biol.* 10, 538–549. doi: 10.1038/nrm2729

Peyrollier, K., Hajduch, E., Gray, A., Litherland, G. J., Prescott, A. R., Leslie, N. R., et al. (2000). A role for the actin cytoskeleton in the hormonal and growth-factor-mediated activation of protein kinase B. *Biochem. J.* 352, 617–622. doi: 10.1042/0264-6021:3520617

Plant, P. J., Fawcett, J. P., Lin, D. C., Holdorf, A. D., Binns, K., Kulkarni, S., et al. (2003). A polarity complex of mPar-6 and atypical PKC binds, phosphorylates and regulates mammalian Lgl. *Nat. Cell Biol.* 5, 301–308. doi: 10.1038/ncb948

Pollen, A. A., Nowakowski, T. J., Chen, J., Retallack, H., Sandoval-Espinosa, C., Nicholas, C. R., et al. (2015). Molecular identity of human outer radial glia during cortical development. *Cell* 163, 55–67. doi: 10.1016/j.cell.2015.09.004

Polleux, F., Morrow, T., and Ghosh, A. (2000). Semaphorin 3A is a chemoattractant for cortical apical dendrites. *Nature* 404, 567–573. doi: 10.1038/35007001

Postiglione, M. P., and Hippenmeyer, S. (2014). Monitoring neurogenesis in the cerebral cortex: an update. *Fut. Neurol.* 9, 323–340. doi: 10.2217/fnl.14.18

Rakic, P. (1972). Mode of cell migration to the superficial layers of fetal monkey neocortex. *J. Comp. Neurol.* 145, 61–83. doi: 10.1002/cne.901450105

Rakic, P. (1974). Neurons in rhesus monkey visual cortex: systematic relation between time of origin and eventual disposition. *Science* 183, 425–427. doi: 10.1126/science.183.4123.425

Reichardt, L. F. (2006). Neurotrophin-regulated signalling pathways. *Philos. Trans. R. Soc. Lond. B Biol. Sci.* 361, 1545–1564. doi: 10.1098/rstb.2006.1894

Rodriguez-Viciana, P., Warne, P. H., Dhand, R., Vanhaesebroeck, B., Gout, I., Fry, M. J., et al. (1994). Phosphatidylinositol-3-OH kinase as a direct target of Ras. *Nature* 370, 527–532. doi: 10.1038/370527a0

Rossman, K. L., Der, C. J., and Sondek, J. (2005). GEF means go: turning on RHO GTPases with guanine nucleotide-exchange factors. *Nat. Rev. Mol. Cell Biol.* 6, 167–180. doi: 10.1038/nrm1587

Sapir, T., Sapoznik, S., Levy, T., Finkelshtein, D., Shmueli, A., Timm, T., et al. (2008). Accurate balance of the polarity kinase MARK2/Par-1 is required for proper cortical neuronal migration. *J. Neurosci.* 28, 5710–5720. doi: 10.1523/JNEUROSCI.0911-08.2008

Sapkota, G. P., Kieloch, A., Lizcano, J. M., Lain, S., Arthur, J. S., Williams, M. R., et al. (2001). Phosphorylation of the protein kinase mutated in Peutz-Jeghers cancer syndrome, LKB1/STK11, at Ser431 by p90(RSK) and cAMP-dependent protein kinase, but not its farnesylation at Cys(433), is essential for LKB1 to suppress cell growth. *J. Biol. Chem.* 276, 19469–19482. doi: 10.1074/jbc.M009953200

Sasaki, A. T., Chun, C., Takeda, K., and Firtel, R. A. (2004). Localized Ras signaling at the leading edge regulates PI3K, cell polarity, and directional cell movement. *J. Cell Biol.* 167, 505–518. doi: 10.1083/jcb.200406177

Sasaki, T., Sasaki, J., Sakai, T., Takasuga, S., and Suzuki, A. (2007). The physiology of phosphoinositides. *Biol. Pharm. Bull.* 30, 1599–1604. doi: 10.1248/bpb.30.1599

Schaar, B. T., Kinoshita, K., and McConnell, S. K. (2004). Doublecortin microtubule affinity is regulated by a balance of kinase and phosphatase activity at the leading edge of migrating neurons. *Neuron* 41, 203–213. doi: 10.1016/s0896-6273(03)00843-2

Schlesinger, A., Shelton, C. A., Maloof, J. N., Meneghini, M., and Bowerman, B. (1999). Wnt pathway components orient a mitotic spindle in the early *Caenorhabditis elegans* embryo without requiring gene transcription in the responding cell. *Genes Dev.* 13, 2028–2038. doi: 10.1101/gad.13.15.2028

Schwamborn, J. C., and Püschel, A. W. (2004). The sequential activity of the GTPases Rap1B and Cdc42 determines neuronal polarity. *Nat. Neurosci.* 7, 923–929. doi: 10.1038/nn1295

Sekine, K., Honda, T., Kawauchi, T., Kubo, K., and Nakajima, K. (2011). The outermost region of the developing cortical plate is crucial for both the switch of the radial migration mode and the Dab1-dependent "inside-out" lamination in the neocortex. *J. Neurosci.* 31, 9426–9439. doi: 10.1523/JNEUROSCI.0650-11.2011

Sekine, K., Kubo, K., and Nakajima, K. (2014). How does Reelin control neuronal migration and layer formation in the developing mammalian neocortex? *Neurosci. Res.* 86, 50–58. doi: 10.1016/j.neures.2014.06.004

Shelly, M., Cancedda, L., Heilshorn, S., Sumbre, G., and Poo, M. M. (2007). LKB1/STRAD promotes axon initiation during neuronal polarization. *Cell* 129, 565–577. doi: 10.1016/j.cell.2007.04.012

Shelly, M., Cancedda, L., Lim, B. K., Popescu, A. T., Cheng, P. L., Gao, H., et al. (2011). Semaphorin3A regulates neuronal polarization by suppressing axon formation and promoting dendrite growth. *Neuron* 71, 433–446. doi: 10.1016/j.neuron.2011.06.041

Shelly, M., and Poo, M. M. (2011). Role of LKB1-SAD/MARK pathway in neuronal polarization. *Dev. Neurobiol.* 71, 508–527. doi: 10.1002/dneu.20884

Shi, S. H., Jan, L. Y., and Jan, Y. N. (2003). Hippocampal neuronal polarity specified by spatially localized mPar3/mPar6 and PI 3-kinase activity. *Cell* 112, 63–75. doi: 10.1016/s0092-8674(02)01249-7

Shi, Y., and Massagué, J. (2003). Mechanisms of TGF-β signaling from cell membrane to the nucleus. *Cell* 113, 685–700. doi: 10.1016/s0092-8674(03)00432-x

Shitamukai, A., Konno, D., and Matsuzaki, F. (2011). Oblique radial glial divisions in the developing mouse neocortex induce self-renewing progenitors outside the germinal zone that resemble primate outer subventricular zone progenitors. *J. Neurosci.* 31, 3683–3695. doi: 10.1523/JNEUROSCI.4773-10.2011

Shitamukai, A., and Matsuzaki, F. (2012). Control of asymmetric cell division of mammalian neural progenitors. *Dev. Growth Differ.* 54, 277–286. doi: 10.1111/j.1440-169X.2012.01345.x

Srinivasan, S., Wang, F., Glavas, S., Ott, A., Hofmann, F., Aktories, K., et al. (2003). Rac and Cdc42 play distinct roles in regulating PI(3,4,5)P3 and polarity during neutrophil chemotaxis. *J. Cell Biol.* 160, 375–385. doi: 10.1083/jcb.200208179

Stancik, E. K., Navarro-Quiroga, I., Sellke, R., and Haydar, T. F. (2010). Heterogeneity in ventricular zone neural precursors contributes to neuronal fate diversity in the postnatal neocortex. *J. Neurosci.* 30, 7028–7036. doi: 10.1523/JNEUROSCI.6131-09.2010

Sun, Y., Fei, T., Yang, T., Zhang, F., Chen, Y. G., Li, H., et al. (2010). The suppression of CRMP2 expression by bone morphogenetic protein (BMP)-SMAD gradient signaling controls multiple stages of neuronal development. *J. Biol. Chem.* 285, 39039–39050. doi: 10.1074/jbc.M110.168351

Swiercz, J. M., Kuner, R., Behrens, J., and Offermanns, S. (2002). Plexin-B1 directly interacts with PDZ-RhoGEF/LARG to regulate RhoA and growth cone morphology. *Neuron* 35, 51–63. doi: 10.1016/s0896-6273(02)00750-x

Tabata, H., and Nakajima, K. (2003). Multipolar migration: the third mode of radial neuronal migration in the developing cerebral cortex. *J. Neurosci.* 23, 9996–10001.

Tabata, H., and Nakajima, K. (2008). Labeling embryonic mouse central nervous system cells by *in utero* electroporation. *Dev. Growth Differ.* 50, 507–511. doi: 10.1111/j.1440-169x.2008.01043.x

Tahirovic, S., Hellal, F., Neukirchen, D., Hindges, R., Garvalov, B. K., Flynn, K. C., et al. (2010). Rac1 regulates neuronal polarization through the WAVE complex. *J. Neurosci.* 30, 6930–6943. doi: 10.1523/JNEUROSCI.5395-09.2010

Taverna, E., Götz, M., and Huttner, W. B. (2014). The cell biology of neurogenesis: toward an understanding of the development and evolution of the neocortex. *Annu. Rev. Cell Dev. Biol.* 30, 465–502. doi: 10.1146/annurev-cellbio-101011-155801

Terabayashi, T., Itoh, T. J., Yamaguchi, H., Yoshimura, Y., Funato, Y., Ohno, S., et al. (2007). Polarity-regulating kinase partitioning-defective 1/microtubule affinity-regulating kinase 2 negatively regulates development of dendrites on hippocampal neurons. *J. Neurosci.* 27, 13098–13107. doi: 10.1523/JNEUROSCI.3986-07.2007

Thompson, B. J. (2013). Cell polarity: models and mechanisms from yeast, worms and flies. *Development* 140, 13–21. doi: 10.1242/dev.083634

Timm, T., von Kries, J. P., Li, X., Zempel, H., Mandelkow, E., and Mandelkow, E. M. (2011). Microtubule affinity regulating kinase activity in living neurons was examined by a genetically encoded fluorescence resonance energy transfer/fluorescence lifetime imaging-based biosensor: inhibitors with therapeutic potential. *J. Biol. Chem.* 286, 41711–41722. doi: 10.1074/jbc.M111.257865

Trepat, X., Chen, Z., and Jacobson, K. (2012). Cell migration. *Compr. Physiol.* 2, 2369–2392. doi: 10.1002/cphy.c110012

Tsai, J. W., Chen, Y., Kriegstein, A. R., and Vallee, R. B. (2005). LIS1 RNA interference blocks neural stem cell division, morphogenesis and motility at multiple stages. *J. Cell Biol.* 170, 935–945. doi: 10.1083/jcb.200505166

Tsai, J. W., and Vallee, R. B. (2011). Live microscopy of neural stem cell migration in brain slices. *Methods Mol. Biol.* 750, 131–142. doi: 10.1007/978-1-61779-145-1_9

Turing, A. M. (1990). The chemical basis of morphogenesis. *Bull. Math. Biol.* 52, 153–197; discussion 119–152. doi: 10.1007/BF02459572

Vaz, W. L. C., Goodsaid-Zalduondo, F., and Jacobson, K. (1984). Lateral diffusion of lipids and proteins in bilayer membranes. *FEBS Lett.* 174, 199–207. doi: 10.1016/0014-5793(84)81157-6

Voss, A. K., Britto, J. M., Dixon, M. P., Sheikh, B. N., Collin, C., Tan, S. S., et al. (2008). C3G regulates cortical neuron migration, preplate splitting and radial glial cell attachment. *Development* 135, 2139–2149. doi: 10.1242/dev.016725

Wang, F. (2009). The signaling mechanisms underlying cell polarity and chemotaxis. *Cold Spring Harb. Perspect. Biol.* 1:a002980. doi: 10.1101/cshperspect.a002980

Wang, F., Herzmark, P., Weiner, O. D., Srinivasan, S., Servant, G., and Bourne, H. R. (2002). Lipid products of PI(3)Ks maintain persistent cell polarity and directed motility in neutrophils. *Nat. Cell Biol.* 4, 513–518. doi: 10.1038/ncb810

Wang, T., Liu, Y., Xu, X. H., Deng, C. Y., Wu, K. Y., Zhu, J., et al. (2011). Lgl1 activation of rab10 promotes axonal membrane trafficking underlying neuronal polarization. *Dev. Cell* 21, 431–444. doi: 10.1016/j.devcel.2011.07.007

Wang, X., Tsai, J. W., LaMonica, B., and Kriegstein, A. R. (2011). A new subtype of progenitor cell in the mouse embryonic neocortex. *Nat. Neurosci.* 14, 555–561. doi: 10.1038/nn.2807

Wang, X., Tsai, J. W., Imai, J. H., Lian, W. N., Vallee, R. B., and Shi, S. H. (2009). Asymmetric centrosome inheritance maintains neural progenitors in the neocortex. *Nature* 461, 947–955. doi: 10.1038/nature08435

Watabe-Uchida, M., John, K. A., Janas, J. A., Newey, S. E., and Van Aelst, L. (2006). The Rac activator DOCK7 regulates neuronal polarity through local phosphorylation of stathmin/Op18. *Neuron* 51, 727–739. doi: 10.1016/j.neuron.2006.07.020

Wedlich-Soldner, R., and Li, R. (2003). Spontaneous cell polarization: undermining determinism. *Nat. Cell Biol.* 5, 267–270. doi: 10.1038/ncb0403-267

Wennekamp, S., Mesecke, S., Nédélec, F., and Hiiragi, T. (2013). A self-organization framework for symmetry breaking in the mammalian embryo. *Nat. Rev. Mol. Cell Biol.* 14, 452–459. doi: 10.1038/nrm3602

Whitman, M., Kaplan, D. R., Schaffhausen, B., Cantley, L., and Roberts, T. M. (1985). Association of phosphatidylinositol kinase activity with polyoma middle-T competent for transformation. *Nature* 315, 239–242. doi: 10.1038/315239a0

Witte, H., Neukirchen, D., and Bradke, F. (2008). Microtubule stabilization specifies initial neuronal polarization. *J. Cell Biol.* 180, 619–632. doi: 10.1083/jcb.200707042

Wu, P. R., Tsai, P. I., Chen, G. C., Chou, H. J., Huang, Y. P., Chen, Y. H., et al. (2011). DAPK activates MARK1/2 to regulate microtubule assembly, neuronal differentiation and tau toxicity. *Cell Death Differ.* 18, 1507–1520. doi: 10.1038/cdd.2011.2

Wynshaw-Boris, A., Pramparo, T., Youn, Y. H., and Hirotsune, S. (2010). Lissencephaly: mechanistic insights from animal models and potential therapeutic strategies. *Semin. Cell Dev. Biol.* 21, 823–830. doi: 10.1016/j.semcdb.2010.07.008

Xu, C., Funahashi, Y., Watanabe, T., Takano, T., Nakamuta, S., Namba, T., et al. (2015). Radial glial cell-neuron interaction directs axon formation at the opposite side of the neuron from the contact site. *J. Neurosci.* 35, 14517–14532. doi: 10.1523/jneurosci.1266-15.2015

Yamanaka, T., Horikoshi, Y., Suzuki, A., Sugiyama, Y., Kitamura, K., Maniwa, R., et al. (2001). PAR-6 regulates aPKC activity in a novel way and mediates cell-cell contact-induced formation of the epithelial junctional complex. *Genes Cells* 6, 721–731. doi: 10.1046/j.1365-2443.2001.00453.x

Yang, H. W., Shin, M. G., Lee, S., Kim, J. R., Park, W. S., Cho, K. H., et al. (2012). Cooperative activation of PI3K by Ras and Rho family small GTPases. *Mol. Cell* 47, 281–290. doi: 10.1016/j.molcel.2012.05.007

Yi, J. J., Barnes, A. P., Hand, R., Polleux, F., and Ehlers, M. D. (2010). TGF-β signaling specifies axons during brain development. *Cell* 142, 144–157. doi: 10.1016/j.cell.2010.06.010

Yingling, J., Youn, Y. H., Darling, D., Toyo-Oka, K., Pramparo, T., Hirotsune, S., et al. (2008). Neuroepithelial stem cell proliferation requires LIS1 for precise spindle orientation and symmetric division. *Cell* 132, 474–486. doi: 10.1016/j.cell.2008.01.026

Yoshimura, T., Arimura, N., and Kaibuchi, K. (2006a). Signaling networks in neuronal polarization. *J. Neurosci.* 26, 10626–10630. doi: 10.1523/jneurosci.3824-06.2006

Yoshimura, T., Arimura, N., Kawano, Y., Kawabata, S., Wang, S., and Kaibuchi, K. (2006b). Ras regulates neuronal polarity via the PI3-kinase/Akt/GSK-3beta/CRMP-2 pathway. *Biochem. Biophys. Res. Commun.* 340, 62–68. doi: 10.1016/j.bbrc.2005.11.147

Yoshimura, Y., Terabayashi, T., and Miki, H. (2010). Par1b/MARK2 phosphorylates kinesin-like motor protein GAKIN/KIF13B to regulate axon formation. *Mol. Cell. Biol.* 30, 2206–2219. doi: 10.1128/mcb.01181-09

Zheng, Y. (2001). Dbl family guanine nucleotide exchange factors. *Trends Biochem. Sci.* 26, 724–732. doi: 10.1016/s0968-0004(01)01973-9

Zong, H., Espinosa, J. S., Su, H. H., Muzumdar, M. D., and Luo, L. (2005). Mosaic analysis with double markers in mice. *Cell* 121, 479–492. doi: 10.1016/j.cell.2005.02.012

10

Adapting for Endocytosis: Roles for Endocytic Sorting Adaptors in Directing Neural Development

*Chan Choo Yap * and Bettina Winckler **

Department of Neuroscience, University of Virginia, Charlottesville, VA, USA

Correspondence:
Chan Choo Yap and Bettina Winckler, Department of Neuroscience, University of Virginia, 409 Lane Rd. Extd., MR-4 6116, Charlottesville, VA 22936, USA
cy5x@virginia.edu; bwinckler@virginia.edu

Proper cortical development depends on the orchestrated actions of a multitude of guidance receptors and adhesion molecules and their downstream signaling. The levels of these receptors on the surface and their precise locations can greatly affect guidance outcomes. Trafficking of receptors to a particular surface locale and removal by endocytosis thus feed crucially into the final guidance outcomes. In addition, endocytosis of receptors can affect downstream signaling (both quantitatively and qualitatively) and regulated endocytosis of guidance receptors is thus an important component of ensuring proper neural development. We will discuss the cell biology of regulated endocytosis and the impact on neural development. We focus our discussion on endocytic accessory proteins (EAPs) (such as numb and disabled) and how they regulate endocytosis and subsequent post-endocytic trafficking of their cognate receptors (such as Notch, TrkB, β-APP, VLDLR, and ApoER2).

Keywords: clathrin, signaling endosomes, TrkB, numb, disabled, doublecortin, migration

Introduction

The development of the mammalian brain involves a multitude of precisely coordinated processes, including proliferation and differentiation of neural stem cells followed by migration of newborn neurons from their birthplace to their final destination, elaboration of axons and dendrites, and finally synapse formation (LoTurco and Bai, 2006; Kawauchi and Hoshino, 2008; Liu, 2011; Lewis et al., 2013; Wu et al., 2014). During cortical development, neurons born in the ventricular zone (VZ) migrate radially by moving along radial glia fibers to form proper cortical layers. Interneurons also migrate long distances, but follow a tangential migratory route that does not involve migration along radial glia processes (Guo and Anton, 2014). Defective neuronal migration causes neurodevelopmental disorders such as mental retardation, Lissencephaly, epilepsy, and others (Jamuar and Walsh, 2014). Other cell types in the brain also migrate to reach their final distribution, including oligodendrocyte precursor cells (Choe et al., 2014) and microglia (Arnò et al., 2014), but less is known about the cues and receptors that guide their movements.

Directional migration in any cell type requires cell polarization and regulated cycles of adhesion and de-adhesion (Vicente-Manzanares and Horwitz, 2011). Multiple extracellular ligands and their receptors mediate the elaboration of polarized cell morphology and of directional protrusions by dynamically regulating linkages to cytoskeletal elements. Cadherins are often implicated in cell-cell contact mediated guidance (such as might occur for radial migration along radial glial fibers) whereas integrins are well known to mediate migratory behavior for cell-extracellular matrix interactions (such as migrating along basement membranes). In addition, polarized membrane addition and removal contributes to directional motility (Vitriol and Zheng, 2012). Because migratory behavior is mediated by membrane receptors, their intracellular trafficking is essential for regulating the responsiveness of migratory cells to extracellular guidance cues. This is also true for neuronal migration. Precise sorting of membrane guidance receptors to specific regions in migratory neurons, regulating surface levels via endocytic trafficking of the receptors, as well as decisions to recycle or degrade receptors post-endocytically are crucial for brain development, but most of the detailed mechanisms are still poorly understood. Since ligand-receptor systems continue to play important roles past the migratory stage for axon and dendrite growth and for synaptogenesis, understanding membrane traffic in brain development will shed light on many normal brain processes as well as on dysfunctions of the nervous system (Yap and Winckler, 2012).

Not surprisingly, multiple genes important for proper brain development have molecular roles in endocytic membrane traffic. One prominent example is numb, an evolutionary conserved protein originally identified as a cell fate determinant during peripheral and CNS development in *Drosophila* (Uemura et al., 1989). The molecular role of Numb is as an endocytic co-adaptor that interacts with cargos and with endocytic machinery, such as the clathrin adaptor AP-2 and the endocytic accessory proteins Eps15. It thus associates with the clathrin complex for clathrin-dependent endocytosis of membrane proteins (Salcini et al., 1997; Santolini et al., 2000; Smith et al., 2004; McGill et al., 2009). How exactly is neural development regulated by an endocytic adaptor, such as numb? The mechanisms involve regulating the endocytosis, trafficking, and signaling of developmentally relevant receptors. Which other endocytic adaptors play roles in receptor endocytosis during neural development? Which receptors require which co-adaptor (numb or another co-adaptor) for endocytosis and how is their endocytosis important for normal development? Are endocytic co-adaptors also involved in post-endocytic trafficking of the receptor? These are some of the question we will explore in this review. In particular, we will discuss co-adaptor proteins that are involved in clathrin-mediated pathways via AP-2, such as Numb, Dab family proteins, and DCX, and explore their respective roles in brain development.

Clathrin-Mediated Endocytosis: The Basic Process

Many excellent reviews have been published about clathrin-mediated endocytosis, and we only want to briefly summarize the most important facts here. Most endocytosis of receptors in mammalian cells is mediated by assembling a multimeric complex between membrane receptors (i.e., cargos), adaptor protein complexes (AP-2, in particular) and a coat lattice composed of many trimers ("triskelions") of clathrin (McMahon, 1999; McMahon and Boucrot, 2011; Merrifield and Kaksonen, 2014). Due to better and better imaging, the sequence of events in assembling this multimeric complex at the plasma membrane (called a "clathrin-coated pit", or CCP) is becoming better understood on a mechanistic level: A nucleation complex (including FCHO proteins, Eps15, and intersectins) associates with the plasma membrane via PIP(4, 5)P_2 binding and initiates CCP formation. The tetrameric AP-2 adaptor is recruited to the nucleation sites and serves as a major hub for recruiting other accessory proteins as well as cargos to the forming CCP. As clathrin coat assembly progresses, the membrane is increasingly deformed into a larger clathrin-coated invagination that accumulates cargos. Ultimately, the invaginating membrane cup fissions to bud a clathrin-coated vesicle into the cell interior. The clathrin coat is rapidly removed by uncoating enzymes, and the endocytic vesicle delivers its cargos into the endosomal system by fusion with early endosomes. In addition to the essential core components of cargo, AP-2 adaptor, and clathrin, many other endocytic accessory proteins (EAPs) or "co-adaptors" associate with CCPs and aid in cargo selection, in the efficiency of cargo enrichment at the CCP, and in execution of subsequent membrane deformation, fission, uncoating, and endosomal fusion events. In addition to clathrin-mediated endocytosis, there are non-clathrin endocytosis pathways that are less well understood. It was found recently that in a mammalian cell line 95% of cargos enter the cells via clathrin-mediated endocytosis (Bitsikas et al., 2014). Surprisingly, this includes GPI-linked proteins, which had been thought to enter primarily via non-clathrin pathways. If this overwhelming preponderance of clathrin- vs. non-clathrin pathways also holds in the nervous system remains to be seen.

Tetrameric Adaptor Complexes

To date, five tetrameric adaptor complexes (AP-1 through AP-5) have been identified in mammals. Each adaptor complex consists of two large (α, γ, δ, ε, ζ and β1–5), one medium (μ1–5), and one small subunit (σ1–5) (Fölsch, 2008; Hirst et al., 2011). The large subunits mediate binding to the target membrane (via specific phosphoinsoitide lipids), to clathrin, and to other accessory proteins (Brodsky et al., 2001). The medium subunit (μ) directly interacts with the "tyrosine-based" sorting signals (YXXΦ) in the cytoplasmic tail of cargo molecules ["X" means any amino acid can be at that position whereas "Φ" means an amino acid with a bulky hydrophobic side chain can be at that position.]. The small σ subunits are involved in the recognition of "dileucine-based" sorting motifs ([DE]XXXL[LI]) [square brackets mean that either of the bracketed amino acids can be at that position], such as the one found in the cation-independent mannose 6-phosphate receptor (CI-M6PR). AP-1 and AP-2 are both components of clathrin-coated vesicles, either for sorting at the trans-Golgi network (TGN)/endosomes (AP-1) or for endocytosis from the plasma membrane (AP-2). Both AP-3 and AP-4 are associated with TGN/endosomal membranes, and either mediate endosome/lysosome delivery (AP3 and AP4) or the biogenesis of specialized secretory vesicles in neurons (AP3) from the TGN (Faúndez et al., 1998; Mullins and Bonifacino, 2001; Robinson and Bonifacino, 2001). AP-3 also binds clathrin, whereas AP-4 is not significantly enriched in clathrin-coated vesicles and has no clathrin box consensus motif in its β4 subunit, suggesting it acts independently of clathrin (Simpson et al., 1996; Dell'Angelica et al., 1997, 1998;

Hirst and Robinson, 1998; Hirst et al., 1999; Barois and Bakke, 2005). AP-5 was only recently identified and shown to associate with late endosomal/lysosomal compartments and might regulate the sorting from early endosome to lysosomes (Hirst et al., 2011). Importantly, mutations in adaptor protein complexes have been implicated in several neurodevelopmental disorders, such as Mednik syndrome (which manifests with abnormal Copper metabolism due to a copper transporter defect) and hereditary spastic paraplegia (HSP; Hirst et al., 2013).

Clathrin-Mediated Endocytosis Via AP-2: Constitutive or Regulated?

Much of the regulation of endocytosis likely involves regulating when and where to form a coated pit and which cargo proteins to recruit into it. Developmental processes that rely on endocytosis of specific receptors are thus subject to regulation of cargo/adaptor/coat interactions. Some of these regulatory mechanisms have been worked out, and many others will certainly be discovered in the future (Traub and Bonifacino, 2013). For example, AP-2 recruitment to the plasma membrane requires PI(4, 5)P_2 clustering, and can be inhibited by phosphorylation of $\mu 2$ by the kinase AAK (Conner and Schmid, 2002; Ricotta et al., 2002). Upon binding to PI(4, 5)P_2, AP-2 undergoes a large conformational change that exposes the binding sites on the $\mu 2$ subunit for tyrosine-based endocytic signals on cargo receptors. Phosphorylation of tyrosine-based signals on the cargos similarly inhibits their binding to AP-2. Endocytosis of receptors is thus regulated from two ends: regulating receptor affinity for endocytic adaptors, and regulating affinity of the adaptor for the sorting signal on the receptor. Endocytosis of receptors is thus far from constitutive, but rather highly regulated.

AP-2 Function in Neurons

AP-2 has been implicated in clathrin-mediated endocytosis of membrane proteins important for synaptic plasticity and neurotransmission (Kononenko et al., 2014). In addition, clathrin-mediated endocytosis is needed during development for axon and dendrite outgrowth and for pathfinding. Clathrin/AP-2 mediated endocytosis has been associated to play an important role in adhesion disassembly during cell migration. For example, clathrin coated pits are enriched at adhesive contacts with matrix substrates and co-localized with adhesion receptors in migratory neurons. Inhibition of dynamin or clathrin function impaired neuronal migration both *in vivo* and *in vitro*, and coincided with a shift in the distribution of adhesion proteins from the original region proximal to the cell body to the rear of the cells (Shieh et al., 2011). In addition, AP-2 also interacts with the tyrosine-based motif of L1-CAM to mediate its endocytosis at axonal growth cones, a process crucial for its local recycling and detachment from adhesive environment to promote axon elongation and outgrowth (Kamiguchi et al., 1998). Additionally, endocytosis of L1-CAM in dendrites is also essential for targeting L1-CAM to axons via an indirect transcytosis pathway (Wisco et al., 2003; Yap et al., 2008).

Monomeric Endocytic Co-Adaptors

Different endocytic cargos have different endocytic signals and can be endocytosed via different molecular assemblies. Since AP-2 is the best studied of the clathrin adaptors, we also understand those endocytic signals best that directly bind to AP-2 itself. Among those signals are short linear signals, in particular the tyrosine-based motifs that bind $\mu 2$ as well as the di-leucine motifs that bind to the interface of $\sigma 2$ and α-subunits of AP-2 (Bonifacino and Traub, 2003; Traub and Bonifacino, 2013). Other endocytic signals do not bind directly to AP-2, but require accessory proteins or "co-adaptors". For instance, the "NPXY" motif ([YF]XNPX[YF]) binds to the PTB domain ["PTB" stands for "phospho-tyrosine binding" but PTB domains can bind other motifs as well] of a number of EAPs, including ARH, numb, and Dab2. These additional accessory proteins are often referred to as "CLASPs" (clathrin-associated sorting proteins), "EAPs", or "co-adaptors". [Note to reader: There is also a class of microtubule-associated proteins named CLASP (cytoplasmic linker associated protein) which are not clathrin-associated proteins. To avoid confusion, we will use the terms "EAP" or "co-adaptor" in this review]. EAPs can be subdivided into several categories depending on their binding interactions. A full adaptor has four direct interactions: with lipids, with cargo, with clathrin, and with additional accessory endocytic proteins (Reider and Wendland, 2011). The AP-2 complex itself falls into this category. Other EAPs/co-adaptors contain only a subset of these binding sites and require additional binding partners to supply the rest of the interactions. For example, Eps15 has been shown to bind ubiquitinated cargos (via its UIM domains) and accessory proteins (via its EH domain), but to date direct binding to lipids or clathrin is not known (Reider and Wendland, 2011).

A Large Arsenal of EAPs Enables Regulated Cargo- and Cell Type-Specific Endocytosis

What might be some of the physiological consequences of having multiple "full" adaptors and/or various "partial" co-adaptors expressed in the same cell? In fact, up to 60 different proteins can participate in the various steps of clathrin-mediated endocytosis (Merrifield and Kaksonen, 2014). Deletion of many of the EAPs does not completely disrupt clathrin-mediated endocytosis. In fact, clathrin-mediated endocytosis is notoriously robust, and continues or compensates rapidly for the loss of a single component. This likely represents the cooperative nature of building a large multimeric assembly from many components that are partially redundant (McMahon, 1999). Surprisingly, under some circumstances even AP-2 itself is dispensable. A large number of EAPs thus endows cells with endocytic robustness. This robustness creates experimental challenges in terms of testing the involvement of specific EAPs in the endocytosis of a cargo of interest (see McMahon and Boucrot, 2011) for a good discussion). In fact, global interference approaches might not be optimally suited to uncover the detailed molecular roles of individual EAPs. New technological advances have given rise to approaches that allow the analysis of the formation of single coated pits and their maturation in relation to the recruitment levels of individual EAPs. These approaches have shown that the kinetics of CCP formation and the concerted maturation to a productive coated pit are regulated by a multi-step cascade. In addition, compensatory mechanisms can be detected, allowing the analysis of phenotypes even when bulk transferrin uptake is not significantly impaired. This has led to a new framework of a concerted molecular checkpoint cascade that regulates CCP maturation. These new approaches with better signal-to-noise detection demonstrate that EAPs binding to the ear domain of α-adaptin are required for the concerted and regulated maturation of CCPs (Aguet et al., 2013).

Another consequence of having cargo-specific EAPs is that it allows cells to endocytose cargos with greatly differing cell surface abundance without competing for potentially limiting cargo binding sites on AP-2 itself (McMahon, 1999; McMahon and Boucrot, 2011). Increasing the abundance of cargo-specific EAPs, thus, leads to increased endocytosis of its specific cognate receptor cargos (containing the specific binding motif) without affecting overall endocytic levels of non-cognate cargos (not containing the specific binding motif).

Another physiological consequence of the large number of EAPs it that many are expressed in a cell-type restricted fashion, resulting in a versatile arsenal for regulating cargo selectivity. For some of them, multiple isoforms exist that can further expand the repertoire of combinatorial players. For the tetrameric AP adaptors themselves, several subunits have multiple isoforms. Some of these are expressed in a cell-type restricted fashion, including in neurons. For example, both the ubiquitously expressed AP-3A (subunit composition δ–β3A–μ3A–σ3) and the neuron-specific AP-3B (subunit composition δ–β3B–μ3B–σ3) complexes are expressed in the brain. AP-3 has been implicated in sorting synaptic vesicle membrane proteins to synaptic terminals (Danglot and Galli, 2007). Loss of the neuronal-specific AP-3B in μ3B mutant mice results in spontaneous epileptic seizure and impairment of GABA release due to a reduction in vesicular GABA transporters (Nakatsu et al., 2004). In humans, Hermansky–Pudlak syndrome (HPS) is associated with mutations in the gene encoding AP3-β3A and is characterized by albinism and defects in lysosome-related organelles (Starcevic et al., 2002). The lack of neurological defects reported in human HPS is most likely due to the presence of functional AP-3B (using the β3B subunit) in neurons. It thus appears that expression of cell type-restricted EAPs provides tissues with a versatile arsenal from which to choose in order to achieve exquisitely precise control over which receptor is endocytosed when and where. Our own attention was directed towards exploring the roles that the "EAP arsenal" might play in neuronal development after we made some surprising observations, first with regard to the neuronal- and cargo-specific roles that the ubiquitous EHD proteins play (Yap et al., 2010), and second with regard to the previously unknown role that doublecortin (DCX) plays in the regulated endocytosis of neurofascin (Yap et al., 2012).

Many genes have been identified over the past decades for their roles in various aspects of neural development. Many of them were first identified in *Drosophila* and *C. elegans*, but mammalian homologs exist and play crucial roles. The inventory list of genes involved in any particular developmental process is ever growing and sheds light on the genetic networks that regulate development. In addition, creating this inventory is a crucial steppingstone to proceed towards a molecular and mechanistic understanding of the identified gene products and their function in a complex network of proteins. Identifying the exact molecular role of each protein in the genetic network is an arduous and slow process, but exciting new discoveries are continuously being reported. The need to regulate endocytosis for proper neural development is highlighted by the fact that "famous" neurodevelopmental genes, such as numb, are now known to be EAPs. We will first discuss the functions of two EAPs with known neurodevelopmental roles, numb and disabled (Dab), and subsequently explore what is currently known about some other EAPs in regulating neuronal endocytosis for a specific subset of cargos.

Numb—A Monomeric EAP Regulating Neural Development

In vertebrates, there are two genes encoding for the related Numb and numb-like (numbl) proteins (Zhong et al., 1996, 1997; Salcini et al., 1997). Numb is a peripheral membrane-associated protein with an amino-terminal phosphotyrosine-binding domain (PTB) and a C-terminal proline rich region (PRR), as well as EH-domain-binding motifs (two DPF and one NPF motif) (**Figure 1**). Numb binds its cargos via its PTB domain, binds the α-adaptin subunit of AP-2 via the C-terminal DPF motif, and binds other accessory proteins, such as Eps15 and EHD1 and 4, via the NPF motif. Numb thus meets the criteria for being an endocytic EAP. There are four spliced isoforms of numb (Dho et al., 1999; Verdi et al., 1999) which differ in the length of the PTB (either including or lacking a 11 aa insert) and PRR domains (including or lacking). Numb-like shares high sequence homology with Numb (**Figure 1**): it contains a PTB domain, the EH-binding motifs but lacks the PRR region and has an additional specific poly-glutamine repeat which is absent in Numb (Zhong et al., 1997). This isoform diversity adds additional variety into the cellular toolbox. The PTB region and the EH-binding motifs are conserved in vertebrate and *Drosophila* numb, suggesting these two regions are functionally relevant and that the roles of numb may be similar across vertebrate and invertebrate species.

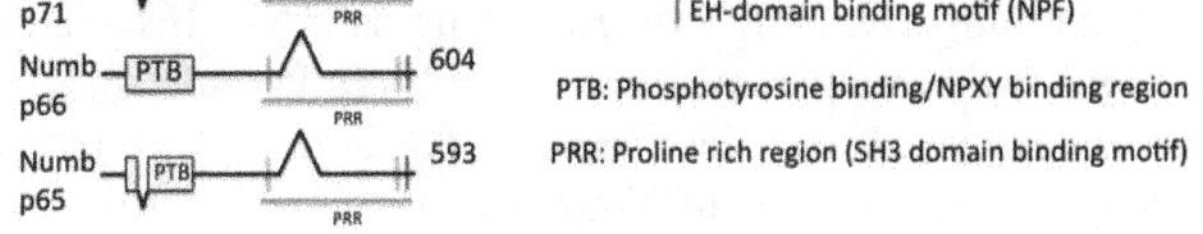

FIGURE 1 | Domain structure of numb and its isoforms. The domain structure of full length numb (p72) and three splice isoforms is depicted. Binding regions are indicated by color bars.

What are the Roles for Numb in Neural Development?

Numb has multiple functions in the nervous system and has been implicated in a dazzling number of processes, including cell fate determination, proliferation, neurogenesis, cell migration, cell adhesion, and axon outgrowth (Gulino et al., 2010). In the mouse embryo, Numb is expressed in all layers of the cortical plate, as well as the progenitor cells of the VZ (Zhong et al., 1997). During cortical neurogenesis and cell division, numb is asymmetrically localized to the apical membrane of the dividing cells, and subsequently segregated to the apical daughter cells that remain progenitors. A numb-knockout mouse displays premature neuronal differentiation in the forebrain, implying numb functions in maintaining progenitor cell numbers (Verdi et al., 1999; Zhong et al., 2000; Shen et al., 2002). In other contexts, Numb appears to be involved in promoting neurogenesis and differentiation instead. In fact, whereas at earlier stages (E10) the daughter cell inheriting numb remains a progenitor, later on in corticogenesis (E13) the daughter inheriting numb becomes a neuron (Shen et al., 2002). Studies from different numb knockout mouse models have given rise to conflicting results pointing to the diverse functions and complex regulation of Numb. For instance, in a second numb knockout mouse model, no premature differentiation phenotype was observed in forebrain, while impaired differentiation was detected in hindbrain and in cerebellum (Zilian et al., 2001; Klein et al., 2004), further suggesting that numb might also play a role in neurogenesis.

Numb has also been reported to play a critical role in cerebellar granule cell polarization during migration (Zhou et al., 2011): Conditional ablation of numb/numbl using the transcription factor math1-cre system in cerebellar granule cell precursors (GCPs) impairs BDNF-induced GCP migration both *in vitro* and *in vivo*. How can numb play so many, sometimes contradictory roles? Since numb is an endocytic adaptor, its particular role depends on the cargos whose trafficking numb regulates in different cellular contexts. Among the known numb cargos are receptors with well established roles in regulating developmental processes: Notch1, βAPP, β1 integrin, and TrkB. numb binds to the conserved NPXY sorting motifs in the cytoplasmic tail of these cargos and mediates their endocytosis. What is the current evidence that the brain phenotypes of numb knockouts are due to impaired endocytosis of a numb cargo?

Numb-Mediated Endocytosis of Receptors Controls Neural Development

Notch

Numb was originally identified as an antagonist of Notch. Notch signaling regulates numerous developmental decisions and patterning events from worms to human. Notch signaling promotes radial glial identity and controls cell fate specification during development of the neocortex (Gaiano et al., 2000). It is likely that endocytosis of Notch receptor *per se* is regulated by Numb because the PTB domain of Numb binds the ram23 and the PEST regions of the Notch cytoplasmic tail directly, and numb-mediated inhibition of Notch requires the AP-2 specific subunit α-adaptin (Guo et al., 1996; Berdnik et al., 2002). The endocytic removal of Notch via numb reduces Notch receptor levels on the surface and reduces Notch signaling. Reduced Notch signaling then affects cell fate.

Additional molecular roles of numb are becoming apparent as well. Numb was found to have additional interacting partners, such as Par3 and atypical protein kinase C (aPKC), protein complexes which function in polarized cell migration. Knockdown of mPar-3 reduces Notch signaling activity and causes premature depletion of progenitor cells from the VZ (Bultje et al., 2009). Conversely, depletion of Numb/numblike abolishes this effect and increases Notch signaling activity. Numb and Numblike are thus required for mPar-3 function in regulating Notch signaling and neocortical neurogenesis.

TrkB

Granule cell precursors in the cerebellum migrate towards a source of the neurotrophin BDNF via activation of the BDNF receptor TrkB at the leading process of the cell (Zhou et al., 2007). Neurotrophin signaling via Trk receptors is well established to require endocytosis into endosomes. These endosomes contain activated Trk receptors and recruit a variety of signaling components, including PI3K, Ras-MAPK, and PLC-γ pathway components. Other cascades, such as PKA via elevated cAMP, have also been implicated in BDNF signaling. High levels of signaling takes place on these so-called "signaling endosomes" (Cosker and Segal, 2014). For some forms of signaling (such as long-range survival signaling by NGF), the signaling endosomes travel long distances back to the cell soma where they continue to signal and regulate transcription. There are also more locally restricted signaling events downstream of Trk receptor activation close to the sites of initial endocytosis that regulate axon growth and polarized mobility of migratory neuronal precursors. Neurotrophin signaling thus is one of the best-documented examples of an endocytosis-dependent signaling event.

How is endocytosis of activated TrkB and the subsequent signaling from signaling endosomes regulated in time and space? Numb is an endocytic co-adaptor for activated TrkB (**Figure 2**): Numb colocalizes with α-adaptin and TrkB in the leading processes, it interacts with the NPXY motif on TrkB after activation (via the numb PTB domain), and it promotes TrkB endocytosis and polarized localization to the leading process of migrating GCPs. Depletion of Numb either by shRNA or conditional knockout impairs BDNF-induced TrkB endocytosis and polarized localization of TrkB to leading processes of migrating GCPs. The polarized localization of numb leads to enhanced endocytosis of activated TrkB at the leading process, increased generation and accumulation of signaling endosomes locally in the leading process of GCPs, and consequently increased activation of downstream signaling cascades that promote local membrane trafficking (such as increased BDNF exocytosis) and cytoskeletal rearrangements that drive directional protrusions and mobility (Zhou et al., 2011; see **Figure 3**).

In addition to promoting local endocytosis of activated TrkB, numb also serves as an adaptor to recruit signaling components, such as aPKC, a well known regulator of polarized cellular events upstream of cytoskeletal rearrangements. Genetic deletion

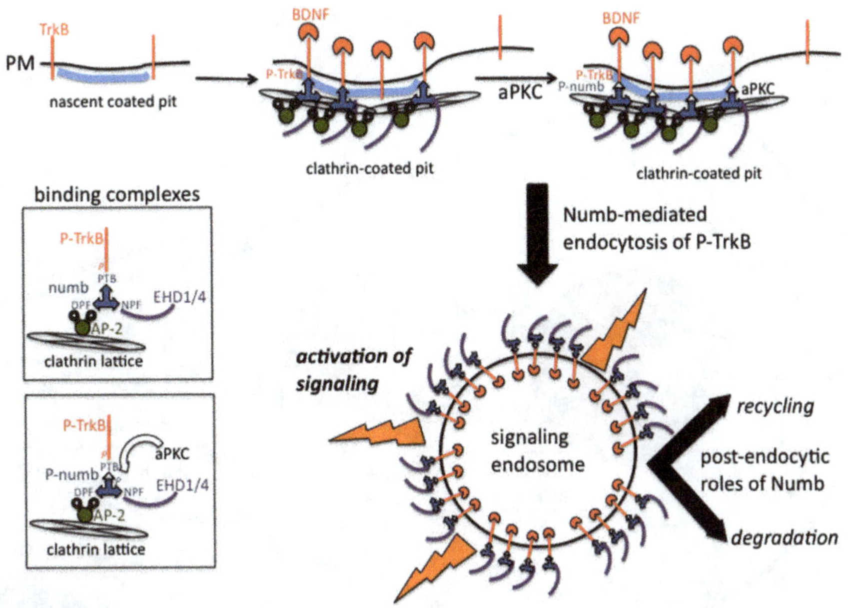

FIGURE 2 | Binding complexes of numb during clathrin-mediated endocytosis of TrkB receptors. Activated TrkB binds to the PTB domain of numb which recruits AP-2, EHD proteins to the forming coated pit. Clathrin is recruited via AP-2 and leads to formation of a clathrin-coated endocytic vesicle. Numb also recruits other signaling effectors such as atypical protein kinase C (aPKC) and par3 (not depicted). Signaling downstream of activated TrkB commences at the plasma membrane and continues after endocytosis from signaling endosomes. Numb continues to play post-endocytic roles and might also regulate recycling vs. degradation trafficking.

of numb/numbl impairs BDNF-induced aPKC activation in GCPs, suggesting BDNF stimulation of TrkB recruits Numb, which in turn acts as an adaptor to recruit and activate aPKC via the PTB region. In BDNF knockout mice, polarization of Numb at the front of GCPs and its interaction with aPKC are significantly decreased, suggesting BDNF regulates the polarization of Numb and its interaction with aPKC in migrating GCPs. Interestingly, Numb is also itself a target of aPKC. BDNF-induced phosphorylation of numb by aPKC increases its binding to TrkB and promotes the chemotactic response to BDNF. Taken together, Numb acts as an adaptor linking BDNF, an extracellular cue, to intrinsic cellular polarity machinery, including aPKC, via TrkB endocytosis and serves as a feed-forward loop to promote BDNF-induced directed GCP migration (Zhou et al., 2011; see **Figure 3**).

L1

Numb is also expressed in postmitotic neurons and functions in axonal outgrowth. Numb accumulates at the tip of growing axons in cultured hippocampal neurons and mediates endocytosis of L1/NgCAM for axon growth (Nishimura et al., 2003). Internalization of L1/NgCAM occurs preferentially in the central domain of migrating growth cones, followed by anterograde transport of L1/NgCAM-containing vesicles and subsequent recycling near the leading edge. Numb has been reported to co-localize with L1/NgCAM at the central region of growth cones, suggesting numb plays a role in regulating local L1/NgCAM internalization and maybe recycling for growth cone advance (Nishimura et al., 2003). Numb co-immunoprecipitates in a complex with L1 and AP-2 and is important for efficient endocytosis of L1/NgCAM. The PTB domain of numb is required for L1/NgCAM internalization, but L1/NgCAM does not itself contain an NPXY motif. It is currently not known if numb binds directly to L1/NgCAM and if so, via what binding motif. The regulation of L1/NgCAM endocytosis on numb is surprising since L1/NgCAM has its own tyrosine-based motif that binds directly to μ2 of the AP-2 tetrameric adaptor complex (Kamiguchi et al., 1998). It will be interesting to determine what aspects of L1/NgCAM function and signaling might be additionally influenced by numb.

How is the Polarized Distribution of Numb Regulated?

In many cell types, numb localization is highly polarized to one side of the cell. This polarized distribution of numb is ideally suited to promote non-uniform endocytosis of numb cargos (see also Section TrkB). How is the polarized distribution of numb regulated? Some evidence points to important roles of the numb interacting polarity proteins par3 and aPKC. For example, numb mediates the endocytosis of integrins via binding of the PTB domain of numb to the NPXY motif in the cytoplasmic tail of integrins (Calderwood et al., 2003; Nishimura and Kaibuchi, 2007). In migrating ECV304 and HeLa cells, Numb polarizes toward the leading edge, accumulates around focal adhesions, and localizes to clathrin-coated structures at the substratum-facing surface of the leading edge. Its localization to clathrin-coated structures is α-adaptin dependent. Depletion of Numb by RNAi impairs both integrin endocytosis and cell migration.

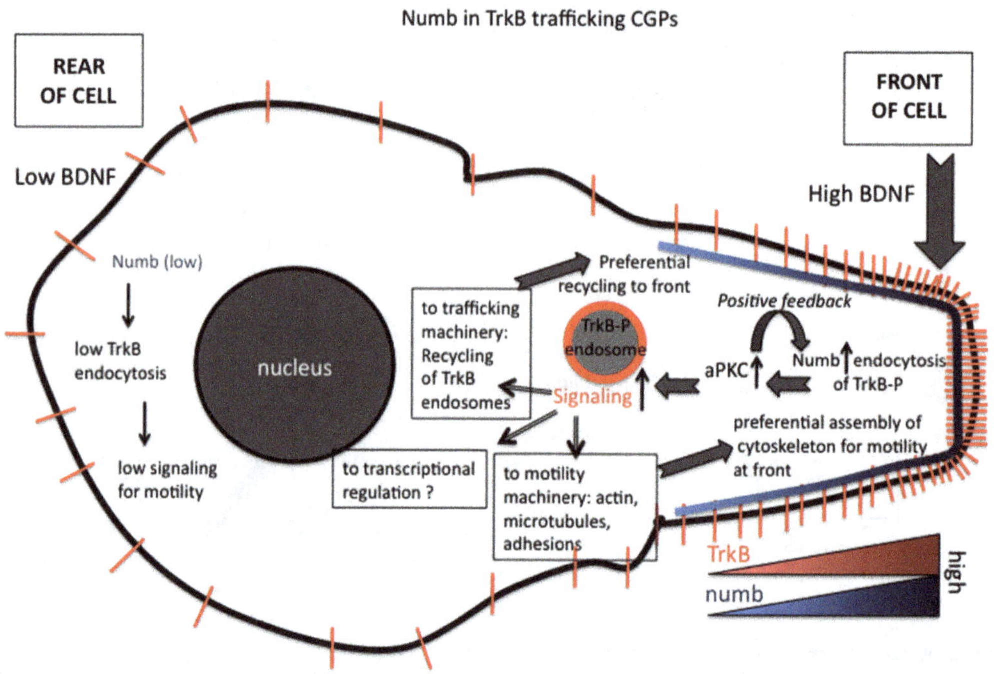

FIGURE 3 | Roles of numb in polarizing signaling responses downstream of BDNF in migrating granule cell precursors (GCPs) in cerebellar development. Polarized distribution of numb at the leading process of a migrating GCP creates a positive feed-forward loop for directional migration. The following steps are proposed (based on Zhou et al., 2011). (1) Higher BDNF in front of migrating GCP. (2) Higher activation of TrkB. (3) Higher recruitment of numb. (4) Higher recruitment of downstream effectors, such as aPKC. (5) Higher numb leads to higher TrkB-P endocytosis via clathrin/AP-2. (6) Higher TrkB endocytosis leads to more TrkB-P in endosomes. (7) More TrkB-P in endosomes recruits more signaling effectors to endosomes. (8) Higher activation of Tiam and Rac to promote more actin assembly in front of cell. (9) Higher signaling promotes preferential recycling of TrkB back to surface at front. (10) TrkB distribution becomes more polarized near front.

Par3-dependent phosphorylation by aPKC regulates the polarized localization of numb and its association with clathrin coated structures. Phosphorylated numb is released from the clathrin-coated structures and no longer binds integrin, suggesting aPKC negatively regulated functions of numb with respect to integrins. However, aPKC is required for polarized subcellular localization of Numb as knockdown of aPKC mislocalizes Numb to both the apical and basal surface leading to less enrichment in leading processes of the cells. Taken together, these results suggested that the polarized numb phosphorylation regulated by aPKC/Par3 complex is important for integrin endocytosis and integrin-substrate based cell migration (Nishimura and Kaibuchi, 2007). This is in contrast to the effects of aPKC phosphorylation on numb-TrkB binding which is increased by phosphorylation of numb (see Section TrkB).

Similarly in dividing sensory organ precursor (SOP) cells in Drosophila, a numb mutant with five PKC phosphorylation–deficient sites is mislocalized to both anterior and posterior sides of the cell. The results suggested that aPKC-mediated phosphorylation of numb regulates the asymmetric localization of numb in dividing cells (Smith et al., 2007), and that overall Numb functions relies on its phosphorylation status which determines its subcellular localization. Similarly, hyper-phosphorylated Numb after treatment with the phosphatase inhibitor calyculin-A dissociates from the AP-2 and Eps15 complex, indicating that phosphorylation at certain sites of numb negatively regulates its endocytic functions (Krieger et al., 2013). Interestingly, phosphorylation of Numb by Ca2+/calmodulin-dependent protein kinase I at positions S264 and S283 prevents Numb binding to AP-2, but promotes its interaction with 14-3-3 proteins (Tokumitsu et al., 2006), pointing to the participation of numb phospho-isoforms in distinct molecular complexes with presumably distinct functions in the cell. In addition, the recruitment of numb to endosomes is also regulated: phosphorylation of numb by AAK1 at position T102 redistributed numb from the plasma membrane to perinuclear endosomes (Sorensen and Conner, 2008).

There is thus strong evidence that numb participates in endocytosis and subsequent endosomal trafficking of NPXY-motif containing cargos during multiple processes in neural development, such as maintaining proper neurogenesis via regulated Notch trafficking, cerebellar migration via regulated TrkB trafficking, and axon growth via regulated L1 endocytosis. Since numb is localized in a polarized manner to only a part of the cell, endocytosis would be preferentially occurring on one side leading to polarized surface distribution of the numb cargo. This leads to changed signaling (for Notch or TrkB) or reduced adhesion (for integrin) or both, and changed cellular behavior. Since most of the numb cargos are signaling receptors that continue to signal after internalization, numb-mediated endocytosis of such a receptor would not stop signaling immediately, but allow signaling from endosomes. Furthermore, numb itself provides a scaffold for signaling components and thus participates directly in determining signaling output from its cargos. Subsequently, these receptors can be recycled to the surface for another round of ligand-binding and signaling (i.e., continued signaling) or be trafficked for degradation (i.e., termination of signaling).

Multiple Splice Isoforms with Different Domain Structure Play Different Roles

In mammalian cells, numb isoforms are expressed in cell type-specific manner and localized differentially subcellularly dependent on the insert in the PTB domain. For instance, the absence of the 11 aa in the PTB domain results in more cytosolic and less membrane-associated Numb (Dho et al., 1999). The Numb isoform with long PRR domain is expressed transiently during early brain development and disappears prior to cell differentiation in P19 embryonic carcinoma cells, suggesting the isoform may function in promoting proliferation of progenitor cells. Conversely, the isoform with short PRR domain is expressed throughout neurogenesis in the developing brain and in adult brain, and during the course of retinoic acid-induced P19 cell differentiation (Dho et al., 1999; Verdi et al., 1999; Toriya et al., 2006). Expression of the short PRR Numb isoform in the outer optic anlage of the *Drosophila* larvae brain also promotes neuronal differentiation and reduces the levels of nuclear-localized Notch (Toriya et al., 2006), implying this short PRR isoform might mediate neuronal differentiation by regulating the endocytic sorting of Notch. Thus, different Numb isoforms might function in different developmental stages dependent on the time of expression and their respective subcellular localization.

Other Co-Adaptor Proteins for NPXY-Motifs Involved in Signaling During Brain Development: Disabled Proteins

The NPXY motif is not only recognized by numb, but also by another set of co-adaptors, the Disabled (Dab) family of proteins. In addition, NPXY motifs bind to other adaptors, such as sorting nexins (SNX), Fe65, and X11/Mint (Uhlik et al., 2005; Stolt and Bock, 2006). Is there specificity of endocytic adaptors to a subset of NPXY-containing cargos, or do multiple endocytic adaptors play roles (either redundant or distinct) in trafficking the same cargos? Participation of a particular adaptor in cargo sorting would largely depend on cell-type expression, and on subcellular localization of the cargo.

The Discovery of Disabled (Dab)

One of the best studied "full" EAPs (i.e., binding sites for cargo, lipid, AP-2, and clathrin) is disabled (Dab), in particular the mammalian isoform Dab2 (**Figure 4**). Dab was first isolated from *Drosophila* in screens for mutations in genes that enhanced phenotypes of Abl-/- (Abelson tyrosine kinase, a non receptor tyrosine kinase) (Gertler et al., 1989, 1993). Although a later study showed that Dab is not the *bona fide* enhancer of Abl

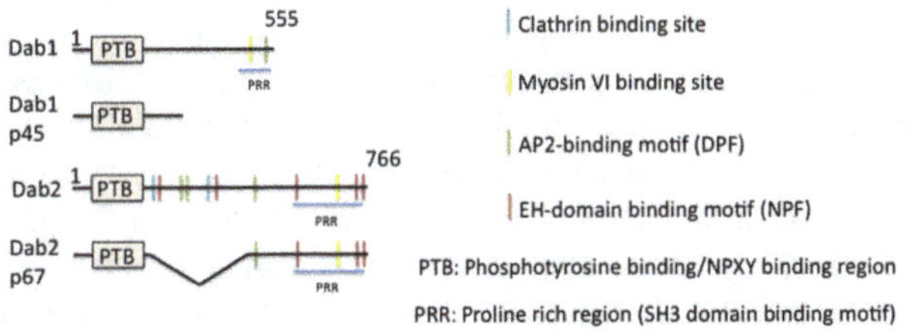

FIGURE 4 | Domain structure of mammalian disabled (Dab) and its isoforms. The domain structure of disabled and of its isoforms is depicted. Binding regions are indicated by color bars.

(Liebl et al., 2003), Dab is still a positive regulator of the Abl signaling pathway. Null mutations of Dab in *Drosophila* causes defects in motor axon patterning and epithelial morphogenesis, phenotypes resembling those of Abl mutants. Genetically, Dab acts in conjunction with Abl for proper growth and guidance of motor axons (Song et al., 2010). While it is not well established which cargos might undergo Dab-mediated endocytosis during axon guidance, a clear role for a clathrin-associated role for *Drosophila* Dab was shown by Kawasaki et al. in mature neurons: a novel Dab mutant that has a nonsense mutation within the conserved N-terminal PTB domain exhibits impaired synaptic function. The experiments indicated that Dab is involved in clathrin-mediated endocytosis for rapid clearance of neurotransmitter release sites, which is important for subsequent vesicle priming and refilling of the readily releasable pool (Kawasaki et al., 2011).

In mammals, the situation is more complicated. There are two members of the Dab family identified thus far, Dab1 and Dab2. Dab is most closely homologous to Dab2. Dab1 was originally isolated as a Src-binding protein (Howell et al., 1997a), whereas Dab2 was identified as a phosphoprotein regulated by colony-stimulating factor CSF1 (Xu et al., 1995). Dab1 is highly neuron-enriched and functions in cell positioning during brain development, whereas Dab2 regulates endodermal cell organization during embryogenesis (Howell et al., 1997b, 1999a; Morris et al., 2002; Yang et al., 2002) and is widely expressed. Dab1 and Dab2 are multi-domain cytoplasmic adaptor proteins and function in mediating several signaling pathways. Structurally, Dab1 contains a PTB-domain, clathrin adaptor AP-2-, SH3 domain-, and myosin-binding sites at its unique C-terminus (**Figure 4**). Similarly to Dab1, Dab2 is composed of an N-terminal PTB domain which is 63% identical to that of Dab1. The Dab2 C-terminus contains clathrin- and EH-domain-binding sites, which are absent in Dab1, in addition to AP-2-, SH3-domain-, and myosin VI-binding sites, which are shared with Dab1. The Dab N-terminal PTB domain is known to bind preferably to non-phosphorylated NPXY internalization motifs present in the cytoplasmic tails of βAPP and LDL-related family proteins, such as LDLR/VLDLR, LRP, ApoER2, and megalin (Trommsdorff et al., 1998, 1999; Howell et al., 1999b; Oleinikov et al., 2000). Additionally, the PTB domain is required for recruitment to the plasma membrane by binding to phospholipids.

Dab2 as an Endocytic Adaptor

Most studies of Dab2 highlight its roles in clathrin-mediated endocytosis. For instance, loss of Dab2 results in decreased endocytosis of transferrin within visceral endoderm and fewer early endosomes in conditional Dab2 knockout mice. Other tissues, such as the kidney, are also affected. In NIH3T3 cells, Dab2 localizes very close to the plasma membrane at CCPs that are also positive for AP-2, but is absent from early endosomal and lysosomal compartments. Its localization to clathrin-coated vesicles is dependent on the clathrin- and AP2-binding sites located in the C-terminus as the Dab2 p67 isoform lacking the binding sites (**Figure 4**) do not associate with CCPs and is defective for receptor endocytosis (Morris and Cooper, 2001; Mishra et al., 2002; Maurer and Cooper, 2006). Mishra at al. demonstrated that Dab2 interacts directly with clathrin independently of AP-2 association, and engages soluble clathrin trimers via its multiple clathrin binding sites to assemble complete polyhedral clathrin cages. Importantly, clathrin recruitment by Dab2 does not affect its interaction with AP-2 (Mishra et al., 2002). Many lines of evidence thus demonstrate that Dab2 is a *bona fide* endocytic co-adaptor in clathrin-mediated endocytosis of NPXY-containing cargos, such as members of the LDL receptor family.

Disabled in the Mammalian Nervous System: Dab1 Regulates Neural Development

There is great interest in Dab1 among developmental neuroscientists since it is highly expressed in neurons, and it has been linked to signaling of major developmental receptors pathways, including reelin (via the reelin receptors ApoER2 and VLDLR), and βAPP. Two mutant mice arising from spontaneous mutations in Dab1, Scrambler and yotari (Sweet et al., 1996; Yoneshima et al., 1997), display inverted cortical lamination, abnormal positioning of neurons, and aberrant orientation of cell bodies and fibers, similar to the reeler mouse which lacks the ligand reelin itself (Falconer, 1951; Goffinet, 1979; Sheldon et al., 1997; Ware et al., 1997). A targeted disruption of the PTB domain of Dab1 resulted in a Dab1 null with no Dab1 mRNA detectable. This Dab1 null mouse also exhibits identical phenotypes to the reeler mouse (Howell et al., 1997b). The Dab1 null mouse is ataxic and dies prematurely between P20 to P30. No clear lamination into layers could be distinguished in either the cerebral cortex or hippocampus. Similarly, the development of the cerebellum is severely affected, unfoliated and small in size. The mutant Purkinje cells are present in the central mass with their dendrites oriented randomly. This suggested that interaction of Dab1 with reelin receptors is essential for reelin-dab1-mediated neuronal migration. Since the phenotypes of the Dab1 null mouse resembles those of the reeler mouse, Dab1 and reelin are part of a single genetic signaling pathway (Rice and Curran, 2001).

The Mechanism of Dab1 Regulation of Reelin Signaling

The PTB domain of Dab1 directly interacts with the NPXY motifs located in the cytoplasmic tails of the reelin receptors VLDLR and ApoER2 (Trommsdorff et al., 1999). Reelin-signaling is initiated by direct binding of reelin to the extracellular domains of VLDLR and ApoER2 (D'Arcangelo et al., 1999; Hiesberger et al., 1999; Rice and Curran, 2001) and subsequently leads to increased levels of phosphorylated Dab1. Reelin-induced phosphorylation of Dab1 leads Src family of non-receptor tyrosine kinases and recruitment of Crk family adaptor proteins (Park and Curran, 2008) which trigger downstream intracellular signaling cascades, such as activation of AKT, PI3K and Erk1/2. Tyrosine phosphorylation of Dab1 at baseline level prior to reelin stimulation is essential for the subsequent reelin-induced activation of Src (Arnaud et al., 2003; Bock and Herz, 2003). VLDLR and ApoER2 are two essential components of the Reelin-signaling pathway. The VLDLR–knockout mouse has smaller cerebellum, whereas the ApoER2-deficient mouse displays two layers of CA1 region. Importantly, the VLDLR and ApoER2 double knockout mouse exhibits identical phenotypes to that observed in reeler/scrambler mice (Trommsdorff et al., 1999). Howell et al. (2000) identified several tyrosine phosphorylation sites clustered close to the PTB domain of Dab1 that are important for cell positioning during brain development. They demonstrated that a mutant mouse with all the identified potential phosphorylation sites mutated display phenotypes identical to those observed in reeler/Dab1-null mice (Howell et al., 2000).

Surprisingly, despite the fact that Dab1 binds the NPXY motif and contains an AP-2 binding site, evidence for a direct role in endocytosis is lacking, and no detailed study demonstrating its association with clathrin-AP2 complex in the regulation of reelin/ApoER2/VLDLR endocytosis exists. Similarly, the endocytic trafficking routes of reelin/receptor-bound Dab1 signaling complex remain poorly understood. Whether phosphorylation affects the function of Dab1 in the endocytic trafficking of reelin-ApoER2 complex, such as dissociation of phosphorylated Dab1 from the complex, remains to be answered. So far there are only a handful of papers showing Dab1-signaling complex in endosomal-like structures. Brian Howell was the first to show Dab1 diffusely in the cell soma and enriched in the axon where it co-localizes with βAPP in small vesicular-like structures (Howell et al., 1999b). Subsequently, Curran's group showed Dab1 co-localization with APLP1 in membrane ruffles and vesicular structures (Homayouni et al., 2001). Although Hiesberger and D'Arcangelo both reported that binding of reelin to VLDLR/ApoER2 on the cell surface mediates its internalization into vesicles (D'Arcangelo et al., 1999; Hiesberger et al., 1999), it is not clear whether vesicles that are positive for internalized reelin also contain Dab1. Similarly, Leeb et al. did not show the presence of Dab1 in EEA1-positive early endosomes colocalizing with clusterin ligand-bound ApoER2/VLDLR complexes (Leeb et al., 2014).

In 2002, it was reported that deletion of the C-terminal region of Dab1 (corresponding to the p45 isoform) (**Figure 4**) has no affect on cortical neuronal migration *in vivo* (Herrick and Cooper, 2002), and the isoform still appears to be phosphorylated, indicating that the AP-2 and SH-domain binding sites are not crucial for activation of reelin-Dab1 signaling during migration. This result argued strongly that

Dab1 works in endocytosis-independent pathways during corticogenesis downstream of reelin signaling. However, a mutant mouse expressing only a single copy of the p45-Dab1 isoform (Dab1$^{p45/-}$, i.e., p45 hemizygote) displays disrupted neocortex and hippocampus development, where the marginal zone of the neocortex shows the presence of late-born neurons, while the CA1 region of hippocampus is separated into two layers. The same paper showed that a mouse carrying one copy of full length p80-Dab1 (Dab1$^{p80/-}$, i.e., p80 hemizygote) shows no migration defect. This observation suggested that the C-terminus of Dab1 might have important functions required for signaling in specific neurons during later stages of brain development.

Is there evidence for or against a role of Dab1 in clathrin-mediated endocytosis? A report by Morimura et al. revealed that tyrosine phosphorylated Dab1 is recruited to the plasma membrane and co-localizes with reelin/receptor complexes in puncta on the cell periphery of cortical neurons of reeler mice after addition of reelin (Morimura et al., 2005). They observed that two minutes after reelin wash-out, phosphorylated Dab1 still co-localizes with reelin in puncta. However, the phosphorylated Dab1 appears to dissociate from the receptor complex 20 min after removal of unbound reelin, the time point when endocytosis is presumably completed, suggesting phosphorylated Dab1 does not traffic extensively with the endocytosed reelin/receptor complex after internalization. Importantly, inhibition of Dab1 phosphorylation by the src kinase inhibitor PP2 prevents internalization of reelin, leaving reelin co-localized with Dab1 near the plasma membrane for a prolonged period. The study concluded that Dab1 regulates cell surface expression of reelin receptors by promoting translocation of the receptors to the plasma membrane, and that phosphorylation of Dab1 initiates intracellular trafficking of reelin/receptor complex in neurons. It is not known whether the puncta positive for reelin and Dab1 at the two-minute time point are on the cell surface or whether they are endocytosed vesicles as the immunostaining for reelin and Dab1 was done after permeabilization. Since endocytosis can be extremely fast, the two-minute time point might include Dab1 on endosomes. This remains to be established more firmly.

In addition, Dab1 has been implicated in regulating the processing and trafficking of βAPP and ApoER2, but this might be during post-endocytic trafficking. A study by Rebeck's group demonstrated that interaction with Dab1 increases the cell surface levels of ApoER2 and βAPP, increases cleavage and secretion of the extracellular domain of the proteins and decreases levels of βAPP C-terminal fragments (Hoe et al., 2006). The effects are NPXY motif- and PTB domain-dependent. Treatment with reelin increases the interaction between Dab1 and βAPP or ApoER2 and significantly lowers the levels of secreted Aβ (Hoe et al., 2006). Notably, Dab1 KO mice have higher levels of Aβ compared to littermate controls, implicating the Dab1-βAPP interaction in regulating Aβ production. Overall the data indicated that Dab1 is involved in regulating the intracellular trafficking and processing of βAPP and of ApoER2 facilitated by reelin. The question of whether Dab1 acts as a scaffold/stabilizer for βAPP/ApoER2 on the cell surface to prevent the proteins from being sorted into endosomal compartments that facilitate Aβ production, or as an adaptor to ensure correct endocytic sorting remains to be investigated.

In addition to direct binding of Dab1 to endocytic machinery, there might also be Dab1 interactions with additional co-adaptors that mediate endocytosis of Dab1 cargos. For example, Fuchigami et al. demonstrated that Dab1 co-localizes with ApoER2 and CIN85 in vesicle-like structures at the plasma membrane (Fuchigami et al., 2013). CIN85 is an adaptor protein involved in endocytosis of receptors including EGFR and dopamine receptor (Dikic, 2003; Shimokawa et al., 2010) by binding to the cbl-EGFR complex via its SH3 domains and to endophilins via its PRR domain. In addition, CIN85 interacts with the PRR region of Dab1. Treatment with a reelin fragment containing the ApoER2/VLDLR binding sites (called the "reelin-repeats") in the presence of Dab1 induced CIN85 localization to early endosomes which contained EEA1, the reelin-repeat fragment and ApoER2 in neurons. Since CIN85 binds phosphorylated Dab1, it is highly possible that interaction of Dab1 with Cin85 might facilitate Dab1-mediated internalization of the receptor complex and possibly trafficking to early endosomal compartments.

Endocytosis Regulation in Neurons—What Other Players are Known?

Numb plays crucial role in the nervous system but is expressed widely outside the nervous system and plays important roles in many places. Are there also neuronal-specific EAPs that might play neuronal-specific roles? And how are cargos with different endocytosis signals endocytosed? What other EAPs and co-adaptors have functions in nervous system development? There are likely many still undiscovered and their roles are largely unknown. We will discuss below the identification of one putative neuronal endocytic co-adaptor, namely doublecortin.

Doublecortin (DCX): A Critical Regulator of Cell Migration and Axon Tract Formation

Doublecortin (DCX) was first identified as the major gene causing X-linked subcortical laminar heterotopia in female and lissencephaly syndrome in male patients (des Portes et al., 1998a,b). These defects manifest as cortical and hippocampal layering defects, leading to phenotypes including epilepsy and mental retardation. The layering defects are due to problems with proper neuronal migration. DCX has two closely related homologs, DCLK1 and DCLK2, both of which contain a kinase-domain at their C-termini, absent in DCX (**Figure 5**). DCX is prominently expressed in young postmitotic neurons, with transient expression detected during adult neurogenesis. Unlike DCX, DCLKs are expressed across the nervous system throughout adulthood. Although DCX is the causative gene for X-linked Lissencephaly in humans, DCX knockout mice display only mild neurodevelopmental delays in the cortex, and cortical lamination in the adult DCX KO mouse is indistinguishable from wild type. In contrast, severe lamination defects are observed in the CA3 region of the hippocampus (Corbo et al., 2002). However, DCX/DCLK1 double KO mice exhibit severely disrupted lamination in the cortical plate, suggesting

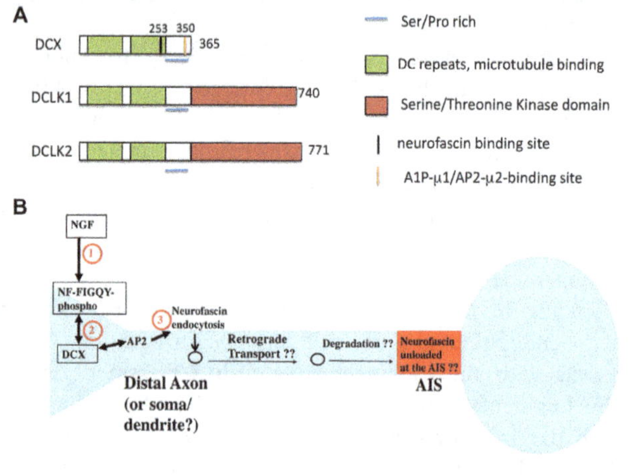

FIGURE 5 | Domain structure of DCX and related proteins DCLK1 and 2. (A) The domain structure of DCX and DCLK1/2 is depicted. Binding regions are indicated by color bars. **(B)** Model of DCX as an endocytic adaptor (based on Yap et al., 2012). DCX binds to the phosphorylated FIGQY motif of the adhesion receptor neurofascin. DCX can bind to AP-2 via its C-terminal YLPL motif and mediate endocytosis of phospho-neurofascin. Neurofascin endocytosis reduces its levels on soma and dendrites and contributes to its gradual accumulation on the axon initial segment (AIS). If endocytosed neurofascin is subsequently degraded or recycled to the AIS is not known.

compensation from DCLK1 might have contributed to the mild cortical phenotypes observed in the DCX KO mouse. Since DCX and DCLK1 are highly related in protein sequence (**Figure 5**), functional redundancy between the two proteins is very likely. In addition, cooperative functions of both proteins in axon outgrowth and in mediating fiber tract decussation have been reported (Deuel et al., 2006; Koizumi et al., 2006; Tanaka et al., 2006). Study on an allelic series of DCX/DCLK1 KO mice with cresyl violet staining reveals a dosage-dependent effect on cortical lamination. Disorganized cytoarchitetonics with dispersion of layer2/3 in the cortex was observed in DCX mutant mice with one copy of DCLK removed. Similar phenotypic defects were detected in DCLK1 mutant mice lacking a copy of DCX. In addition, Koizumi et al. (2006) observed a dosage-dependent interaction between DCX and DCLK1 in commissural fiber tract formation. Removal of one copy of DCLK1 in DCX-null mice causes hypoplastic corpus callosum and thin anterior commissures, whereas anterior commissures are hypoplastic in DCLK1 mutant mice lacking a copy of DCX. On the other hand, deletion of all four copies of DCX and DCLK1 results in disappearance of the corpus callosum, anterior commissures and hippocampus commissures.

Microtubule-Based Roles for DCX

On the molecular level, DCX binds microtubules (MTs) via its two DC repeats to stabilize MTs and promote MT polymerization (**Figure 5A**). DCX has been reported to function with Lis1 and dynein to mediate nucleus-centrosome coupling in neuronal migration. Depletion of DCX in neurons results in delayed centrosomal-nuclear movement, whereas DCX overexpression is able to rescue the nucleus-centrosome coupling defect caused by dynein inhibition and increases the migration rates (Tanaka et al., 2004). These defects are largely attributed to the microtubule-binding activity of DCX. Similar to Dabs, DCX is a phosphoprotein and is known to be a substrate for kinases such as PKA, Cdk5, MAPK8 (aka JNK1), and others. Phosphorylation of DCX regulates its MT binding activity and its localization at the leading processes of migrating neurons: Cdk5-mediated phosphorylation of DCX at Ser297 increases DCX binding to MTs, leading to MT stabilization and promotion of tubulin polymerization, events crucial for neuronal migration (Tanaka et al., 2004).

In addition to microtubule binding, DCX also binds several other proteins (Caspi et al., 2000; Friocourt et al., 2001; Kizhatil et al., 2002; Tanaka et al., 2004; Liu et al., 2012). The roles of these binding interactions are still under investigation. Analysis of double knockout mice for DCX and DCLK1 have uncovered a previously unsuspected role for the DCX proteins in axon outgrowth and dendrite branching and demonstrated aberrant trafficking of synaptic vesicle proteins (Deuel et al., 2006). In neurons cultured from DCLK1 KO with additional DCX knockdown, VAMP2 and synaptophysin accumulate in the cell body, but are completely absent from axons, a drastic contrast from the WT where both proteins are detected in the cell body and the axons. In a follow-up study by Liu et al., the VAMP2 transport defect found in DCX/DCLK1-deficient neurons is caused by the mislocalization of Kif1a. Interestingly, a disease-associated DCX mutation impairs Kif1a motility and disrupts Kif1a-mediated VAMP2 transport from the soma to the neurites. The finding suggested that DCX/DCLK1 is involved in neuronal migration and axonal outgrowth via its interaction with Kif1a on the microtubules for transport regulation (Liu et al., 2012).

DCX as an Endocytic Co-Adaptor for Cell Adhesion Molecules

Several of the other reported defects in DCX deficiencies have led to suggestions that DCX is involved in vesicle trafficking. Defects in synaptic vesicles and synaptic vesicle proteins (such as VAMP2) have all been found (Friocourt et al., 2003; Deuel et al., 2006). The exact molecular mechanisms of such putative trafficking effects of DCX, though, are not known, nor are the cargos. We recently found that DCX might act as an endocytic adaptor and modulate the surface distribution of the cell adhesion molecule neurofascin in developing cultured rat neurons (Yap et al., 2012). DCX binds directly to the cytoplasmic tail of neurofascin via a binding site dependent on residue G253 in DCX (Kizhatil et al., 2002). In contrast to numb and Dab2 which interact with the α subunit of AP-2, DCX associates with the AP2-μ2 subunit via a YLPL motif located in the DCX C-terminus (Friocourt et al., 2001; **Figure 5A**). The YLPL motif conforms to the YXXΦ class of tyrosine-based sorting motifs and is absent in DCLK1/2. Since DCX had been reported to bind to neurofascin (Kizhatil et al., 2002), we tested if DCX mediated the endocytosis of neurofascin. In fact, depletion of DCX diminishes endocytosis of endogenous neurofascin in cultured neurons (Yap et al., 2012). It was previously shown that a cytoplasmic motif in neurofascin (FIGQY) binds to ankyrin when unphosphorylated. In contrast, the phosphorylated FIGQY motif has low affinity for ankyrin, but high affinity for DCX (Kizhatil et al., 2002). Signaling of neurotrophins leads to phosphorylation of the FIGQY motif in the cytoplasmic tail of neurofascin, thereby increasing its affinity for DCX. We proposed (Yap et al., 2012) that local signaling via NGF leads to phosphorylation of the FIGQY motif in neurofascin, which can then bind to DCX locally. Neurofascin is then endocytosed in a DCX-dependent manner from the neuronal plasma membrane, especially in the soma and dendrites (**Figure 5B**). The endocytic machinery required for this event is not yet clear but may involve AP-2 clathrin adaptors. Since we observed the most robust endocytosis of neurofascin in young neurons, DCX-mediated modulation of neurofascin levels could play a role during development. Whether DCX interacts with and modulates sorting of other cargos via clathrin/AP-2 mediated endocytic trafficking remains to be investigated.

Postendocytic Trafficking—Same Signals, Different Machinery?

Given the fact that the μ-subunits of tetrameric AP complexes recognize and interact with similar cytoplasmic motifs in cargos, it is believed that endocytic trafficking of a cargo involves several AP complexes to act in conjunction with each other in a sequential manner for sorting a cargo to its final destination. Yuzaki's group showed that NMDA-induced AMPAR trafficking to the late endosome requires sequential interactions of stargazin, a transmembrane AMPA receptor regulatory protein (aka TARP-γ2), with AP-2 followed by AP-3 during NMDA-dependent long-term depression. Stargazin promotes association of AMPAR with AP-2 and AP-3, and mediates formation of ternary complexes containing AMPAR and the AP complexes. Inhibition of the stargazin interaction with AP-2 impairs NMDA-induced AMPAR endocytosis, whereas inhibition of the stargazin interaction with AP-3 disrupts late endosomal/lysosomal trafficking of AMPAR, thereby leading to recycling of AMPAR back to the cell surface (Matsuda et al., 2013). Similarly, Schachner's group showed that NCAM promotes switching of synaptic vesicles recycling from an AP-3 to an AP-2–dependent mechanism during synapse maturation (Shetty et al., 2013). Both studies suggested that the sequential interaction of a cargo with different AP complexes for its sorting from one endosomal compartment to the subsequent compartment along the endocytic pathway is essential for proper functions in neurons.

Post-Endocytic Roles of Numb

Numb localizes not only to the plasma membrane where it can aid endocytosis, but also to endocytic organelles as well as the TGN, and co-traffics to endosomes with endocytosed receptors (Santolini et al., 2000). In addition to its function in clathrin/AP2-mediated internalization, growing evidence thus implicates Numb in regulating endosomal sorting of receptors post-endocytosis. This is not surprising since many adaptor binding proteins bind more than one of the 5 tetrameric adaptors, such as AP-1 and AP-2. In fact, *Drosophila* numb physically interacts with the AP-1 complex by co-immunoprecipitation (Cotton et al., 2013).

Notch

Numb has been implicated in regulating the post-endocytic trafficking of Notch1. Endocytosis is required to maintain the steady state level of Notch receptors (Le Borgne et al., 2005). Mammalian Notch1 is known to constitutively internalize and traffic to recycling and late endosomal compartments. Despite the fact that numb-mediated inhibition of Notch signaling requires α-adaptin, it is still unknown whether Numb directly regulates the endocytosis or it regulates the endocytic trafficking of Notch after internalization via its association with Eps15 and α-adaptin (Le Borgne et al., 2005). What is known is that interaction of numb with the intracellular domain of Notch (Notch ICD) recruits the E3-ubiquitin ligase itch to the membrane-tethered Notch and leads to polyubiquitination and degradation of Notch ICD. In a study using mammalian cell lines, overexpression of Numb promotes trafficking and degradation of Notch 1, whereas depletion of numb facilitates recycling of Notch1. Numb mutants defective for binding to Itch, Eps15 or adaptin, fail to promote Notch 1 degradation, suggesting Numb suppresses Notch activity by regulating post-endocytic sorting pathways that lead to the degradation of Notch (McGill and McGlade, 2003; McGill et al., 2009).

Sanpodo

In *Drosophila*, interaction of Numb with α-adaptin is required for numb-mediated asymmetric cell division. During asymmetric cell division of SOPs, numb distributes asymmetrically between two daughter cells (called pIIa and pIIb), which is important for the subsequent binary cell fate decision. Hutterer et al reported that internalization of Sanpodo, a transmembrane protein required for Notch signaling in *Drosophila*, is mediated by α-adaptin via interaction with Numb (Hutterer and Knoblich, 2005). However, two recent studies demonstrated that Numb is not essential for the internalization of Sanpodo. The bulk of AP-2-dependent Sanpodo endocytosis still occurs in Numb mutant SOPs (Cotton et al., 2013; Couturier et al., 2013a,b). The studies proposed that Numb interacts with the sanpodo-Notch complex at early endosomes in concert with AP-1 to regulate the endosomal trafficking of the complex. The interaction of numb with sanpodo blocks the recycling of Notch back to the plasma membrane, leading to the asymmetric distribution of Notch along the pIIa-pIIb cell contact interface. A recent finding by Couturier et al. (2014) using dual GFP/cherry-tagged sensors in live SOP cells further confirmed that sanpodo is internalized into early/sorting endosomes in the Numb-inheriting daughter cell and sorted toward late endosomes, a process which is dependent on Numb. Similar to mammalian cells then, numb in flies mediates inhibition of Notch via its regulation of cargo sorting towards late endosomes and inhibition of recycling (Couturier et al., 2014). Some of the seemingly disparate roles of numb on Notch signaling might thus be due to differential post-endocytic sorting of numb cargos towards either recycling or degradative pathways. Depending on the cell type or developmental timing, numb-dependent Notch trafficking could either lead to increased signaling (via recycling) or decreased signaling (via degradation).

Cadherins

Cadherins are required for adhesion and polarity of radial glia cells (RGCs) in the cortex as depletion of cadherins by shRNA results in loss of end-feet and of bipolar morphology. Numb and Numbl are required for the maintenance of cadherin-mediated radial glial adherens junctions (Rasin et al., 2007). EM analysis demonstrated that Numb was enriched just basally of the apical end-feet of interphase RGCs and localized to internalized cadherin-containing Rab11-positive endosomes. Numb physically interacts with the cadherin/catenin complex via its PTB and C-terminal domains, and proper localization of cadherins requires Numb/numbl. Inactivation of Numb and Numbl in conditional double knockout mice decreases basolateral insertion of cadherins and mislocalizes cadherins to the cytoplasm and to apical membrane regions of RGCs. The changed cadherin distribution is likely the reason for the disrupted adherens junctions and loss of polarity observed in the mice. This results in progenitor cells dispersion and disorganized cortical lamination. In contrast, overexpression of Numb and numbl prolongs cadherin-dependent RGC apical attachment and polarization. Thus, Numb plays a critical role in ensuring correct trafficking of cadherins, a process required for the maintenance of adherens junctions during neurogenesis (Rasin et al., 2007).

Sorting Nexin 17 (SNX17): Regulating Post-Endocytic Trafficking of ApoER2

In addition to binding to Dab1, ApoER2 has recently been reported to interact with SNX17 via its cytoplasmic NPXY motif for its endocytic trafficking and receptor signaling (Sotelo et al., 2014). SNX17 is a cytosolic protein that is highly expressed in mouse brain and localized to early endosomes. SNX17 is involved in the endocytic trafficking of membrane proteins, including LRP1, integrins, and P-selectin. For instance, SNX17 has been reported to mediate recycling of integrins. SNX17 binds integrin and prevents degradation in lysosomes (Böttcher et al., 2012; Steinberg et al., 2012). Similarly, SNX17 co-localizes with endocytosed ApoER2 and facilitates the trafficking from early endosomes to recycling endosomes (Sotelo et al., 2014). Depletion of SNX17 causes retention of ApoER2 in Rab5-positive early endosome compartments, leading to a decrease of ApoER2 in Rab11 recycling endosomes. The defect in ApoER2 recycling causes low surface level of ApoER2 and leads to dendritic outgrowth defects. Interestingly, accumulation of ApoER2 in the early endosome of SNX17-deficient neurons promotes proteolytic cleavage of its C-terminal domain. Furthermore, downregulation of SNX17 also promotes reelin-induced degradation of ApoER2, and dampens the activation of downstream reelin effectors, such as the phosphorylation of Dab1. The data suggested that SNX17 is an endosomal adaptor that regulates the post-endocytic trafficking and recycling of ApoER2. It is via this post-endocytic role that SNX17 participates in reelin-receptor signaling (Sotelo et al., 2014). Therefore, in neurons some co-adaptors such as Numb (and possibly Dab1) regulate endocytosis of NPXY-containing cargos at the plasma membrane as well as their postendocytic sorting. Other co-adaptors, such as SNX and likely other still unidentified co-adaptors, might be additionally involved in the subsequent steps of sorting following endocytosis.

Conclusions

In this review, we laid out some of the emerging themes of how regulating the endocytosis and endosomal trafficking of critical receptors contributes to orchestrating developmental decisions in the nervous system. We highlighted some of the better understood endocytic co-adaptors, but many other pathways are similarly coordinated by endocytic regulation. For instance, Wnt signaling via disshevelled is dependent on endocytosis (Onishi et al., 2013). In particular, we discussed examples highlighting the following concepts:

(1) Monomeric EAPs enable interactions of their cognate cargos with the AP-2/clathrin machinery via binding sites that are distinct from endocytic signal binding sites on AP-2 itself. They do thus not compete with cargos using different signals or distinct EAPs. Changing the expression levels of one EAP can therefore change the endocytic rate of just the cognate cargos without affecting other non-cognate cargos.
(2) NPXY-containing cargos can interact with more than one monomeric co-adaptor. The consequences of which co-adaptors binds to which cargo include differential recruitment of different effector cascades, decision to recycle or degrade, effects on residence time in endosomes which affects signaling strength.
(3) EAPs do more than promote endocytosis of their cognate cargos. They can participate in multiple distinct complexes while bound to their cargos and thus regulate signaling. They are regulated scaffolds that can recruit signaling effectors.
(4) Distinct isoforms of EAPs have distinct functions and can affect the ultimate signaling output from the cognate ligand-receptor system.
(5) Many monomeric co-adaptors act at multiple steps along the endocytic-endosomal pathways and sequentially engage distinct set of tetrameric AP complexes as well as other machinery.

Given the large number of receptor pathways, we look forward to many more exciting discoveries of the diverse roles of EAPs in neural development.

References

Aguet, F., Antonescu, C. N., Mettlen, M., Schmid, S. L., and Danuser, G. (2013). Advances in analysis of low signal-to-noise images link dynamin and AP2 to the functions of an endocytic checkpoint. *Dev. Cell* 26, 279–291. doi: 10.1016/j.devcel.2013.06.019

Arnaud, L., Ballif, B. A., Förster, E., and Cooper, J. A. (2003). Fyn tyrosine kinase is a critical regulator of disabled-1 during brain development. *Curr. Biol.* 13, 9–17. doi: 10.1016/s0960-9822(02)01397-0

Arnò, B., Grassivaro, F., Rossi, C., Bergamaschi, A., Castiglioni, V., Furlan, R., et al. (2014). Neural progenitor cells orchestrate microglia migration and positioning into the developing cortex. *Nat. Commun.* 5:5611. doi: 10.1038/ncomms6611

Barois, N., and Bakke, O. (2005). The adaptor protein AP-4 as a component of the clathrin coat machinery: a morphological study. *Biochem. J.* 385(Pt. 2), 503–510. doi: 10.1042/bj20041010

Berdnik, D., Török, T., González-Gaitán, M., and Knoblich, J. A. (2002). The endocytic protein alpha-Adaptin is required for numb-mediated asymmetric cell division in *Drosophila. Dev. Cell* 3, 221–231. doi: 10.1016/s1534-5807(02)00215-0

Bitsikas, V., Correa, I. R. Jr., and Nichols, B. J. (2014). Clathrin-independent pathways do not contribute significantly to endocytic flux. *Elife* 3:e03970. doi: 10.7554/eLife.03970

Bock, H. H., and Herz, J. (2003). Reelin activates SRC family tyrosine kinases in neurons. *Curr. Biol.* 13, 18–26. doi: 10.1016/s0960-9822(02)01403-3

Bonifacino, J. S., and Traub, L. M. (2003). Signals for sorting of transmembrane proteins to endosomes and lysosomes. *Annu. Rev. Biochem.* 72, 395–447. doi: 10.1146/annurev.biochem.72.121801.161800

Böttcher, R. T., Stremmel, C., Meves, A., Meyer, H., Widmaier, M., Tseng, H. Y., et al. (2012). Sorting nexin 17 prevents lysosomal degradation of α1 integrins by binding to the α1-integrin tail. *Nat. Cell Biol.* 14, 584–592. doi: 10. 1038/ncb2501

Brodsky, F. M., Chen, C. Y., Knuehl, C., Towler, M. C., and Wakeham, D. E. (2001). Biological basket weaving: formation and function of clathrin-coated vesicles. *Annu. Rev. Cell Dev. Biol.* 17, 517–568. doi: 10.1146/annurev.cellbio. 17.1.517

Bultje, R. S., Castaneda-Castellanos, D. R., Jan, L. Y., Jan, Y. N., Kriegstein, A. R., and Shi, S. H. (2009). Mammalian Par3 regulates progenitor cell asymmetric division via notch signaling in the developing neocortex. *Neuron* 63, 189–202. doi: 10.1016/j.neuron.2009.07.004

Calderwood, D. A., Fujioka, Y., de Pereda, J. M., García-Alvarez, B., Nakamoto, T., Margolis, B., et al. (2003). Integrin beta cytoplasmic domain interactions with phosphotyrosine-binding domains: a structural prototype for diversity in integrin signaling. *Proc. Natl. Acad. Sci. U S A* 100, 2272–2277. doi: 10. 1073/pnas.262791999

Caspi, M., Atlas, R., Kantor, A., Sapir, T., and Reiner, O. (2000). Interaction between LIS1 and doublecortin, two lissencephaly gene products. *Hum. Mol. Genet.* 9, 2205–2213. doi: 10.1093/oxfordjournals.hmg.a018911

Choe, Y., Huynh, T., and Pleasure, S. J. (2014). Migration of oligodendrocyte progenitor cells is controlled by transforming growth factor β family proteins during corticogenesis. *J. Neurosci.* 34, 14973–14983. doi: 10.1523/JNEUROSCI. 1156-14.2014

Conner, S. D., and Schmid, S. L. (2002). Identification of an adaptor-associated kinase, AAK1, as a regulator of clathrin-mediated endocytosis. *J. Cell Biol.* 156, 921–929. doi: 10.1083/jcb.200108123

Corbo, J. C., Deuel, T. A., Long, J. M., LaPorte, P., Tsai, E., Wynshaw-Boris, A., et al. (2002). Doublecortin is required in mice for lamination of the hippocampus but not the neocortex. *J. Neurosci.* 22, 7548–7557.

Cosker, K. E., and Segal, R. A. (2014). Neuronal signaling through endocytosis. *Cold Spring Harb. Perspect. Biol.* 6:a020669. doi: 10.1101/cshperspect. a020669

Cotton, M., Benhra, N., and Le Borgne, R. (2013). Numb inhibits the recycling of Sanpodo in *Drosophila* sensory organ precursor. *Curr. Biol.* 23, 581–587. doi: 10.1016/j.cub.2013.02.020

Couturier, L., Mazouni, K., and Schweisguth, F. (2013a). Inhibition of Notch recycling by Numb: relevance and mechanism(s). *Cell Cycle* 12, 1647–1648. doi: 10.4161/cc.24983

Couturier, L., Mazouni, K., and Schweisguth, F. (2013b). Numb localizes at endosomes and controls the endosomal sorting of notch after asymmetric division in *Drosophila. Curr. Biol.* 23, 588–593. doi: 10.1016/j.cub.2013. 03.002

Couturier, L., Trylinski, M., Mazouni, K., Darnet, L., and Schweisguth, F. (2014). A fluorescent tagging approach in *Drosophila* reveals late endosomal trafficking of Notch and Sanpodo. *J. Cell Biol.* 207, 351–363. doi: 10.1083/jcb.201407071

Danglot, L., and Galli, T. (2007). What is the function of neuronal AP-3?. *Biol. Cell* 99, 349–361. doi: 10.1042/bc20070029

D'Arcangelo, G., Homayouni, R., Keshvara, L., Rice, D. S., Sheldon, M., and Curran, T. (1999). Reelin is a ligand for lipoprotein receptors. *Neuron* 24, 471–479. doi: 10.1016/s0896-6273(00)80860-0

Dell'Angelica, E. C., Klumperman, J., Stoorvogel, W., and Bonifacino, J. S. (1998). Association of the AP-3 adaptor complex with clathrin. *Science* 280, 431–434. doi: 10.1126/science.280.5362.431

Dell'Angelica, E. C., Ohno, H., Ooi, C. E., Rabinovich, E., Roche, K. W., and Bonifacino, J. S. (1997). AP-3: an adaptor-like protein complex with ubiquitous expression. *EMBO J.* 16, 917–928. doi: 10.1093/emboj/16.5.917

des Portes, V., Francis, F., Pinard, J. M., Desguerre, I., Moutard, M. L., Snoeck, I., et al. (1998a). Doublecortin is the major gene causing X-linked Subcortical Laminar Heterotopia (SCLH). *Hum. Mol. Genet.* 7, 1063–1070. doi: 10. 1093/hmg/7.7.1063

des Portes, V., Pinard, J. M., Billuart, P., Vinet, M. C., Koulakoff, A., Carrié, A., et al. (1998b). A novel CNS gene required for neuronal migration and involved in X-linked subcortical laminar heterotopia and lissencephaly syndrome. *Cell* 92, 51–61. doi: 10.1016/s0092-8674(00)80898-3

Deuel, T. A., Liu, J. S., Corbo, J. C., Yoo, S. Y., Rorke-Adams, L. B., and Walsh, C. A. (2006). Genetic interactions between doublecortin and doublecortin-like kinase in neuronal migration and axon outgrowth. *Neuron* 49, 41–53. doi: 10. 1016/j.neuron.2005.10.038

Dho, S. E., French, M. B., Woods, S. A., and McGlade, C. J. (1999). Characterization of four mammalian numb protein isoforms. Identification of cytoplasmic and membrane-associated variants of the phosphotyrosine binding domain. *J. Biol. Chem.* 274, 33097–33104. doi: 10.1074/jbc.274.46.33097

Dikic, I. (2003). Mechanisms controlling EGF receptor endocytosis and degradation. *Biochem. Soc. Trans.* 31(Pt. 6), 1178–1181. doi: 10. 1042/bst0311178

Falconer, D. S. (1951). Two new mutants, 'trembler' and 'reeler', with neurological actions in the house mouse (Mus musculus L.). *J. Genet.* 50, 192–201. doi: 10. 1007/BF02996215

Faúndez, V., Horng, J. T., and Kelly, R. B. (1998). A function for the AP3 coat complex in synaptic vesicle formation from endosomes. *Cell* 93, 423–432. doi: 10.1016/s0092-8674(00)81170-8

Fölsch, H. (2008). Regulation of membrane trafficking in polarized epithelial cells. *Curr. Opin. Cell Biol.* 20, 208–213. doi: 10.1016/j.ceb.2008.01.003

Friocourt, G., Chafey, P., Billuart, P., Koulakoff, A., Vinet, M. C., Schaar, B. T., et al. (2001). Doublecortin interacts with μ subunits of clathrin adaptor complexes in the developing nervous system. *Mol. Cell Neurosci.* 18, 307–319. doi: 10. 1006/mcne.2001.1022

Friocourt, G., Koulakoff, A., Chafey, P., Boucher, D., Fauchereau, F., Chelly, J., et al. (2003). Doublecortin functions at the extremities of growing neuronal processes. *Cereb. Cortex* 13, 620–626. doi: 10.1093/cercor/13.6.620

Fuchigami, T., Sato, Y., Tomita, Y., Takano, T., Miyauchi, S. Y., Tsuchiya, Y., et al. (2013). Dab1-mediated colocalization of multi-adaptor protein CIN85 with Reelin receptors, ApoER2 and VLDLR, in neurons. *Genes Cells* 18, 410–424. doi: 10.1111/gtc.12045

Gaiano, N., Nye, J. S., and Fishell, G. (2000). Radial glial identity is promoted by Notch1 signaling in the murine forebrain. *Neuron* 26, 395–404. doi: 10. 1016/s0896-6273(00)81172-1

Gertler, F. B., Bennett, R. L., Clark, M. J., and Hoffmann, F. M. (1989). *Drosophila* abl tyrosine kinase in embryonic CNS axons: a role in axonogenesis is revealed through dosage-sensitive interactions with disabled. *Cell* 58, 103–113. doi: 10. 1016/0092-8674(89)90407-8

Gertler, F. B., Hill, K. K., Clark, M. J., and Hoffmann, F. M. (1993). Dosage-sensitive modifiers of *Drosophila* abl tyrosine kinase function: prospero, a regulator of axonal outgrowth and disabled, a novel tyrosine kinase substrate. *Genes Dev.* 7, 441–453. doi: 10.1101/gad.7.3.441

Goffinet, A. M. (1979). An early development defect in the cerebral cortex of the reeler mouse. A morphological study leading to a hypothesis concerning the action of the mutant gene. *Anat. Embryol. (Berl)* 157, 205–216. doi: 10. 1007/bf00305160

Gulino, A., Di Marcotullio, L., and Screpanti, I. (2010). The multiple functions of Numb. *Exp. Cell Res.* 316, 900–906. doi: 10.1016/j.yexcr.2009.11.017

Guo, J., and Anton, E. S. (2014). Decision making during interneuron migration in the developing cerebral cortex. *Trends Cell Biol.* 24, 342–351. doi: 10.1016/j. tcb.2013.12.001

Guo, M., Jan, L. Y., and Jan, Y. N. (1996). Control of daughter cell fates during asymmetric division: interaction of Numb and Notch. *Neuron* 17, 27–41. doi: 10.1016/S0896-6273(00)80278-0

Herrick, T. M., and Cooper, J. A. (2002). A hypomorphic allele of dab1 reveals regional differences in reelin-Dab1 signaling during brain development. *Development* 129, 787–796.

Hiesberger, T., Trommsdorff, M., Howell, B. W., Goffinet, A., Mumby, M. C., Cooper, J. A., et al. (1999). Direct binding of Reelin to VLDL receptor and

ApoE receptor 2 induces tyrosine phosphorylation of disabled-1 and modulates tau phosphorylation. *Neuron* 24, 481–489. doi: 10.1016/s0896-6273(00)80861-2

Hirst, J., Barlow, L. D., Francisco, G. C., Sahlender, D. A., Seaman, M. N., Dacks, J. B., et al. (2011). The fifth adaptor protein complex. *PLoS Biol.* 9:e1001170. doi: 10.1371/journal.pbio.1001170

Hirst, J., Bright, N. A., Rous, B., and Robinson, M. S. (1999). Characterization of a fourth adaptor-related protein complex. *Mol. Biol. Cell* 10, 2787–2802. doi: 10.1091/mbc.10.8.2787

Hirst, J., Irving, C., and Borner, G. H. (2013). Adaptor protein complexes AP-4 and AP-5: new players in endosomal trafficking and progressive spastic paraplegia. *Traffic* 14, 153–164. doi: 10.1111/tra.12028

Hirst, J., and Robinson, M. S. (1998). Clathrin and adaptors. *Biochim. Biophys. Acta* 1404, 173–193. doi: 10.1016/S0167-4889(98)00056-1

Hoe, H. S., Tran, T. S., Matsuoka, Y., Howell, B. W., and Rebeck, G. W. (2006). DAB1 and Reelin effects on amyloid precursor protein and ApoE receptor 2 trafficking and processing. *J. Biol. Chem.* 281, 35176–35185. doi: 10.1074/jbc.m602162200

Homayouni, R., Rice, D. S., and Curran, T. (2001). Disabled-1 interacts with a novel developmentally regulated protocadherin. *Biochem. Biophys. Res. Commun.* 289, 539–547. doi: 10.1006/bbrc.2001.5998

Howell, B. W., Gertler, F. B., and Cooper, J. A. (1997a). Mouse disabled (mDab1): a Src binding protein implicated in neuronal development. *EMBO J.* 16, 121–132. doi: 10.1093/emboj/16.1.121

Howell, B. W., Hawkes, R., Soriano, P., and Cooper, J. A. (1997b). Neuronal position in the developing brain is regulated by mouse disabled-1. *Nature* 389, 733–737. doi: 10.1038/39607

Howell, B. W., Herrick, T. M., and Cooper, J. A. (1999a). Reelin-induced tyrosine [corrected] phosphorylation of disabled 1 during neuronal positioning. *Genes Dev.* 13, 643–648. doi: 10.1101/gad.13.6.643

Howell, B. W., Herrick, T. M., Hildebrand, J. D., Zhang, Y., and Cooper, J. A. (2000). Dab1 tyrosine phosphorylation sites relay positional signals during mouse brain development. *Curr. Biol.* 10, 877–885. doi: 10.1016/s0960-9822(00)00608-4

Howell, B. W., Lanier, L. M., Frank, R., Gertler, F. B., and Cooper, J. A. (1999b). The disabled 1 phosphotyrosine-binding domain binds to the internalization signals of transmembrane glycoproteins and to phospholipids. *Mol. Cell. Biol.* 19, 5179–5188.

Hutterer, A., and Knoblich, J. A. (2005). Numb and alpha-Adaptin regulate Sanpodo endocytosis to specify cell fate in *Drosophila* external sensory organs. *EMBO Rep.* 6, 836–842. doi: 10.1038/sj.embor.7400500

Jamuar, S. S., and Walsh, C. A. (2014). Somatic mutations in cerebral cortical malformations. *N. Engl. J. Med.* 371, 2037–2038. doi: 10.1056/NEJMc1411784

Kamiguchi, H., Long, K. E., Pendergast, M., Schaefer, A. W., Rapoport, I., Kirchhausen, T., et al. (1998). The neural cell adhesion molecule L1 interacts with the AP-2 adaptor and is endocytosed via the clathrin-mediated pathway. *J. Neurosci.* 18, 5311–5321.

Kawasaki, F., Iyer, J., Posey, L. L., Sun, C. E., Mammen, S. E., Yan, H., et al. (2011). The DISABLED protein functions in CLATHRIN-mediated synaptic vesicle endocytosis and exoendocytic coupling at the active zone. *Proc. Natl. Acad. Sci. U S A* 108, E222–E229. doi: 10.1073/pnas.1102231108

Kawauchi, T., and Hoshino, M. (2008). Molecular pathways regulating cytoskeletal organization and morphological changes in migrating neurons. *Dev. Neurosci.* 30, 36–46. doi: 10.1159/000109850

Kizhatil, K., Wu, Y. X., Sen, A., and Bennett, V. (2002). A new activity of doublecortin in recognition of the phospho-FIGQY tyrosine in the cytoplasmic domain of neurofascin. *J. Neurosci.* 22, 7948–7958.

Klein, A. L., Zilian, O., Suter, U., and Taylor, V. (2004). Murine numb regulates granule cell maturation in the cerebellum. *Dev. Biol.* 266, 161–177. doi: 10.1016/j.ydbio.2003.10.017

Koizumi, H., Tanaka, T., and Gleeson, J. G. (2006). Doublecortin-like kinase functions with doublecortin to mediate fiber tract decussation and neuronal migration. *Neuron* 49, 55–66. doi: 10.1016/j.neuron.2005.10.040

Kononenko, N. L., Puchkov, D., Classen, G. A., Walter, A. M., Pechstein, A., Sawade, L., et al. (2014). Clathrin/AP-2 mediate synaptic vesicle reformation from endosome-like vacuoles but are not essential for membrane retrieval at central synapses. *Neuron* 82, 981–988. doi: 10.1016/j.neuron.2014.05.007

Krieger, J. R., Taylor, P., Gajadhar, A. S., Guha, A., Moran, M. F., and McGlade, C. J. (2013). Identification and selected reaction monitoring (SRM) quantification of endocytosis factors associated with Numb. *Mol. Cell. Proteomics* 12, 499–514. doi: 10.1074/mcp.M112.020768

Le Borgne, R., Bardin, A., and Schweisguth, F. (2005). The roles of receptor and ligand endocytosis in regulating Notch signaling. *Development* 132, 1751–1762. doi: 10.1242/dev.01789

Leeb, C., Eresheim, C., and Nimpf, J. (2014). Clusterin is a ligand for apolipoprotein E receptor 2 (ApoER2) and very low density lipoprotein receptor (VLDLR) and signals via the Reelin-signaling pathway. *J. Biol. Chem.* 289, 4161–4172. doi: 10.1074/jbc.M113.529271

Lewis, T. L. Jr., Courchet, J., and Polleux, F. (2013). Cell biology in neuroscience: cellular and molecular mechanisms underlying axon formation, growth and branching. *J. Cell Biol.* 202, 837–848. doi: 10.1083/jcb.201305098

Liebl, E. C., Rowe, R. G., Forsthoefel, D. J., Stammler, A. L., Schmidt, E. R., Turski, M., et al. (2003). Interactions between the secreted protein Amalgam, its transmembrane receptor Neurotactin and the Abelson tyrosine kinase affect axon pathfinding. *Development* 130, 3217–3226. doi: 10.1242/dev.00545

Liu, J. S. (2011). Molecular genetics of neuronal migration disorders. *Curr. Neurol. Neurosci. Rep.* 11, 171–178. doi: 10.1007/s11910-010-0176-5

Liu, J. S., Schubert, C. R., Fu, X., Fourniol, F. J., Jaiswal, J. K., Houdusse, A., et al. (2012). Molecular basis for specific regulation of neuronal kinesin-3 motors by doublecortin family proteins. *Mol. Cell* 47, 707–721. doi: 10.1016/j.molcel.2012.06.025

LoTurco, J. J., and Bai, J. (2006). The multipolar stage and disruptions in neuronal migration. *Trends Neurosci.* 29, 407–413. doi: 10.1016/j.tins.2006.05.006

Matsuda, S., Kakegawa, W., Budisantoso, T., Nomura, T., Kohda, K., and Yuzaki, M. (2013). Stargazin regulates AMPA receptor trafficking through adaptor protein complexes during long-term depression. *Nat. Commun.* 4:2759. doi: 10.1038/ncomms3759

Maurer, M. E., and Cooper, J. A. (2006). The adaptor protein Dab2 sorts LDL receptors into coated pits independently of AP-2 and ARH. *J. Cell Sci.* 119(Pt. 20), 4235–4246. doi: 10.1242/jcs.03217

McGill, M. A., Dho, S. E., Weinmaster, G., and McGlade, C. J. (2009). Numb regulates post-endocytic trafficking and degradation of Notch1. *J. Biol. Chem.* 284, 26427–26438. doi: 10.1074/jbc.M109.014845

McGill, M. A., and McGlade, C. J. (2003). Mammalian numb proteins promote Notch1 receptor ubiquitination and degradation of the Notch1 intracellular domain. *J. Biol. Chem.* 278, 23196–23203. doi: 10.1074/jbc.m302827200

McMahon, H. T. (1999). Endocytosis: an assembly protein for clathrin cages. *Curr. Biol.* 9, R332–R335. doi: 10.1016/s0960-9822(99)80206-1

McMahon, H. T., and Boucrot, E. (2011). Molecular mechanism and physiological functions of clathrin-mediated endocytosis. *Nat. Rev. Mol. Cell Biol.* 12, 517–533. doi: 10.1038/nrm3151

Merrifield, C. J., and Kaksonen, M. (2014). Endocytic accessory factors and regulation of clathrin-mediated endocytosis. *Cold Spring Harb. Perspect. Biol.* 6:a016733. doi: 10.1101/cshperspect.a016733

Mishra, S. K., Keyel, P. A., Hawryluk, M. J., Agostinelli, N. R., Watkins, S. C., and Traub, L. M. (2002). Disabled-2 exhibits the properties of a cargo-selective endocytic clathrin adaptor. *EMBO J.* 21, 4915–4926. doi: 10.1093/emboj/cdf487

Morimura, T., Hattori, M., Ogawa, M., and Mikoshiba, K. (2005). Disabled1 regulates the intracellular trafficking of reelin receptors. *J. Biol. Chem.* 280, 16901–16908. doi: 10.1074/jbc.m409048200

Morris, S. M., and Cooper, J. A. (2001). Disabled-2 colocalizes with the LDLR in clathrin-coated pits and interacts with AP-2. *Traffic* 2, 111–123. doi: 10.1034/j.1600-0854.2001.020206.x

Morris, S. M., Tallquist, M. D., Rock, C. O., and Cooper, J. A. (2002). Dual roles for the Dab2 adaptor protein in embryonic development and kidney transport. *EMBO J.* 21, 1555–1564. doi: 10.1093/emboj/21.7.1555

Mullins, C., and Bonifacino, J. S. (2001). The molecular machinery for lysosome biogenesis. *Bioessays* 23, 333–343. doi: 10.1002/bies.1048

Nakatsu, F., Okada, M., Mori, F., Kumazawa, N., Iwasa, H., Zhu, G., et al. (2004). Defective function of GABA-containing synaptic vesicles in mice lacking the AP-3B clathrin adaptor. *J. Cell Biol.* 167, 293–302. doi: 10.1083/jcb.200405032

Nishimura, T., Fukata, Y., Kato, K., Yamaguchi, T., Matsuura, Y., Kamiguchi, H., et al. (2003). CRMP-2 regulates polarized Numb-mediated endocytosis for axon growth. *Nat. Cell Biol.* 5, 819–826. doi: 10.1038/ncb1039

Nishimura, T., and Kaibuchi, K. (2007). Numb controls integrin endocytosis for directional cell migration with aPKC and PAR-3. *Dev. Cell* 13, 15–28. doi: 10.1016/j.devcel.2007.05.003

Oleinikov, A. V., Zhao, J., and Makker, S. P. (2000). Cytosolic adaptor protein Dab2 is an intracellular ligand of endocytic receptor gp600/megalin. *Biochem. J.* 347(Pt. 3), 613–621. doi: 10.1042/0264-6021:3470613

Onishi, K., Shafer, B., Lo, C., Tissir, F., Goffinet, A. M., and Zou, Y. (2013). Antagonistic functions of Dishevelleds regulate Frizzled3 endocytosis via filopodia tips in Wnt-mediated growth cone guidance. *J. Neurosci.* 33, 19071–19085. doi: 10.1523/JNEUROSCI.2800-13.2013

Park, T. J., and Curran, T. (2008). Crk and Crk-like play essential overlapping roles downstream of disabled-1 in the Reelin pathway. *J. Neurosci.* 28, 13551–13562. doi: 10.1523/JNEUROSCI.4323-08.2008

Rasin, M. R., Gazula, V. R., Breunig, J. J., Kwan, K. Y., Johnson, M. B., Liu-Chen, S., et al. (2007). Numb and Numbl are required for maintenance of cadherin-based adhesion and polarity of neural progenitors. *Nat. Neurosci.* 10, 819–827. doi: 10.1038/nn1924

Reider, A., and Wendland, B. (2011). Endocytic adaptors–social networking at the plasma membrane. *J. Cell Sci.* 124(Pt. 10), 1613–1622. doi: 10.1242/jcs.073395

Rice, D. S., and Curran, T. (2001). Role of the reelin signaling pathway in central nervous system development. *Annu. Rev. Neurosci.* 24, 1005–1039. doi: 10.1146/annurev.neuro.24.1.1005

Ricotta, D., Conner, S. D., Schmid, S. L., von Figura, K., and Honing, S. (2002). Phosphorylation of the AP2 mu subunit by AAK1 mediates high affinity binding to membrane protein sorting signals. *J. Cell Biol.* 156, 791–795. doi: 10.1083/jcb.200111068

Robinson, M. S., and Bonifacino, J. S. (2001). Adaptor-related proteins. *Curr. Opin. Cell Biol.* 13, 444–453. doi: 10.1016/s0955-0674(00)00235-0

Salcini, A. E., Confalonieri, S., Doria, M., Santolini, E., Tassi, E., Minenkova, O., et al. (1997). Binding specificity and *in vivo* targets of the EH domain, a novel protein-protein interaction module. *Genes Dev.* 11, 2239–2249. doi: 10.1101/gad.11.17.2239

Santolini, E., Puri, C., Salcini, A. E., Gagliani, M. C., Pelicci, P. G., Tacchetti, C., et al. (2000). Numb is an endocytic protein. *J. Cell Biol.* 151, 1345–1352. doi: 10.1083/jcb.151.6.1345

Sheldon, M., Rice, D. S., D'Arcangelo, G., Yoneshima, H., Nakajima, K., Mikoshiba, K., et al. (1997). Scrambler and yotari disrupt the disabled gene and produce a reeler-like phenotype in mice. *Nature* 389, 730–733. doi: 10.1038/39601

Shen, Q., Zhong, W., Jan, Y. N., and Temple, S. (2002). Asymmetric Numb distribution is critical for asymmetric cell division of mouse cerebral cortical stem cells and neuroblasts. *Development* 129, 4843–4853.

Shetty, A., Sytnyk, V., Leshchyns'ka, I., Puchkov, D., Haucke, V., and Schachner, M. (2013). The neural cell adhesion molecule promotes maturation of the presynaptic endocytotic machinery by switching synaptic vesicle recycling from adaptor protein 3 (AP-3)- to AP-2-dependent mechanisms. *J. Neurosci.* 33, 16828–16845. doi: 10.1523/JNEUROSCI.2192-13.2013

Shieh, J. C., Schaar, B. T., Srinivasan, K., Brodsky, F. M., and McConnell, S. K. (2011). Endocytosis regulates cell soma translocation and the distribution of adhesion proteins in migrating neurons. *PLoS One* 6:e17802. doi: 10.1371/journal.pone.0017802

Shimokawa, N., Haglund, K., Holter, S. M., Grabbe, C., Kirkin, V., Koibuchi, N., et al. (2010). CIN85 regulates dopamine receptor endocytosis and governs behaviour in mice. *EMBO J.* 29, 2421–2432. doi: 10.1038/emboj.2010.120

Simpson, F., Bright, N. A., West, M. A., Newman, L. S., Darnell, R. B., and Robinson, M. S. (1996). A novel adaptor-related protein complex. *J. Cell Biol.* 133, 749–760. doi: 10.1083/jcb.133.4.749

Smith, C. A., Dho, S. E., Donaldson, J., Tepass, U., and McGlade, C. J. (2004). The cell fate determinant numb interacts with EHD/Rme-1 family proteins and has a role in endocytic recycling. *Mol. Biol. Cell* 15, 3698–3708. doi: 10.1091/mbc.e04-01-0026

Smith, C. A., Lau, K. M., Rahmani, Z., Dho, S. E., Brothers, G., She, Y. M., et al. (2007). aPKC-mediated phosphorylation regulates asymmetric membrane localization of the cell fate determinant Numb. *EMBO J.* 26, 468–480. doi: 10.1038/sj.emboj.7601495

Song, J. K., Kannan, R., Merdes, G., Singh, J., Mlodzik, M., and Giniger, E. (2010). Disabled is a bona fide component of the Abl signaling network. *Development* 137, 3719–3727. doi: 10.1242/dev.050948

Sorensen, E. B., and Conner, S. D. (2008). AAK1 regulates Numb function at an early step in clathrin-mediated endocytosis. *Traffic* 9, 1791–1800. doi: 10.1111/j.1600-0854.2008.00790.x

Sotelo, P., Farfán, P., Benitez, M. L., Bu, G., and Marzolo, M. P. (2014). Sorting nexin 17 regulates ApoER2 recycling and reelin signaling. *PLoS One* 9:e93672. doi: 10.1371/journal.pone.0093672

Starcevic, M., Nazarian, R., and Dell'Angelica, E. C. (2002). The molecular machinery for the biogenesis of lysosome-related organelles: lessons from Hermansky-Pudlak syndrome. *Semin. Cell Dev. Biol.* 13, 271–278. doi: 10.1016/s1084952102000563

Steinberg, F., Heesom, K. J., Bass, M. D., and Cullen, P. J. (2012). SNX17 protects integrins from degradation by sorting between lysosomal and recycling pathways. *J. Cell Biol.* 197, 219–230. doi: 10.1083/jcb.201111121

Stolt, P. C., and Bock, H. H. (2006). Modulation of lipoprotein receptor functions by intracellular adaptor proteins. *Cell. Signal.* 18, 1560–1571. doi: 10.1016/j.cellsig.2006.03.008

Sweet, H. O., Bronson, R. T., Johnson, K. R., Cook, S. A., and Davisson, M. T. (1996). Scrambler, a new neurological mutation of the mouse with abnormalities of neuronal migration. *Mamm. Genome* 7, 798–802. doi: 10.1007/s003359900240

Tanaka, T., Koizumi, H., and Gleeson, J. G. (2006). The doublecortin and doublecortin-like kinase 1 genes cooperate in murine hippocampal development. *Cereb. Cortex* 16(Suppl. 1), i69–i73. doi: 10.1093/cercor/bhk005

Tanaka, T., Serneo, F. F., Higgins, C., Gambello, M. J., Wynshaw-Boris, A., and Gleeson, J. G. (2004). Lis1 and doublecortin function with dynein to mediate coupling of the nucleus to the centrosome in neuronal migration. *J. Cell Biol.* 165, 709–721. doi: 10.1083/jcb.200309025

Tokumitsu, H., Hatano, N., Yokokura, S., Sueyoshi, Y., Nozaki, N., and Kobayashi, R. (2006). Phosphorylation of Numb regulates its interaction with the clathrin-associated adaptor AP-2. *FEBS Lett.* 580, 5797–5801. doi: 10.1016/j.febslet.2006.09.043

Toriya, M., Tokunaga, A., Sawamoto, K., Nakao, K., and Okano, H. (2006). Distinct functions of human numb isoforms revealed by misexpression in the neural stem cell lineage in the *Drosophila* larval brain. *Dev. Neurosci.* 28, 142–155. doi: 10.1159/000090760

Traub, L. M., and Bonifacino, J. S. (2013). Cargo recognition in clathrin-mediated endocytosis. *Cold Spring Harb. Perspect. Biol.* 5:a016790. doi: 10.1101/cshperspect.a016790

Trommsdorff, M., Borg, J. P., Margolis, B., and Herz, J. (1998). Interaction of cytosolic adaptor proteins with neuronal apolipoprotein E receptors and the amyloid precursor protein. *J. Biol. Chem.* 273, 33556–33560. doi: 10.1074/jbc.273.50.33556

Trommsdorff, M., Gotthardt, M., Hiesberger, T., Shelton, J., Stockinger, W., Nimpf, J., et al. (1999). Reeler/Disabled-like disruption of neuronal migration in knockout mice lacking the VLDL receptor and ApoE receptor 2. *Cell* 97, 689–701. doi: 10.1016/s0092-8674(00)80782-5

Uemura, T., Shepherd, S., Ackerman, L., Jan, L. Y., and Jan, Y. N. (1989). Numb, a gene required in determination of cell fate during sensory organ formation in *Drosophila* embryos. *Cell* 58, 349–360. doi: 10.1016/0092-8674(89)90849-0

Uhlik, M. T., Temple, B., Bencharit, S., Kimple, A. J., Siderovski, D. P., and Johnson, G. L. (2005). Structural and evolutionary division of phosphotyrosine binding (PTB) domains. *J. Mol. Biol.* 345, 1–20. doi: 10.1016/j.jmb.2004.10.038

Verdi, J. M., Bashirullah, A., Goldhawk, D. E., Kubu, C. J., Jamali, M., Meakin, S. O., et al. (1999). Distinct human NUMB isoforms regulate differentiation vs. proliferation in the neuronal lineage. *Proc. Natl. Acad. Sci. U S A* 96, 10472–10476. doi: 10.1073/pnas.96.18.10472

Vicente-Manzanares, M., and Horwitz, A. R. (2011). Cell migration: an overview. *Methods Mol. Biol.* 769, 1–24. doi: 10.1007/978-1-61779-207-6_1

Vitriol, E. A., and Zheng, J. Q. (2012). Growth cone travel in space and time: the cellular ensemble of cytoskeleton, adhesion and membrane. *Neuron* 73, 1068–1081. doi: 10.1016/j.neuron.2012.03.005

Ware, M. L., Fox, J. W., González, J. L., Davis, N. M., Lambert de Rouvroit, C., Russo, C. J., et al. (1997). Aberrant splicing of a mouse disabled homolog, mdab1, in the scrambler mouse. *Neuron* 19, 239–249. doi: 10.1016/s0896-6273(00)80936-8

Wisco, D., Anderson, E. D., Chang, M. C., Norden, C., Boiko, T., Fölsch, H., et al. (2003). Uncovering multiple axonal targeting pathways in hippocampal neurons. *J. Cell Biol.* 162, 1317–1328. doi: 10.1083/jcb.200307069

Wu, Q., Liu, J., Fang, A., Li, R., Bai, Y., Kriegstein, A. R., et al. (2014). The dynamics of neuronal migration. *Adv. Exp. Med. Biol.* 800, 25–36. doi: 10.1007/978-94-007-7687-6_2

Xu, X. X., Yang, W., Jackowski, S., and Rock, C. O. (1995). Cloning of a novel phosphoprotein regulated by colony-stimulating factor 1 shares a domain with the *Drosophila* disabled gene product. *J. Biol. Chem.* 270, 14184–14191. doi: 10.1074/jbc.270.23.14184

Yang, D. H., Smith, E. R., Roland, I. H., Sheng, Z., He, J., Martin, W. D., et al. (2002). Disabled-2 is essential for endodermal cell positioning and structure formation during mouse embryogenesis. *Dev. Biol.* 251, 27–44. doi: 10.1006/dbio.2002.0810

Yap, C. C., Lasiecka, Z. M., Caplan, S., and Winckler, B. (2010). Alterations of EHD1/EHD4 protein levels interfere with L1/NgCAM endocytosis in neurons and disrupt axonal targeting. *J. Neurosci.* 30, 6646–6657. doi: 10.1523/JNEUROSCI.5428-09.2010

Yap, C. C., Vakulenko, M., Kruczek, K., Motamedi, B., Digilio, L., Liu, J. S., et al. (2012). Doublecortin (DCX) mediates endocytosis of neurofascin independently of microtubule binding. *J. Neurosci.* 32, 7439–7453. doi: 10.1523/JNEUROSCI.5318-11.2012

Yap, C. C., and Winckler, B. (2012). Harnessing the power of the endosome to regulate neural development. *Neuron* 74, 440–451. doi: 10.1016/j.neuron.2012.04.015

Yap, C. C., Wisco, D., Kujala, P., Lasiecka, Z. M., Cannon, J. T., Chang, M. C., et al. (2008). The somatodendritic endosomal regulator NEEP21 facilitates axonal targeting of L1/NgCAM. *J. Cell Biol.* 180, 827–842. doi: 10.1083/jcb.200707143

Yoneshima, H., Nagata, E., Matsumoto, M., Yamada, M., Nakajima, K., Miyata, T., et al. (1997). A novel neurological mutant mouse, yotari, which exhibits reeler-like phenotype but expresses CR-50 antigen/reelin. *Neurosci. Res.* 29, 217–223. doi: 10.1016/s0168-0102(97)00088-6

Zhong, W., Feder, J. N., Jiang, M. M., Jan, L. Y., and Jan, Y. N. (1996). Asymmetric localization of a mammalian numb homolog during mouse cortical neurogenesis. *Neuron* 17, 43–53. doi: 10.1016/S0896-6273(00)80279-2

Zhong, W., Jiang, M. M., Schonemann, M. D., Meneses, J. J., Pedersen, R. A., Jan, L. Y., et al. (2000). Mouse numb is an essential gene involved in cortical neurogenesis. *Proc. Natl. Acad. Sci. U S A* 97, 6844–6849. doi: 10.1073/pnas.97.12.6844

Zhong, W., Jiang, M. M., Weinmaster, G., Jan, L. Y., and Jan, Y. N. (1997). Differential expression of mammalian Numb, Numblike and Notch1 suggests distinct roles during mouse cortical neurogenesis. *Development* 124, 1887–1897.

Zhou, P., Alfaro, J., Chang, E. H., Zhao, X., Porcionatto, M., and Segal, R. A. (2011). Numb links extracellular cues to intracellular polarity machinery to promote chemotaxis. *Dev. Cell* 20, 610–622. doi: 10.1016/j.devcel.2011.04.006

Zhou, P., Porcionatto, M., Pilapil, M., Chen, Y., Choi, Y., Tolias, K. F., et al. (2007). Polarized signaling endosomes coordinate BDNF-induced chemotaxis of cerebellar precursors. *Neuron* 55, 53–68. doi: 10.1016/j.neuron.2007.05.030

Zilian, O., Saner, C., Hagedorn, L., Lee, H. Y., Säuberli, E., Suter, U., et al. (2001). Multiple roles of mouse Numb in tuning developmental cell fates. *Curr. Biol.* 11, 494–501. doi: 10.1016/s0960-9822(01)00149-x

11

Lost Highway(s): Barriers to Postnatal Cortical Neurogenesis and Implications for Brain Repair

Aslam Abbasi Akhtar [1,2] *and Joshua J. Breunig* [1,2,3]*

[1] *Board of Governors Regenerative Medicine Institute, Cedars-Sinai Medical Center, Los Angeles, CA, USA,* [2] *Department of Biomedical Sciences, Cedars-Sinai Medical Center, Los Angeles, CA, USA,* [3] *Samuel Oschin Comprehensive Cancer Institute, Cedars-Sinai Medical Center, Los Angeles, CA, USA*

***Correspondence:**
Joshua J. Breunig,
Board of Governors Regenerative Medicine Institute, Cedars-Sinai Medical Center, AHSP A8109, Los Angeles, CA 90048, USA
joshua.breunig@cshs.org

The genesis of the cerebral cortex is a highly complex and tightly-orchestrated process of cell division, migration, maturation, and integration. Developmental missteps often have catastrophic consequences on cortical function. Further, the cerebral cortex, in which neurogenesis takes place almost exclusively prenatally, has a very poor capacity for replacement of neurons lost to injury or disease. A multitude of factors underlie this deficit, including the depletion of radial glia, the gliogenic switch which mitigates continued neurogenesis, diminished neuronal migratory streams, and inflammatory processes associated with disease. Despite this, there are glimmers of hope that new approaches may allow for more significant cortical repair. Herein, we review corticogenesis from the context of regeneration and detail the strategies to promote neurogenesis, including interneuron transplants and glial reprogramming. Such strategies circumvent the "lost highways" which are critical for cortical development but are absent in the adult. These new approaches may provide for the possibility of meaningful clinical regeneration of elements of cortical circuitry lost to trauma and disease.

Keywords: reprogramming, transdifferentiation, regeneration, neurogenesis, brain repair, ventricular zone, gliogenesis

Introduction

Comprising 10–26 billion neurons and a similar number of glia (Azevedo et al., 2009; Herculano-Houzel, 2009), and possessing roughly a trillion synapses per cubic centimeter (Drachman, 2005), the mammalian cerebral cortex is one of the most complex structures known to man. Through tightly orchestrated interactions between these neurons and glia, along with communication to and from other brain regions, the cortex mediates higher-order cognition, coordinates motor function, visual perception, somatosensory perception, memory, and a host of other processes (Shipp, 2007). Because of this complexity, developmental disorders often lead to lifelong impairment or disability (Francis et al., 2006). Further, trauma or disease resulting in neurodegeneration in the cortex almost inevitably leads to impairment of psychosocial, cognitive, motor, visual or somatosensory function, depending on the age of the individual and site(s) of neuronal loss (Van Hoesen et al., 1991; Johansson, 2000; Rosema et al., 2015).

To compound this, the primate cortex has almost no proclivity for de novo neurogenesis after birth (Rakic, 1985, 2002a,c; Kornack and Rakic, 2001; Spalding et al., 2005; Bhardwaj et al., 2006). The evidence for and against postnatal neurogenesis in the cortex of primates and other mammals has been extensively reviewed elsewhere and less recent findings will not be discussed here

(Rakic, 2002b; Breunig et al., 2007, 2011; Feliciano and Bordey, 2013). Nevertheless, despite the contradictory data from model organisms, carbon-14 dating of human cortical neurons under normal and post stroke conditions indicates that these cells are born prenatally (Huttner et al., 2014), though adult neurogenesis was detected with similar methods in the human hippocampus where it had been previously observed (Eriksson et al., 1998; Spalding et al., 2013). Therefore, cortical neurogenesis is unlikely to significantly contribute to plasticity after cortical injury.

Taken together, directed regeneration of cortical circuitry, however difficult the prospect may be, is one of the few approaches available to potentially ameliorate functional deficits due to cortical neurodegeneration. Though, it is possible that functional recovery after neurodegeneration may turn out to be a matter of generating the appropriate cell numbers and types; developmental cortical disorders such as those seen in *Reeler* mutants—where neurons are generated normally but migrate inappropriately, resulting in mental retardation—suggests that a more meticulous reconstruction of circuitry, one that mimics the pattern of normal development may be necessary (Caviness and Rakic, 1978). Here we review cortical development in this context and describe emerging approaches to generate cortical neurons for cell therapy or *in situ* replacement.

Cortical Development

The majority of cortical neurons and glia arise from radial glia stem cells which reside along the ventricle (**Figure 1A**) and provide highway-like migratory substrates from the ventricle to the pial surface (Rakic, 1972; Noctor et al., 2001; Breunig et al., 2011). During neurogenesis, radial glia divide asymmetrically

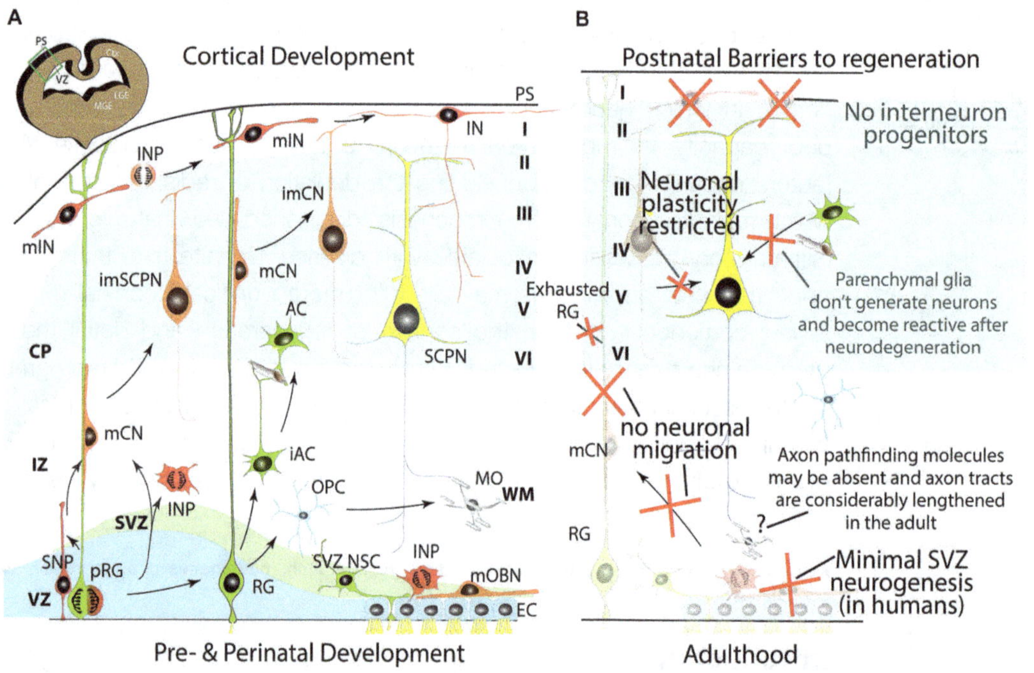

FIGURE 1 | Cortical development and barriers to regeneration. **(A)** Schematic representation of neocortical development from neurogenesis through postnatal stages. Approximate location denoted by green box in coronal brain. Proliferative radial glia (pRG) asymmetrically divide to generate intermediate progenitors (INPs) and short neural precursors (SNPs) which proliferate and contribute to the migratory cortical neuron (mCN) population. This population migrates along radial glia and into the cortical plate (CP), where they exit the RG fiber and begin the maturation process. As neurogenesis procedes, progressively more superficial layers are generated (i.e., Layer VI, then Layer V, etc.) Depicted here is the generation of Layer V subcortical projection neurons (SCPN) and the later generation of an upper layer immature callosal neuron (imCN). (Other layers are not depicted for the sake of space and clarity). In parallel, migrating interneurons (mINs) from the ventral telencephalon invade and can proliferate locally prior to maturation into functional interneurons (INs). After neurogenesis ceases, gliogenesis commences en force with the conversion of some RG into immature and subsequently mature astrocytes (iACs and ACs, respectively). Also, oligodendrocyte progenitor cells (OPCs) are born and differentiate into myelinating oligodendrocytes (MOs) in the white matter (WM). Other RG transition into subventricular zone neural stem cells (NSCs), and ependymal cells (ECs). NSCs can give rise to INPs, which generate migrating olfactory bulb-destined neurons (mOBNs). **(B)** In the postnatal and adult brain, significant barriers to regeneration are present. Radial glia are exhausted and become a "lost highway" to any neuronal migration. Similarly, cortical neurons are no longer generated and thus virtually no neurons can be found migrating into the cortex. Neuronal plasticity becomes significantly attenuated, preventing the type of plasticity observed prior to developmental critical periods. Interneuron progenitors and mINs disappear. Parenchymal glia do not cross lineage boundaries and become reactive after injury and degeneration. Moreover, the axon lengths become many fold longer in the adult due to the growth of the organism. For example, a SCPN may reach almost a meter in length while the initial axon started at a few millimeters before progressive lengthening. Finally, in humans there is minimal subventricular zone (SVZ) neurogenesis in the adult, inhibiting strategies which might utilize such cells. Abbreviations: PS, pial surface; IZ, intermediate zone; MGE, medial ganglionic eminence; LGE, lateral ganglionic eminence; Ctx, cortex.

to generate developing neurons which migrate along these scaffolds and exit off into their respective cortical layers (**Figure 1A**; Noctor et al., 2001; Rakic, 2009). The cortex is distinctly organized into six horizontal layers which are generated embryonically in an inside-out fashion (Rakic, 2009). As development progresses, generation of lower layers tapers off into genesis of progressively more superficial layers due to an underlying transcriptional program (Kwan et al., 2012). As neurogenesis completes, the "gliogenic switch" shifts the fate of radial glial stem cells towards the genesis of astrocytes and oligodendrocyte progenitor cells (**Figure 1A**; Rowitch and Kriegstein, 2010). Hence, the majority of cortical neurogenesis occurs prior to birth, while gliogenesis is a perinatal and postnatal phenomenon (Bhardwaj et al., 2006; Yeung et al., 2014).

The majority of neurons in the cortex are glutamatergic while the remaining (roughly 20%) of neurons are GABAergic interneurons (Chu and Anderson, 2015). These interneurons are generated in the subcortical areas of the ventral telencephalon in the rostral forebrain, specifically in the medial ganglionic eminence (MGE) and caudal ganglionic eminence (Anderson et al., 2002; Nery et al., 2002; Wonders and Anderson, 2006; Southwell et al., 2014). Immature interneurons migrate to the developing and neonatal cortex, attain their mature fate (**Figure 1A**), and integrate their circuitry wherein they function to modulate neuronal activity through inhibitory neurotransmission (Nery et al., 2002; Wonders and Anderson, 2006; Hansen et al., 2013). In humans, evidence exists for the local generation of interneurons in the cortical ventricular and subventricular zone (VZ and SVZ), respectively during embryogenesis, but this remains contentious (Letinic et al., 2002; Hansen et al., 2013; Radonjić et al., 2014). Moreover, there is evidence that interneuron progenitors can proliferate extensively during their migration, including in the cortex and, in addition, the tail end of this migrating progenitor population can be observed postnatally (Costa et al., 2007; Inta et al., 2008; Breunig et al., 2012; Levy et al., 2014).

Due to the intricate spatial and temporal cues that orchestrate cortical development, the task of regenerating the cortex in adulthood possesses many challenges (**Figure 1B**). Physically speaking, projection neurons in the cortex reach their respective targets early in development (e.g., the spinal cord for Layer V neurons and the thalamus for Layer VI neurons). After axonal targeting is achieved in embryogenesis, these processes progressively lengthen with age from a distance of millimeters and centimeters to almost a meter for an adult corticospinal projection neuron. Furthermore, the cortical radial glia population is exhausted in early postnatal life leaving no scaffold for migration to respective cortical layers (Tramontin et al., 2003). The absence of a path to cortical layers from the ventricular zone represents a significant "lost highway" that may impede regeneration (**Figure 1B**). Further, neurons are postmitotic cells that do not divide once they have reached their final position in the cortex. And though precursors do exist around the lateral ventricles in the human, akin to development, they largely lose their neurogenic ability *in vivo* (**Figure 1B**; Sanai et al., 2011; discussed in detail below).

Postnatal Forebrain Cell Genesis

The neurogenic niches of the adult brain have received a great deal of attention over the past fifteen years due to their ability to contribute to brain plasticity and serve as a model and perhaps substrate for regeneration. The two neurogenic niches in the adult mammalian brain are the subventricular zone (SVZ) of the lateral ventricles and the subgranular zone (SGZ) of the hippocampus (Song et al., 2002; Alvarez-Buylla and Lim, 2004; Ming and Song, 2011). The SVZ neural stem cells are derived from embryonic and perinatal radial glia (Merkle et al., 2004). As these radial glia transition into neural stem cells of the astrocyte lineage, they lose the long basal process that they possess (and therefore the migratory substrate for neurons to migrate into the parenchyma—the eponymous "lost highway"). These Gfap$^+$ neural precursors also serve to populate the cortex and striatum with astrocytes (Ge et al., 2012) and oligodendrocytes (Menn et al., 2006), as well as seed the olfactory bulb (OB) with neurons (Alvarez-Buylla and Lim, 2004; Ming and Song, 2011). Specifically, SVZ precursors generate transit amplifying cells which proliferate and generate neuroblasts (Doetsch et al., 1999). These neuroblasts migrate in a clustered, tangential fashion to the OB through the rostral migratory stream (RMS), a structure of ensheathing glial fibers and migrating neurons between the lateral ventricle and OB core (Lois et al., 1996). Upon reaching the OB core, the immature neurons migrate radially towards the OB periphery, establish synapses, and mature into OB interneurons (Carleton et al., 2003; Ming and Song, 2011). Importantly, OB neurogenesis does not appear to be lifelong in humans and instead may be supplanted by striatal interneuron genesis, which does not appear to occur in other non-human primates and rodents (Ernst et al., 2014). Unlike neural precursors, the glial subtypes generated by SVZ radial glia extensively divide perinatally throughout the forebrain (Ge et al., 2012; Yeung et al., 2014). Astrocyte turnover attenuates perinatally in rodents, but polydendrocytes of the oligodendrocyte lineage are believed to be the most proliferative cell type in the adult brain (Burns et al., 2009; Geha et al., 2010).

In the postnatal hippocampal SGZ, radial glia-like neural stem cells give rise to intermediate progenitors (INPs) which in turn generate neuroblasts (Seri et al., 2004). These neuroblasts migrate to the inner granule cell layer and differentiate into granule cells which project to the CA3 region of the hippocampus (Ming and Song, 2011). Several studies in mice have associated changes in hippocampal neurogenesis to learning and memory (Deng et al., 2009, 2010; Mu and Gage, 2011) though a new genetically modified rat allowing for ablation of adult neurogenesis failed to find a similar correlation (Groves et al., 2013). Importantly, evidence of human hippocampal neurogenesis is observed late into life (Eriksson et al., 1998; Spalding et al., 2013). Taken together, the adult brain does have active sites of neurogenesis, but postnatal cortical neurogenesis has seemingly been selected against by evolution. Nevertheless, these neurogenic zones have provided insight into the mechanisms of postnatal neurogenesis and have also served as experimental testing platforms for various genetic experiments which aim at using stem cells for postnatal cortical neurogenesis. In particular, the postnatal cortical SVZ is of increased interest due to its proximity to the cortex. Furthermore, in addition to techniques such as viral-mediated transgenesis, which can manipulate progenitors in the SVZ and SGZ (Braun et al., 2013; Zuccotti et al., 2014); novel techniques such as electroporation allow rapid transgenic manipulation of SVZ progenitors pre- and postnatally, without the need of virus generation (Breunig et al., 2007).

Learning from Development

In light of the radial glia-to-cortical neuron development paradigm which exists embryonically, neuroscientists have strived to achieve adult cortical neurogenesis from several angles, namely: (1) the redevelopment of radial glia to serve as substrates for differentiation to cortical neurons or as scaffolds for nascent neurons generated through other means; (2) the transplantation of neural stem and progenitor cells to the cortex; and (3) the analysis of developmental genetic factors which direct stem and progenitor cells to become cortical neurons, and as such, the effect of their misexpression in astrocytes and neurons. Below we detail examples of the work neuroscientists have achieved which show glimpses of postnatal neurogenesis in a region of the brain that was initially thought to be cemented during early development. Due to the numerous reviews present in this field, we will focus on recent findings in respect to cortical regeneration and direct the reader towards other reviews for an in-depth analysis of postnatal neurogenesis (Breunig et al., 2007; Urbán and Guillemot, 2014).

Promoting Radial Glia Reemergence and Alternate Migratory Substrates

Radial glia are necessary for the development of the cortex as they divide asymmetrically to generate immature neurons and are scaffolds for migrating neurons as they travel to their respective layers (Rakic, 2003; Breunig et al., 2011). Efforts have been made to generate radial glia in adulthood to serve as: (1) a source of progenitors for replacing cortical neurons; and (2) scaffolds for migration of neurons into the cortex. In this regard, expression of the tyrosine kinase receptor, ErbB2, in cortical quiescent mature astrocytes for 3 weeks enabled a subset of these astrocytes to assume a radial glia-like phenotype (Ghashghaei et al., 2007). In addition to possessing elongated processes, these "induced radial glia" had increased expression of the Notch 1 ligand which has been shown to be essential for the maintenance of radial glia identity. Other transcription factors required for radial glial maintenance, Sox2, Pax6, and Hes5 (the downstream targets of Notch1) were also upregulated in the induced cells. Interestingly, only astrocytes surrounding the ventricles, but not those in the cortical parenchyma, were able to re-assume their radial glia identity, suggesting that not all astrocytes in the cortex are the same. Induced radial glia were able to give rise to new neurons *in vitro* and *in vivo*, and also supported the migration of transplanted embryonic-day 16 cortical neurons. Similar work was done by Gregg and Weiss (2003) where epidermal growth factor (EGF) expression in cultures of forebrain neural stem cells resulted in an adoption of radial glia morphology, expression of Nestin and RC2, and supported the migration of immature neurons. Infusion of EGF into the adult forebrain lateral ventricle also led to the generation of radial glia-like cells within the adult forebrain ependyma (Gregg and Weiss, 2003). In addition, the endocytic adaptor proteins Numb and Numbl have been identified as regulators of radial glia adhesion and polarity (Rasin et al., 2007). Though originally identified in Drosophila neural progenitors for its role in promoting neuronal cell fate by inhibiting notch signaling, when Numb and Numbl were inactivated in mouse radial glia, adheren junctions and polarity were disrupted through disrupted cadherin trafficking, resulting in progenitor cell dispersion and disordered cortical lamination (Rasin et al., 2007). In contrast, when Numb or cadherin was overexpressed, radial glia were maintained postnatally beyond the standard neurogenic period in the cortex (Rasin et al., 2007).

Investigation into the migrational modalities used by OB neurons may also provide insight regarding different migratory substrates that may potentially be utilized for induced cortical neurogenesis. As previously mentioned, OB neurons are one of the few neuronal populations continuously generated in the adult rodent. These nascent neurons migrate radially from the OB core to the OB periphery. However, the OB does not contain radial glia-like projections or an RMS-like glial sheath to serve as scaffolds for these migrating neurons. Upon investigating the mode of travel of these neurons, it was found that these nascent interneurons use the OB vasculature as a scaffold for migration (Bovetti et al., 2007; Tanaka et al., 2011). This new modality, termed *vasophilic migration* is facilitated through an interaction between the extracellular matrix and perivascular astrocyte end feet (Bovetti et al., 2007). Therefore, it is possible that vasculature in the cortex may serve as a modality for migration of nascent neuronal populations to their respective cortical layers. Indeed, there is evidence that upon focal microlesions, SVZ cells can generate neurons in the cortex (Magavi et al., 2000; Brill et al., 2009) but more recent work failed to find new neurons after employing two different genetic lesion paradigms (Diaz et al., 2013).

Employing Developmental Lessons to Facilitate Transplantation

The creation of induced pluripotent stem cells (iPSCs), which led to Shinya Yamanaka receiving the 2012 Nobel Prize, energized the field of regenerative medicine in several ways. First, the finding that pluripotency can be induced in postmitotic cell types opens the door to myriad possibilities in terms of reprogramming and directed differentiation. Secondly, iPSCs now provide a virtually unlimited source of patient-matched cells for transplantation. Over the last two decades, numerous groups have generated various cortical neuronal subtypes from embryonic and induced pluripotent stem cells *in vitro* (Gaspard et al., 2008; Hansen et al., 2011; Shi et al., 2012; Espuny-Camacho et al., 2013; Michelsen et al., 2015). In parallel with these findings, investigators have also demonstrated that a three-dimensional culture of pluripotent stem cells can "self-organize" into a complex tissue with striking similarities to the cerebral cortex, suggesting that neural stem cells may possess the inherent cues needed for cortical formation (Lancaster et al., 2013). This raises the prospect of transplanted stem cells to replace damaged or diseased neurons in the adult cortex. This possibility would exist *if* the adult cortex maintained the intrinsic *spatial* cues of development in order to direct the differentiation of *temporally* relevant stem cells. In this regard, (Ideguchi et al., 2010) derived mouse embryonic stem (ES) cells from the E4.5 blastocyst and differentiated them for 7 days before transplanting into various regions of the cortex. The cells exhibited region specific projections, with cells transplanted to the motor or visual cortex projecting to their respective targets. In a similar experiment, (Gaspard et al., 2008) transplanted cells were differentiated for 12–17 days (instead of 7) and did not present the region specific projections as all cells projected to visual cortex targets, despite being transplanted to the frontal cortex. This suggests that a variation of 5–10 days of *in vitro* differentiation plays a role in the success of graft integration and specificity, and highlights the need for *temporal* specificity of the transplanted cells. Furthermore, recent work further illustrates the need for matching the areal identity of transplanted neurons (Michelsen et al., 2015). In this study, visual cortex neurons were differentiated from mouse ES cells *in vitro* for 14 days and transplanted into the adult visual cortex after a focal neurotoxic lesion. The transplanted cells integrated into their respective pathways and electrophysiological recordings revealed the cells were responsive to visual stimuli. Similar to previous studies, significant integration and engraftment were not observed when ES cell-derived visual cortex neurons were transplanted into the motor cortex, or when motor cortex neurons were transplanted into the visual cortex, indicating the need for *areal* specificity. Importantly, recent work suggests that *in vitro* differentiation of ES-derived neural progenitors towards cortical fates fails to properly recapitulate *in vivo* development in many aspects, including aberrant progenitor specification and stalled differentiation (Sadegh and Macklis, 2014). It should be noted that this report (Sadegh and Macklis, 2014) used mouse ES cells cultured in a monolayer and allowed to mature in a manner previously used for cortical differentiation. Taken together, these findings suggest that neuronal replacement using pluripotent stem cells combined with specific differentiation protocols holds promise. However, they also suggest that it will be important to spatiotemporally match donor cells for transplantation and this will require a requisite understanding of the mechanisms of areal identity in order to specify the appropriate populations from pluripotent cells. In this regard, much work remains to be done to understand how to appropriately derive specific cortical cells and tissues from pluripotent cell types despite an increasing understanding of how this process occurs during development (Rakic et al., 2009; Kwan et al., 2012; Greig et al., 2013). Clinically, the long-term safety issues of iPSC-based cell therapy will need more thorough evaluation in light of recent findings of oncogenic transformation of iPSC-derived NSCs when transplanted into the spinal cord (Nori et al., 2015). However, the iPSCs from this study were generated using lentivirus (Nori et al., 2015) and it remains to be seen if similar problems will emerge from non-integrating iPSC generation methods where continued transgene mis-expression is unlikely. In the interim, the use of iPSCs for generating neurons for disease modeling and drug screening will likely be of great importance.

Interneuron Transplantation

As previously mentioned, unlike other neuronal subtypes in the cortex which are generated locally from radial glia, interneurons are generated from the ganglionic eminences of the ventral telencephalon and migrate to the cortex (among other regions of the brain) where they mature and integrate into their respective networks (Noctor et al., 2004; Southwell et al., 2014). While projection neurons of the cortex target various intra- and extra-cortical regions, cortical interneurons project onto other neurons in the cortex and inhibit neurotransmission within this region. This balance of inhibitory/excitatory signals is critical for the proper function of the cortex. Conditions such as epilepsy and schizophrenia are thought to be related at least in part to dysfunctional interneurons, giving them the title of "interneuronopathies" (Kato and Dobyns, 2005; Southwell et al., 2014).

As cortical interneurons exhibit a developmental paradigm which involves long distance migration from extra-cortical regions followed by maturation and integration in the cortex, the use of interneuron progenitors in transplant therapy for interneuron replacement may be more feasible compared to transplant efforts aimed at replacing cortical projection neurons. For a detailed review of interneuron transplants, we direct the reader to Alvarez Dolado and Broccoli (2011) and Southwell et al. (2014). Indeed, interneurons do not require radial glia-like scaffolds to migrate from the ganglionic eminences to the cortex, and the neuronal subtypes they project on are not as distant as the respective targets of projection neurons. To this, several groups have achieved promising results transplanting interneurons generated from the embryonic MGE, ES cells, and iPSCs (Tanaka et al., 2011; Maroof et al., 2013; Nicholas et al., 2013; Southwell et al., 2014). Transplanted interneurons migrate from the graft site throughout the cortex and successfully integrate into the young and adult rodent cortex (Maroof et al., 2013; Nicholas et al., 2013). Unlike the transplantation of other cell types which has resulted in decreased transplant survival or a decrease in the native population, which may be detrimental, transplanted interneurons increase the overall pool of cortical interneurons (Southwell et al., 2010). Notably, the cortex has a limit of how many interneurons it can support, which is reported to be roughly 10% more than the native population (Southwell et al., 2010, 2014). Transplanted interneurons display spontaneous and induced synaptic currents and further, transplantation has been shown to increase inhibitory signals in glutamatergic neurons (Southwell et al., 2010; Bráz et al., 2012). Additionally, several groups have reported functional benefits from cortical interneuron transplants in mouse models of epilepsy and schizophrenia (Baraban et al., 2009; Tanaka et al., 2011). Specifically, (Baraban et al., 2009) transplanted precursor cells from the embryonic E13.5 MGE into the postnatal day 2 mouse brain and reported their maturation into GABAergic interneurons when analyzed 30 days after transplantation.

The transplanted cells integrated and dispersed throughout the cortex as indicated by immunohistochemistry, electron microscopy, electrophysiology, and increased GABA-mediated synaptic inhibition on pyramidal neurons. Bilateral grafts of the embryonic MGE cells into experimental epileptic mice reduced the duration and frequency of spontaneous electrographic seizures. (Tanaka et al., 2011) transplanted MGE cells of the same embryonic age (E13.5) into the medial prefrontal cortex and observed similar functional integration as well prevention of phencyclidine-induced cognitive defects.

While diseases that independently affect cortical projection neurons may not directly benefit from the increased inhibition provided by transplanted interneurons, these migratory neurons may be used as a vehicle for delivery of trophic factors. Traditionally, astrocytes have been used in this regard as they have been viewed as a resilient supportive cell type for neurons. Among the characteristics that have made astrocytes more appealing are their ability to divide after transplantation, migrate to sites of injury, ensheathe neurons, and their ease of generation *in vitro* (Svendsen et al., 1997; Behrstock et al., 2006, 2008; Suzuki et al., 2007). However, recent reports of successful interneuron generation from iPSCs, engraftment after transplantation, and transgenic manipulation may suggest interneurons as tools for factor delivery to areas of the cortex (Southwell et al., 2014).

Genetic Engineering and Reprogramming

Over the last decade, "direct reprogramming" or "transdifferentiation" has allowed for terminally differentiated cells to directly assume fate of another differentiated cell type without having to go through a state of pluripotency. Direct reprogramming of neurons from a host of different terminally differentiated cells such as fibroblasts, pericytes, hepatocytes, and other neural cells has been described (Heinrich et al., 2010, 2014; Vierbuchen et al., 2010; Marro et al., 2011; Karow et al., 2012). Much of the discovery and success of these direct reprogramming experiments have come to fruition due to our increasing knowledge of the molecular control of neurogenesis and the advances in transcriptomics over the last decade. For example, neurogenesis follows a general pattern (**Figure 2A**) whereby a neuronal progenitor is generated by Notch-mediated asymmetric cell division of a neural stem cell (Ables et al., 2011). Among the resulting pair of cells after mitosis, the Notch^{High} cell will remain a stem cell and the Notch^{Low} cell will subsequently upregulate proneural genes such as *Neurog1* and *Neurog2* (or *Ascl1* in other regions) and become an intermediate progenitor (**Figure 2A**; Bertrand et al., 2002; Ables et al., 2011). This progenitor will continue to terminally differentiatiate under the regulation of basic helix-loop-helix transcription factors such as NeuroD1 (**Figure 2A**) until later maturation (Guillemot,

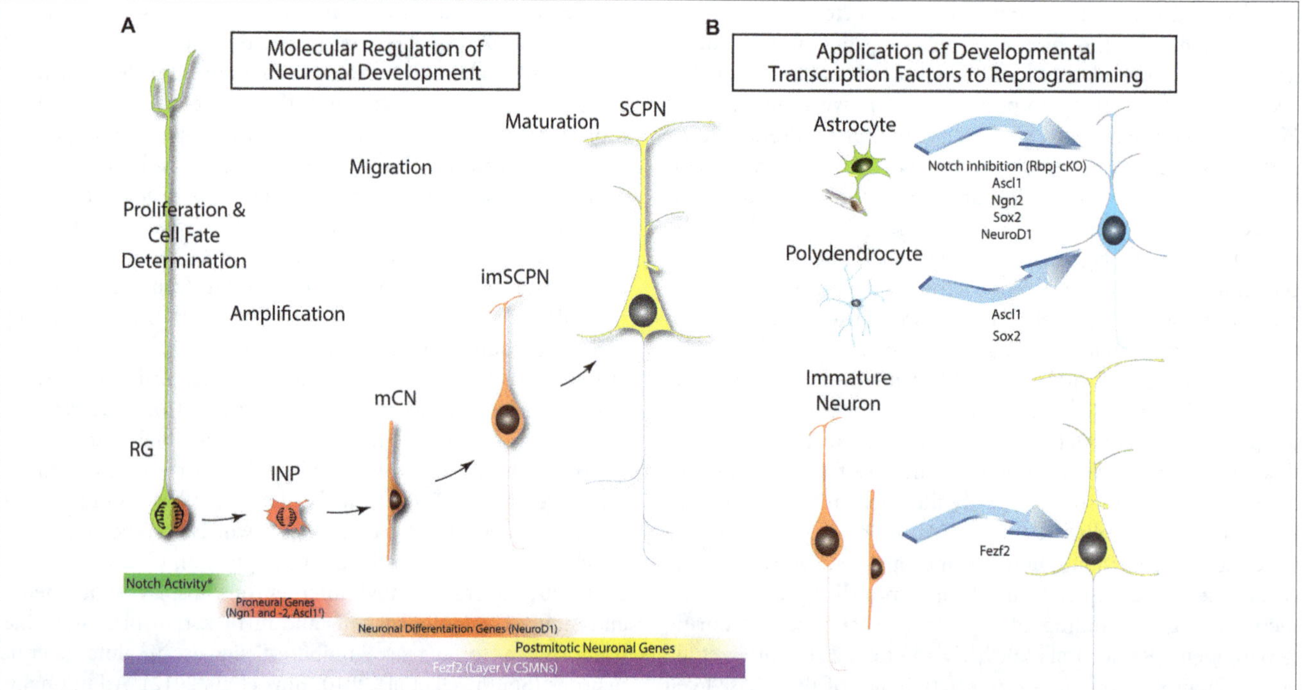

FIGURE 2 | Molecular control of neurogenesis and its use in reprogramming. (A) Radial glia utilize Notch signaling to self-renew during mitosis. (*-during asymmetric division the cell inheriting the basal process exhibits high Notch activity while the other daughter displays diminished Notch activity). Neuronal daughter cells upregulate proneural genes such as Ngn1 and Ngn2 in the cortex. (†-Ascl1 is the predominant proneural gene in the ventral telencephalon among other regions). Basic helix-loop-helix (bhlh) transcription factors such as NeuroD1 regulate the terminal differentiation of migrating neurons into mature projection neurons. Fezf2 cooperates with all of these factors in the specification of subcortical projection neurons (SCPNs), leading to the eventual expression of a diverse array of transcription factors involved in the postmitotic identity of this neuronal subtype. **(B)** Transgenic misexpression strategies for reprogramming of disparate cell types to neurons.

2007). Finally, any number of transcription factors involved in neuronal subtype specification will be expressed to control neuronal identity (Kwan et al., 2012). Transcriptomics has led to the discovery of several "master regulators" which specify particular neuronal subtypes (Kwan et al., 2012; Greig et al., 2013) such as Fezf2 (discussed in detail below). As mature cortical projection neurons cannot be transplanted, the ability to directly differentiate or reprogram other cell types into precise neuronal subtypes with the end goal of replacing neurons lost due to damage or neurodegenerative disease would be invaluable. Below we discuss the burgeoning field devoted to directed differentiation of neurons.

Glia to Neuron Reprogramming

The reasoning behind using cortical glia as substrates for reprogramming to neurons stems from several characteristics of glial cells. Glial cells are plentiful in the cortex (Azevedo et al., 2009) and are actively generated throughout life (Colodner et al., 2005; Geha et al., 2010; Yeung et al., 2014). Therefore, a lack of substrate cells is not an issue. Furthermore, in response to injury and disease, glial cells become reactive and increasingly proliferative, allowing for an increased number of cells to reprogram at the injury site.

One of the first studies that investigated the ability of single transcription factors to induce directed differentiation of cortical astroglia to specific neuronal subtypes was done by isolating cortical glia from postnatal day 5–7 mice followed by retrovirus-induced expression of *Neurog2* or *Dlx2* (Heinrich et al., 2010). As mentioned above, *Neurog2* is a proneural gene that regulates the early differentiation of glutamatergic neurons (Hevner et al., 2006; Heng et al., 2008; Zhang et al., 2013). In contrast, the *Dlx2* homeobox protein is normally expressed in progenitor cells derived from the ventral telencephalon and has been shown to promote the generation of GABAergic interneurons (Petryniak et al., 2007; de Chevigny et al., 2012). Expression of *Neurog2* in astroglial cultures led to the generation of glutamatergic-like neurons which expressed Tbr1 and Tbr2, the T-box transcription factors expressed by glutamatergic neurons in the forebrain. The *Neurog2*-induced neurons also generated synapses, expressed vGluT1 around their soma and MAP2^{+} processes, and acquired projection neuron-like morphology. In contrast, the *Dlx2*-induced neurons expressed markers of GABAergic interneuron lineage GAD67 and vGAT, and generated functional synapses. Interestingly, the *Dlx2*-mediated reprogramming was not as efficient as *Neurog2*-induced reprogramming.

The majority of glia to neuron conversion studies in the brain have been reported in regions other than the cortex. Several groups have reported successful conversion of glia to neurons in the striatum by the expression (or knockout) of various factors (Niu et al., 2013; Torper et al., 2013; Magnusson et al., 2014). The expression of *Brn2a*, *Ascl1*, and *Mytl1* (also known as BAM factors) was previously shown to convert fibroblasts and hepatocytes to neurons *in vitro* (Vierbuchen et al., 2010; Marro et al., 2011). Expression of the BAM-factors mediated by a Cre-inducible lentiviral injection into the striatum of GFAP-Cre heterozygous mice converted striatal glia to neurons. These induced neurons expressed NeuN and had neuronal morphology; however the functionality of the induced neurons was not assessed (Torper et al., 2013).

Notch signaling is involved in various stages of cortical neurogenesis and generally functions to inhibit neuronal differentiation (Ables et al., 2011). A recent study has shown that an experimental model of middle cerebral artery occlusion-induced stroke results in transient neurogenesis in striatal astrocytes (Magnusson et al., 2014). Notch1 signaling was reduced in striatal astrocytes after stroke while ectopic activation in astrocytes inhibited stroke-induced neuroblast production. Furthermore, blocking notch signaling in the absence of stroke promoted astrocytes in the striatum and medial cortex to enter a neurogenic program and express markers of immature and mature neurons, such as Ascl1, Dcx, and NeuN (Magnusson et al., 2014). Taken together, this suggests that Notch signaling actively suppresses the neurogenic potential of parenchymal astrocytes in the striatum (**Figure 2B**). Lastly, several studies have shown that single factors can convert glia to neurons after injury (Guo et al., 2014; Heinrich et al., 2014). These are discussed below.

Cortical Neurogenesis after Inflammation and Injury

Over the last decade, plentiful information has been discovered about the relationship between inflammation and neurodegenerative disease. Previous dogma understood neuroinflammation to always have a negative role in disease progression. However, recent studies have shown that certain aspects of the immune system are beneficial to the host in neurodegenerative conditions such as amyotrophic lateral sclerosis (ALS), Alzheimer's disease and multiple sclerosis (McCombe and Henderson, 2011; Weitz and Town, 2012; Breunig et al., 2013; Guillot-Sestier and Town, 2013; Hussain et al., 2014). In respect to cortical neurogenesis, neuroinflammation is a double-edged sword. Numerous groups have reported that inflammation promotes cortical neurogenesis and conversion of various cell types to neurons in the cortex (Guo et al., 2014; Heinrich et al., 2014; Magnusson et al., 2014). As mentioned above, several groups reported that laser-induced injury and apoptosis in deep layers of the cortex can stimulate precursors *in situ* to increase division and differentiation into glutamatergic neurons (Magavi et al., 2000; Brill et al., 2009). However, a follow up study which used a neuronal promoter-driven caspase as well as a neuronal promoter-driven diphtheria toxin method of induced apoptosis reported increased proliferation of microglia, but did not promote generation of glutamatergic neurons (Diaz et al., 2013). In respect to transgene-induced conversion, the retrovirus-mediated misexpression of *Sox2* in the adult mouse cortex following stab wound injury induced the conversion of NG2 cells to interneuron-like cells (**Figure 2B**), whereas misexpression under normal (non-stab wound) conditions did not result in conversion (Heinrich et al., 2014). The resulting induced neurons exhibited voltage-and time-dependent conductance and received synaptic connections from endogenous GABAergic neurons. This study used NG2 glia cells as a substrate, a cell type that is abundant and proliferating in the adult brain

(Dimou and Gotz, 2014). Other studies have shown that NG2 cells are recruited to the site of injury and may be equally or more permissive to conversion than astrocytes, suggesting that future reprogramming efforts should not look over this cell type (Buffo et al., 2005, 2008; Hughes et al., 2013). Interestingly, (Buffo et al., 2005) reported that stab wound injury increased expression of *Olig2* by immunohistochemistry and mRNA expression, and 26% of these *Olig2*$^+$ cells were NG2 cells. Furthermore, increased *Olig2* expression after stab wound was accompanied by decreased *Pax6* expression. This *Pax6-Olig2* relationship is also seen in the developing spinal cord and subependymal zone (Mizuguchi et al., 2001; Hack et al., 2005). Inhibition of *Olig2* by retrovirus encoding a dominant-negative form of *Olig2* two days after stab wound resulted in increased *Pax6* expression and increased neurogenesis as evidenced by the generation of Dcx$^+$ neuroblasts. The retroviral-mediated overexpression of *Pax6* two days after stab wound injury also resulted in similar increases in *Pax6* expression and neurogenesis.

It was also reported that retroviral expression of *NeuroD1* in the cortex of adult stab wound-injured mice resulted in conversion of: (1) astrocytes to glutamatergic neurons; and (2) NG2 cells to GABAergic and glutamatergic neurons (**Figure 2B**; Guo et al., 2014). Electrophysiology performed on slice cultures revealed that the *NeuroD1*-converted neurons exhibited spontaneous and evoked synaptic responses. Similar results were seen in the cortex of Alzheimer's disease mice, but not in control (un-injured or non-diseased) mice (Guo et al., 2014). Similar work was done *in vitro* where adult cortical astrocytes where isolated after stab wound injury and converted to glutamatergic neurons by *Neurog2* or GABAergic interneurons by *Dlx2* as previously discussed (Heinrich et al., 2010). Taken together, these reports suggest the importance of the neuroinflammatory response for conversion to neuronal subtypes in the adult mouse cortex under certain conditions.

Of increased interest in the Heinrich et al. (2014) and Guo et al. (2014) reports, is the idea that transcription factors can exhibit opposing roles depending on the context. Developmentally, *Sox2* promotes self-renewal in neural stem cells and prevents their differentiation into neurons (Graham et al., 2003). However, when *Sox2* is expressed in NG2 cells after injury, it promotes their reprogramming to interneuron-like cells as described above Heinrich et al. (2014). A similar study in the adult mouse striatum reported the conversion of astrocytes to other neuronal subtypes upon induction of *Sox2* (Niu et al., 2013). The mechanism of these differential responses remains to be determined. It may reflect different expression levels of the transgene, the epigenetic state of the transduced cells, or extrinsic cues associated with the neuroinflammatory state of the substrate cells and their microenvironment. Going forward, an integrated analysis of genome-wide binding sites, interacting proteins (e.g., other transcription factors and co-factors), chromatin configuration, and other epigenetic marks in these varied spatiotemporal contexts will likely illuminate the disparate responses to transcription factor misexpression (Amador-Arjona et al., 2015).

Interestingly, the majority of *in vivo* glia-to-neuron conversion studies have been carried out in an inflamed neocortex. Importantly, the activation of the immune system in response to injury or disease usually results in perpetuated and chronic neuroinflammation, which eventually leads to neurotoxicity. The glial scar is an example of this as the resulting activated astrocytes after injury are initially beneficial but eventually form a chronic scar which serves as a barrier to neuronal regeneration (Sofroniew, 2009; Cregg et al., 2014). In respect to the examples discussed above regarding expression of *Sox2* or *NeuroD1* in NG2 cells (Guo et al., 2014; Heinrich et al., 2014), future studies will need to determine what exactly is different in the NG2 cells or their environment after injury that allows for their reprogramming. Is it only that they are cycling more rapidly? Is the inflammatory microenvironment transiently more permissive to reprogramming in the cortex? And if so, can these features be mimicked in the un-inflamed cortex for a more translatable approach to replacing cortical neurons? Indeed there is some indication that activation of innate immunity is necessary for reprogramming. Specifically, it was noted that TLR3 pathway activation induced notable epigenetic changes leading to chromatin alterations which enhanced the pluripotent stem cell conversion of fibroblasts by four reprogramming factors (Li et al., 2009, c-Myc; Lee et al., 2012). When TLR3 (or its adaptor protein TRIF) was knocked down, reprogramming efficiencies decreased. Interestingly, the authors noted that conventional retroviral methods of transgene expression activate the TLR3 pathway, and non-viral methods of transgene expression complemented with ectopic TLR3 activation increased reprogramming efficiencies. Specifically, a change in the methylation status of the *Oct4* and *Sox2* promoters was observed. These authors claim that there is an optimal window of immune activation necessary for reprogramming (Cooke et al., 2014). They term this the "Goldilocks zone." A greater understanding of such a phenomenon in the context of neuronal reprogramming might yield more powerful control over the process. In this regard, it is also possible that the neuroinflammatory state present in the successful neuronal reprogramming experiments discussed above involve an activated TLR3 pathway resulting in an open, "pro-reprogramming" chromatin configuration.

Other Cell Types

Reprograming strategies in cell types other than neurons and glia may also show promise for cortical neurogenesis. (Brill et al., 2009) isolated human pericytes from the adult cerebral cortex and converted them to neurons by the misexpression of *Ascl1* and *Sox2*. Pericytes are involved in regulation of blood flow in the brain and the establishment and maintenance of the blood brain barrier (Armulik et al., 2011). Interestingly, they have also been reported to be multipotent mesenchymal stem cell-like and can give rise to cartilage, muscle, and bone lineages (Armulik et al., 2011). Since these cells are dispersed throughout the cortex and are more abundant than neural stem cells, they may be an attractive substrate for *in vivo* reprogramming to cortical neurons.

Neuron to Neuron Reprogramming

While the above studies provide important insight into the phenomenon of neuronal reprogramming, they all employ transcription factors broadly expressed in diverse types of neurons (**Table 1**). And while it is clear that neurons are generated, detailed characterization awaits. Given these facts, the precise nature of the resulting reprogrammed populations are hard to predict and may be extremely heterogeneous. For example, this approach might yield the types of populations seen after differentiation of pluripotent cell types, namely many neurons exhibiting "stalled" phenotypes and aberrant expression of phenotypic markers (Sadegh and Macklis, 2014). Going forward, it may be necessary to employ additional specific factors to direct the differentiation of precise subtypes. One such example of a protein which may be utilized is the transcription factor Fezf2. During embryogenesis, *Fezf2* is necessary for the specification of corticospinal motor neurons and *Fezf2*$^{-/-}$ mice lack corticospinal motor neurons (Chen et al., 2005a,b; Molyneaux et al., 2005). Embryonically, forced expression of *Fezf2* is sufficient to reprogram progenitors destined to generate upper layer neurons or striatal neurons to corticospinal motor neurons (Chen et al., 2005b; Molyneaux et al., 2005; Rouaux and Arlotta, 2010). Elegant work by Rouaux and Arlotta (2013) has shown that early postnatal overexpression of *Fezf2* in postmitotic Layer 2/3 callosal projection neurons which typically project interhemispherically via the corpus callosum, results in reprogramming to Layer 5-like corticofugal neurons (**Figure 2B**). The newly generated neurons acquired the molecular properties of Layer 5 neurons expressing markers ER81 and CRYM, and downregulating CUX1. Axonal projections in the newly reprogrammed cells were also re-directed from interhemispherical targets to subcortical targets. (De la Rossa et al., 2013) has shown that early postnatal overexpression of *Fezf2* in Layer 4 spiny neurons changes their identity to Layer 5-like corticofugal neurons. Taken together, these two reports indicate that postmitotic neurons, which are already in their respective cortical layer and have defined their projections, still maintain a sense of plasticity to reprogramming catalyzed by single transcription factor overexpression in early postnatal life. However, both groups reported decreased reprogramming efficiencies at postnatal day 21, suggesting that the plasticity of these postmitotic neurons declines with age and will likely be absent in the adult brain. Interestingly, when *Fezf2* is expressed in SVZ progenitors destined to become OB GABAergic interneurons, it directs fate towards a glutamatergic phenotype (Zuccotti et al., 2014). The resulting *Fezf2*-respecified OB neurons have features akin to pyramidal cells including larger cell bodies, elaborative dendritic trees, and pyramidal neuron-like electrophysiological outputs. However, the reprogramming reported does not appear to be as complete as is seen in the studies performed embryonically or perinatally. Interestingly, a recent study has also reported high Fezf2 expression in a subset of callosal neurons in the adult cortex, suggesting that Fezf2 expression may not be restricted solely to corticospinal motor neuron fate (Tantirigama et al., 2014). Taken together, the findings of the reprogramming studies discussed above suggest a reduction in reprogramming ability by *Fezf2* with age. Given the complex combinatorial transcriptional co-regulation of neuronal specification during development (Kwan et al., 2012; Greig et al., 2013), this is perhaps not surprising.

Furthermore, as suggested by various examples discussed above, a single transcription factor may have several respective roles and its expression may result in different outcomes depending on the time and context of its expression. For example, *Sox2* promotes self-renewal in neural stem cells and is one of the Yamanaka factors for induced pluripotency (Graham et al., 2003). However, when *Sox2* is expressed in NG2 cells after stab-wound injury or in adult astrocytes in the striatum, these cells can be reprogrammed to interneuron-like cells (Heinrich et al., 2014) or neuroblasts respectively (Niu et al., 2013). These results suggest the need to carefully sculpt strategies for directed differentiation by incorporating developmental logic, knowledge of the donor cell properties, knowledge of the host tissue, and forethought in avoiding situations which might be deleterious clinically (e.g., tumor growth due to transgene misexpression; Nori et al., 2015). Employing such developmental metrics combined with precise tools for genetic manipulation will likely be increasingly necessary in bolstering reprogramming efficiencies to generate precise neuronal subtypes (Victor et al., 2014; Akhtar et al., 2015). Lastly, the use of accurate

TABLE 1 | Reported examples of transcription factor-mediated postnatal cortical neuronal conversion.

Factor(s)	Gene introduction	Age of animal	Region	Substrate cell	End cell (similar to)	Reference
Fezf2	Electroporation	Neonate	Layer 2/3 cortex	Callosal projection neuron	Corticofugal projection neuron	Rouaux and Arlotta (2013)
Fezf2	Iontoporation	Neonate	Layer 4 cortex	Spiny neuron	Corticofugal projection neuron	De la Rossa et al. (2013)
Fezf2	Lentivirus	Neonate/Adult	Lateral ventricle	SVZ progenitor	Glutamatergic pyrimidal Neuron in OB	Zuccotti et al. (2014)
RBP-Jk	Conditional KO	Adult	Medial cortex	Astrocyte	Dcx+ neuron	Magnusson et al. (2014)
dn-Olig2	Retrovirus	Adult	Stab wound injured cortex	Olig2+ cell	Dcx+ neuron	Buffo et al. (2005)
Sox2	Retrovirus	Adult	Stab wound injured cortex	NG2 cell	Dcx+ neuron	Heinrich et al. (2014)
Neurod1	Retrovirus	Adult	Stab wound injured cortex	Astrocytes	Glutamatergic neuron	Guo et al. (2014)
Neurod1	Retrovirus	Adult	Stab wound injured cortex	NG2 cell	Glutamatergic and GABAergic neurons	Guo et al. (2014)

disease-specific models systems and transplant hosts—including aged genetically modified rodents, non-human primates, and potentially human organoids—will likely be of the utmost importance to assess the translational capacity of potential novel therapies.

Conclusions

Grafting and transplantation of neuronal tissue has proceeded for decades with little or no progress towards clinical therapies for cortical trauma and degeneration. However, a critical mass of findings in multiple subfields promises to improve this situation. The development of iPSC technology has reformatted our conception of cell differentiation. Moreover, this technology provides virtually unlimited "starting material" for the generation of cells for transplant. Our knowledge of cortical development has greatly informed our ability to rationally direct differentiation of neurons from pluripotent stem cells. Specifically, employing developmental paradigms to direct neuron subtype differentiation holds the promise of enabling mix and match generation of neurons lost to injury and disease. Nevertheless, as we have detailed, meaningful clinical replacement of cortical circuitry will be among the most difficult problems for modern science to solve. Generating the appropriate cell types will only partially solve this challenge. The next step is to bridge the gap between the precise specificity of circuits created during development with our ability to transplant or reprogram cell types in a manner that allows for the recapitulation of these circuits. With a trillion synapses per centimeter of lost tissue, this will be no small feat. However, given the lack of alternatives, we have no choice but to "beat on, boats against the current," in attempting to rise to the challenge of creating efficacious clinical treatments for those who would otherwise suffer lifelong disability.

Acknowledgments

We apologize to colleagues whose work we could not include due to space constraints. We thank P. Rakic and N. Sestan for many insightful discussions on these subjects and assistance with figure elements. We thank M. Dutra-Clarke for critical review. JJB was supported by funding from the Samuel Oschin Comprehensive Cancer Institute Cancer Research Forum Award and the Board of Governors Regenerative Medicine Institute of Cedars-Sinai.

References

Ables, J. L., Breunig, J. J., Eisch, A. J., and Rakic, P. (2011). Not(ch) just development: Notch signalling in the adult brain. *Nat. Rev. Neurosci.* 12, 269–283. doi: 10.1038/nrn3024

Akhtar, A. A., Molina, J., Dutra-Clarke, M., Kim, G. B., Levy, R., Schreiber-Stainthorp, W., et al. (2015). A transposon-mediated system for flexible control of transgene expression in stem and progenitor-derived lineages. *Stem Cell Reports* 4, 323–331. doi: 10.1016/j.stemcr.2015.01.013

Alvarez-Buylla, A., and Lim, D. A. (2004). For the long run: maintaining germinal niches in the adult brain. *Neuron* 41, 683–686. doi: 10.1016/S0896-6273(04)00111-4

Alvarez Dolado, M., and Broccoli, V. (2011). GABAergic neuronal precursor grafting: implications in brain regeneration and plasticity. *Neural Plast.* 2011:384216. doi: 10.1155/2011/384216

Amador-Arjona, A., Cimadamore, F., Huang, C. T., Wright, R., Lewis, S., Gage, F. H., et al. (2015). SOX2 primes the epigenetic landscape in neural precursors enabling proper gene activation during hippocampal neurogenesis. *Proc. Natl. Acad. Sci. U S A* 112, E1936–E1945. doi: 10.1073/pnas.1421480112

Anderson, S. A., Kaznowski, C. E., Horn, C., Rubenstein, J. L., and McConnell, S. K. (2002). Distinct origins of neocortical projection neurons and interneurons *in vivo*. *Cereb. Cortex* 12, 702–709. doi: 10.1093/cercor/12.7.702

Armulik, A., Genové, G., and Betsholtz, C. (2011). Pericytes: developmental, physiological and pathological perspectives, problems and promises. *Dev. Cell* 21, 193–215. doi: 10.1016/j.devcel.2011.07.001

Azevedo, F. A., Carvalho, L. R., Grinberg, L. T., Farfel, J. M., Ferretti, R. E., Leite, R. E., et al. (2009). Equal numbers of neuronal and nonneuronal cells make the human brain an isometrically scaled-up primate brain. *J. Comp. Neurol.* 513, 532–541. doi: 10.1002/cne.21974

Baraban, S. C., Southwell, D. G., Estrada, R. C., Jones, D. L., Sebe, J. Y., Alfaro-Cervello, C., et al. (2009). Reduction of seizures by transplantation of cortical GABAergic interneuron precursors into Kv1.1 mutant mice. *Proc. Natl. Acad. Sci. U S A* 106, 15472–15477. doi: 10.1073/pnas.0900141106

Behrstock, S., Ebert, A. D., Klein, S., Schmitt, M., Moore, J. M., and Svendsen, C. N. (2008). Lesion-induced increase in survival and migration of human neural progenitor cells releasing GDNF. *Cell Transplant.* 17, 753–762. doi: 10.3727/096368908786516819

Behrstock, S., Ebert, A., McHugh, J., Vosberg, S., Moore, J., Schneider, B., et al. (2006). Human neural progenitors deliver glial cell line-derived neurotrophic factor to parkinsonian rodents and aged primates. *Gene Ther.* 13, 379–388. doi: 10.3410/f.1030023.349469

Bertrand, N., Castro, D. S., and Guillemot, F. (2002). Proneural genes and the specification of neural cell types. *Nat. Rev. Neurosci.* 3, 517–530. doi: 10.1038/nrn874

Bhardwaj, R. D., Curtis, M. A., Spalding, K. L., Buchholz, B. A., Fink, D., Björk-Eriksson, T., et al. (2006). Neocortical neurogenesis in humans is restricted to development. *Proc. Natl. Acad. Sci. U S A* 103, 12564–12568. doi: 10.1073/pnas.0605177103

Bovetti, S., Hsieh, Y. C., Bovolin, P., Perroteau, I., Kazunori, T., and Puche, A. C. (2007). Blood vessels form a scaffold for neuroblast migration in the adult olfactory bulb. *J. Neurosci.* 27, 5976–5980. doi: 10.1523/jneurosci.0678-07.2007

Braun, S. M., Machado, R. A., and Jessberger, S. (2013). Temporal control of retroviral transgene expression in newborn cells in the adult brain. *Stem Cell Reports* 1, 114–122. doi: 10.1016/j.stemcr.2013.06.003

Bráz, J. M., Sharif-Naeini, R., Vogt, D., Kriegstein, A., Alvarez-Buylla, A., Rubenstein, J. L., et al. (2012). Forebrain GABAergic neuron precursors integrate into adult spinal cord and reduce injury-induced neuropathic pain. *Neuron* 74, 663–675. doi: 10.1016/j.neuron.2012.02.033

Breunig, J. J., Arellano, J. I., Macklis, J. D., and Rakic, P. (2007). Everything that glitters isn't gold: a critical review of postnatal neural precursor analyses. *Cell Stem Cell* 1, 612–627. doi: 10.1016/j.stem.2007.11.008

Breunig, J. J., Gate, D., Levy, R., Rodriguez, J. Jr., Kim, G. B., Danielpour, M., et al. (2012). Rapid genetic targeting of pial surface neural progenitors and immature neurons by neonatal electroporation. *Neural Dev.* 7:26. doi: 10.1186/1749-8104-7-26

Breunig, J. J., Guillot-Sestier, M. V., and Town, T. (2013). Brain injury, neuroinflammation and Alzheimer's disease. *Front. Aging Neurosci.* 5:26. doi: 10.3389/fnagi.2013.00026

Breunig, J. J., Haydar, T. F., and Rakic, P. (2011). Neural stem cells: historical perspective and future prospects. *Neuron* 70, 614–625. doi: 10.1016/j.neuron.2011.05.005

Brill, M. S., Ninkovic, J., Winpenny, E., Hodge, R. D., Ozen, I., Yang, R., et al. (2009). Adult generation of glutamatergic olfactory bulb interneurons. *Nat. Neurosci.* 12, 1524–1533. doi: 10.1038/nn.2416

Buffo, A., Rite, I., Tripathi, P., Lepier, A., Colak, D., Horn, A. P., et al. (2008). Origin and progeny of reactive gliosis: a source of multipotent cells in the injured brain. *Proc. Natl. Acad. Sci. U S A* 105, 3581–3586. doi: 10.1073/pnas.0709002105

Buffo, A., Vosko, M. R., Ertürk, D., Hamann, G. F., Jucker, M., Rowitch, D., et al. (2005). Expression pattern of the transcription factor Olig2 in response to brain injuries: implications for neuronal repair. *Proc. Natl. Acad. Sci. U S A* 102, 18183–18188. doi: 10.1073/pnas.0506535102

Burns, K. A., Murphy, B., Danzer, S. C., and Kuan, C. Y. (2009). Developmental and post-injury cortical gliogenesis: a genetic fate-mapping study with Nestin-CreER mice. *Glia* 57, 1115–1129. doi: 10.1002/glia.20835

Carleton, A., Petreanu, L. T., Lansford, R., Alvarez-Buylla, A., and Lledo, P. M. (2003). Becoming a new neuron in the adult olfactory bulb. *Nat. Neurosci.* 6, 507–518. doi: 10.1038/nn1048

Caviness, V. S., and Rakic, P. (1978). Mechanisms of cortical development: a view from mutations in mice. *Annu. Rev. Neurosci.* 1, 297–326. doi: 10.1146/annurev.ne.01.030178.001501

Chen, J. G., Rasin, M. R., Kwan, K. Y., and Sestan, N. (2005b). Zfp312 is required for subcortical axonal projections and dendritic morphology of deep-layer pyramidal neurons of the cerebral cortex. *Proc. Natl. Acad. Sci. U S A* 102, 17792–17797. doi: 10.1073/pnas.0509032102

Chen, B., Schaevitz, L. R., and McConnell, S. K. (2005a). Fezl regulates the differentiation and axon targeting of layer 5 subcortical projection neurons in cerebral cortex. *Proc. Natl. Acad. Sci. U S A* 102, 17184–17189. doi: 10.1073/pnas.0508732102

Chu, J., and Anderson, S. A. (2015). Development of cortical interneurons. *Neuropsychopharmacology* 40, 16–23. doi: 10.1038/npp.2014.171

Colodner, K. J., Montana, R. A., Anthony, D. C., Folkerth, R. D., De Girolami, U., and Feany, M. B. (2005). Proliferative potential of human astrocytes. *J. Neuropathol. Exp. Neurol.* 64, 163–169.

Cooke, J. P., Sayed, N., Lee, J., and Wong, W. T. (2014). Innate immunity and epigenetic plasticity in cellular reprogramming. *Curr. Opin. Genet. Dev.* 28, 89–91. doi: 10.1016/j.gde.2014.11.002

Costa, M. R., Kessaris, N., Richardson, W. D., Götz, M., and Hedin-Pereira, C. (2007). The marginal zone/layer I as a novel niche for neurogenesis and gliogenesis in developing cerebral cortex. *J. Neurosci.* 27, 11376–11388. doi: 10.1523/jneurosci.2418-07.2007

Cregg, J. M., DePaul, M. A., Filous, A. R., Lang, B. T., Tran, A., and Silver, J. (2014). Functional regeneration beyond the glial scar. *Exp. Neurol.* 253, 197–207. doi: 10.1016/j.expneurol.2013.12.024

de Chevigny, A., Core, N., Follert, P., Wild, S., Bosio, A., Yoshikawa, K., et al. (2012). Dynamic expression of the pro-dopaminergic transcription factors Pax6 and Dlx2 during postnatal olfactory bulb neurogenesis. *Front. Cell. Neurosci.* 6:6. doi: 10.3389/fncel.2012.00006

De la Rossa, A., Bellone, C., Golding, B., Vitali, I., Moss, J., Toni, N., et al. (2013). *In vivo* reprogramming of circuit connectivity in postmitotic neocortical neurons. *Nat. Neurosci.* 16, 193–200. doi: 10.1038/nn.3299

Deng, W., Aimone, J. B., and Gage, F. H. (2010). New neurons and new memories: how does adult hippocampal neurogenesis affect learning and memory? *Nat. Rev. Neurosci.* 11, 339–350. doi: 10.1038/nrn2822

Deng, W., Saxe, M. D., Gallina, I. S., and Gage, F. H. (2009). Adult-born hippocampal dentate granule cells undergoing maturation modulate learning and memory in the brain. *J. Neurosci.* 29, 13532–13542. doi: 10.1523/jneurosci.3362-09.2009

Diaz, F., McKeehan, N., Kang, W., and Hébert, J. M. (2013). Apoptosis of glutamatergic neurons fails to trigger a neurogenic response in the adult neocortex. *J. Neurosci.* 33, 6278–6284. doi: 10.1523/JNEUROSCI.5885-12.2013

Dimou, L., and Gotz, M. (2014). Glial cells as progenitors and stem cells: new roles in the healthy and diseased brain. *Physiol. Rev.* 94, 709–737. doi: 10.1152/physrev.00036.2013

Doetsch, F., Caillé, I., Lim, D. A., Garcia-Verdugo, J. M., and Alvarez-Buylla, A. (1999). Subventricular zone astrocytes are neural stem cells in the adult mammalian brain. *Cell* 97, 703–716. doi: 10.1016/s0092-8674(00)80783-7

Drachman, D. A. (2005). Do we have brain to spare? *Neurology* 64, 2004–2005. doi: 10.1212/01.wnl.0000166914.38327.bb

Eriksson, P. S., Perfilieva, E., Björk-Eriksson, T., Alborn, A. M., Nordborg, C., Peterson, D. A., et al. (1998). Neurogenesis in the adult human hippocampus. *Nat. Med.* 4, 1313–1317. doi: 10.1038/3305

Ernst, A., Alkass, K., Bernard, S., Salehpour, M., Perl, S., Tisdale, J., et al. (2014). Neurogenesis in the striatum of the adult human brain. *Cell* 156, 1072–1083. doi: 10.1016/j.cell.2014.01.044

Espuny-Camacho, I., Michelsen, K. A., Gall, D., Linaro, D., Hasche, A., Bonnefont, J., et al. (2013). Pyramidal neurons derived from human pluripotent stem cells integrate efficiently into mouse brain circuits *in vivo*. *Neuron* 77, 440–456. doi: 10.1016/j.neuron.2012.12.011

Feliciano, D. M., and Bordey, A. (2013). Newborn cortical neurons: only for neonates? *Trends Neurosci.* 36, 51–61. doi: 10.1016/j.tins.2012.09.004

Francis, F., Meyer, G., Fallet-Bianco, C., Moreno, S., Kappeler, C., Socorro, A. C., et al. (2006). Human disorders of cortical development: from past to present. *Eur. J. Neurosci.* 23, 877–893. doi: 10.1111/j.1460-9568.2006.04649.x

Gaspard, N., Bouschet, T., Hourez, R., Dimidschstein, J., Naeije, G., van den Ameele, J., et al. (2008). An intrinsic mechanism of corticogenesis from embryonic stem cells. *Nature* 455, 351–357. doi: 10.1038/nature07287

Ge, W. P., Miyawaki, A., Gage, F. H., Jan, Y. N., and Jan, L. Y. (2012). Local generation of glia is a major astrocyte source in postnatal cortex. *Nature* 484, 376–380. doi: 10.1038/nature10959

Geha, S., Pallud, J., Junier, M. P., Devaux, B., Leonard, N., Chassoux, F., et al. (2010). NG2+/Olig2+ cells are the major cycle-related cell population of the adult human normal brain. *Brain Pathol.* 20, 399–411. doi: 10.1111/j.1750-3639.2009.00295.x

Ghashghaei, H. T., Weimer, J. M., Schmid, R. S., Yokota, Y., McCarthy, K. D., Popko, B., et al. (2007). Reinduction of ErbB2 in astrocytes promotes radial glial progenitor identity in adult cerebral cortex. *Genes Dev.* 21, 3258–3271. doi: 10.1101/gad.1580407

Graham, V., Khudyakov, J., Ellis, P., and Pevny, L. (2003). SOX2 functions to maintain neural progenitor identity. *Neuron* 39, 749–765. doi: 10.1016/s0896-6273(03)00497-5

Gregg, C., and Weiss, S. (2003). Generation of functional radial glial cells by embryonic and adult forebrain neural stem cells. *J. Neurosci.* 23, 11587–11601.

Greig, L. C., Woodworth, M. B., Galazo, M. J., Padmanabhan, H., and Macklis, J. D. (2013). Molecular logic of neocortical projection neuron specification, development and diversity. *Nat. Rev. Neurosci.* 14, 755–769. doi: 10.1038/nrn3586

Groves, J. O., Leslie, I., Huang, G. J., McHugh, S. B., Taylor, A., Mott, R., et al. (2013). Ablating adult neurogenesis in the rat has no effect on spatial processing: evidence from a novel pharmacogenetic model. *PLoS Genet.* 9:e1003718. doi: 10.1371/journal.pgen.1003718

Guillemot, F. (2007). Spatial and temporal specification of neural fates by transcription factor codes. *Development* 134, 3771–3780. doi: 10.1242/dev.006379

Guillot-Sestier, M. V., and Town, T. (2013). Innate immunity in Alzheimer's disease: a complex affair. *CNS Neurol. Disord. Drug Targets* 12, 593–607. doi: 10.2174/1871527311312050008

Guo, Z., Zhang, L., Wu, Z., Chen, Y., Wang, F., and Chen, G. (2014). *In Vivo* direct reprogramming of reactive glial cells into functional neurons after brain injury and in an Alzheimer's disease model. *Cell Stem Cell* 14, 188–202. doi: 10.1016/j.stem.2013.12.001

Hack, M. A., Saghatelyan, A., de Chevigny, A., Pfeifer, A., Ashery-Padan, R., Lledo, P. M., et al. (2005). Neuronal fate determinants of adult olfactory bulb neurogenesis. *Nat. Neurosci.* 8, 865–872. doi: 10.1038/nn1479

Hansen, D. V., Lui, J. H., Flandin, P., Yoshikawa, K., Rubenstein, J. L., Alvarez-Buylla, A., et al. (2013). Non-epithelial stem cells and cortical interneuron production in the human ganglionic eminences. *Nat. Neurosci.* 16, 1576–1587. doi: 10.1038/nn.3541

Hansen, D. V., Rubenstein, J. L., and Kriegstein, A. R. (2011). Deriving excitatory neurons of the neocortex from pluripotent stem cells. *Neuron* 70, 645–660. doi: 10.1016/j.neuron.2011.05.006

Heinrich, C., Bergami, M., Gascon, S., Lepier, A., Vigano, F., Dimou, L., et al. (2014). Sox2-mediated conversion of NG2 glia into induced neurons in the injured adult cerebral cortex. *Stem Cell Reports* 3, 1000–1014. doi: 10.1016/j.stemcr.2014.10.007

Heinrich, C., Blum, R., Gascón, S., Masserdotti, G., Tripathi, P., Sánchez, R., et al. (2010). Directing astroglia from the cerebral cortex into subtype specific functional neurons. *PLoS Biol.* 8:e1000373. doi: 10.1371/journal.pbio.1000373

Heng, J. I., Nguyen, L., Castro, D. S., Zimmer, C., Wildner, H., Armant, O., et al. (2008). Neurogenin 2 controls cortical neuron migration through regulation of Rnd2. *Nature* 455, 114–118. doi: 10.1038/nature07198

Herculano-Houzel, S. (2009). The human brain in numbers: a linearly scaled-up primate brain. *Front. Hum. Neurosci.* 3:31. doi: 10.3389/neuro.09.031.2009

Hevner, R. F., Hodge, R. D., Daza, R. A., and Englund, C. (2006). Transcription factors in glutamatergic neurogenesis: conserved programs in neocortex, cerebellum and adult hippocampus. *Neurosci. Res.* 55, 223–233. doi: 10.1016/j.neures.2006.03.004

Hughes, E. G., Kang, S. H., Fukaya, M., and Bergles, D. E. (2013). Oligodendrocyte progenitors balance growth with self-repulsion to achieve homeostasis in the adult brain. *Nat. Neurosci.* 16, 668–676. doi: 10.1038/nn.3390

Hussain, R. Z., Hayardeny, L., Cravens, P. C., Yarovinsky, F., Eagar, T. N., Arellano, B., et al. (2014). Immune surveillance of the central nervous system in multiple sclerosis—relevance for therapy and experimental models. *J. Neuroimmunol.* 276, 9–17. doi: 10.1016/j.jneuroim.2014.08.622

Huttner, H. B., Bergmann, O., Salehpour, M., Rácz, A., Tatarishvili, J., Lindgren, E., et al. (2014). The age and genomic integrity of neurons after cortical stroke in humans. *Nat. Neurosci.* 17, 801–803. doi: 10.1038/nn.3706

Ideguchi, M., Palmer, T. D., Recht, L. D., and Weimann, J. M. (2010). Murine embryonic stem cell-derived pyramidal neurons integrate into the cerebral cortex and appropriately project axons to subcortical targets. *J. Neurosci.* 30, 894–904. doi: 10.1523/jneurosci.4318-09.2010

Inta, D., Alfonso, J., von Engelhardt, J., Kreuzberg, M. M., Meyer, A. H., van Hooft, J. A., et al. (2008). Neurogenesis and widespread forebrain migration of distinct GABAergic neurons from the postnatal subventricular zone. *Proc. Natl. Acad. Sci. U S A* 105, 20994–20999. doi: 10.1073/pnas.0807059105

Johansson, B. B. (2000). Brain plasticity and stroke rehabilitation. The Willis lecture. *Stroke* 31, 223–230. doi: 10.1161/01.str.31.1.223

Karow, M., Sánchez, R., Schichor, C., Masserdotti, G., Ortega, F., Heinrich, C., et al. (2012). Reprogramming of pericyte-derived cells of the adult human brain into induced neuronal cells. *Cell Stem Cell* 11, 471–476. doi: 10.1016/j.stem.2012.07.007

Kato, M., and Dobyns, W. B. (2005). X-linked lissencephaly with abnormal genitalia as a tangential migration disorder causing intractable epilepsy: proposal for a new term, "interneuronopathy". *J Child Neurol.* 20, 392–397. doi: 10.1177/08830738050200042001

Kornack, D. R., and Rakic, P. (2001). Cell proliferation without neurogenesis in adult primate neocortex. *Science* 294, 2127–2130. doi: 10.1126/science.1065467

Kwan, K. Y., Sestan, N., and Anton, E. S. (2012). Transcriptional co-regulation of neuronal migration and laminar identity in the neocortex. *Development* 139, 1535–1546. doi: 10.1242/dev.069963

Lancaster, M. A., Renner, M., Martin, C. A., Wenzel, D., Bicknell, L. S., Hurles, M. E., et al. (2013). Cerebral organoids model human brain development and microcephaly. *Nature* 501, 373–379. doi: 10.1038/nature12517

Lee, J., Sayed, N., Hunter, A., Au, K. F., Wong, W. H., Mocarski, E. S., et al. (2012). Activation of innate immunity is required for efficient nuclear reprogramming. *Cell* 151, 547–558. doi: 10.1016/j.cell.2012.09.034

Letinic, K., Zoncu, R., and Rakic, P. (2002). Origin of GABAergic neurons in the human neocortex. *Nature* 417, 645–649. doi: 10.1038/nature00779

Levy, R., Molina, J., Danielpour, M., and Breunig, J. J. (2014). Neonatal pial surface electroporation. *J. Vis. Exp.* 7:e51319. doi: 10.3791/51319

Li, H., Collado, M., Villasante, A., Strati, K., Ortega, S., Cañamero, M., et al. (2009). The Ink4/Arf locus is a barrier for iPS cell reprogramming. *Nature* 460, 1136–1139. doi: 10.1038/nature08290

Lois, C., García-Verdugo, J. M., and Alvarez-Buylla, A. (1996). Chain migration of neuronal precursors. *Science* 271, 978–981. doi: 10.1126/science.271.5251.978

Magavi, S. S., Leavitt, B. R., and Macklis, J. D. (2000). Induction of neurogenesis in the neocortex of adult mice. *Nature* 405, 951–955. doi: 10.1038/35016083

Magnusson, J. P., Göritz, C., Tatarishvili, J., Dias, D. O., Smith, E. M., Lindvall, O., et al. (2014). A latent neurogenic program in astrocytes regulated by Notch signaling in the mouse. *Science* 346, 237–241. doi: 10.1126/science.346.6206.237

Maroof, A. M., Keros, S., Tyson, J. A., Ying, S. W., Ganat, Y. M., Merkle, F. T., et al. (2013). Directed differentiation and functional maturation of cortical interneurons from human embryonic stem cells. *Cell Stem Cell* 12, 559–572. doi: 10.1016/j.stem.2013.04.008

Marro, S., Pang, Z. P., Yang, N., Tsai, M. C., Qu, K., Chang, H. Y., et al. (2011). Direct lineage conversion of terminally differentiated hepatocytes to functional neurons. *Cell Stem Cell* 9, 374–382. doi: 10.1016/j.stem.2011.09.002

McCombe, P. A., and Henderson, R. D. (2011). The role of immune and inflammatory mechanisms in ALS. *Curr. Mol. Med.* 11, 246–254. doi: 10.2174/156652411795243450

Menn, B., Garcia-Verdugo, J. M., Yaschine, C., Gonzalez-Perez, O., Rowitch, D., and Alvarez-Buylla, A. (2006). Origin of oligodendrocytes in the subventricular zone of the adult brain. *J. Neurosci.* 26, 7907–7918. doi: 10.1523/jneurosci.1299-06.2006

Merkle, F. T., Tramontin, A. D., García-Verdugo, J. M., and Alvarez-Buylla, A. (2004). Radial glia give rise to adult neural stem cells in the subventricular zone. *Proc. Natl. Acad. Sci. U S A* 101, 17528–17532. doi: 10.1073/pnas.0407893101

Michelsen, K. A., Acosta-Verdugo, S., Benoit-Marand, M., Espuny-Camacho, I., Gaspard, N., Saha, B., et al. (2015). Area-specific reestablishment of damaged circuits in the adult cerebral cortex by cortical neurons derived from mouse embryonic stem cells. *Neuron* 85, 982–997. doi: 10.1016/j.neuron.2015.02.001

Ming, G. L., and Song, H. (2011). Adult neurogenesis in the mammalian brain: significant answers and significant questions. *Neuron* 70, 687–702. doi: 10.1016/j.neuron.2011.05.001

Mizuguchi, R., Sugimori, M., Takebayashi, H., Kosako, H., Nagao, M., Yoshida, S., et al. (2001). Combinatorial roles of olig2 and neurogenin2 in the coordinated induction of pan-neuronal and subtype-specific properties of motoneurons. *Neuron* 31, 757–771. doi: 10.1016/s0896-6273(01)00413-5

Molyneaux, B. J., Arlotta, P., Hirata, T., Hibi, M., and Macklis, J. D. (2005). Fezl is required for the birth and specification of corticospinal motor neurons. *Neuron* 47, 817–831. doi: 10.1016/j.neuron.2005.08.030

Mu, Y., and Gage, F. H. (2011). Adult hippocampal neurogenesis and its role in Alzheimer's disease. *Mol. Neurodegener.* 6:85. doi: 10.1186/1750-1326-6-85

Nery, S., Fishell, G., and Corbin, J. G. (2002). The caudal ganglionic eminence is a source of distinct cortical and subcortical cell populations. *Nat. Neurosci.* 5, 1279–1287. doi: 10.1038/nn971

Nicholas, C. R., Chen, J., Tang, Y., Southwell, D. G., Chalmers, N., Vogt, D., et al. (2013). Functional maturation of hPSC-derived forebrain interneurons requires an extended timeline and mimics human neural development. *Cell Stem Cell* 12, 573–586. doi: 10.1016/j.stem.2013.04.005

Niu, W., Zang, T., Zou, Y., Fang, S., Smith, D. K., Bachoo, R., et al. (2013). *In vivo* reprogramming of astrocytes to neuroblasts in the adult brain. *Nat. Cell Biol.* 15, 1164–1175. doi: 10.1038/ncb2843

Noctor, S. C., Flint, A. C., Weissman, T. A., Dammerman, R. S., and Kriegstein, A. R. (2001). Neurons derived from radial glial cells establish radial units in neocortex. *Nature* 409, 714–720. doi: 10.1038/35055553

Noctor, S. C., Martínez-Cerdeño, V., Ivic, L., and Kriegstein, A. R. (2004). Cortical neurons arise in symmetric and asymmetric division zones and migrate through specific phases. *Nat. Neurosci.* 7, 136–144. doi: 10.1038/nn1172

Nori, S., Okada, Y., Nishimura, S., Sasaki, T., Itakura, G., Kobayashi, Y., et al. (2015). Long-term safety issues of iPSC-based cell therapy in a spinal cord injury model: oncogenic transformation with epithelial-mesenchymal transition. *Stem Cell Reports* 4, 360–373. doi: 10.1016/j.stemcr.2015.01.006

Petryniak, M. A., Potter, G. B., Rowitch, D. H., and Rubenstein, J. L. (2007). Dlx1 and Dlx2 control neuronal versus oligodendroglial cell fate acquisition in the developing forebrain. *Neuron* 55, 417–433. doi: 10.1016/j.neuron.2007.06.036

Radonjić, N. V., Ayoub, A. E., Memi, F., Yu, X., Maroof, A., Jakovcevski, I., et al. (2014). Diversity of cortical interneurons in primates: the role of the dorsal proliferative niche. *Cell Rep.* 9, 2139–2151. doi: 10.1016/j.celrep.2014.11.026

Rakic, P. (1972). Mode of cell migration to the superficial layers of fetal monkey neocortex. *J. Comp. Neurol.* 145, 61–83. doi: 10.1002/cne.901450105

Rakic, P. (1985). Limits of neurogenesis in primates. *Science* 227, 1054–1056. doi: 10.1126/science.3975601

Rakic, P. (2002a). Adult neurogenesis in mammals: an identity crisis. *J. Neurosci.* 22, 614–618.

Rakic, P. (2002b). Neurogenesis in adult primate neocortex: an evaluation of the evidence. *Nat. Rev. Neurosci.* 3, 65–71. doi: 10.1038/nrn700

Rakic, P. (2002c). Neurogenesis in adult primates. *Prog. Brain Res.* 138, 3–14. doi: 10.1016/s0079-6123(02)38067-1

Rakic, P. (2003). Developmental and evolutionary adaptations of cortical radial glia. *Cereb. Cortex* 13, 541–549. doi: 10.1093/cercor/13.6.541

Rakic, P. (2009). Evolution of the neocortex: a perspective from developmental biology. *Nat. Rev. Neurosci.* 10, 724–735. doi: 10.1038/nrn2719

Rakic, P., Ayoub, A. E., Breunig, J. J., and Dominguez, M. H. (2009). Decision by division: making cortical maps. *Trends Neurosci.* 32, 291–301. doi: 10.1016/j.tins.2009.01.007

Rasin, M. R., Gazula, V. R., Breunig, J. J., Kwan, K. Y., Johnson, M. B., Liu-Chen, S., et al. (2007). Numb and Numbl are required for maintenance of cadherin-based adhesion and polarity of neural progenitors. *Nat. Neurosci.* 10, 819–827. doi: 10.3410/f.1087494.540615

Rosema, S., Muscara, F., Anderson, V., Godfrey, C., Hearps, S. J., and Catroppa, C. (2015). The trajectory of long-term psychosocial development 16 years following childhood traumatic brain injury. *J. Neurotrauma* doi: 10.1089/neu.2014.3567 [Epub ahead of print].

Rouaux, C., and Arlotta, P. (2010). Fezf2 directs the differentiation of corticofugal neurons from striatal progenitors *in vivo*. *Nat. Neurosci.* 13, 1345–1347. doi: 10.1038/nn.2658

Rouaux, C., and Arlotta, P. (2013). Direct lineage reprogramming of post-mitotic callosal neurons into corticofugal neurons *in vivo*. *Nat. Cell Biol.* 15, 214–221. doi: 10.1038/ncb2660

Rowitch, D. H., and Kriegstein, A. R. (2010). Developmental genetics of vertebrate glial-cell specification. *Nature* 468, 214–222. doi: 10.1038/nature09611

Sadegh, C., and Macklis, J. D. (2014). Established monolayer differentiation of mouse embryonic stem cells generates heterogeneous neocortical-like neurons stalled at a stage equivalent to midcorticogenesis. *J. Comp. Neurol.* 522, 2691–2706. doi: 10.1002/cne.23628

Sanai, N., Nguyen, T., Ihrie, R. A., Mirzadeh, Z., Tsai, H. H., Wong, M., et al. (2011). Corridors of migrating neurons in the human brain and their decline during infancy. *Nature* 478, 382–386. doi: 10.1038/nature10487

Seri, B., García-Verdugo, J. M., Collado-Morente, L., McEwen, B. S., and Alvarez-Buylla, A. (2004). Cell types, lineage and architecture of the germinal zone in the adult dentate gyrus. *J. Comp. Neurol.* 478, 359–378. doi: 10.1002/cne.20288

Shi, Y., Kirwan, P., Smith, J., Robinson, H. P., and Livesey, F. J. (2012). Human cerebral cortex development from pluripotent stem cells to functional excitatory synapses. *Nat. Neurosci.* 15, 477–486. doi: 10.1038/nn.3041

Shipp, S. (2007). Structure and function of the cerebral cortex. *Curr. Biol.* 17, R443–R449. doi: 10.1016/j.cub.2007.03.044

Sofroniew, M. V. (2009). Molecular dissection of reactive astrogliosis and glial scar formation. *Trends Neurosci.* 32, 638–647. doi: 10.1016/j.tins.2009.08.002

Song, H. J., Stevens, C. F., and Gage, F. H. (2002). Neural stem cells from adult hippocampus develop essential properties of functional CNS neurons. *Nat. Neurosci.* 5, 438–445. doi: 10.1038/nn844

Southwell, D. G., Froemke, R. C., Alvarez-Buylla, A., Stryker, M. P., and Gandhi, S. P. (2010). Cortical plasticity induced by inhibitory neuron transplantation. *Science* 327, 1145–1148. doi: 10.1126/science.1183962

Southwell, D. G., Nicholas, C. R., Basbaum, A. I., Stryker, M. P., Kriegstein, A. R., Rubenstein, J. L., et al. (2014). Interneurons from embryonic development to cell-based therapy. *Science* 344:1240622. doi: 10.1126/science.1240622

Spalding, K. L., Bergmann, O., Alkass, K., Bernard, S., Salehpour, M., Huttner, H. B., et al. (2013). Dynamics of hippocampal neurogenesis in adult humans. *Cell* 153, 1219–1227. doi: 10.1016/j.cell.2013.05.002

Spalding, K. L., Bhardwaj, R. D., Buchholz, B. A., Druid, H., and Frisén, J. (2005). Retrospective birth dating of cells in humans. *Cell* 122, 133–143. doi: 10.1016/j.cell.2005.04.028

Suzuki, M., McHugh, J., Tork, C., Shelley, B., Klein, S. M., Aebischer, P., et al. (2007). GDNF secreting human neural progenitor cells protect dying motor neurons, but not their projection to muscle, in a rat model of familial ALS. *PloS One* 2:e689. doi: 10.1371/journal.pone.0000689

Svendsen, C. N., Caldwell, M. A., Shen, J., ter Borg, M. G., Rosser, A. E., Tyers, P., et al. (1997). Long-term survival of human central nervous system progenitor cells transplanted into a rat model of Parkinson's disease. *Exp. Neurol.* 148, 135–146. doi: 10.1006/exnr.1997.6634

Tanaka, D. H., Toriumi, K., Kubo, K., Nabeshima, T., and Nakajima, K. (2011). GABAergic precursor transplantation into the prefrontal cortex prevents phencyclidine-induced cognitive deficits. *J. Neurosci.* 31, 14116–14125. doi: 10.1523/jneurosci.2786-11.2011

Tantirigama, M. L., Oswald, M. J., Duynstee, C., Hughes, S. M., and Empson, R. M. (2014). Expression of the developmental transcription factor Fezf2 identifies a distinct subpopulation of layer 5 intratelencephalic-projection neurons in mature mouse motor cortex. *J. Neurosci.* 34, 4303–4308. doi: 10.1523/jneurosci.3111-13.2014

Torper, O., Pfisterer, U., Wolf, D. A., Pereira, M., Lau, S., Jakobsson, J., et al. (2013). Generation of induced neurons via direct conversion *in vivo*. *Proc. Natl. Acad. Sci. U S A* 110, 7038–7043. doi: 10.1073/pnas.1303829110

Tramontin, A. D., García-Verdugo, J. M., Lim, D. A., and Alvarez-Buylla, A. (2003). Postnatal development of radial glia and the ventricular zone (VZ): a continuum of the neural stem cell compartment. *Cereb. Cortex* 13, 580–587. doi: 10.1093/cercor/13.6.580

Urbán, N., and Guillemot, F. (2014). Neurogenesis in the embryonic and adult brain: same regulators, different roles. *Front. Cell. Neurosci.* 8:396. doi: 10.3389/fncel.2014.00396

Van Hoesen, G. W., Hyman, B. T., and Damasio, A. R. (1991). Entorhinal cortex pathology in Alzheimer's disease. *Hippocampus* 1, 1–8. doi: 10.1002/hipo.450010102

Victor, M. B., Richner, M., Hermanstyne, T. O., Ransdell, J. L., Sobieski, C., Deng, P. Y., et al. (2014). Generation of human striatal neurons by microRNA-dependent direct conversion of fibroblasts. *Neuron* 84, 311–323. doi: 10.1016/j.neuron.2014.10.016

Vierbuchen, T., Ostermeier, A., Pang, Z. P., Kokubu, Y., Sudhof, T. C., and Wernig, M. (2010). Direct conversion of fibroblasts to functional neurons by defined factors. *Nature* 463, 1035–1041. doi: 10.1038/nature08797

Weitz, T. M., and Town, T. (2012). Microglia in Alzheimer's disease: it's all about context. *Int. J. Alzheimers Dis.* 2012:314185. doi: 10.1155/2012/314185

Wonders, C. P., and Anderson, S. A. (2006). The origin and specification of cortical interneurons. *Nat. Rev. Neurosci.* 7, 687–696. doi: 10.1038/nrn1954

Yeung, M. S., Zdunek, S., Bergmann, O., Bernard, S., Salehpour, M., Alkass, K., et al. (2014). Dynamics of oligodendrocyte generation and myelination in the human brain. *Cell* 159, 766–774. doi: 10.1016/j.cell.2014.10.011

Zhang, Y., Pak, C., Han, Y., Ahlenius, H., Zhang, Z., Chanda, S., et al. (2013). Rapid single-step induction of functional neurons from human pluripotent stem cells. *Neuron* 78, 785–798. doi: 10.1016/j.neuron.2013.05.029

Zuccotti, A., Le Magueresse, C., Chen, M., Neitz, A., and Monyer, H. (2014). The transcription factor Fezf2 directs the differentiation of neural stem cells in the subventricular zone toward a cortical phenotype. *Proc. Natl. Acad. Sci. U S A* 111, 10726–10731. doi: 10.1073/pnas.1320290111

12

Lipidome of Midbody Released from Neural Stem and Progenitor Cells During Mammalian Cortical Neurogenesis

Yoko Arai †*, Julio L. Sampaio, Michaela Wilsch-Bräuninger, Andreas W. Ettinger* †*, Christiane Haffner and Wieland B. Huttner* *

Max Planck Institute of Molecular Cell Biology and Genetics, Dresden, Germany

Correspondence:
Wieland B. Huttner,
Max Planck Institute of Molecular Cell Biology and Genetics,
Pfotenhauerstrasse 108,
D-01307 Dresden, Germany
huttner@mpi-cbg.de

*† **Present Address:***
Yoko Arai,
Institut Jacques Monod, Centre National de la Recherche Scientifique UMR 7592, Université Paris Diderot, Sorbonne Paris Cité, Paris, France;
Andreas W. Ettinger,
University of California, San Francisco, San Francisco, CA, USA

Midbody release from proliferative neural progenitor cells is tightly associated with the neuronal commitment of neural progenitor cells during the progression of neurogenesis in the mammalian cerebral cortex. While the central portion of the midbody, a cytoplasmic bridge between nascent daughter cells, is engulfed by one of the daughter cell by most cells *in vitro*, it is shown to be released into the extracellular cerebrospinal fluid (CF) *in vivo* in mouse embryos. Several proteins have been involved in midbody release; however, few studies have addressed the participation of the plasma membrane's lipids in this process. Here, we show by Shotgun Lipidomic analysis that phosphatydylserine (PS), among other lipids, is enriched in the released midbodies compared to lipoparticles and cellular membranes, both collected from the CF of the developing mouse embryos. Moreover, the developing mouse embryo neural progenitor cells released two distinct types of midbodies carrying either internalized PS or externalized PS on their membrane. This strongly suggests that phagocytosis and an alternative fate of released midbodies exists. HeLa cells, which are known to mainly engulf the midbody show almost no PS exposure, if any, on the outer leaflet of the midbody membrane. These results point toward that PS exposure might be involved in the selection of recipients of released midbodies, either to be engulfed by daughter cells or phagocytosed by non-daughter cells or another cell type in the developing cerebral cortex.

Keywords: neural stem cells, midbody, shotgun lipidomic analysis, phosphatydylserine, mammalian cortical neurogenesis

Introduction

At the end of mitosis, after the ingression of the cleavage furrow, a dividing cell is partitioned into two daughter cells that remain connected through a cytoplasmic bridge, the midbody, which is composed of the remnants of the central spindle including a set of microtubule interacting proteins (Glotzer, 2009; Chen et al., 2013). Physical separation of daughter cells is achieved by abscission, which completes cell division/cytokinesis by severing the midbody-bridge, bypassing the central portion of the midbody that contains a dense matrix of antiparallel microtubules and electron-dense material (Buck and Tidsale, 1962). Accumulating *in vitro* evidence from induced pluripotent stem and cancer-derived immortalized cells indicates that the post-abscission midbody, with its characteristic matrix composition, is subsequently either retracted asymmetrically by a daughter cell (single abscission) (Kuo et al., 2011) or released into the extracellular space (double abscission). Alternatively, released midbodies could get attached to the surface of a daughter cell and consequently be engulfed (Ettinger et al., 2011; Crowell et al., 2014). In culture cells, neural stem cells, embryonic stem cells, or cancer-derived cells, which are still responsive to differentiation agents, showed midbody-release into the extracellular space (Ettinger et al., 2011). Potentially, these midbodies might be taken up by non-daughter cells, which could result in a long-range dispersion of midbodies. A similar phenomenon is observed in neuroepithelial cells during mouse cortical development (Marzesco et al., 2005; Dubreuil et al., 2007).

At the onset of neurogenesis, neuroepithelial cells divide asymmetrically and preferentially release their midbody (NE midbody in short) into the extracellular ventricular fluid (Marzesco et al., 2005). The NE midbody release showed a strong correlation with the increase of neurogenesis (Dubreuil et al., 2007). Therefore, an efficient release of midbodies from neuroepithelial cells was postulated as a mechanism to reduce proliferative capacity of neuroepithelial cells. Midbody release ultimately results in loss of both the cytoplasmic and membraneous components present in the midbody including lipids from neuroepithelial cells. While the mechanism of the midbody release from neuroepithelial cells had been addressed through protein functions (Dubreuil et al., 2007), it is still unclear what is the fate of the NE midbody during neurogenesis.

In this study, we characterized the NE midbody for the first time through lipidome analysis, where we observed enrichments of specific classes of phosphatidylserine (PS), phosphatidylethanolamine (PE), and specific species of ceramide (Cer), and triacylglycerols (TAGs). Among these, PS was strikingly enriched in NE midbody. It has been proposed that midbodies with PS, particularly carrying externalized PS on their membrane bilayer, are cleaned up by phagocytes in *Caenorhabditis elegans* (Chai et al., 2012). This observation suggests that the PS status on the membrane bilayer is associated with the fate of the NE midbody, which may allow deducing its fate. Our data regarding PS status suggests at least two different categories of recipients, either a daughter cell for an engulfment pathway or non-daughter cells for phagocytosis. The distinct subtype of NE midbodies released upon differentiation (Dubreuil et al., 2007; Ettinger et al., 2011) and carry a stem cell marker (Marzesco et al., 2005; Corbeil et al., 2010) may be a novel cue in and contribute to the complexity of the proliferative territories in the developing cerebral cortex.

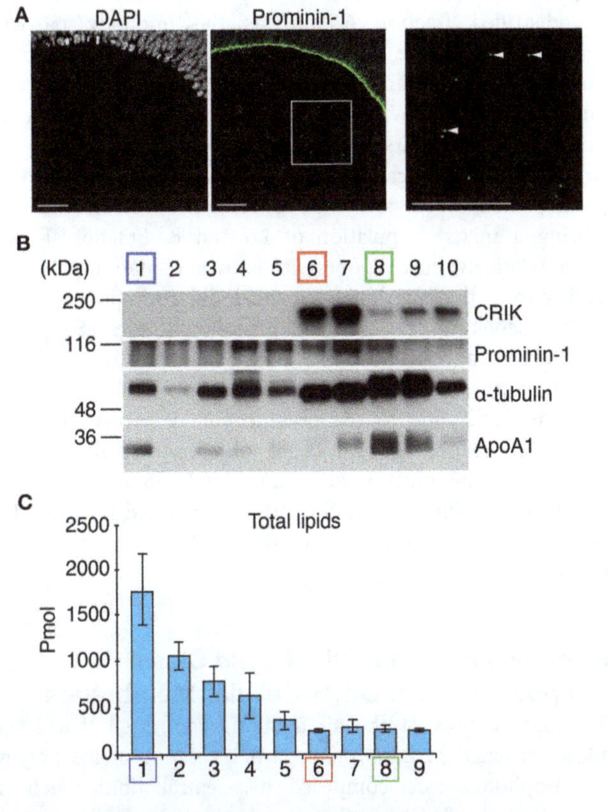

FIGURE 1 | Midbody enrichment from the E11.5 mouse embryonic cerebrospinal fluid. (A) Immunofluorescence for prominin-1 (green) combined with DAPI staining (white) of a coronal cryosection (single optical section) of E11.5 dorsal telencephalon. A white box is shown at high magnification in corresponding right panels. Examples of prominin-1-positive midbodies are shown (white arrowheads). Prominin-1-positive midbodies are released into the cerebrospinal fluid. Scale bars, 50 μm. **(B)** Analysis of mouse embryonic cerebrospinal fluid by velocity sucrose density gradient centrifugation and immunoblotting. The lightest density fraction (containing small lipid particles) is indicated as 1 and the densest fraction (containing large materials including likely cell debris and skin tissue fragments) is indicated as 10. Half of each fraction was subjected to immunoblot analysis for CRIK (~197 kDa), Prominin-1 (~115 kDa), α-tubulin (~50 kDa), and Apolipoprotein A1 (~28 kDa). The positions of molecular weight markers are indicated. **(C)** Total lipid quantified from cerebrospinal fluid of E11.5 mouse embryos present in the individual fractions 1–9 after velocity sucrose density gradient.

Results

Midbody Enrichment for Lipidomic Characterization

To enrich midbodies released from neural progenitor cells of the developing mouse embryo ("NE midbody" in short), we collected the ventricular fluid [embryonic cerebrospinal fluid (CF)] of mouse embryos at E11.5 (the number of midbodies is high at this stage) (Marzesco et al., 2005) (**Figure 1A**). In order to separate the midbody particles (~500 nm) from the biggest lipid "contaminant," the lipoprotein particles (~50 nm), which are both present in the ventricular fluid (Marzesco et al., 2005), we subjected the sample to a velocity sucrose gradient. We analyzed all fractions from the gradient by immunoblotting for marker proteins prior lipid analysis in order to check for the quality of the separation (**Figure 1B**). We used the midbody markers: citron rho-interacting kinase (CRIK) (Madaule et al., 1998), prominin-1 and α-tubulin (Dubreuil et al., 2007) in order to identify the fraction enriched in midbody particles in the sucrose fractions. Lipoparticles enriched fractions were identified with the marker apolipoprotein A1 (Furbee et al., 2002) (**Figure 1B**).

Comparing all fractions in terms of abundance of all markers, we were able to fractionate midbodies (L6) from lipoprotein particles (L1) and cell membranes (L8) (**Figure 1B**). We identified fraction 6 (L6) as the midbody particle-enriched fraction due to the relative enrichment of midbody markers CRIK, prominin-1 and α-tubulin and the absence of apolipoprotein A1. While fraction 7 (L7) was also enriched with midbody markers, we did not present this fraction as a midbody fraction because of the increased contamination by apolipoprotein A1 as compared to fraction L6, and considered it being a mixed population of L6 and 8. Fraction 1 (L1) was a relatively pure lipoprotein particle-containing fraction judging from the enrichment of α-tubulin and apolipoprotein A1 and depletion of CRIK and prominin-1. Fraction 8 (L8) was used as a reference of a mixed fraction that included low amounts of midbody and plasma membrane of neural progenitor cells due to the presence of all protein markers (**Figure 1B**). Moreover, we could observe that lipoproteins were by far the most predominant lipid-containing entities present in the ventricular fluid where its purified fraction (L1) outweighs the midbody fraction (L6) by more than seven-fold (**Figure 1C**).

Midbodies Have a Distinct Lipid Class Composition from Other Cellular Membranes

The lipid analysis of the all fractions confirmed that L1 is indeed enriched in lipoprotein particles. Lipoproteins possess a hydrophobic core composed by neutral lipids such as triacylglycerols (TAG) and cholesterol ester (CE) (Willnow et al., 2007) and we observe that this fraction is the most enriched in these lipid classes (**Figure 2A**). We then see a continuous decrease in the total lipid amount in lower gradient fractions that is accompanied by changes in several lipid classes (**Figures 1C, 2A**). As expected from fractions more depleted from lipoprotein particles, CEs and TAGs decrease in lower gradient fractions as well as sphingomyelin (SM) (**Figure 2A**). Most importantly, we observe a sharp increase in phosphatidylethanolamine (PE) and phosphatidylserine (PS) in lower gradient fractions that peak precisely at fraction L6 where we observe the purest midbody fraction (L6) followed by a sharp decrease in the following fractions (**Figure 2A**). It is important to note that in the fractions below L6, we also observe a dramatic decrease in TAGs and PE plasmalogens (PE O-) and a slight increase in PC (phosphatidylcholine) suggesting high specificity in terms of lipid class composition of the midbody containing fraction compared to the remaining cell membrane fragments. Importantly, the mean PS amount in L6 was 27-fold higher than in L1 (L6, 2.64 ± 1.26; L1, 0.098 ± 0.11, **Figure 2B**) and 2.4-fold when L6 was compared to the intermediate fraction L8 (L8, 1.11 ± 0.8, **Figure 2B**). Respective to the amount of PE, the mean PE amount in L6 was 9.3 and four times higher than in L1 and L8, respectively (L6, 2.05 ± 0.66; L1, 0.22 ± 0.13; L8, 0.51 ± 0.15, **Figure 2B**).

In summary, we observe high specificity of lipid class composition in the midbody-enriched fraction most notably, PS and PE are highly enriched in the midbody-containing fraction compared to that of lipoprotein and cell membrane mixed fractions.

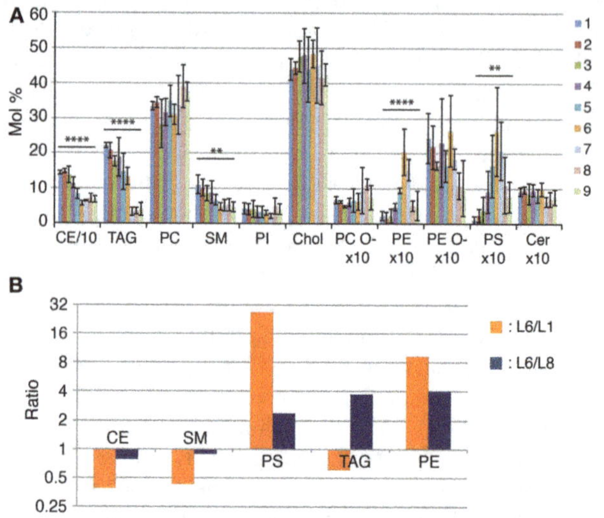

FIGURE 2 | The Lipidome of NE midbodies. (A) Lipid class profile of all sucrose fraction. The content of individual lipid classes was determined by summing up absolute abundances of all identified species and is expressed as mol %. We consider 100% to be all the membrane lipids, meaning that CE and TAG are excluded from the normalization. CE and TAG amounts are also normalized to the total membrane lipids. *P*-values were estimated by One-Way ANOVA; $^{**}P < 0.01$, $^{****}P < 0.0001$. Error bars correspond to SD ($n = 3$). CE amounts are divided by 10 and PC O-, PE, PE O-, PS, and Cer are multiplied by 10 for visualization purposes. CE, cholesterol ester; TAG, triacylglycerol; PC, phosphatidylcholine; SM, sphingomyelin; PI, phosphatidylinositol; Chol, Cholesterol; PC O- and PE O-, plasmalogens; PE, phosphatidylethanolamine; PS, phosphatidylserine, Cer, ceramide. **(B)** Enrichment of lipid constituency in layer 6 (L6) compared to layer 1 (L1) (L6/L1) and layer 8 (L8) (L6/L8), respectively. The *y*-axis is on a $\log_2$ scale.

Specific Lipid Species are Enriched in Midbodies Compared to Other Cellular Membranes

It has been previously reported that midbodies collected from HeLa cells ("HeLa midbody" in short) showed the specific accumulation of lipid species of C22–24 ceramides, TAG [16:1, 12:0, 18:1] and PS [18:0–20:4] when compared to cells in cytokinesis (Atilla-Gokcumen et al., 2014). In agreement with the result of the HeLa midbody lipidome, the NE midbody lipidome displays an enrichment of TAG [46:2] in the midbody fraction and a specific enrichment of PS [38:4] and ceramides but in our case, we observed instead a specific increase in C16–18 ceramides, Cer [36:1:2] (**Figure 3A**). Importantly, we could observe many more species enriched in the midbody fraction. Not only we found TAG [46:2] enriched in the midbody fraction, but also many other TAGs with similar short chain fatty acid compositions (C12–18) in different putative combinations, TAG [46:0], TAG [46:1], TAG [46:2], and TAG [50:4] (**Figure 3A**). We could also observe that most lipid species belonging to PS and PE irrespective of the fatty acid saturation and chain length level display a strong enrichment in the midbody fraction (**Figures 3B,C**). Interestingly, specific PE O- species, namely with longer and more unsaturated fatty acids, PE O- [38:6] and PE O- [40:6] are enriched in the midbody fraction (**Figure 3C**). Although PC as a class is not changing significantly between the different fractions, we can observe some changes in lipid

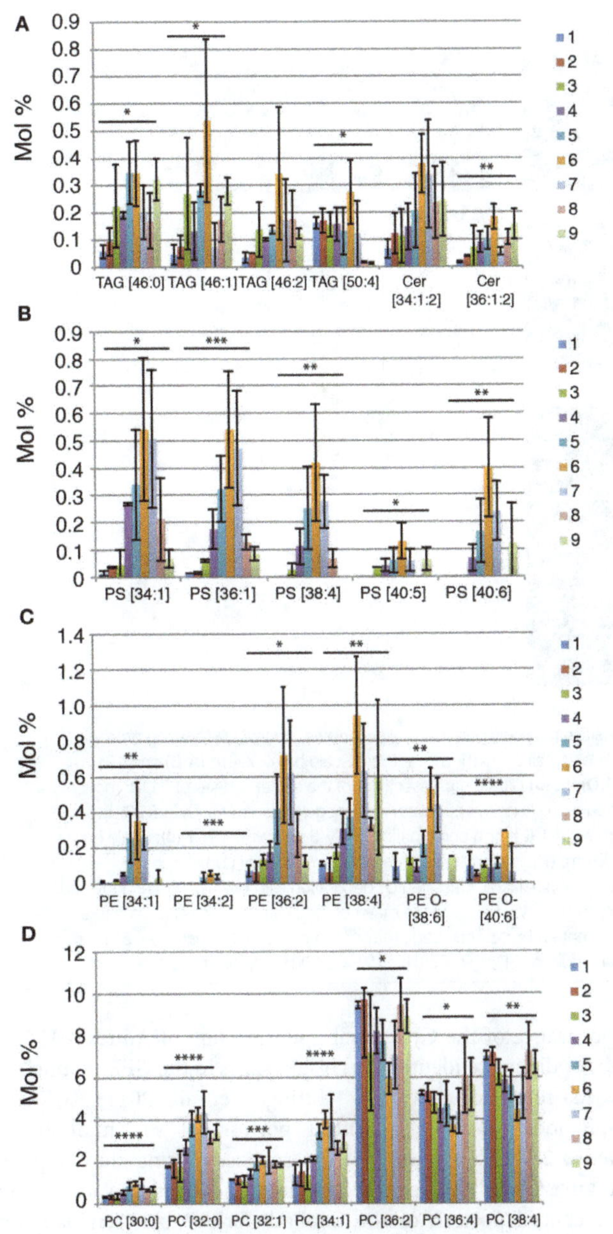

FIGURE 3 | Lipid species that correlate with the presence of NE midbodies. (A–D) Lipid species relative abundance (mol %) across the sucrose fractions. Each lipid species is shown as the sum of number of carbon atoms and double bonds present in the long chain base and/or fatty acids. *P*-values were estimated by One-Way ANOVA; $^*P < 0.05$, $^{**}P < 0.01$, $^{***}P < 0.001$ and $^{****}P < 0.0001$. Error bars correspond to SD ($n = 3$).

species. Shorter and more saturated PC lipid species (C30–34) are enriched in midbodies, PC [30:0], PC [32:0], PC [32:1], and PC [34:1], while longer and more unsaturated lipid species are depleted in the midbody fraction, PC [36:2], PC [36:4], and PC [38:4] (**Figure 3D**).

In conclusion, we could reproduce the previous published results on lipids enriched in the midbody of Hela cells but identified new midbobody specific lipids, namely within Cer, PS and TAG lipid classes, PE as a lipid class and long and unsaturated PE O- and a remodeling of the PC lipid class to shorter and more saturated lipid species in the midbody.

NE Midbodies Carry Internalized and Externalized PS

From the lipidome analysis, we observed that mainly PC is the most depleted membrane lipid classes (aprox. 8 mol %) while PS and PE are the most enriched lipid classes in NE midbody (almost 5 mol % in total) compared to cell membranes (L8) (**Figures 3B–D**). If we take into consideration the plasma membrane lipid asymmetry where PC is on the extracellular leaflet of the plasma membrane at the cell surface, and both PS and PE face the cytoplasmic leaflet (Verkleij et al., 1973), it raises the interesting possibility that PS and/or PE might be externalized to keep the membrane integrity. In *C. elegans*, externalization of PS on midbodies released from Q neuroblasts was shown to be an engulfment signal for the midbody via clearance by phagocytes (Chai et al., 2012). These lines of evidence suggest that the status of PS externalization on the midbody might be a mark to infer the fate and/or recipient cell of released midbodies.

Therefore, we assessed the leaflet localization of PS in midbody membranes, taking advantage of its specific interacting partner, Annexin V (Schutte et al., 1998). To this end, we injected Annexin V directly coupled with Cy5 (Annexin V-Cy5) into the cerebral fluid of mouse embryos at the level of the forming cortex (E11.5), allowing binding for 30 min, followed by fixation and analysis by immunofluorescence. At this early stage of neurogenesis, the fluid filling the ventricular space contains a high amount of released NE midbodies. In this experimental setup, binding of Annexin V-Cy5 to particles is expected only if PS was externalized on the outer leaflet of the membrane bilayer. We confirmed Annexin V-Cy5 positive particles in the ventricular fluid as NE midbodies by a counterstaining with prominin-1, a midbody marker (Marzesco et al., 2005) (**Figures 4A–D**). In addition to particles in the lumen, we also detected Annexin V-Cy5 staining at the apical plasma membrane of neuroepithelial cells, which is the site of cytokinesis midbody formation between nascent daughter cells (**Figure 4C**). The presence of Annexin V-Cy5 and prominin-1 double positive midbody structures on the apical surface was confirmed by immunogold labeling and electron microscopy (**Figures 4E–J**). We found comparably electron-dense, ~500 nm–large structures labeled individually or together by antibodies against prominin-1 or Cy5 (**Figures 4E–J**). These results indicate that PS externalization could occur at the end of cytokinesis of neuronal progenitor cells.

NE midbodies show three distinct populations defined by their decoration with Annexin V-Cy5 and presence of prominin-1. At the apical surface of the ventricular zone, we observed prominin-1 positive and Annexin V-Cy5 negative particles as a major population (57%, **Supplementary Figure 1**) and prominin-1 and Annexin V-Cy5 double positive particles as a second population (41%, **Supplementary Figure 1**). A third minor population (2%) contained only Annexin V-Cy5. Interestingly, in the CF, prominin-1, and Annexin V-Cy5 double positive particles became the major population (55%, **Figure 4K**)

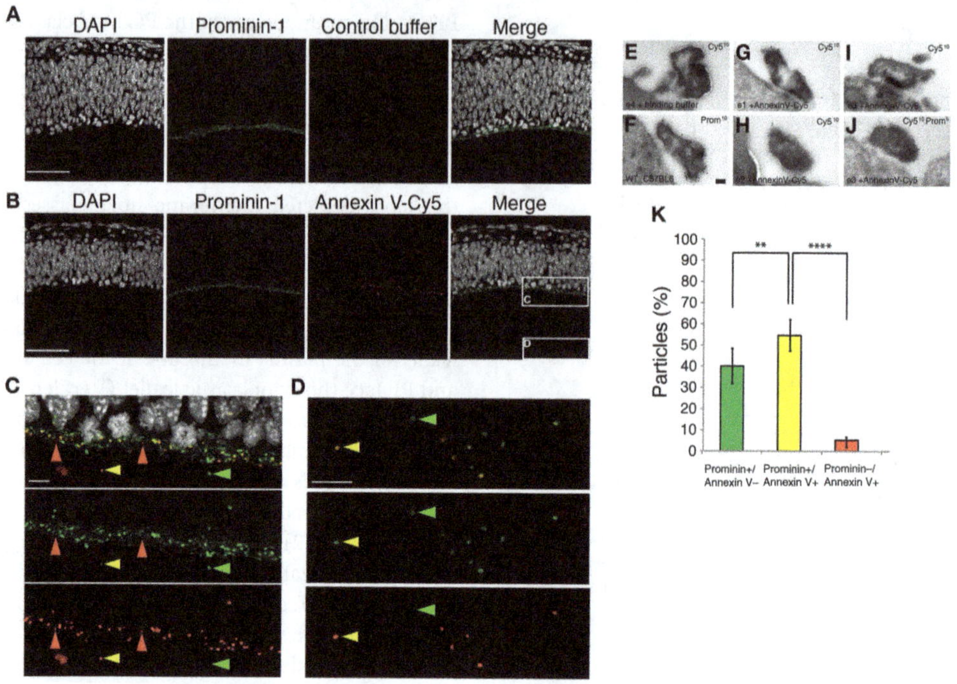

FIGURE 4 | Phosphatidylserine is on the outer-leaflet of the plasma membrane of the released midbody. (A–D) Micrographs of mouse embryonic E11.5 coronal cryosections of dorsal telencephalon injected with either Annexin V binding buffer alone **(A)** or containing Annexin V-Cy5 **(B–D)**. Sections were consecutively stained by immunofluorescence for prominin-1 (green) and counterstained with DAPI (white). Images are z-projections of 32 consecutive 0.38-μm optical sections. **(C,D)** Higher magnifications of either the apical plasma membrane of the ventricular zone **(C)** or particles in the cerebrospinal fluid **(D)** [regions indicated by the boxes in **(B)**]. Red arrows, Annexin V-Cy5 single positive particles, green arrows, prominin-1 single positive midbody particles, yellow arrows, Annexin V-Cy5 and prominin-1 double positive midbody particles. Scale bars, 50 μm **(A,B)** and 10 μm **(C,D)**. **(E–J)** Ultrathin cryosections of the apical surface of E11.5 mouse telencephalic neuroepithelium immunogold labeled for Cy-5 **(E,G–I)**, prominin-1 **(F)**, or a combination of Cy-5 and prominin-1 **(J)**. Scale bar, 100 nm. **(K)** Percentage of three different types of particles in the cerebrospinal fluid, classified by decoration with prominin-1 antibody and Annexin V-Cy5. Data are the mean of six 213-μm wide fields from three different embryos and litters; total number of counted particles, 581; error bars indicate SD; $^{**}P < 0.01$, $^{****}P < 0.0001$; unpaired *t*-test.

and the prominin-1 positive and Annexin V-Cy5 negative particles were the second population (40%, **Figure 4K**). The third minor population (5%) contained only Annexin V-Cy5 was still observed. Taken together, these results strongly suggest that a fraction of neural progenitor cell midbodies externalized PS prior to their release in the ventricular fluid and ultimately both PS-externalized and -internalized midbodies were found after cytokinesis.

PS Flipping Occurs Upon the Detachment of the Midbody after Cytokinesis

In order to determine the dynamics of flipping of PS on the membrane, we analyzed dividing neuroblastoma cells (Neuro-2a), which have been shown to have the capacity of both releasing and engulfing midbodies (Ettinger et al., 2011). We performed live-cell time-lapse microscopy using a transgenic Neuro-2a cell line expressing GFP- tagged mitotic kinesin-like protein-1 (MKLP1) (Poser et al., 2008; Ettinger et al., 2011), a core midbody and central spindle protein (Hu et al., 2012). This cell line allows the visualization of the forming and released midbody (Neuro2a midbody, in short). To visualize externalized PS, we added Annexin V-Cy5 to the culture medium at the beginning of the movie. We assessed PS externalization by appearance of the Cy5 signal upon binding of Annexin V-Cy5. Midbodies were identified as bright spots in the GFP channel.

As reported previously (Ettinger et al., 2011), MKLP1-GFP localized to the central portion of the midbody in Neuro-2a cells. PS was not externalized during the telophase (**Figure 5A**, "T"). The midbody was subsequently detached from the central portion of the midbody bridge between daughter cells after either a first or second abscission event of the cytoplasmic membrane. This detachment was identified by the displacement of the midbody from the point of contact of the daughter cell to one of the two daughter cells and PS was externalized at this moment, as determined from appearance of a Cy5 spot (**Figure 5A**, "A"). Approximately 1 h after the detachment, the midbody was released from a daughter cell (**Figure 5A**, "R"). These results indicate that PS was flipped out and exposed to the extracellular space at the end of the cytokinesis before midbody release (see Supplementary Movie 1).

We quantified Annexin V and MKLP1-GFP double positive midbodies in Neuro-2a MKLP1-GFP cell cultures in order to understand how widespread this phenomenon is (**Figures 5B–E**). During late telophase, a midbody bridge is formed between the nascent daughter cells. MKLP1-GFP was recruited to the

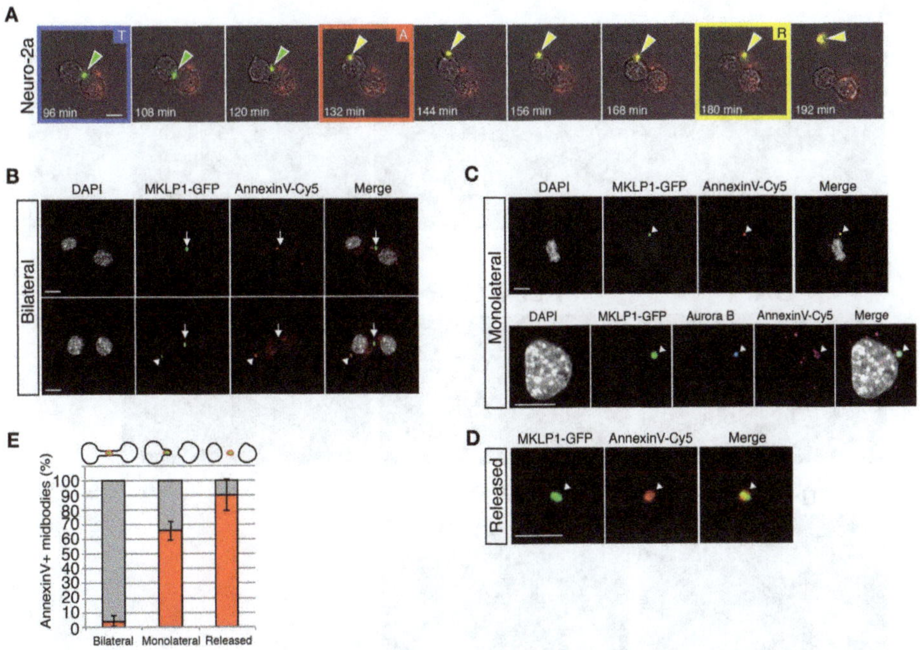

FIGURE 5 | Phosphatidylserine is maintained on the outer-leaflet of the plasma membrane of retained and released midbodies in MKLP1-GFP Neuro-2a cells. (A) Individual frames of live-cell time-lapse video microscopy of a MKLP1-GFP stable expressing Neuro-2a cell line recoded at 12 min intervals (Supplementary Movie 1). Selected images of combined bright-field and epifluorescence channels are shown. Green-white arrows show the position of MKLP1-GFP positive midbodies. Yellow-white arrows indicate midbodies that bound to Annexin V-Cy5, which has been added to the medium and interacts with exposed PSs. "T" with blue frame, telophase; "A" with red frame, appearance of a Cy5 spot; "R" with yellow frame, released midbody. Scale bar, 10 μm. **(B–D)** MKLP1-GFP Neuro-2a cells were incubated with AnnexinV-Cy5 for 10 min in culture medium. Images are obtained as z-stacks every 0.38-μm and are maximum intensity projections. Scale bars, 10 μm. **(B)** Examples of bilateral midbodies. Fluorescence for MKLP1-GFP (green) and AnnexinV-Cy5 (red) combined with DAPI staining (white). White arrowheads show Annexin V-Cy5 positive midbodies and white arrows show Annexin V-Cy5 negative midbody. **(C)** Examples of monolateral midbodies. Upper panels, fluorescence for MKLP1-GFP (green), Annexin V-Cy5 (red), and DAPI (white). Lower panels, fluorescence for MKLP1-GFP (green), Aurora B kinase (blue), Annexin V-Cy5 (red), and DAPI (white). White arrowheads, Annexin V-Cy5 positive midbody. **(D)** Example of a released Annexin V-Cy5 positive midbody. Fluorescence for MKLP1-GFP (green) and AnnexinV-Cy5 (red). **(E)** Quantification of MKLP1-GFP and Annexin V-Cy5 colocalization (red columns) vs. non-colocalization (gray columns), expressed as percentage of total number of MKLP1-GFP+ midbodies. Data are the mean four independent experiments, counted in at least 20 randomly chosen fields (total number of counted particles, 243 for bilateral, 234 for monolateral and 137 for released); error bars indicate SD.

central portion of the midbody (**Figure 5B**) as confirmed by immunostaining for α-tubulin to highlight the central spindle microtubules and for Aurora B kinase which localizes to the midzone in anaphase and decorates the inner part of the central spindle in telophase (**Supplementary Figure 2A**) (Hu et al., 2012). We almost never detected Annexin V-Cy5 staining in these newly formed midbodies (about 3.5% of total bilateral midbodies, **Figures 5B,E**). Instead, Annexin V was present in midbodies either adhering to one of the daughter cells after a first abscission or on interphase cells (**Figures 5B,C**, white arrowheads and see **Supplementary Figure 2B**). The majority of such monolateral midbodies were Annexin V-Cy5 positive (≈66% of total monolateral midbodies, **Figure 5E**). Fully released Neuro2a midbodies contained Annexin V-Cy5 in the majority of cases (≈90% of total released GFP positive particles, **Figures 5D,E**). Taken together, PS exposure occurred before the complete release of the midbody and it likely occurred after the first abscission step.

PS Status on HeLa Midbodies

A previous study indicated that half of the total Neuro-2a midbodies are retained on daughter cells and the rest are released into the extracellular space (Ettinger et al., 2011). Conversely, in HeLa cells, midbodies were described to be engulfed by a daughter cell (Crowell et al., 2014). Therefore, we asked whether HeLa midbodies carry externalized PS. Similarly to the analysis of Neuro2a cells, we used a transgenic HeLa cell line expressing MKLP1-GFP to follow the midbody and determined the presence of PS in the outer leaflet of the midbody membrane with Annexin V-Cy5 (**Figure 6**). Midbody bridges formed during telophase were identified by recruitment of MKLP1-GFP and confirmed by immunostaining for α-tubulin and Aurora B (**Supplementary Figure 3**). In both monolateral inherited midbodies (**Figure 6A**) and in newly formed/bilateral midbodies (**Figure 6B**), we hardly detected PS externalization. These results suggest that PS exposure to the extracellular environment is a characteristic feature of neural-related cell lines and neuronal progenitor cells.

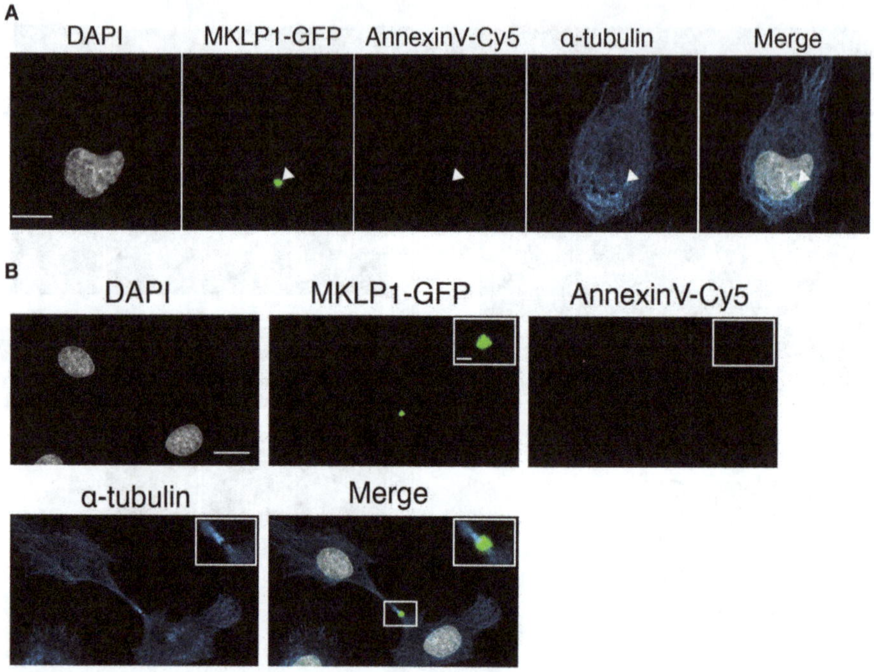

FIGURE 6 | No AnnexinV-Cy5 colocalization with midbody markers in MKLP1-GFP HeLa cells. (A,B) MKLP1-GFP HeLa cells were incubated with AnnexinV-Cy5 for 10 min in culture medium. Images were obtained as z-stacks every 0.38-μm and are maximum intensity projections. Shown are individual channels and merge for MKLP1-GFP (green), AnnexinV-Cy5 (red), immunofluorescence for α-tubulin (blue), and DAPI staining (white). Scale bars, 10 μm. **(A)** Example for monolateral midbody. White arrow heads indicate the MKLP1-GFP positive midbody. **(B)** Example for bilateral midbody. Inset, magnification of boxed region in merged channel. Scale bar, 1 μm.

Discussion

The present study is the first quantitative analysis of the lipid composition of released NE midbodies from mouse embryonic CF. A comparison of lipidome data from HeLa and NE midbodies showed a common enrichment of several lipid species (Atilla-Gokcumen et al., 2014). Among them, the enrichment in specific PS, TAG and Cer species was observed both in NE and HeLa midbodies compared to both lipoprotein particles and dividing cells. In comparison to midbodies from HeLa cells, NE midbodies displayed a wider extent of enrichment of other lipid classes and specific lipid species. This apparent divergence may reflect the functional complexity of the NE midbody in developing mouse embryos, in contrast to cancer-derived, cultured cells like HeLa. It has been shown previously that cultured cells showed a re-arrangement of protein levels involved in metabolic pathways at the expense of other pathways as compared to primary cells, which seems to be required for the adaptation to the cultured conditions (Pan et al., 2009). Particularly relevant for this study is the down-regulation of proteins involved in fatty acid metabolism in cell lines (Pan et al., 2009), a fact that can explain why we identified more varying lipid species in NE midbody when compared to HeLa midbody.

What could be the relevance of the combined enrichment of all the reported lipids for the midbody structure and function? Interestingly, both Ceramide species (C16 and C24-ceramide) identified in our and the previous study (Atilla-Gokcumen et al., 2014), respectively have been shown to contribute for apoptosis (Seumois et al., 2007). Moreover, the enrichment and exposure of PS to the outer leaflet of plasma membrane, a feature observed in midbody membranes, is a common feature of many apoptotic cells (Fadok et al., 1998). These two observations put together suggest that released midbody membranes might contain a potent apoptotic signal and, upon its releasing from the neural stem and progenitor cells and its engulfment by neighboring cells, it might alter the cell fate of both. The strong enrichment in unsaturated PE species in the midbody, is in line with its recognized fusogenic properties and the finding that PE species are exposed on the cell surface specifically at the cleavage furrow during late telophase of cytokinesis (Emoto et al., 1996). PE, due to its unique geometry (inverted cone) which is enhanced by the increase of the degree of unsaturation, in that it forms a non-bilayer structure, is thought to promote rapid phospholipid trans-bilayer movement (Ellens et al., 1989) and stalk membrane formation (Markin et al., 1984) facilitating membrane fusion and fission processes in cellular membranes a process required for midbody release after cytokinesis.

Cells in cytokinesis have been shown to possess more resilient cell membranes requiring three-fold higher forces to provoke their disruption when compared to cells in interphase (Atilla-Gokcumen et al., 2014). This observation is in line with the increase in relative saturation of the most abundant phospholipid in mammalian cells, PC (**Figure 2D**). We observe enrichment in PC species containing 0 and 1 unsaturations and a decrease in

PC species containing two or more unsaturations (**Figure 2D**). Unsaturation level of lipids is known to alter dramatically the physical properties of cell membranes by changing the membrane fluidity and order [Gennis RB, Biomembranes: Molecular structure and function (Springer Advanced Texts in Chemistry), 1989]. The specific enrichment in short chain TAGs is intriguing. TAGs in general are known to be metabolic energetic reservoirs in cells but the putative different functions of TAGs with specific fatty acid composition are still unknown.

Together, the lipid specificity observed in midbodies, seems to be intimately related to its structure and function. From it, we can conclude that midbodies possess relatively sturdy membranes due to the decrease of saturation of PC species, they are enriched in fusogenic lipids, unsaturated PEs, which facilitate fission and release of midbody, and are also enriched in potent signaling lipids, specific Ceramides and PS species that might influence neighboring cells if engulfed by them. All these observations put together highlight the importance of lipid compositional complexity, specificity and cellular localization in cell biology and how it can be directly associated with structural and functional aspects of cellular processes (Simons and Sampaio, 2011).

Although differences in lipid composition exist, common lipid species suggest shared characteristics between NE and HeLa midbodies. In HeLa cells, midbodies are known to be engulfed by a daughter cell through an actin-dependent phagocytosis-like mechanism (Crowell et al., 2014) while the release of midbody from neural-derived cells (Ettinger et al., 2011) seems not compatible with the engulfment by one of the daughter cells. PS is a structural phospholipid, which exists in the cytoplasmic leaflet of the plasma membrane bilayer and whose externalization has been associated with phagocytosis during apoptotic body clearance (Fadok et al., 1998), retinal rod and cone photoreceptors clearance (Kevany and Palczewski, 2010) and also in midbody clearance in *C. elegans* (Chai et al., 2012). In above examples, the phagocytosis of PS-externalized midbodies was carried out by non-daughter cells. Hence, it is possible that PS-externalized NE midbodies may be engulfed by phagocytes in the developing mouse embryo. It has been proposed, however, that other cell types in the developing mouse central nervous system such as microglia, astrocytes and even neural progenitor cells or neurons have the potential to behave as phagocytes due to the expression of phagocytic receptors (Sokolowski and Mandell, 2011). One of the phagocytic receptors, Gas6, which binds to PS, is indeed expressed highly in proliferative neural progenitor cells compared to neurogenic progenitor cells (Arai and Huttner, unpublished data). These lines of evidence support the idea that PS-externalized NE midbodies could be phagocytosed by sister neural progenitor cells through a phagocytosis-related mechanism using Gasp6 signaling. We previously reported that midbodies carrying the stem cell marker prominin-1 (Marzesco et al., 2005) were released from proliferative neural progenitor cells, which may contribute to their loss of stemness (Dubreuil et al., 2007). One possibility is that PS-externalized midbody could be engulfed by proliferative neural progenitor cells to maintain a balance for the stem cell capacity or serving as a means of communicating between the proliferative territories of the developing mouse brain. In addition to the PS externalized NE midbody, we also observed PS internalized NE midbodies (**Figure 4K**), which may reflect the heterogeneity of neural progenitor cells providing these two different types of midbodies. With the progression of neurogenesis, proliferative neural progenitor cells give rise to neuronally committed neurogenic progenitor cells (Haubensak et al., 2004). It would be interesting to identify which type of neural progenitor cells preferentially release either PS-externalized or -internalyzed midbodies.

What could be the fate of the biological components of NE midbodies after cells take them up? The engulfed midbody should be digested in lysosomes into monomolecular species, which are recycled if necessary. Fatty acids from the PS species of the NE midbody could also be recycled, if any, it participates on any metabolic pathways. Amongst the PS species identified in our lipidomics, the presence of omega-3 and 6 fatty acids that cannot be produced *de novo* have been strongly suggested, for instance, (PS [38:4] = PS [18:0–20:4], arachidonic acid [20:4]) (Sampaio et al., 2011). Therefore, the recycling of midbodies could participate to the essential lipid metabolism during cortical development, participating to the maintenance of a lipid species pool for controlling proper neurogenesis.

Methods

Animals

All mouse embryos used were wildtype C57BL/six mice obtained by overnight mating of wildtype C57BL/six males and females. Noon of the day on which the vaginal plug was observed was defined as embryonic day (E) 0.5. All animal studies were conducted in accordance with German animal welfare legislation, and the necessary licenses obtained from the regional Ethical Commission for Animal Experimentation of Dresden, Germany.

Enrichment of the Midbody Fraction Using Velocity Sucrose Density Gradient Centrifugation

E11.5 C57BL/6 mouse embryos were dissected in ice-cold 150 mM NH_4Ac dissolved in lipid mass spectrometry-grade water (Merck; LiChrosolv grade). CF was collected as described (Marzesco et al., 2005). 1–2 μl of CF per embryo were collected and pooled in a 1.5 ml Eppendorf tube (Eppendorf) on ice. Seventy-six micro liter of CF were mixed with 4 μl of 100x proteinase inhibitor mix (Roche) and 320 μl of 2.5 M sucrose in water to yield a total of 400 μl of CF mixture at a final concentration of 2 M sucrose. The CF mix was transferred into the bottom of an ultraclean ultracentrifugation tube (Beckman coulter). The gradient was prepared by adding layers of less dense sucrose solutions (400 μl of 1.6 M, 400 μl of 1 M, 300 μl of 0.3 M, and 300 μl of 0.1 M) upon one another. The samples were centrifuged in a TLS55 swinging rotor (Beckman coulter) at 50,000 rpm for 18 h at 4°C with a no deceleration profile. Immediately after the centrifugation, 180 μl fractions were collected into 1.5 ml Eppendorf tubes on ice. Ten micro liter of each fraction were used to determine the sucrose concentration in the fraction, 85 μl were used each for Western blotting and lipid mass spectrometry. In case of electron microscopy (EM) analysis, 10 μl of each fraction were fixed overnight at 4°C in 0.5% of EM grade glutaraldehyde/4%

paraformaldehyde in 0.12 M sodium phosphate buffer, pH 7.2.

Protein and Lipid Precipitations from Sucrose Samples

For immunoblotting, samples were subjected to methanol-chloroform precipitation by mixing samples in 1:4:1:3 ratio (sample:methanol:chloroform:water). Protein was precipitated by gently vortexing the tube followed by centrifugation at 13,000 rpm for 5 min at room temperature (r.t.). The upper layer was removed without touching the interface layer. Two-hundred and fifty-five liter of methanol were added (3 × volume of the original sample volume, 85 μl). Proteins were pelleted by centrifugation at 13,000 rpm for 5 min at r.t. and resuspended in 2x concentrated SDS Laemmli sample buffer. Protein samples were denatured by boiling at 95°C for 5 min and stored at −20°C.

For lipid extraction, 85 μl sample from each fraction were transferred into a 1.5 ml Eppendorf tube filled with 157 mM of ammonium bicarbonate (NH_4HCO_3) up to 1.5 ml. Particles were pelleted in the TLA55 fixed-angle rotor (Beckman coulter) at 30,000 rpm for 4 h at 4°C. Removed NH_4HCO_3 and pelleted lipid samples were frozen in liquid nitrogen and stored at −80°C.

Lipid Extraction for Lipid Mass Spectrometry

Lipid samples were mixed with 200 μl of 157 mM of NH4HCO3 and vortexed at 1400 rpm at 4°C. Ten micro liter of an internal standard lipid mix (Avanti Polar lipids; PC, PE, PS, PG, PA, Cer, SM, GalCer, LacCer, Chol, and DAG) was added to each sample. To extract all lipids, 1 ml of a 2.75:1 mixture of chloroform/methanol was added to each tube and vortexed at 1400 rpm for 1 h at 4°C. Fractions with high sucrose content (>1 M) were "pre-washed" with 200 μl of MS grade water before the extraction to remove excess sucrose. After extraction, sample tubes were centrifuged at 1000 g for 2 min at 4°C. Bottom phases were transferred into fresh 1.5 ml Eppendorf tubes (10:1 lipid fraction). The organic solvent was evaporated using a vacuum centrifuge. Dried samples were re-suspended with 100 μl of a 1:2 mixture of chloroform/methanol and vortexed for 10 min at 4°C. This re-suspension solution was mixed with MS compatible polarity specific buffers to optimize for ionization of specific lipids as described previously (Carvalho, 2012). The data was acquired on a LTQ-Orbitrap using high mass resolution $R_{m-z=400} = 100,000$ and the spectra was analyzed with LipidXplorer software (Herzog et al., 2011, 2012).

Immunofluorescence, Electron Microscopy, Annexin V-Cy5 Injection, and Image Acquisition

Living embryos at E11.5 were dissected out of the uterus with the placenta intact and transferred into 1x Tyrode solution (Sigma-Aldrich). AnnexinV-Cy5 solution (BioVision) was diluted to 1:300 in 1x binding buffer (10 mM Hepes-NaOH pH7.4 containing 140 mM NaCl and 2.5 mM $CaCl_2$) and injected into telencephalic vesicles of living embryos (1x concentrated binding buffer was used as control). Injected embryos were incubated at r.t. for 30 min (room air and protected from light). Whole embryos were fixed for 20–25 h at 4°C in 4% paraformaldehyde in 0.12 M sodium phosphate buffer, pH 7.2. For cryosectioning, embryos were equilibrated for 12–24 h at 4°C in 30% sucrose in PBS, embedded in Tissue-Tek O.C.T compound (Sakura Finetek), and stored at −20°C. Cryostat sections (10 μm) were rehydrated with PBS, quenched with 50 mM NH_4CL for 30 min, washed with 0.01% Digitonin (Sigma-Aldrich) in PBS for 30 min and blocked with 3% BSA in 0.01% Digitonin/PBS for 30 min at r.t. Sections were washed with 1% BSA in 0.01% Digitonin/PBS and incubated overnight at 4°C with first primary antibody, followed by incubation for 1 h at r.t. with fluorescently labeled secondary antibodies and DAPI (4′,6-diamidino-2-phenylindole, Roche) in 1% BSA in 0.01% Digitonin/PBS. Sections were mounted in Mowiol. For electron microscopy, E11.5 dorsal telencephalon was analyzed by transmission EM, with pre- or post-embedding prominin-1 immunolabeling.

The following primary antibodies were used: rabbit anti-Prominin-1 [αD, MPI-CBG; 1:20,000 for immunoblotting (IB)]; goat antibody against apolipoprotein A1 (Biodesign; 1:1000); mouse monoclonal antibodies against CRIK [BD bioscience; 1:200 for immunofluorescence (IF) and 1:4000 for IB], α-tubulin (Sigma; 1:300 for IF and 1:60,000 for IB) and Aurora B (BD bioscience; 1:300) and rat anti-Prominin-1 (13A4, MPI-CBG; 1:300 for IF). Secondary antibodies were: horseradish peroxidase-coupled antibodies (Jackson laboratory), Alexa Fluor 488, 555, and 647 labeled IgG antibodies (Invitrogen).

Fluorescence images were acquired by confocal microscopy (Zeiss LSM 700) and images were acquired with a Zeiss Plan-Apochromat 20x, 0.8 NA and a Zeiss C-Apochromat 40x, 1.2 NA objectives.

Live-cell Time-lapse Microscopy

The protocol for this time-lapse microscopy has been described previously (Ettinger et al., 2011). Briefly, Neuro-2a MKLP1-GFP cells were grown on chambered coverslips (Lab-Tek, Nunc) in DMEM-GlutaMax medium supplemented with 10% FCS and incubated for 24 h at 37°C with 5% CO_2. The medium was replaced with Annexin V-Cy5 containing medium (1:5000) and cells were imaged with a Zeiss Axiovert 200 M inverted epifluorescence microscope equipped with a motorized stage, incubator, humidifier, and carbon dioxide supply (Visitron Systems, Germany). Bright-field and fluorescence images were acquired using a C-Apochromat 40x water immersion objective (NA 1.4) and recorded with a Roper Scientific Cool SNAP ES CCD camera using MetaMorph software. Multiple fields were acquired in parallel per experiment at 12 min intervals for up to 24 h.

Annexin V-Cy5 Incubation with the Neuro-2a-MKLP1 Transgenic Cell Line

Neuro-2a MKLP1-GFP cells were grown on poly-L-lysine coated coverslips in DMEM-GlutaMax medium supplemented with 10% FCS and incubated for 24 h at 37°C with 5% CO_2. The medium was replaced with Annexin V-Cy5 containing medium (1:2500), incubated for 10 min at r.t. protected from light, and fixed with 4% paraformaldehyde in 0.12 M sodium phosphate buffer, pH 7.2. Cells were further processed for immunofluorescence like sections of mouse embryos.

Author Contributions

YA designed and performed the experiments, analyzed the data and co-wrote the manuscript, JS designed and performed lipid mass spectrometry, analyzed the data and co-wrote the manuscript, MB performed EM and co-wrote the manuscript, AE helped and performed time-lapse imaging, and co-wrote the manuscript, CH performed experiments and WH analyzed data, co-wrote the manuscript and supervised project. The authors declare that they have no competing financial interests.

Acknowledgments

We thank the animal and light microscopy facilities of MPI-CBG for excellent support, Drs. Vitary Matiash, Dominik Schwudke, Andrej Shevchenko, and Kai Simons for helpful discussion at the beginning of the lipid mass spectrometry and project. YA was supported by ARC (Association pour la Recherche sur le Cancer), FRM (Fondation pour la Recherche Médicale), and JSPS (Japan Society for the Promotion of Science) and WH was supported by grants from the DFG (SFB 655, A2; TRR 83, Tp6) by the DFG-funded Center for Regenerative Therapies Dresden, the Fonds der Chemischen Industrie and ERC.

Supplementary Material

Supplementary Figure 1 | Phosphatidylserine is on the outer-leaflet of the apical plasma membrane of the neuronal progenitor cells. (A,B) Micrographs of mouse embryonic E11.5 coronal cryosections of dorsal telencephalon injected with Annexin V-Cy5 binding buffer. Sections were consecutively stained by immunofluorescence for prominin-1 (green) and counterstained with DAPI (white). Images are z-projections of 32 consecutive 0.38-μm optical sections. **(B)** Higher magnifications of the apical plasma membrane of the ventricular zone [boxed region indicated in **(A)**]. Red-white arrows, Annexin V-Cy5 single positive particles, green arrows, prominin-1 single positive midbody particles, yellow arrows, Annexin V-Cy5 and prominin-1 double positive midbody particles. Scale bars, 50 μm **(A)** and 10 μm **(B)**. **(C)** Percentage of three different types of particles on the apical plasma membrane of the ventricular zone, classified by decoration with prominin-1 positive and Annexin V-Cy5 positive signal. Data are the mean of six 213-μm wide fields from three different embryos and litters; total number of counted particles, 455 for prominin+ AnnexinV–, 354 for prominin+ AnnexinV+ and 16 for prominin– AnnexinV+; error bars indicate SD; $^{*}P < 0.05$, $^{****}P < 0.0001$; unpaired *t*-test.

Supplementary Figure 2 | Expression of midbody markes in MKLP1-GFP Neuro-2a cells. (A,B) Fluorescence for MKLP1-GFP (green), immunofluorescence for α-tubulin and Aurora B kinase (red) in Neuro-2a MKLP1-GFP cells during telophase **(A)** and interphase **(B)** combined with DAPI staining (white). Images are maximum intensity projections of z-stacks of optical sections taken every 0.38 μm. Insets, magnifications of bilateral **(A)** and monolateral **(B)** midbodies. Scale bars, 10 μm and 1 μm (inset).

Supplementary Figure 3 | Expression of midbody markers in MKLP1-GFP HeLa cells. (A) Fluorescence for MKLP1-GFP (green) and immunofluorescence for α-tubulin in telophase (2 upper panels) and interphase (lower panels) cells combined with DAPI staining (white). Scale bars, 10 μm. **(B)** Fluorescence for MKLP1-GFP (green) and immunofluorescence for Aurora B kinase in telophase (upper panels) and interphase (lower panels) cells having midbody combined with DAPI staining (white). Scale bars, 10 μm. Insets, magnifications of newly formed midbodies with telophase-bridge between the two daughter cells intact [upper panels in **(A,B)**] or inherited, monolateral midbodies with no apparent cytoplasmic bridge to the other daughter cell [lower panels in **(A,B)**]. Scale bars, 1 μm.

References

Atilla-Gokcumen, G. E., Muro, E., Relat-Goberna, J., Sasse, S., Bedigian, A., Coughlin, M. L., et al. (2014). Dividing cells regulate their lipid composition and localization. *Cell* 156, 428–439. doi: 10.1016/j.cell.2013.12.015

Buck, R. C., and Tidsale, J. M. (1962). An electron microscopic study of the cleavage furrow in mammalian cells. *J. Cell Biol.* 13, 117–125. doi: 10.1083/jcb.13.1.117

Carvalho, V. M. (2012). The coming of age of liquid chromatography coupled to tandem mass spectrometry in the endocrinology laboratory. *J. Chromatogr. B Analyt. Technol. Biomed. Life. Sci.* 883–884, 50–58. doi: 10.1016/j.jchromb.2011.08.027

Chai, Y., Tian, D., Yang, Y., Feng, G., Cheng, Z., Li, W., et al. (2012). Apoptotic regulators promote cytokinetic midbody degradation in *C. elegans*. *J. Cell Biol.* 199, 1047–1055. doi: 10.1083/jcb.201209050

Chen, C.-T., Ettinger, A. W., Huttner, W. B., and Doxsey, S. J. (2013). Resurrecting remnants: the lives of post-mitotic midbodies. *Trends Cell Biol.* 23, 118–128. doi: 10.1016/j.tcb.2012.10.012

Corbeil, D., Marzesco, A.-M., Wilsch-Bräuninger, M., and Huttner, W. B. (2010). The intriguing links between prominin-1 (CD133), cholesterol-based membrane microdomains, remodeling of apical plasma membrane protrusions, extracellular membrane particles, and (neuro)epithelial cell differentiation. *FEBS Lett.* 584, 1659–1664. doi: 10.1016/j.febslet.2010.01.050

Crowell, E. F., Gaffuri, A.-L., Gayraud-Morel, B., Tajbakhsh, S., and Echard, A. (2014). Engulfment of the midbody remnant after cytokinesis in mammalian cells. *J. Cell Sci.* 127, 3840–3851. doi: 10.1242/jcs.154732

Dubreuil, V., Marzesco, A.-M., Corbeil, D., Huttner, W. B., and Wilsch-Bräuninger, M. (2007). Midbody and primary cilium of neural progenitors release extracellular membrane particles enriched in the stem cell marker prominin-1. *J. Cell Biol.* 176, 483–495. doi: 10.1083/jcb.200608137

Ellens, H., Siegel, D. P., Alford, D., Yeagle, P. L., Boni, L., Lis, L. J., et al. (1989). Membrane fusion and inverted phases. *Biochemistry* 28, 3692–3703. doi: 10.1021/bi00435a011

Emoto, K., Kobayashi, T., Yamaji, A., Aizawa, H., Yahara, I., Inoue, K., et al. (1996). Redistribution of phosphatidylethanolamine at the cleavage furrow of dividing cells during cytokinesis. *Proc. Natl. Acad. Sci. U.S.A.* 93, 12867–12872. doi: 10.1073/pnas.93.23.12867

Ettinger, A. W., Wilsch-Bräuninger, M., Marzesco, A.-M., Bickle, M., Lohmann, A., Maliga, Z., et al. (2011). Proliferating versus differentiating stem and cancer cells exhibit distinct midbody-release behaviour. *Nat. Commun.* 2, 503. doi: 10.1038/ncomms1511

Fadok, V. A., Bratton, D. L., Frasch, S. C., Warner, M. L., and Henson, P. M. (1998). The role of phosphatidylserine in recognition of apoptotic cells by phagocytes. *Cell Death Differ.* 5, 551–562. doi: 10.1038/sj.cdd.4400404

Furbee, J. W., Francone, O., and Parks, J. S. (2002). *In vivo* contribution of LCAT to apolipoprotein B lipoprotein cholesteryl esters in LDL receptor and apolipoprotein E knockout mice. *J. Lipid Res.* 43, 428–437.

Glotzer, M. (2009). The 3Ms of central spindle assembly: microtubules, motors and MAPs. *Nat. Rev. Mol. Cell Biol.* 10, 9–20. doi: 10.1038/nrm2609

Haubensak, W., Attardo, A., Denk, W., and Huttner, W. B. (2004). Neurons arise in the basal neuroepithelium of the early mammalian telencephalon: a major site of neurogenesis. *Proc. Natl. Acad. Sci. U.S.A.* 101, 3196–3201. doi: 10.1073/pnas.0308600100

Herzog, R., Schuhmann, K., Schwudke, D., Sampaio, J. L., Bornstein, S. R., Schroeder, M., et al. (2012). LipidXplorer: a software for consensual cross-platform lipidomics. *PLoS ONE* 7:e29851. doi: 10.1371/journal.pone.0029851

Herzog, R., Schwudke, D., Schuhmann, K., Sampaio, J. L., Bornstein, S. R., Schroeder, M., et al. (2011). A novel informatics concept for high-throughput shotgun lipidomics based on the molecular fragmentation query language. *Genome Biol.* 12:R8. doi: 10.1186/gb-2011-12-1-r8

Hu, C.-K., Coughlin, M., and Mitchison, T. J. (2012). Midbody assembly and its regulation during cytokinesis. *Mol. Biol. Cell* 23, 1024–1034. doi: 10.1091/mbc.E11-08-0721

Kevany, B. M., and Palczewski, K. (2010). Phagocytosis of retinal rod and cone photoreceptors. *Physiology (Bethesda)* 25, 8–15. doi: 10.1152/physiol.00038.2009

Kuo, T.-C., Chen, C.-T., Baron, D., Onder, T. T., Loewer, S., Almeida, S., et al. (2011). Midbody accumulation through evasion of autophagy contributes to cellular reprogramming and tumorigenicity. *Nat. Cell Biol.* 13, 1214–1223. doi: 10.1038/ncb2332

Madaule, P., Eda, M., Watanabe, N., Fujisawa, K., Matsuoka, T., Bito, H., et al. (1998). Role of citron kinase as a target of the small GTPase Rho in cytokinesis. *Nature* 394, 491–494. doi: 10.1038/28873

Markin, V. S., Kozlov, M. M., and Borovjagin, V. L. (1984). On the theory of membrane fusion. The stalk mechanism. *Gen. Physiol. Biophys.* 3, 361–377.

Marzesco, A.-M., Janich, P., Wilsch-Bräuninger, M., Dubreuil, V., Langenfeld, K., Corbeil, D., et al. (2005). Release of extracellular membrane particles carrying the stem cell marker prominin-1 (CD133) from neural progenitors and other epithelial cells. *J. Cell Sci.* 118, 2849–2858. doi: 10.1242/jcs.02439

Pan, C., Kumar, C., Bohl, S., Klingmueller, U., and Mann, M. (2009). Comparative proteomic phenotyping of cell lines and primary cells to assess preservation of cell type-specific functions. *Mol. Cell. Proteomics* 8, 443–450. doi: 10.1074/mcp.M800258-MCP200

Poser, I., Sarov, M., Hutchins, J. R. A., Hériché, J.-K., Toyoda, Y., Pozniakovsky, A., et al. (2008). BAC TransgeneOmics: a high-throughput method for exploration of protein function in mammals. *Nat. Methods* 5, 409–415. doi: 10.1038/nmeth.1199

Sampaio, J. L., Gerl, M. J., Klose, C., Ejsing, C. S., Beug, H., Simons, K., et al. (2011). Membrane lipidome of an epithelial cell line. *Proc. Natl. Acad. Sci. U.S.A.* 108, 1903–1907. doi: 10.1073/pnas.1019267108

Schutte, B., Nuydens, R., Geerts, H., and Ramaekers, F. (1998). Annexin V binding assay as a tool to measure apoptosis in differentiated neuronal cells. *J. Neurosci. Methods* 86, 63–69. doi: 10.1016/S0165-0270(98)00147-2

Seumois, G., Fillet, M., Gillet, L., Faccinetto, C., Desmet, C., François, C., et al. (2007). *De novo* C16- and C24-ceramide generation contributes to spontaneous neutrophil apoptosis. *J. Leukoc. Biol.* 81, 1477–1486. doi: 10.1189/jlb.0806529

Simons, K., and Sampaio, J. L. (2011). Membrane organization and lipid rafts. *Cold Spring Harb. Perspect. Biol.* 3:a004697. doi: 10.1101/cshperspect.a004697

Sokolowski, J. D., and Mandell, J. W. (2011). Phagocytic clearance in neurodegeneration. *Am. J. Pathol.* 178, 1416–1428. doi: 10.1016/j.ajpath.2010.12.051

Verkleij, A. J., Zwaal, R. F., Roelofsen, B., Comfurius, P., Kastelijn, D., and van Deenen, L. L. (1973). The asymmetric distribution of phospholipids in the human red cell membrane. A combined study using phospholipases and freeze-etch electron microscopy. *Biochim. Biophys. Acta* 323, 178–193. doi: 10.1016/0005-2736(73)90143-0

Willnow, T. E., Hammes, A., and Eaton, S. (2007). Lipoproteins and their receptors in embryonic development: more than cholesterol clearance. *Developement* 134, 3239–3249. doi: 10.1242/dev.004408

13

High-Mobility Group Box 1 Contributes to Cerebral Cortex Injury in a Neonatal Hypoxic-Ischemic Rat Model by Regulating the Phenotypic Polarization of Microglia

Yanyan Sun[1], Mingyan Hei[2], Zhihui Fang[3], Zhen Tang[1], Bo Wang[2] and Na Hu[1]*

[1] Department of Pediatrics, The Third Xiangya Hospital of Central South University, Changsha, China, [2] Neonatal Center, Beijing Children's Hospital, Capital Medical University, Beijing, China, [3] Department of Nuclear Medicine, The Second Xiangya Hospital of Central South University, Changsha, China

***Correspondence:**
Mingyan Hei
heimingyan@bch.com.cn

Neonatal hypoxic-ischemic (HI) encephalopathy is a severe disease for which there is currently no curative treatment. Recent evidence suggests that high-mobility group box 1 (HMGB1) protein can promote neuroinflammation after stroke in adult rodents, but its role in perinatal hypoxic-ischemic brain damage (HIBD) remains largely uninvestigated. In the present work, the potential role of HMGB1 in the pathogenesis of HIBD was explored. A HIBD model was established in postpartum day 7 rat pups. HMGB1 expression, the cellular distribution of HMGB1, and microglial activation were all evaluated. Glycyrrhizin (GL), an inhibitor of HMGB1, was used to investigate whether the inhibition of HMGB1 modulated microglial M1/M2 polarization or attenuated brain damage after HI. HAPI microglial cells and primary neurons were cultured *in vitro* and an oxygen-glucose deprivation model was established to evaluate the effects of different microglial-conditioned media on neurons using GL and recombinant HMGB1. Results showed that the expression of HMGB1 was increased in both the ipsilateral cortex and peripheral blood 72 h after HI. Immunofluorescence analyses showed that HMGB1 in the cortex was primarily expressed in neurons. This increase in cortical HMGB1 expression 72 h after HI was characterized by increased co-expression with microglia, rather than neurons or astrocytes. The expression of both M1 and M2 microglia was upregulated 72 h after HI. The administration of GL significantly suppressed M1 microglial polarization and promoted M2 microglial polarization. Meanwhile, GL pretreatment significantly alleviated brain edema and cerebral infarction. *In vitro* experimentation showed that HMGB1-induced M1-conditioned media aggravated neuronal damage, but this effect was neutralized by GL. These findings suggest that HMGB1 may result in an imbalance of M1/M2 microglial polarization in the cortex and thus cause neuronal injury. Pharmacological blockade of HMGB1 signaling may attenuate this imbalanced polarization of microglia and thus could be used as a therapeutic strategy against brain injury in HIBD.

Keywords: hypoxic-ischemic (HI), HMGB1, microglia, polarization, cerebral cortex injury, neonatal

INTRODUCTION

Although neonatal resuscitation has been strongly promoted in recent years, moderate to severe hypoxic-ischemic brain damage (HIBD) still occurs after asphyxia (Barkhuizen et al., 2017). The pathogenesis of HIBD is complex, and there currently exists no effective treatment except for hypothermia. Even with timely hypothermia, more than 40% of neonates who experience severe asphyxia in the perinatal period still exhibit adverse outcomes, or even die as a result (Wu et al., 2016).

The expression of pro-inflammatory factors is higher in the developing brain than in the mature brain (Kaur et al., 2017). Given that HIBD is a pathological condition of the developing brain, it is hypothesized that inflammation, primarily mediated by microglia, may play an important role in HIBD after perinatal asphyxia. Microglia-related neuroinflammation is reported to be associated with the release of cytokines and additional inflammatory mediators, leading to secondary neuronal injury (Umekawa et al., 2015). Microglia can be classified into two main forms: M1-type (pro-inflammatory) and M2-type (anti-inflammatory) (Colton, 2009). M1 microglia promote neuronal death by expressing pro-inflammatory mediators, such as interleukin-6 (IL-6), tumor necrosis factor-α (TNF-α), and inducible nitric oxide synthase (iNOS). In contrast, M2 microglia promote tissue repair and support neuronal survival through the secretion of anti-inflammatory cytokines such as transforming growth factor-β (TGF-β), interleukin-10 (IL-10), and arginase-1 (Olah et al., 2011; Patel et al., 2013). Normally, there exists a careful balance of pro-inflammatory M1 and anti-inflammatory M2 microglia (Jin et al., 2019). Both *in vitro* and *in vivo* experiments have proved that correction of a polarization imbalance of M1/M2 microglia can inhibit the release of pro-inflammatory cytokines and decrease neurotoxicity (Weinstein et al., 2010; Xia et al., 2015; Zhou et al., 2019). *In vivo* studies have reported an imbalance of microglial M1/M2 polarization after hypoxic-ischemic (HI) exposure (Weinstein et al., 2010; Bhalala et al., 2014). However, the exact mechanism underlying this M1/M2 microglia imbalance after HI in neonatal models remains unclear.

High-mobility group box 1 (HMGB1) is a chromatin-associated protein widely expressed in the nuclei of brain cells, which, under physiological conditions, promotes neurite outgrowth and thus brain development (Merenmies et al., 1991; Guazzi et al., 2003; Liu et al., 2010). Under pathological conditions, HMGB1 can act as a pro-inflammatory factor, promoting brain damage (Wang et al., 1999; Zhang et al., 2011; Andersson et al., 2018). Studies have demonstrated that HMGB1 is involved in the pathogenesis of ischemic stroke in adult rodents, activating microglia and promoting neuroinflammation (Ye et al., 2019). In immature animal models, it was reported that HMGB1 translocated from nuclear to cytosolic compartments after HI (Zhang et al., 2016), and the translocation of HMGB1 was primarily in neurons along with release from apoptotic cells (Chen et al., 2019). This translocation may enable the action of HMGB1 as a proinflammatory cytokine that contributes to HI injury in the developing brain (Zhang et al., 2016). Unfortunately, the above studies mainly explored the cellular localization changes of HMGB1 after HI, further mechanism by which HMGB1 aggravates brain injury in HIBD is still unclear.

The objective of the present study was to explore whether HMGB1 played an important role in regulating the phenotypic balance of M1/M2 microglia in the cortex of neonatal SD rats after HI exposure, and whether the HMGB1 inhibitor, glycyrrhizin (GL), could modulate microglial M1/M2 polarization after HI *in vivo* and *in vitro*. We found that HMGB1 was upregulated in microglia after HI. Furthermore, HMGB1 was able to regulate the M1/M2 phenotypic polarization of microglia, leading to cortical injury.

MATERIALS AND METHODS

Animals and Ethical Permission

All experiments were performed in accordance with the guidelines for experimental animal use of Central South University. The protocol was approved by the ethics committee of the Third Xiangya Hospital of Central South University (No. 2016-S006). Perinatal Sprague-Dawley (SD) rats were purchased from Central South University (China). All rats were housed in a 12-h light/dark cycled facility with free access to food and water.

HIBD Animal Model and Drug Administration

The Rice and Vannucci HIBD model was induced with minor modifications in postpartum day 7 (P7) rat pups of both genders. In brief, rat pups were anesthetized with isoflurane and the left common carotid artery was permanently ligated with 5–0 silk sutures. Pups were returned to the dam for a 2 h recovery before initiation of a 2 h hypoxia exposure (37°C, 8% O_2/92% N_2). The sham-operation control animals were given only a small incision on the left side of the neck and the left common carotid artery was isolated without artery ligation or hypoxia treatment.

SD rat pups were randomly divided into three groups: sham + PBS, HI + PBS, and HI + GL. In the HI + GL group, GL was administered 1 h before artery ligation (20 mg/kg, i.p.). In the other two groups, an equal volume of 0.01M PBS was administered.

Primary Neuron Cultures and Microglial-Conditioned Media Treatment

Cells from the microglia-like cell line HAPI (highly aggressive proliferating cell type) were seeded into 6-well plates at 1×10^5/mL and incubated overnight in high-glucose Dulbecco's Modified Eagle Medium (DMEM) containing 10% fetal bovine serum (FBS). Then, an oxygen-glucose deprivation (OGD) model was established to mimic the *in vivo* HI process. HAPI cells were divided into the following three groups: OGD + PBS, OGD + GL, and OGD + r-HMGB1. In brief, PBS (0.01M), GL (55 μM), and recombinant HMGB1 (r-HMGB1, 10 ng/mL) were added to the respective cell groups for 2 h. The cells' medium was then replaced with glucose-free Earle's balanced salt solution, and they were placed in an oxygen- deprived incubator

(93% N_2/5% CO_2/2% O_2) at 37°C for 12 h. Finally, the culture supernatant was collected, one part was used for an ELISA, and the other was used as a conditioned medium (CM) for primary neurons.

Primary cortical neurons were obtained from P1 rat pups. In brief, the cortices of P1 rats were isolated, digested by trypsin, and filtered using a 50 µm sterile nylon filter. Cells were then placed in 24-well plates pre-coated with poly-L-lysine in a neurobasal medium with 10% FBS and B27 supplement. The cells were placed in an incubator (37°C, 5% CO_2) to differentiate for 7 days. At this point, the neuronal medium was removed and substituted with the aforementioned CM from HAPI microglial cells. To analyze the effects of CM on cell viability, neurons were cultured with this microglial CM for 24 h.

Cell Viability and Neurite Length Measurement

Primary cortical neurons were seeded in 96-well plates at a density of 5×10^3 cells/well. After culturing with microglial CM for 24 h, a cell viability assay was performed using a cell-counting kit (CCK-8; Beyotime, China). The optical density was read at a wave length of 450nm using an EnVision Xcite microplate reader (PerkinElmer, United States). Cell viability was calculated using the following formula:

$$Cell\ viability\ (\%) = \frac{optical\ density\ of\ treated\ group}{optical\ density\ of\ control\ group} \times 100$$

For neurite length measurement, three digital images were taken per well after microtubule-associated protein 2 (MAP-2) and 4′, 6′- diamidino-2-phenylindole (DAPI) immunostaining. Using the plugins NeuronJ and ImageScience, Image J software was then used to calculate the average neurite length of MAP-2- positive neurons in every image following the instructions provided.

Western Blotting

Western blotting was used to assess the expression of HMGB1, ionized calcium-binding adaptor molecule 1 (Iba-1), and β-actin in the cortex. Briefly, frozen cortex samples were completely homogenized in lysis buffer containing Phenylmethanesulfonyl fluoride (PMSF, Beyotime, China, ST505) and Radio Immunoprecipitation Assay (RIPA, Beyotime, China, P0013B) and centrifuged at 12,000 rpm for 15 min at 4°C. The supernatant was collected and contained the total protein extracted from the tissue. The quantity of protein in the samples was determined using a BCA protein assay kit (Beyotime, China), according to the manufacturer's instructions. Samples (30 µg per lane) were separated by 12% sodium dodecyl sulfate polyacrylamide gel electrophoresis (SDS-PAGE) and transferred to polyvinylidene fluoride (PVDF) membranes. Membranes were blocked with 5% defatted milk for 2 h at room temperature (temperature of 20–25°C) and, then incubated overnight at 4°C with primary antibodies: rabbit anti-HMGB1 (1:1000 dilution, Abcam, ab18256), rabbit anti-Ibal (1:100 dilution, Abcam, ab178847), and rabbit anti-β-actin (1:2000 dilution, Proteintech, 14395-1-AP). After three washes in PBST (0.01M PBS containing 0.1% Tween-20), the membranes were incubated with secondary antibodies (goat anti-rabbit IgG, IRDye® 800CW Conjugated, 1:5000 dilution) at room temperature for 2 h. Finally, visualization of the blotted protein bands was accomplished using an infrared laser imaging system (Odyssey CLx, LI-COR, United States) and was quantified by densitometry. The relative expression levels of protein were normalized by the ratio of target protein (HMGB1 and Iba-1) to β-actin.

Enzyme-Linked Immunosorbent Assay (ELISA)

Under anesthesia, whole blood samples were collected from the left ventricles of the rats before transcardial perfusion. Subsequently, samples were centrifuged at 3000 rpm for 10 min at room temperature. The supernatants were collected and frozen at −80°C for further analyses. Before analysis, the samples were centrifuged again, and the supernatant was used for the ELISA assay. HMGB1 concentration was determined using an HMGB1 ELISA kit (Chondrex, United States, 6160), following the manufacturer's protocol.

For the *in vitro* experiment, the culture supernatant from HAPI microglia was collected for the ELISA. The concentrations of TNF-α, IL-1β, and IL-10 were determined using the following ELISA kits: TNF-α (Thermo Fisher, United States, 88-7340-22), IL-1β (R&D Systems, United States, DY501-05), and IL-10 (Abcam, United States, ab218796). All measurements were performed following the manufacturers' protocols.

Immunofluorescence Staining

Animals were anesthetized and, transcardially perfused with 0.01M PBS and 4% paraformaldehyde (PFA). The brains were then removed and post-fixed in 4% PFA immediately. After dehydration with a sucrose gradient, 20 serial coronal sections were cut across the middle of hemisphere. Sections were then washed three times with 0.01M PBS, blocked with 5% bovine serum albumin (BSA), and used for active HMGB1, Ibal, neuronal nuclei (NeuN), glial fibrillary acidic protein (GFAP), CD86, and CD206 staining. The sections were then incubated overnight at 4°C with the following primary antibodies: rabbit anti-Ibal (1:100 dilution, Abcam, ab178847), rabbit anti-NeuN (1:300 dilution, Abcam, ab177487), mouse anti-HMGB1 (1:500 dilution, Gene Tex, GT348), mouse anti-GFAP (1:300 dilution, Cell Signaling, 3670T), rabbit anti-HMGB1 (1:1000 dilution, Abcam, ab18256), rabbit anti-CD86 (1:200 dilution, Proteintech, 13395-1-AP), rabbit anti-CD206 (1:500 dilution, Abcam, ab125028), and mouse anti- Ibal (1:500 dilution, Abcam, ab15690). After three washes in 0.01M PBS, the sections were incubated with Cy3-conjugated goat anti-rabbit IgG (1:2000 dilution, Boster Biological Technology, BA1032) or FITC-conjugated goat anti-mouse IgG (1:2000 dilution, Boster Biological Technology, BA1101) for 1 h at room temperature. After three washes in 0.01M PBS, these were then covered with diamidino-2-phenylindole (DAPI, 1:1000, Beyotime, C1002) for 5 min. For each staining, five non-overlapping digital microscopic images of cortical areas were randomly captured using a fluorescence microscope (IX71, OLYMPUS, Japan). The number of positive cells was determined using Image-Pro Plus 6.0 (Media Cybernetics, United States).

The cultured cortical neurons were fixed with 4% PFA for 24 h after culturing in microglial-CM. They were then incubated with rabbit anti-MAP2 antibodies (1:200 dilution, Proteintech, 17490-1-AP) overnight at 4°C. After three washes in 0.01M PBS, they were incubated with Cy3-conjugated goat anti-rabbit IgG (1:2000 dilution, Boster Biological Technology, BA1032) and then covered with DAPI. Digital microscopic images were taken using the aforementioned IX71 fluorescence microscope.

Reverse Transcription and qRT-PCR

Under deep anesthesia, the brains of the rats were removed and the cerebral cortex was rapidly separated and snap-frozen in liquid nitrogen. Total RNA was isolated using TRIzol reagent (Invitrogen, United States). The first-strand cDNA was synthesized using the Reverse Transcription System (Toyobo, Osaka, Japan), according to the manufacturer's protocol. The relative expression level of mRNA was then assessed using the SYBR Green Real-time PCR Master Mix Kit (Toyobo, Osaka, Japan) and quantified using the Mastercycler® ep realplex qRT-PCR system (Eppendorf, Germany) with glyceraldehyde 3-phosphate dehydrogenase (GAPDH) as the reference gene. All primers used in the qRT-PCR reactions were purchased from Sangon Biotech (China). The sequences of the primer pairs are described as follows: TNF-α (forward: 5′-GCA TGA TCC GAG ATG TGG AAC TGG-3′; reverse: 5′-CGC CAC GAG CAG GAA TGA GAA G-3′); IL-6 (forward: 5′-AGG AGT GGC TAA GGA CCA AGA CC-3′; reverse: 5′-TGC CGA GTA GAC CTC ATA GTG ACC-3′); IL-1β (forward: 5′-ATC TCA CAG CAT CTC GAC AAG-3′; reverse: 5′-CAC ACT AGC AGG TCG TCA TCC-3′); iNOS (forward: 5′-AGA TCC CGA AAC GCT ACA CTT-3′; reverse: 5′-TGC GGC TGG ACT TCT CAC TC-3′); arginase-1 (forward: 5′-ACA TCA ACA CTC CGC TGA CAA CC-3′; reverse: 5′-GCC GAT GTA CAC GAT GTC CTT GG-3′); TGF-β (forward: 5′-GGC ACC ATC CAT GAC ATG AAC CG-3′; reverse: 5′-GCC GTA CAC AGC AGT TCT CTG-3′); IL-4 (forward: 5′-CAA GGA ACA CCA CGG AGA ACG AG-3′; reverse: 5′-CTT CAA GCA CGG AGG TAC ATC ACG-3′); GAPDH (forward: 5′-GAC ATG CCG CCT GGA GAA AC-3′; reverse: 5′-AGC CCA GGA TGC CCT TTA GT-3′). The relative expression of mRNA was calculated using the $2^{-\Delta\Delta Ct}$ method.

Infarct Ratio Calculation

The rat brains were rapidly removed 3 days post-HI and frozen in a freezer at −20°C for 20 min. They were then taken out and four 1.5 mm thick sections were sliced. These sections were placed in 2% TTC staining solution, and incubated at 37°C for 20 min in the dark. Finally, the stained brain slices were placed on a drape for photographing. The aforementioned Image-Pro Plus 6.0 software was used to calculate the volume of each section. The following formula was used to calculate infarct ratio:

$$Ratio\ of\ infarct = \frac{infarct\ volume}{total\ section\ volume} \times 100$$

Brain Water Content

Rats were sacrificed under anesthesia24 h after HI. The brains were bisected to generate two hemispheres (ipsilateral and contralateral to the injury) which were then immediately weighed (wet weight). The hemispheres were then put in an oven (105°C)

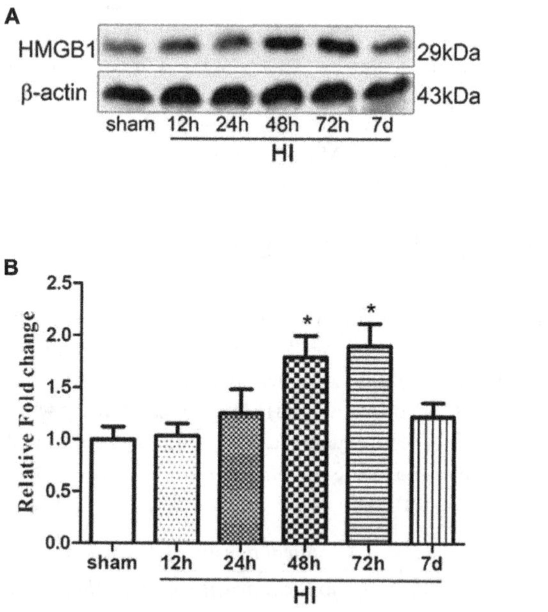

FIGURE 1 | Expression of HMGB1 in the cerebral cortex after HI. **(A)** Western blot bands of HMGB1 expression in the cerebral cortex of P7 SD rats at different time points from 12 h to 7 days after HI. **(B)** Quantitative analyses of the western blot bands (relative OD value) at different time points from 12 h to 7 days after HI, comparing to the sham group ($n = 5$ for each group). The expression of HMGB1 dramatically increased 24 h after HI and peaked 72 h after HI. Bars represent the mean ± SEM. *$P < 0.05$ compared to the sham group.

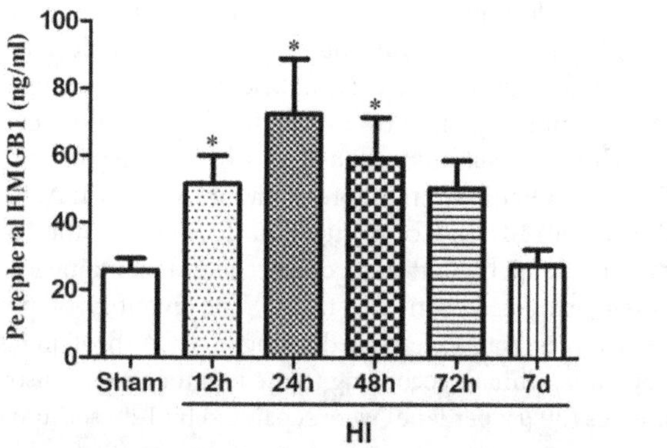

FIGURE 2 | Expression of HMGB1 in serum after HI. HMGB1 level in the peripheral blood detected by ELISA was increased significantly 12, 24, and 48 h after HI exposure with a peak level 24 h after HI comparing to the sham group ($n = 10$ for each group except $n = 9$ for the 12 and 24 h group). The serum level of HMGB1 7 days after HI was decreased to a similar level of the sham group. Bars represent the mean ± SEM. *$P < 0.05$ compared to the sham group.

for 48 h and weighed again (dry weight). The following formula was used to calculate brain water content:

$$\text{Brain water content } (\%) = \left[\frac{\text{wet weight} - \text{dry weight}}{\text{wet weight}}\right] \times 100$$

Statistical Analysis

All data are shown as means ± SEM. Data from the different experimental groups were analyzed using one-way ANOVA and the Tukey test for *post hoc* comparisons. Statistical Package for the Social Sciences 19.0 (SPSS, IBM, United States) and GraphPad Prism 5.0 (GraphPad, San Diego, CA, United States) were used for this statistical analysis. A p-value < 0.05 was considered statistically significant.

RESULTS

HMGB1 Was Upregulated in Both the Cerebral Cortex and Serum After HI

To investigate the effect of HI on HMGB1, we examined the expression of HMGB1 in the ipsilateral cerebral cortex and peripheral blood by western blotting and ELISA, respectively. Western blot analysis revealed that the expression of HMGB1 was increased in the ipsilateral cerebral cortex 48 h after HI, peaked 72 h after HI, and subsequently decreased to baseline level compared to the sham group (both $p < 0.05$) (**Figures 1A,B**). ELISA results revealed that the expression of HMGB1 was rapidly up-regulated in serum after HI, peaking at 24 h and gradually returning to a normal level (51.72 ± 8.32, 72.43 ± 16.38,

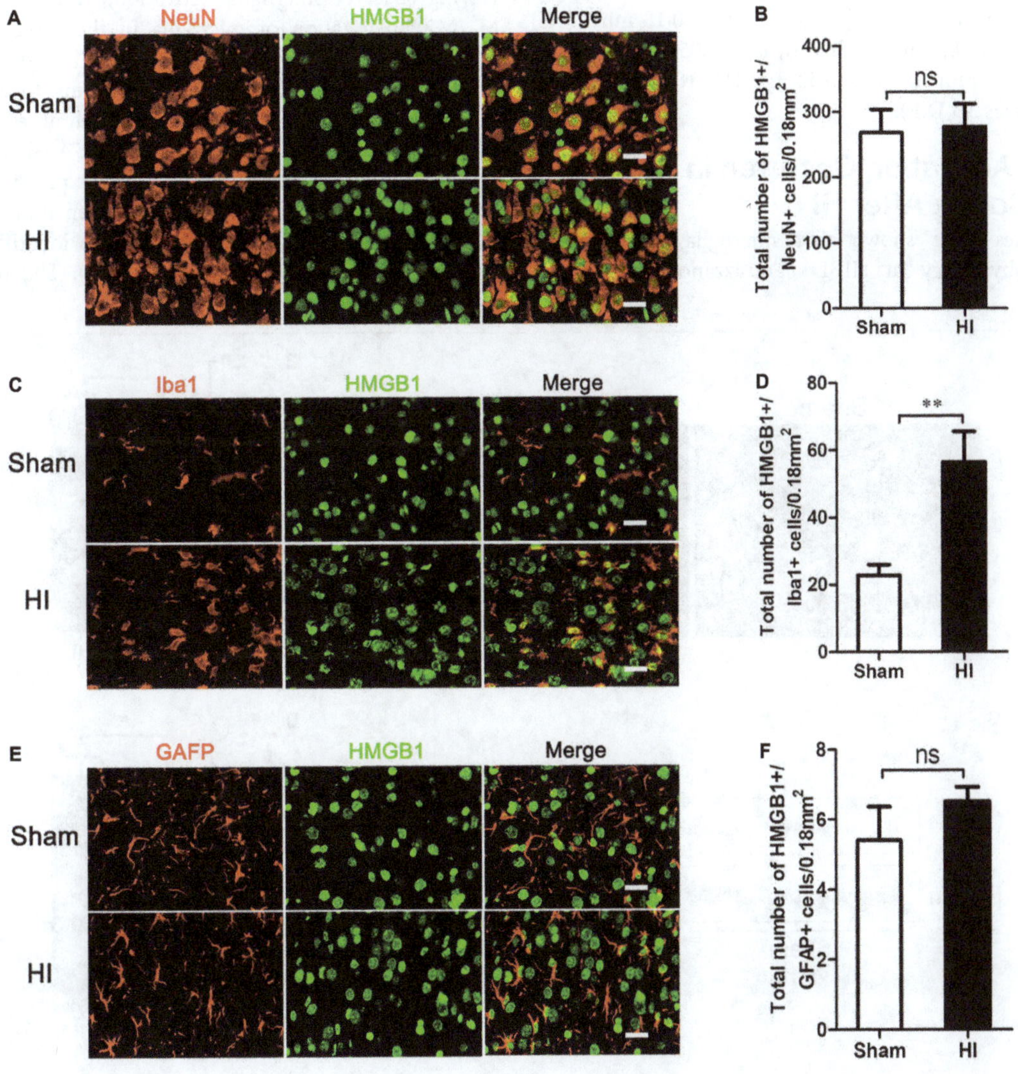

FIGURE 3 | Co-expression of HMGB1 and neural cells in the cerebral cortex after HI. **(A,C,E)** Double immunofluorescent labeling for HMGB1 with NeuN **(A)**, Iba-1 **(C)** and GFAP **(E)** in the cerebral cortex 72 h after HI. Scale bars = 20 μm. NeuN, Iba-1 and GFAP positive cells are red, HMGB1 positive cells are green and merged cells are yellow. **(B,D,F)** Statistical results of NeuN+/HMGB1+, Iba-1+/HMGB1+ and GFAP+/HMGB1+ cell numbers in 0.18 mm^2 area (n = 6 for each group). Iba-1+/HMGB1+ cell numbers significantly increased after HI. There were no significant changes in NeuN+/HMGB1+ and GFAP+/HMGB1+ cell numbers after HI compared to the sham group. Bars represent the mean ± SEM. $^{**}P < 0.01$, ns, no significance compared to the sham group.

59.32 ± 12.18 vs. 25.78 ± 3.58 ng/mL at 12, 24, 48 h post-HI compared to sham group respectively; all $p < 0.05$) (**Figure 2**).

Cortical HMGB1 Expression Was Increased in Microglia, but Not in Neurons or Astrocytes

As HMGB1 is widely expressed in the brain, we then explored in which type of cells HMGB1 was up-regulated. Double-labeled immunofluorescence of HMGB1 was performed in neurons, microglia, and astrocytes. In the sham group, cortical HMGB1 was primarily expressed in neurons (NeuN+/HMGB1+) (267.40 ± 36.04/0.18 mm^2), with low expression in microglia (Iba1+/HMGB1+) (22.72 ± 3.17/0.18 mm^2) and astrocytes (GFAP+/HMGB1+) (5.40 ± 0.97/0.18 mm^2) (**Figures 3A,C,E**). However, 72 h after HI, HMGB1 was increased in microglia [56.36 ± 9.13/0.18 mm^2 (HI) vs. 22.72 ± 3.17/0.18 mm^2 (Sham), $p < 0.01$], but not in neurons [267.40 ± 36.04/0.18 mm^2 (HI) vs. 276.90 ± 34.98/0.18 mm^2 (Sham), $p > 0.05$] or astrocytes [(5.40 ± 0.97/0.18 mm^2 (HI) vs. 6.52 ± 0.41/0.18 mm^2 (Sham), $p > 0.05$] (**Figures 3B,D,F**).

Microglial Activation Occurred in the Cerebral Cortex After HI

Previous studies have shown that microglia are activated in the pathophysiology of HIBD (Ferrazzano et al., 2013; Cengiz et al., 2019), and HMGB1, a pro-inflammatory factor, is upregulated in these activated microglia. Therefore, we explored whether microglial activation was induced in the cerebral cortex after HI. Immunofluorescence (**Figures 4A,B**) and western blot (**Figures 4C,D**) experiments showed that 72 h after HI injury, the expression of Iba-1, a marker of microglia, was significantly higher in the HI group than in the sham group ($p < 0.01$ and, $p < 0.05$, respectively). Meanwhile, microglial morphology changed from branch to amoeba-like after HI exposure. These changes demonstrated that cortical microglia were activated 72 h after HI.

HMGB1 Inhibition Altered M1/M2 Microglial Polarization and Cytokine Transcription

Having observed microglial activation, we further analyzed the M1/M2 polarization of microglia in the cerebral cortex and investigated if this was affected by GL, a specific inhibitor of HMGB1. We first used western blotting to detect whether the expression of HMGB1 in the cerebral cortex could be inhibited by GL pretreatment (**Figures 5A,B**). It was showed that GL could effectively attenuate the expression of HMGB1 in the cerebral cortex 72 h after HI. Then Iba1+/CD86+ and Iba1+/CD206+ co-staining were used to identify M1 and M2 phenotypes, respectively (**Figures 6A–D**). The results showed

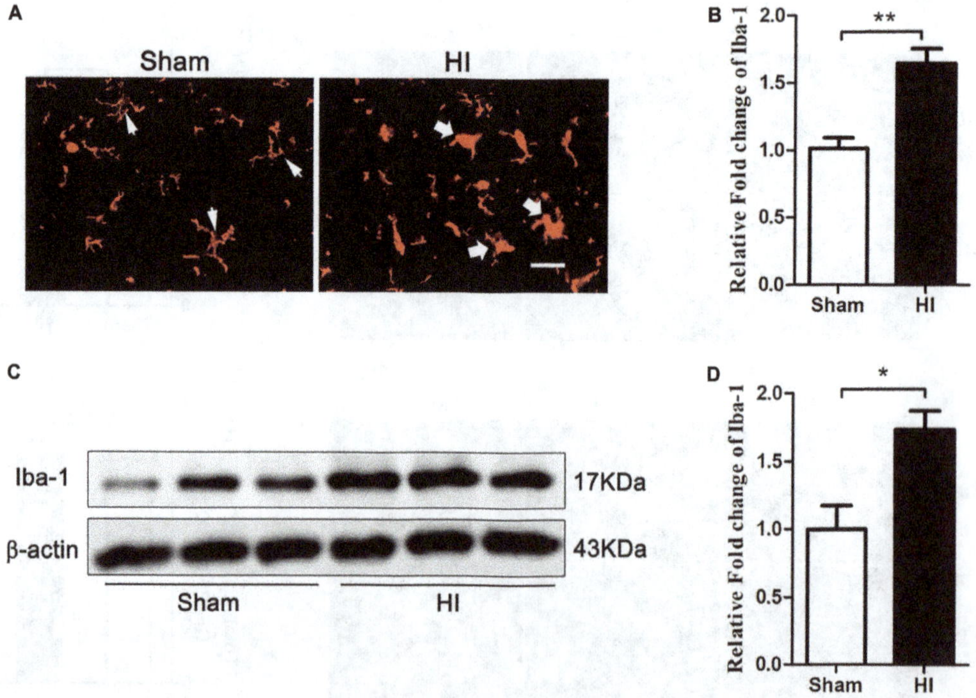

FIGURE 4 | Expression of microglia in the cerebral cortex after HI. **(A)** Immunofluorescent labeling of microglia (Iba-1) in the cerebral cortex 72 h after HI. The morphology of microglia changed from branch in sham group (white narrow arrows) to ameba-like in HI group (white wide arrows) after HI exposure. Scale bar = 20 μm. **(B)** Quantitative analyses of Iba-1 fluorescence intensity (relative OD value) showed that there was an increased expression of Iba-1 ($n = 6$ for each group). **(C)** The expression of Iba-1 in the cerebral cortex detected by western blot 72 h after HI. **(D)** Quantitative analyses of the western blot bands (relative OD value) revealed that there was a significantly increase in the expression of Iba-1 ($n = 6$ for each group). Bars represent the mean ± SEM. *$P < 0.05$ compared to the sham group, **$P < 0.01$ compared to the sham group.

that the expression of both M1 and M2 phenotypes was significantly increased 72 h after HI [37.00 ± 6.29 cells/0.18mm^2 (Sham + PBS) vs. 126.60 ± 23.74 cells/0.18mm^2 (HI + PBS); 23.60 ± 6.94 cells/0.18mm^2 (Sham + PBS) vs. 61.20 ± 8.12 cells/0.18mm^2 (HI + PBS), $p < 0.01$ and $p < 0.05$, respectively]. When rats were pretreated with GL, the number of M1 microglia (Iba1+/CD86+ cells) significantly reduced [126.60 ± 23.74 cells/0.18 mm^2 (HI + PBS) vs. 56.80 ± 9.12 cells/0.18 mm^2 (HI + GL), $p < 0.05$] (**Figures 6A,B**), while the number of M2 microglia (Iba1+/CD206+ cells) significantly increased [61.20 ± 8.12 cells/0.18 mm^2 (HI + PBS) vs. 127.60 ± 20.60 cells/0.18 mm^2 (HI + GL), $p < 0.05$] (**Figures 6C,D**).

We then detected the mRNA expression of M1 and M2 inflammatory factors using qRT-PCR. Results showed that the mRNA expression of M1 and M2 functional cytokines was significantly increased in the HI + PBS compared to the sham + PBS group 72 h after HI ($p < 0.05$, **Figures 7A,B**). The mRNA expression of M1 functional cytokines (iNOS, TNF-α, and IL-1β) was significantly decreased in the HI + GL group compared to the HI + PBS group (all $p < 0.05$, **Figure 7A**). In contrast, the mRNA expression of M2 functional cytokines (arginase1, IL-4, and TGF-β) was significantly increased in the HI + GL group compared to the HI + PBS group (all $p < 0.05$ except for arginase1, **Figure 7B**).

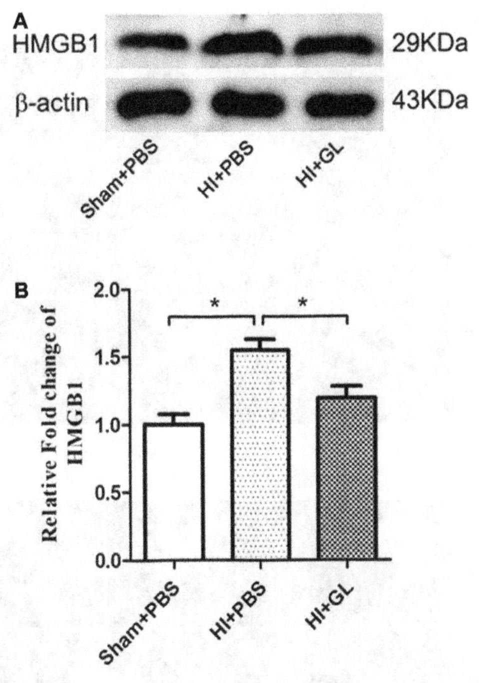

FIGURE 5 | Effect of GL on the expression of HMGB1 in the cerebral cortex after HI. **(A)** Western blot bands of HMGB1 expression in the cerebral cortex 72 h after HI. **(B)** Quantitative analyses of the western blot bands (relative OD value) showed that GL effectively inhibited the expression of HMGB1 in the cerebral cortex 72 h after HI ($n = 5$ for each group). Bars represent the mean ± SEM. $^*P < 0.05$.

HMGB1 Aggravated Microglial-Induced Neurotoxicity *in vitro*

To further elucidate the effect of HMGB1 on microglial phenotype, an OGD model of HAPI microglial cells was established *in vitro.* The effects of r-HMGB1 and its inhibitor GL, on the phenotypic changes of HAPI microglial cells were examined (**Figure 8A**). ELISA analysis showed that GL significantly reduced the expression of the M1-associated inflammatory cytokines TNF-α [66.44 ± 4.84 pg/mL (OGD + PBS) vs. 35.08 ± 2.94 pg/mL (OGD + GL), $p < 0.05$] and IL-1β [113.00 ± 2.99 pg/mL (OGD + PBS) vs. 62.21 ± 2.85 pg/mL (OGD + GL), $p < 0.05$], and significantly increased the expression of the M2-associated inflammatory cytokine IL-10 [97.89 ± 3.08 pg/mL (OGD + PBS) vs. 221.90 ± 5.43 pg/mL (OGD + GL), $p < 0.05$]. In contrast, r-HMGB1 significantly increased the expression of TNF-α [66.44 ± 4.84 pg/mL (OGD + PBS) vs. 119.00 ± 2.70 pg/mL (OGD + r-HMGB1), $p < 0.05$] and IL-1β [113.00 ± 2.99 pg/mL (OGD + PBS) vs. 173.60 ± 2.77 pg/mL (OGD + r-HMGB1), $p < 0.05$], and significantly reduced the expression of IL-10 [97.89 ± 3.08 pg/mL (OGD + PBS) vs. 49.37 ± 3.98 pg/mL (OGD + GL), $p < 0.05$]. These results indicated that under OGD conditions, HMGB1 promoted the polarization of microglia to a M1-like phenotype. In contrast, inhibition of HMGB1 promoted the polarization of microglia to a M2-like phenotype.

Next, the effect of different CM from HAPI microglial cells on neurons was examined (**Figures 8B–D**). We defined CM from M1 and M2-like phenotypes, as M1-CM and M2-CM, respectively. We first used MAP2 as a marker to explore the effects of different CMs on the length of nerve dendrites using an immunofluorescence assay. It was noted that the mean neurite length of MAP2-positive cells significantly decreased in the presence of M1-CM. In contrast, the mean neurite length of MAP2-positive cells significantly increased in the presence of M2-CM (**Figures 8B,C**). The survival of cortical neurons was then evaluated using a CCK-8 assay. This showed that M1-CM from the OGD+ r-HMGB1 group significantly reduced the cell viability of the primary cortical neurons, while M2-CM from the OGD + GL group significantly increased the cell viability of the primary cortical neurons, compared to the OGD + PBS control group (**Figure 8D**). These results suggested that HMGB1 could aggravate microglial-induced neurotoxicity in OGD conditions.

HMGB1 Inhibition Alleviated HI-Induced Brain Injury

As HMGB1 induced microglial polarization to an M1 phenotype, leading to increased neurotoxicity, we then explored whether inhibition of HMGB1 could attenuate HI-induced brain damage using edema assessment and cerebral infarction detection (**Figures 9A–D**). As shown in **Figure 9A**, the ipsilateral side of the brain was visibly edematous 72 h after HI insult. Pretreatment with GL alleviated this edema and morphological damage in the HI group. As shown in **Figure 9B**, the water content of the ipsilateral hemispheres was significantly increased in the HI group compared to the sham group. The inhibition of HMGB1 significantly alleviated the water content of the ipsilateral hemispheres in the HI group ($p < 0.05$). TTC staining

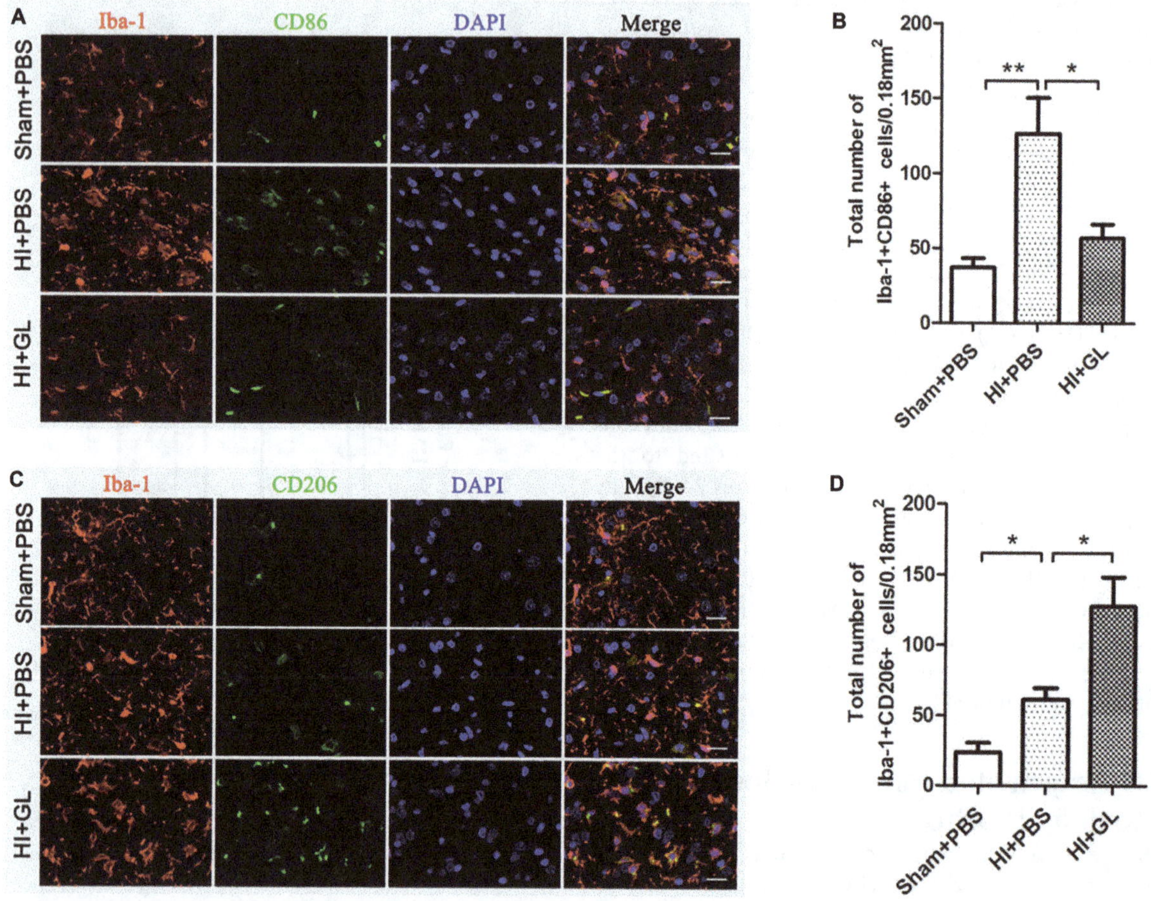

FIGURE 6 | Effect of GL on M1 and M2 phenotypes of microglia in the cerebral cortex after HI. **(A)** Immunofluorescent labeling of M1 phenotype (Iba-1+/CD86+) in the cerebral cortex 72 h after HI. Scale bars = 20 μm, Iba-1 positive cells are red, CD86 positive cells are green, DAPI-stained nuclei are blue and merged cells are yellow. **(B)** The statistical results of Iba-1+/CD86+ cell numbers in 0.18 mm^2 area. The expression of M1 phenotype significantly increased after HI. While it had a decrease in HI + GL group compared to HI + PBS group. **(C)** Immunofluorescent labeling of M2 phenotype (Iba-1+/CD206+) in the cerebral cortex 72 h after HI. Scale bars = 20 μm, Iba-1 positive cells are red, CD206 positive cells are green, DAPI-stained nuclei are blue and merged cells are yellow. **(D)** The statistical results of Iba-1+/CD206+ cell numbers in 0.18 mm^2 area. The expression of M2 phenotype significantly increased after HI and it had an increase in HI + GL group compared to HI + PBS group. $N = 6$ for each group, bars represent the mean ± SEM. $^*P < 0.05$, $^{**}P < 0.01$.

showed that HI insult substantially increased ipsilateral infarct size, which was reversed by pretreatment with HMGB1 inhibition ($p < 0.05$, **Figures 9C,D**). These results suggested that the inhibition of HMGB1 could alleviate HI-induced brain damage.

DISCUSSION

The present study investigated whether HMGB1 has a role in the pathogenesis of neonatal rat HIBD, focusing on the polarization of microglia. It was found that HMGB1 led to an imbalance in M1/M2 microglial polarization in the cortex, thus aggravating brain damage. This was alleviated by inhibiting HMGB1 with GL in HIBD.

HMGB1, a damage-associated protein, mediates neuroinflammation and brain damage in many neurological diseases including ischemic stroke (Angelopoulou et al., 2018; Paudel et al., 2018; Ye et al., 2019). Previous studies demonstrated that HMGB1 increased early at 3 h in serum and decreased in cerebral cortex after HI (Chen et al., 2019). Similarly, we found that HMGB1 was upregulated in peripheral blood after HI insult. But in our study, ipsilateral cortical HMGB1 also increased and serum HMGB1 increased 12 h after HI, inconsistent with the aforementioned results. These different results may be due to the different temperatures and different severity of injury after suffering from HI. It is suggested that pathological change and cerebral metabolic rate are different under different temperatures, and different temperatures can even affect clinical efficacy in hypothermia-treated HIE (Kim et al., 2014). And due to individual variation in animals, different severity of brain injury may occur, which could also lead to the discrepancy above.

Besides the serum and cortical upregulation of HMGB1, we also found that the expression of HMGB1 increased in peripheral blood much earlier than in the brain. There are two potential mechanisms underlying this experimental phenomenon. One possibility is that the early increase of peripheral HMGB1

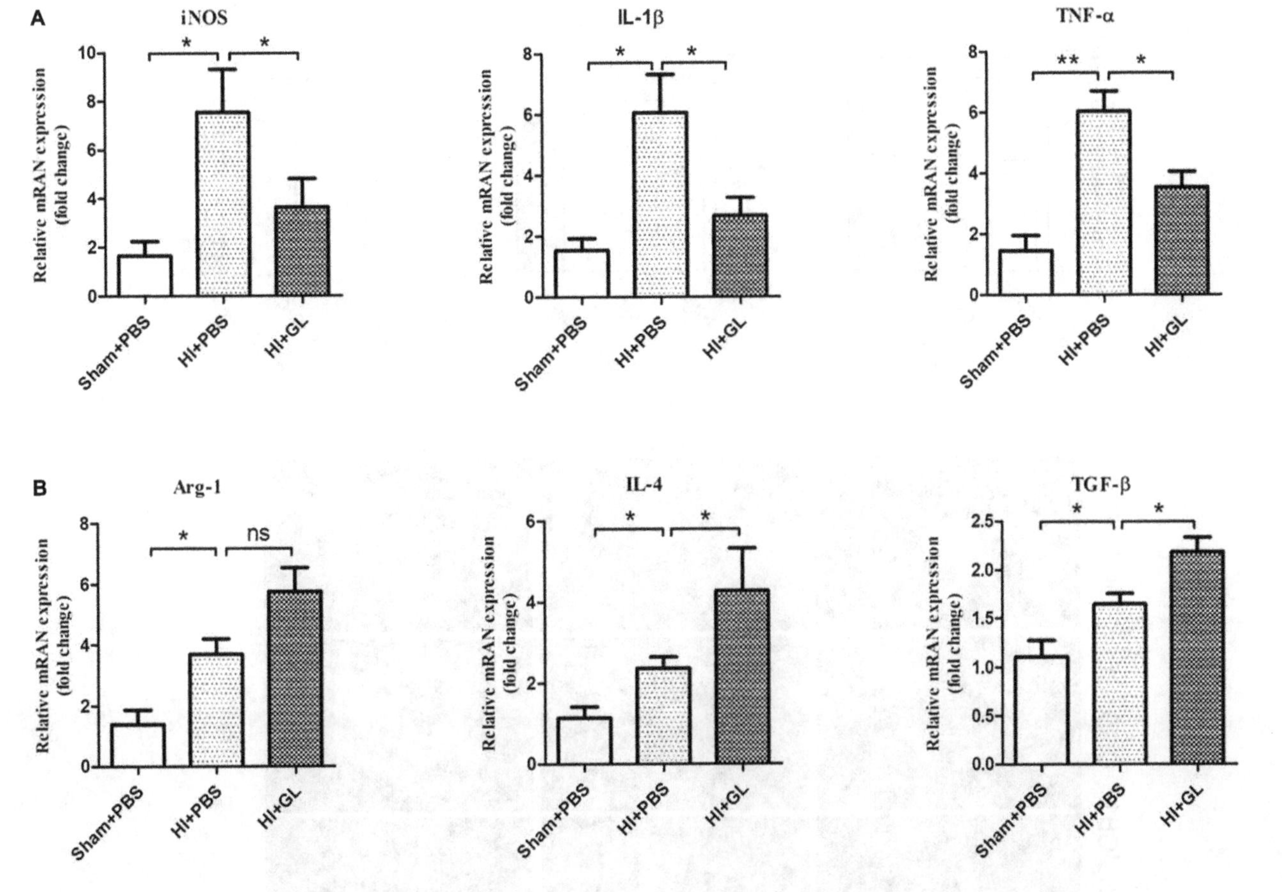

FIGURE 7 | Effect of GL on M1 and M2 functional cytokines in the cerebral cortex after HI. **(A)** The mRNA levels of M1 functional cytokines (iNOS, IL-1β, and TNF-α) were detected using qRT-PCR 72 h after HI. Results showed that the mRNA expression of M1 functional cytokines all increased after HI. While there was a significant decrease in HI + GL group compared to HI + PBS group. **(B)** The mRNA levels of M2 functional cytokines (Arg-1, IL-4, and TGF-β) were detected using qRT-PCR 72h after HI. Results showed that the expression of M2 functional cytokines all increased after HI and there was a higher level in HI + GL group compared to HI + PBS group. *N* = 6 for each group, bars represent the mean ± SEM, $^*P < 0.05$, $^{**}P < 0.01$, ns, no significance.

comes from brain tissue damage. As a typical damage-associated protein, HMGB1 could be released from damaged or necrotic brain tissue after HI insult, directing blood-brain barrier (BBB) breakdown and entering peripheral blood immediately, leading to a rapid increase of peripheral HMGB1 (Faraco et al., 2007; Ye et al., 2019). In addition, stimulation such as surgery and HI insult may have induced the release of HMGB1 from peripheral organs, causing peripheral HMGB1 to increase rapidly (Jellema et al., 2013; Terrando et al., 2016). The increased peripheral HMGB1 could in turn damage BBB and enter the brain, along with HMGB1 from the damaged brain tissue to lead to an increase of cerebral HMGB1. Our previous study showed that serum HMGB1 levels were significantly elevated in persistent pulmonary hypertension of the newborn (PPHN) and decreased dramatically after PPHN resolution (Tang et al., 2019). A meta-analysis by Le et al. (2018) demonstrated that circulating blood HMGB1 levels increased in ischemic stroke, with a higher HMGB1 level indicating a more serious condition. The rapid rise observed in peripheral HMGB1 after HI suggested that HMGB1 is sensitive to HI insult, and may potentially be useful as a biomarker in the early stage of HIBD.

In our study, we found that HMGB1 was widely expressed in the neurons of neonatal rat brains. However, the upregulation of HMGB1 after HI was characterized by an increased expression in microglia, but not in neurons or astrocytes. Several studies have demonstrated that HMGB1 can be transferred from the nucleus of the neuron to the cytoplasm or released extracellularly by stimulation such as brain ischemia (Qiu et al., 2008; Zhang et al., 2016; Chen et al., 2019) and subarachnoid hemorrhage (Sun et al., 2014). Under severe cerebral ischemic conditions, neuronal cells undergo apoptosis or necrosis by the induction of a number of pathways (Thal et al., 2011). As a result, HMGB1 could be released from necrotic neurons and interact with microglia as an extracellular cytokine (Frasch and Nygard, 2017). Based on the above research, it is therefore likely that HMGB1 was transferred extracellularly from neuronal nuclei or released from necrotic neurons after HI insult. This neuronal HMGB1 could then serve as an extracellular factor, binding to microglia and, resulting in the increase of HMGB1+/Iba1+ cells. As a group of innate immune cells in the central nervous system, it is known that microglial-mediated neuroinflammation plays an important role in the pathogenesis of many neurological

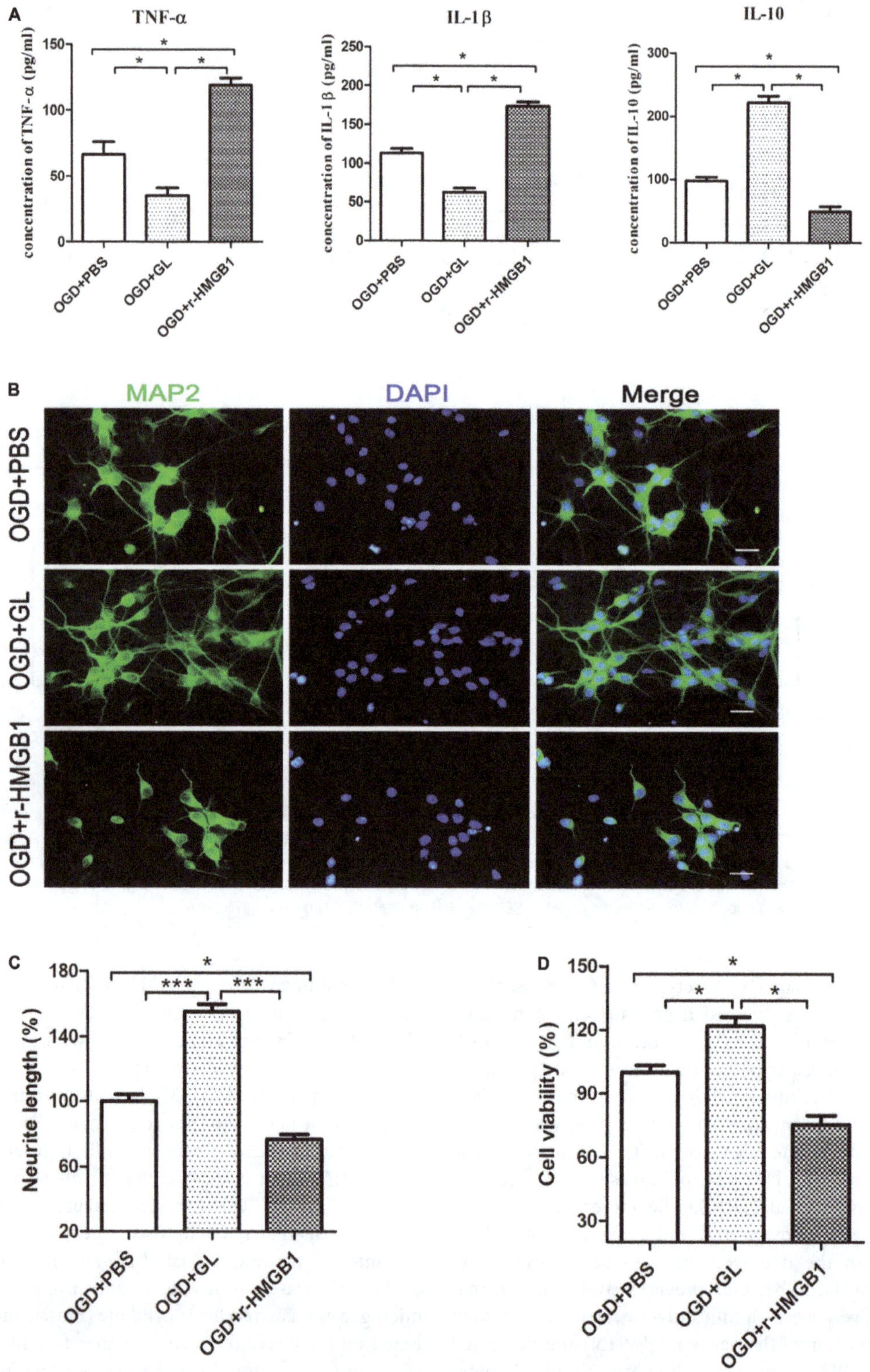

FIGURE 8 | Effect of HMGB1 on microglia-induced neurotoxicity *in vitro*. **(A)** HAPI microglia was pretreated with r-HMGB1 or GL and then undergoing OGD for 24 h. The expression of TNF-α, IL-1β and IL-10 in culture supernatant was measured by ELISA (n = 4 wells per group). **(B)** Immunofluorescent staining of primary cortical neurons (MAP2, green) with DAPI (blue) 48 h after incubation with different CM from HAPI microglial medium. Scale bars = 20 μm. **(C)** Quantitative analyses of relative neurite length of primary neurons after immunofluorescent staining using ImageJ. N = 4 wells for each group, 3 digital microscopic images for each well. **(D)** Cell viability of primary neurons 48 h after incubation with different CM from HAPI microglial medium using CCK8 method (n = 4 wells for each group). Bars represent the mean ± SEM, $^*P < 0.05$, $^{***}P < 0.001$.

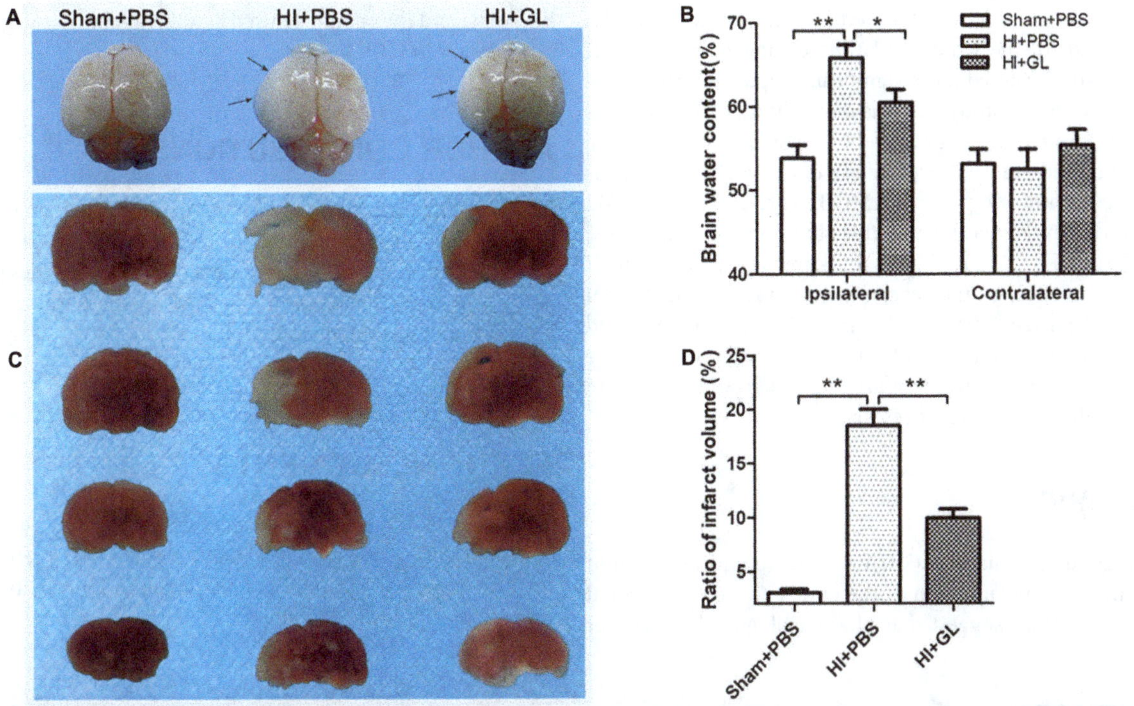

FIGURE 9 | Effect of GL treatment on HI-induced brain injury. **(A)** Whole brain photos showing cerebral edema 24 h after HI. Gray arrows indicate sites of significant edema. Cerebral edema area in HI + GL group was smaller than HI + PBS group. **(B)** The brain water content measurement showed that the ipsilateral brain water content in HI + GL group was significantly lower compared to the HI + PBS group (n = 6 for each group). **(C)** TTC staining of all treatment groups 72 h after HI. Normal tissues were red or pink, while infract tissues were white. The white area in HI + GL group was smaller than HI + PBS group. **(D)** Statistical results showed that the ratio of infract volume in HI + GL group was significantly lower compared to HI + PBS group (n = 5 for each group). Bars represent the mean ± SEM, *$P < 0.05$, **$P < 0.01$.

diseases, including HIBD (Fonken et al., 2016; Zhang et al., 2016; Kigerl et al., 2018). As an important inflammatory factor, the binding of HMGB1 to microglia could further promote this neuroinflammation (Sun et al., 2018), in turn triggering an inflammation cascade response and, aggravating brain damage. Further, the *in vitro* experiments in our study showed that HMGB1 increased the neurotoxicity of neurons under the condition of OGD (**Figure 8**). It is implied that the increase of HMGB1+/Iba1+ cells may result in a decrease of HMGB1+/NeuN+ cells. However, we did not find a decrease in the number of HMGB1+/NeuN+ cells 72 h after HI. Due to the sustained neuroinflammation, there is a great possibility that the number of HMGB1+/NeuN+ cells will decrease after 72 h post HI. Thus, inhibition of HMGB1 expression may help to reduce neuroinflammation.

Studies have shown that microglia can be activated after HI stimulation (Ohsawa and Kohsaka, 2011; Serdar et al., 2019). In our study, HI insult resulted in an increased expression of Iba-1 and a change in microglial morphology from branch to ameba-like. These results indicated that cortical microglia were activated after HI, consistent with previous research (Harry, 2013; Cengiz et al., 2019). Microglia can be differentiated into different subtypes after activation. The two main subtypes are M1 and M2 microglia, characterized by pro-inflammatory (neurotoxic) and anti- inflammatory (neuroprotective) phenotypes, respectively (Olah et al., 2011; Patel et al., 2013). In this study, the HMGB1 inhibitor GL was used to investigate the effect of HMGB1 on the M1/M2 polarization of microglia during the pathogenesis of HIBD. The results showed that the expression of both M1 and M2 microglia was significantly increased 72 h after HI. Inhibition of HMGB1 by GL reduced the expression of the M1 phenotype and promoted the expression of the M2 phenotype, indicating that HMGB1 was involved in the imbalance of M1/M2 microglial polarization in HIBD.

In addition, an *in vitro* experiment was conducted to mimic the HI process *in vivo*. We investigated the polarization state of microglia and the effect of microglia on HMGB1 expression in neurons during the process of OGD. We found that HMGB1 promoted the polarization of microglia to an M1 phenotype, enhancing the expression of pro-inflammatory factors such as TNF-α and IL-1β, and resulting in a decrease in neuronal activity and dendritic length. However, the above phenomenon could be neutralized by inhibiting HMGB1 with GL. We conducted further animal experiments and found that HMGB1 inhibition could reduce brain edema and cerebral infarction area after HI. The above effects of HMGB1 are similar to those reported by Gao et al. (2018) and Sun et al. (2018). Taken together, these findings suggest that HMGB1 may cause neuroinflammation and neuronal damage by inducing an imbalance of M1/M2 microglial polarization, leading to brain damage.

There exists a number of limitations of our study. As different pathological changes occur at different time points after HI (Park et al., 2018), the window of time during which post-HI treatment is administered has a significant impact on prognosis. Unfortunately, in our study, GL was only administered as a pre-treatment before HI and not at different time points after HI. In addition, this study did not explore the underlying mechanisms and specific pathways by which HMGB1 regulates the M1/M2 polarization of microglia. Finally, this study only examined the acute phase of HI (0–72 h), whereas it is known that, perinatal HI has a long-term effect on the development of the nervous system in children (Papazian, 2018; Sanches et al., 2019). This study did not investigate the effects of HMGB1 on the development of the brain in the late phase of HI. The aforementioned points therefore need to be addressed in further research.

CONCLUSION

Our findings suggest that HMGB1 may lead to an imbalance of M1/M2 microglial polarization in the cortex and thus neuronal injury. Such findings suggest that pharmacological blockade of HMGB1 signaling may attenuate this imbalanced polarization of microglia and thus could be used as a therapeutic strategy against brain injury in HIBD.

AUTHOR CONTRIBUTIONS

YS, ZF, and ZT performed the experiments, analyzed the data, and wrote the manuscript. NH and BW performed the experiments and analyzed the data. YS and MH designed the study and revised the manuscript. All of the authors read and approved the final manuscript.

ACKNOWLEDGMENTS

We would like to thank Editage (www.editage.com) for English language editing. We sincerely thank the staff in the central lab of the Third Xiangya Hospital of Central South University for their wonderful support in this study.

REFERENCES

Andersson, U., Yang, H., and Harris, H. (2018). High-mobility group box 1 protein (HMGB1) operates as an alarmin outside as well as inside cells. *Semin. Immunol.* 38, 40–48. doi: 10.1016/j.smim.2018.02.011

Angelopoulou, E., Piperi, C., and Papavassiliou, A. G. (2018). High-mobility group box 1 in Parkinson's disease: from pathogenesis to therapeutic approaches. *J. Neurochem.* 146, 211–218. doi: 10.1111/jnc.14450

Barkhuizen, M., van den Hove, D. L., Vles, J. S., Steinbusch, H. W., Kramer, B. W., and Gavilanes, A. W. (2017). 25 years of research on global asphyxia in the immature rat brain. *Neurosci. Biobehav. Rev.* 75, 166–182. doi: 10.1016/j.neubiorev.2017.01.042

Bhalala, U. S., Koehler, R. C., and Kannan, S. (2014). Neuroinflammation and neuroimmune dysregulation after acute hypoxic-ischemic injury of developing brain. *Front, Pediatr.* 2:144. doi: 10.3389/fped.2014.00144

Cengiz, P., Zafer, D., Chandrashekhar, J. H., Chanana, V., Bogost, J., Waldman, A., et al. (2019). Developmental differences in microglia morphology and gene expression during normal brain development and in response to hypoxia-ischemia. *Neurochem. Int.* 127, 137–147. doi: 10.1016/j.neuint.2018.12.016

Chen, X., Zhang, J., Kim, B., Jaitpal, S., and Meng, S. S. (2019). High-mobility group box-1 translocation and release after hypoxic ischemic brain injury in neonatal rats. *Exp. Neurol.* 311, 1–14. doi: 10.1016/j.expneurol.2018.09.007

Colton, C. A. (2009). Heterogeneity of microglial activation in the innate immune response in the brain. *J. Neuroimmune. Pharmacol.* 4, 399–418. doi: 10.1007/s11481-009-9164-4

Faraco, G., Fossati, S., Bianchi, M. E., Patrone, M., and Pedrazzi, M. (2007). High mobility group box 1 protein is released by neural cells upon different stresses and worsens ischemic neurodegeneration in vitro and in vivo. *J. Neurochem.* 103, 590–603. doi: 10.1111/j.1471-4159.2007.04788.x

Ferrazzano, P., Chanana, V., Uluc, K., Fidan, E., and Akture, E. (2013). Age-dependent microglial activation in immature brains after hypoxia-ischemia. *CNS Neurol. Disord. Drug Targets* 12, 338–349. doi: 10.2174/1871527311312030007

Fonken, L. K., Frank, M. G., Kitt, M. M., D'Angelo, H. M., and Norden, D. M. (2016). The alarmin HMGB1 mediates age-induced neuroinflammatory priming. *J. Neurosci.* 36, 7946–7956. doi: 10.1523/JNEUROSCI.1161-16.2016

Frasch, M. G., and Nygard, K. L. (2017). Location, location, location: appraising the pleiotropic function of HMGB1 in fetal brain. *J. Neuropathol. Exp. Neurol.* 76, 332–334. doi: 10.1093/jnen/nlx004

Gao, T., Chen, Z., Chen, H., Yuan, H., and Wang, Y. (2018). Inhibition of HMGB1 mediates neuroprotection of traumatic brain injury by modulating the microglia/macrophage polarization. *Biochem. Biophys. Res. Commun.* 497, 430–436. doi: 10.1016/j.bbrc.2018.02.102

Guazzi, S., Strangio, A., Franzi, A. T., and Bianchi, M. E. (2003). HMGB1, an architectural chromatin protein and extracellular signalling factor, has a spatially and temporally restricted expression pattern in mouse brain. *Gene. Expr. Patterns* 3, 29–33. doi: 10.1016/s1567-133x(02)00093-5

Harry, G. J. (2013). Microglia during development and aging. *Pharmacol. Ther.* 139, 313–326. doi: 10.1016/j.pharmthera.2013.04.013

Jellema, R. K., Lima, P. V., Zwanenburg, A., Ophelders, D. R., and De Munter, S. (2013). Cerebral inflammation and mobilization of the peripheral immune system following global hypoxia-ischemia in preterm sheep. *J. Neuroinflammation* 10:13. doi: 10.1186/1742-2094-10-13

Jin, X., Liu, M. Y., Zhang, D. F., Zhong, X., Du, K., Qian, P., et al. (2019). Natural products as a potential modulator of microglial polarization in neurodegenerative diseases. *Pharmacol. Res.* 145:104253. doi: 10.1016/j.phrs.2019.104253

Kaur, C., Rathnasamy, G., and Ling, E. A. (2017). Biology of microglia in the developing brain. *J. Neuropathol. Exp. Neurol.* 76, 736–753. doi: 10.1093/jnen/nlx056

Kigerl, K. A., Lai, W., Wallace, L. M., Yang, H., and Popovich, P. G. (2018). High mobility group box-1 (HMGB1) is increased in injured mouse spinal cord and can elicit neurotoxic inflammation. *Brain Behav. Immun.* 72, 22–33. doi: 10.1016/j.bbi.2017.11.018

Kim, J. H., Yun, S. H., Jang, K. H., Park, J., and Han, H. S. (2014). Delayed and prolonged local brain hypothermia combined with decompressive craniectomy: a novel therapeutic strategy that modulates glial dynamics. *Exp. Neurobiol.* 23, 115–123. doi: 10.5607/en.2014.23.2.115

Le, K., Mo, S., Lu, X., Idriss, A. A., Yu, D., and Guo, Y. (2018). Association of circulating blood HMGB1 levels with ischemic stroke: a systematic review and meta-analysis. *Neurol. Res.* 40, 907–916. doi: 10.1080/01616412.2018.1497254

Liu, Y., Prasad, R., and Wilson, S. H. (2010). HMGB1: roles in base excision repair and related function. *Biochim. Biophys. Acta* 1799, 119–130. doi: 10.1016/j.bbagrm.2009.11.008

Merenmies, J., Pihlaskari, R., Laitinen, J., Wartiovaara, J., and Rauvala, H. (1991). 30-KDa heparin-binding protein of brain (amphoterin) involved in neurite outgrowth. Amino acid sequence and localization in the filopodia of the advancing plasma membrane. *J. Biol Chem.* 266, 16722–16729.

Ohsawa, K., and Kohsaka, S. (2011). Dynamic motility of microglia: purinergic modulation of microglial movement in the normal and pathological brain. *Glia* 59, 1793–1799. doi: 10.1002/glia.21238

Olah, M., Biber, K., Vinet, J., and Boddeke, H. W. (2011). Microglia phenotype diversity. *CNS Neurol. Disord. Drug Targets* 10, 108–118. doi: 10.2174/187152711794488575

Papazian, O. (2018). Neonatal hypoxic-ischemic encephalopathy. *Medicina* 78(Suppl. 2), 36–41.

Park, J. H., Noh, Y., Kim, S., Ahn, J. H., and Ohk, T. G. (2018). Time-course changes and new expressions of MIP-3 and its receptor, CCR6, in the gerbil hippocampal CA1 area following transient global cerebral ischemia. *Neurochem. Res.* 43, 2102–2110. doi: 10.1007/s11064-018-2632-6

Patel, A. R., Ritzel, R., McCullough, L. D., and Liu, F. (2013). Microglia and ischemic stroke: a double-edged sword. *Int. J. Physiol. Pathophysiol. Pharmacol.* 5, 73–90.

Paudel, Y. N., Shaikh, M. F., Chakraborti, A., Kumari, Y., and Aledo-Serrano, A. (2018). HMGB1: a common biomarker and potential target for TBI, neuroinflammation, epilepsy, and cognitive dysfunction. *Front. Neurosci.* 12:628. doi: 10.3389/fnins.2018.00628

Qiu, J., Nishimura, M., Wang, Y., Sims, J. R., and Qiu, S. (2008). Early release of HMGB-1 from neurons after the onset of brain ischemia. *J. Cereb. Blood Flow Metab* .28, 927–938. doi: 10.1038/sj.jcbfm.9600582

Sanches, E. F., van de Looij, Y., Toulotte, A., Sizonenko, S. V., and Lei, H. (2019). Mild neonatal brain Hypoxia-Ischemia in very immature rats causes Long-Term behavioral and cerebellar abnormalities at adulthood. *Front. Physiol.* 10:634. doi: 10.3389/fphys.2019.00634

Serdar, M., Kempe, K., Rizazad, M., Herz, J., and Bendix, I. (2019). Early pro-inflammatory microglia activation after inflammation-sensitized hypoxic-ischemic brain injury in neonatal rats. *Front. Cell Neurosci.* 13:237. doi: 10.3389/fncel.2019.00237

Sun, Q., Wu, W., Hu, Y. C., Li, H., and Zhang, D. (2014). Early release of high-mobility group box 1 (HMGB1) from neurons in experimental subarachnoid hemorrhage in vivo and in vitro. *J. Neuroinflammation* 11:106. doi: 10.1186/1742-2094-11-106

Sun, X., Zeng, H., Wang, Q., Yu, Q., and Wu, J. (2018). Glycyrrhizin ameliorates inflammatory pain by inhibiting microglial activation-mediated inflammatory response via blockage of the HMGB1-TLR4-NF-kB pathway. *Exp. Cell Res.* 369, 112–119. doi: 10.1016/j.yexcr.2018.05.012

Tang, Z., Jiang, M., Ou-Yang, Z., Wu, H., Dong, S., and Hei, M. (2019). High mobility group box 1 protein (HMGB1) as biomarker in hypoxia-induced persistent pulmonary hypertension of the newborn: a clinical and in vivo pilot study. *Int. J. Med. Sci.* 16, 1123–1131. doi: 10.7150/ijms.34344

Terrando, N., Yang, T., Wang, X., Fang, J., and Cao, M. (2016). Systemic HMGB1 neutralization prevents postoperative neurocognitive dysfunction in aged rats. *Front. Immunol.* 7:441. doi: 10.3389/fimmu.2016.00441

Thal, S. E., Zhu, C., Thal, S. C., Blomgren, K., and Plesnila, N. (2011). Role of apoptosis inducing factor (AIF) for hippocampal neuronal cell death following global cerebral ischemia in mice. *Neurosci. Lett.* 499, 1–3. doi: 10.1016/j.neulet.2011.05.016

Umekawa, T., Osman, A. M., Han, W., Ikeda, T., and Blomgren, K. (2015). Resident microglia, rather than blood-derived macrophages, contribute to the earlier and more pronounced inflammatory reaction in the immature compared with the adult hippocampus after hypoxia-ischemia. *Glia* 63, 2220–2230. doi: 10.1002/glia.22887

Wang, H., Bloom, O., Zhang, M., Vishnubhakat, J. M., and Ombrellino, M. (1999). HMG-1 as a late mediator of endotoxin lethality in mice. *Science* 285, 248–251. doi: 10.1126/science.285.5425.248

Weinstein, J. R., Koerner, I. P., and Moller, T. (2010). Microglia in ischemic brain injury. *Future Neurol.* 5, 227–246. doi: 10.2217/fnl.10.1

Wu, Y. W., Mathur, A. M., Chang, T., McKinstry, R. C., and Mulkey, S. B. (2016). High-Dose erythropoietin and hypothermia for Hypoxic-Ischemic encephalopathy: a phase II trial. *Pediatrics* 137:e20160191. doi: 10.1542/peds.2016-0191

Xia, C. Y., Zhang, S., Gao, Y., Wang, Z. Z., and Chen, N. H. (2015). Selective modulation of microglia polarization to M2 phenotype for stroke treatment. *Int. Immunopharmacol.* 25, 377–382. doi: 10.1016/j.intimp.2015.02.019

Ye, Y., Zeng, Z., Jin, T., Zhang, H., Xiong, X., and Gu, L. (2019). The role of high mobility group box 1 in ischemic stroke. *Front. Cell Neurosci.* 13:127. doi: 10.3389/fncel.2019.00127

Zhang, J., Klufas, D., Manalo, K., Adjepong, K., and Davidson, J. O. (2016). HMGB1 translocation after ischemia in the ovine fetal brain. *J. Neuropathol. Exp. Neurol.* 75, 527–538. doi: 10.1093/jnen/nlw030

Zhang, J., Takahashi, H. K., Liu, K., Wake, H., and Liu, R. (2011). Anti-high mobility group box-1 monoclonal antibody protects the blood-brain barrier from ischemia-induced disruption in rats. *Stroke* 42, 1420–1428. doi: 10.1161/STROKEAHA.110.598334

Zhou, X., Chu, X., Xin, D., Li, T., and Bai, X. (2019). L-Cysteine-Derived H2S promotes microglia m2 polarization via activation of the AMPK pathway in Hypoxia-Ischemic neonatal mice. *Front. Mol. Neurosci.* 12:58. doi: 10.3389/fnmol.2019.00058

14

Emerging Roles of Axin in Cerebral Cortical Development

*Tao Ye, Amy K. Y. Fu and Nancy Y. Ip**

Division of Life Science, Molecular Neuroscience Center and State Key Laboratory of Molecular Neuroscience, The Hong Kong University of Science and Technology, Hong Kong, China

***Correspondence:**
Nancy Y. Ip,
Division of Life Science, Molecular Neuroscience Center and State Key Laboratory of Molecular Neuroscience, The Hong Kong University of Science and Technology, Clear Water Bay, Hong Kong, China
boip@ust.hk

Proper functioning of the cerebral cortex depends on the appropriate production and positioning of neurons, establishment of axon–dendrite polarity, and formation of proper neuronal connectivity. Deficits in any of these processes greatly impair neural functions and are associated with various human neurodevelopmental disorders including microcephaly, cortical heterotopias, and autism. The application of *in vivo* manipulation techniques such as *in utero* electroporation has resulted in significant advances in our understanding of the cellular and molecular mechanisms that underlie neural development *in vivo*. Axin is a scaffold protein that regulates neuronal differentiation and morphogenesis *in vitro*. Recent studies provide novel insights into the emerging roles of Axin in gene expression and cytoskeletal regulation during neurogenesis, neuronal polarization, and axon formation. This review summarizes current knowledge on Axin as a key molecular controller of cerebral cortical development.

Keywords: Axin, cerebral cortex, neurogenesis, polarization, axon formation, cytoskeletal regulation

Introduction

The mammalian cerebral cortex is characterized by a six-layered laminar structure, which forms the structural basis for higher cognitive function. Each cortical layer contains distinct distributions of neuron types with specific dendritic morphology, electrophysiological properties, and axonal connection with other brain regions. Remarkably, the characteristic distribution and connectivity of cortical neurons originate from a single layer of progenitor cells called the neuroepithelium. During cortical development, neural progenitor cells located in the ventricular zone undergo symmetric cell division to proliferate and maintain a proper progenitor pool; moreover, they utilize asymmetric cell division to differentiate and generate successive waves of neurons. After neuronal differentiation, the postmitotic neurons go through a multipolar stage; they subsequently polarize, taking on a bipolar morphology with a leading process towards the cortical plate and a nascent axon toward the opposite direction. The cell body continues to migrate along radial glial fibers towards the cortical plate and past the existing layers of neurons. Thus, cortical layers are created in an inside-out manner, with the early- and later-born neurons occupying the deeper and superficial layers, respectively.

When the neurons mature at their destination, the leading process spawns the apical dendrite, followed by dendritic arborization and synaptic formation. The nascent axon elongates tangentially, projecting to form synaptic connections with other neurons. Defects in any of these coordinated events can greatly impair neural functions and are implicated in various neurological and psychiatric disorders including lissencephaly, cortical heterotopias, and autism (Ayala et al., 2007). Thus, these steps require the orchestration of various signaling cascades; accordingly, scaffold proteins have emerged as key molecular controls of cortical development owing to their abilities to interact with and regulate a myriad of signaling proteins. This review summarizes the emerging roles of the scaffold protein Axin in the orchestration of the transcriptional program of neurogenesis and cytoskeletal regulation of neural development in the cerebral cortex.

Identification and Regulation of Axin

Axin was initially identified from the analysis of the *Fused* locus, mutations of which cause defects in axis formation in mouse embryos (Zeng et al., 1997). Because of its inhibition of axis formation, the *Fused* gene was named *Axis inhibitor* (*Axin*). Genetic analyses identified Axin as a negative regulator of the canonical Wnt signaling pathway, although its precise roles remained unclear (Kikuchi, 1999). Biochemical studies demonstrated that Axin acts as a scaffold and associates with various components of the canonical Wnt signaling pathway, forming the β-catenin destruction complex, which leads to the GSK3β–dependent phosphorylation of β-catenin (Luo and Lin, 2004).

Axin possesses several functional domains including the Regulators of G protein signaling domain near its N-terminus and the C-terminal DIX domain, which is also found in Disheveled and Dixdc1 (also called Ccd1). In addition, Axin contains domains for interacting with other proteins such as GSK3β and β-catenin (**Figure 1**). In brief, Axin interacts with adenomatosis polyposis coli (APC), GSK3β, and β-catenin via distinct domains to form the β-catenin destruction complex (Furuhashi et al., 2001). Without Wnt ligand stimulation, Axin facilitates GSK3β-mediated phosphorylation of β-catenin, and thus triggers the proteasome-dependent ubiquitination and degradation of β-catenin. Hence, although β-catenin is constitutively expressed in the cytoplasm, its protein level remains relatively low because of destruction complex activity. When the Wnt ligands bind to the receptors Frizzled and LRP5/6, they activate several signaling components such as Disheveled. Disheveled associates with Axin, translocating Axin to the membrane, which leads to Axin degradation. Loss of Axin results in the disassembly of the destruction complex as well as the suppression of β-catenin phosphorylation by GSK3β. Subsequently, β-catenin accumulates and translocates into the nucleus, where it forms a complex with TCF/Lef transcription factors and turns on Wnt-responsive gene transcription (Furuhashi et al., 2001). It should be noted that most of these findings are from studies using different types of cultured cells. Thus, the precise mechanisms *in vivo* are only beginning to be elucidated.

Axin has also emerged as a master scaffold for multiple signaling pathways (Kikuchi, 1999). Axin interacts with and activates MEKK, which activates JNK, suggesting that Axin regulates the JNK pathway (Liu et al., 2006). Axin also functions as a scaffold in the transforming growth factor β (TGF-β) pathway by facilitating the ubiquitin E3 ligase Arkadia-dependent degradation of Smad7 (Zeng et al., 1997). It also directly interacts with Smad3 and promotes its phosphorylation by TGF-β receptors (Furuhashi et al., 2001; Guo et al., 2008).

Coordination of Neurogenesis by Axin-Mediated Signaling

Neurons are generated from neural progenitor cells. Cortical neural progenitors include neuroepithelial progenitors, radial glial progenitors (RGPs; Ever and Gaiano, 2005), and intermediate progenitors (IPs; Farkas and Huttner, 2008). Among them, RGPs in the ventricular zone are responsible for generating most or all neurons during embryonic development (Kriegstein et al., 2002; Götz et al., 2003; Heintz et al., 2004). RGPs enlarge the progenitor pool through symmetric proliferative divisions in order to enable the subsequent rapid increase in neurons (Götz and Huttner, 2005; Huttner and Kosodo, 2005). As development proceeds, RGPs switch to neuronal differentiation, dividing asymmetrically and producing several neurons. RGPs adopt two modes of asymmetric divisions to generate neurons: producing one RGP for self-renewal and either one neuron (direct neurogenesis) or one neurogenic IP (indirect neurogenesis) to enlarge the population of neurons (Noctor et al., 2004; Götz and Huttner, 2005). Consequently, asymmetric cell division of RGPs plays a critical role in generating a proper number of neurons, while at the same time maintaining an adequate pool of neural

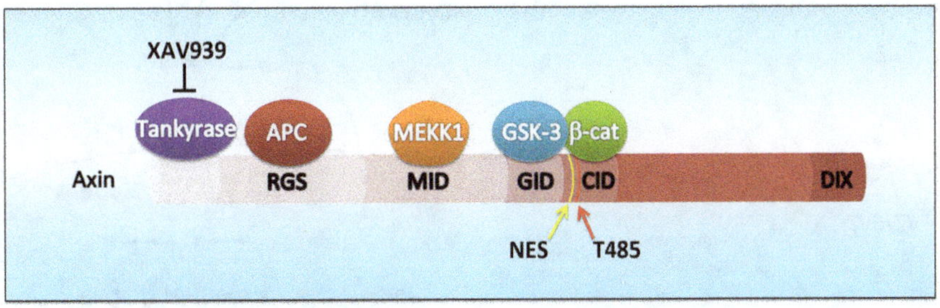

FIGURE 1 | Schematic diagram of Axin domains, molecular interactions and Cdk5-dependent phosphorylation site. Axin possesses functional domains including the Regulators of G protein signaling (RGS which interacts with adenomatosis polyposis coli, APC) and DIX domains. Axin contains domains for interacting with other proteins such as MEKK1 (MID), GSK3β (GID), and β-catenin (CID). A small molecule, XAV939, stabilizes Axin by inhibiting the poly-ADP-ribosylating enzyme tankyrase which stimulates Axin degradation through the ubiquitin-proteasome pathway. It is worth noting that the Cdk5-dependent phosphorylation site (Thr485) is located close to the nuclear export signal (NES) of Axin (amino acids 413–423).

progenitors for self-renewal. IPs that preferentially reside in the subventricular zone are transient neurogenic progenitors with limited amplifying capability (1–3 mitotic cycles). IPs undergo symmetric divisions to produce pairs of IPs that subsequently differentiate into neurons (Pontious et al., 2008; Kowalczyk et al., 2009). Thus, the birthdates and numbers of neurons are dependent on the balance between neural progenitor proliferation and differentiation.

Recent evidence suggests that Axin serves as a master scaffold for coordinating the proliferation and differentiation of neural progenitors during cerebral cortical development (Fang et al., 2013). Our laboratory has demonstrated that the level and subcellular localization of Axin in neural progenitors determine their fate, either self-proliferation or neuronal differentiation. In the presence of proliferating cues such as SHH, the Axin-GSK3β interaction in the cytoplasm is crucial for the proliferation of the intermediate progenitor cells (**Figure 2**). Upon stimulation by neurogenic cues such as WNT, RA, and TGFβ, the Axin-β-catenin interaction in the nucleus promotes neuronal production through the activation of neurogenic transcription factors (**Figure 3**). Of note, Axin phosphorylation at Thr485 (**Figure 1**) by cyclin-dependent kinase-5 (Cdk5) determines the subcellular localization of Axin, which translocates from the cytoplasm to the nucleus upon neural progenitor differentiation, thus serving as a molecular switch that causes IPs to switch from proliferation to differentiation (Fang et al., 2013).

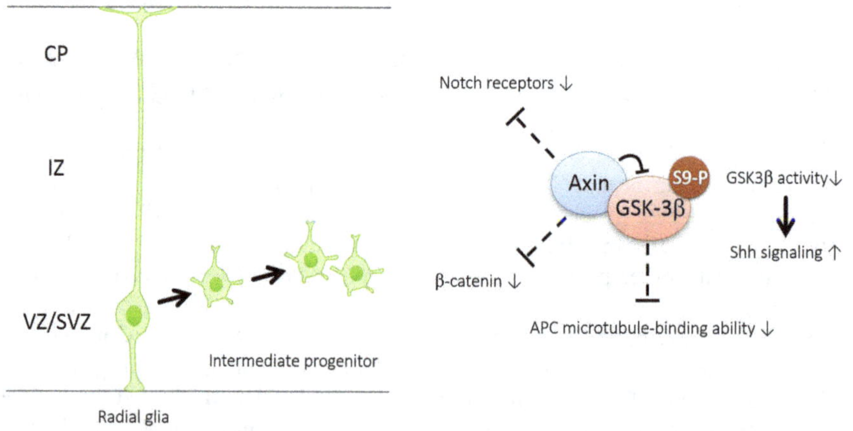

FIGURE 2 | Axin promotes the generation and amplification of intermediate progenitors by interacting with GSK3β in the cytoplasm. Axin is well-characterized as a "master" scaffold for various signaling proteins including GSK3β, β-catenin, Notch and adenomatosis polyposis coli (APC)—all of which are known to control neurogenesis. Interaction with Axin can cause increased Ser9 phosphorylation and subsequent inhibition of GSK3β in the cytoplasm. GSK3β inhibition may enhance intermediate progenitor amplification by activating Shh signaling and repressing the expression levels of Notch receptors and β-catenin, as well as APC-regulated division plane.

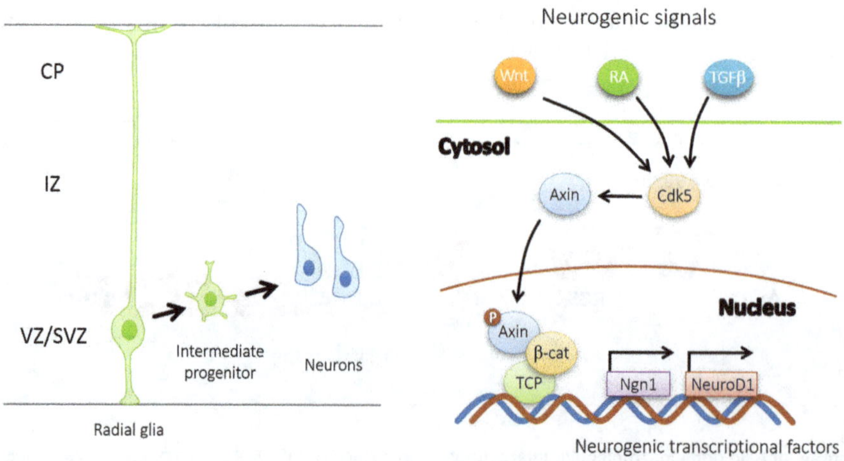

FIGURE 3 | Upon Cdk5 phosphorylation, Axin promotes the differentiation of intermediate progenitors by interacting with β-catenin in the nucleus. In response to neurogenic signals (Wnt, RA, TGFβ, etc.), nuclear Axin forms complex with β-catenin and TCP to activate downstream neurogenic transcriptional factors, such as Ngn1 and NeuroD1.

Axin-GSK3β Signaling in Neuronal Polarization and Migration

Newborn neurons exit the ventricular and subventricular zones, and migrate into the intermediate zone. They initially exhibit a multipolar morphology characterized by several thin processes in various directions but subsequently adopt a bipolar morphology with a leading process pointing toward the apical pia and a trailing process extending toward the ventricle. Directed by their leading processes, neurons migrate toward the cortical (i.e., pial) surface in an orderly progression to occupy their proper positions (Tsai and Gleeson, 2005). Each wave of migrating neurons travels past their predecessors, forming cortical layers of the cortical plate in an inside-out manner, in which the older and younger neurons reside in deeper layers closer to the ventricle and outer layers of the cerebral cortex closer to the pia, respectively (Noctor et al., 2004). Projection neurons generally migrate in two modes: radial glial fiber-independent somal translocation and radial glial fiber-dependent locomotion. Somal translocating neurons attach their long leading processes to the pia through Reelin-mediated cell-matrix adhesion (Sekine et al., 2012) and subsequently shorten them to move their cell bodies to their final positions and detach from the pia to terminate migration (Dulabon et al., 2000). Notably, as the cortical plate is sufficiently thin during the early stage of cortical development, early-generated neurons can extend leading processes to the pia and migrate through somal translocation alone (Nadarajah et al., 2001). On the other hand, locomoting neurons adhere to the radial glial fibers and extend their short leading processes to wrap around the fibers, forming a temporary adhesion that facilitates their migration along the fiber (Noctor et al., 2004; Ayala et al., 2007). Thus, various factors including the polarity and morphology of migrating neurons as well as adhesion with radial glial fibers contribute to the appropriate laminar positioning of neurons.

The first line of evidence suggesting that Axin plays a role in neuronal migration came from the effect of Axin overexpression in migrating neurons (Fang et al., 2013). Notably, a substantial number of Axin-overexpressing neurons are stacked in the intermediate zone, suggesting that Axin has an alternative function in neuronal migration probably through the regulation of GSK3 signaling (Fang et al., 2013). A recent study using mutant mice lacking both GSK3α and GSK3β confirms the *in vivo* role of GSK3 signaling in neuronal migration (Morgan-Smith et al., 2014). Conditional *Gsk3* deletion in cortical neurons under neuron-specific *Neurod6* promoter resulted in dramatic mislocalization of layer 2/3 neurons in deeper layers. In particular, *Gsk3* deletion disrupts the transition of cortical neurons from multipolar migration phase to bipolar migration phase (Morgan-Smith et al., 2014). Since GSK3β but not GSK3α interacts with Axin during neural development (Fang et al., 2011, 2013), these findings collectively suggest that Axin-GSK3β interaction can target the neuronal polarization process to regulate neuronal migration during cerebral cortical development.

How does Axin-GSK3β signaling specify the neuronal polarity? Increasing evidence suggests that GSK3β functions as a critical regulator of neuronal polarization and migration by controlling microtubule dynamics (Hur and Zhou, 2010). Initial studies on neuronal polarization came from cultured dissociated hippocampal neurons. Before polarity establishment, Ser9-phosphorylated GSK3β, which is the inactive form, is universally expressed at the tip of each neurite. Upon neuronal polarization, one of the neurites gives rise to the axon, where phosphorylated GSK3β becomes enriched at the tip of the nascent axon. Therefore, axon specification depends on the local inhibition of GSK3β in one neurite and activation of GSK3β in other neurites. Accordingly, multiple axons are induced when GSK3β activity is globally suppressed by pharmaceutical inhibitors or GSK3β-specific knockdown. In contrast, axon specification is impaired when the constitutive GSK3β-Ser9Ala mutant is overexpressed, and thus neuronal polarization is inhibited. Besides, the instructive role of GSK3β inactivation in axon specification is further demonstrated by the observation that the differentiated dendrite can be transformed into axons after axon-dendrite polarity specification. This evidence collectively indicates that local inhibition of GSK3β is essential for the establishment and maintenance of neuronal polarity (Hur and Zhou, 2010). Notably, we have suggested that the specific Axin-GSK3β interaction ensures the precise localization and inactivation of GSK3β in one neurite during neuronal polarization (Fang et al., 2011).

Cytoskeletal reorganization is required for neurons to undergo morphological changes during polarization and migration. Several substrates of GSK3β have been identified as important downstream effectors in regulating neuronal polarization through microtubule rearrangement (**Figure 4**). These substrates includes microtubule plus-end binding proteins CRMP-2 (Yoshimura et al., 2005), APC (Zumbrunn et al., 2001), and doublecortin DCX (Bilimoria et al., 2010), as well as structural microtubule associated proteins (MAPs) such as MAP1B (Trivedi et al., 2005) and Tau (Johnson and Stoothoff, 2004). In polarizing neurons, plus-end binding proteins CRMP-2 and APC localizes at the tips of immature neurites and later becomes concentrated in the growth cone of the nascent axon (Inagaki et al., 2001; Zumbrunn et al., 2001). Binding of unphosphorylated active forms of CRMP2, DCX, APC, and Tau to microtubules promotes their assembly and stabilization. The microtubule-binding activity of these proteins is abrogated by GSK3β phosphorylation (Hur and Zhou, 2010). Therefore, GSK3β inactivation in the growth cone of the nascent axon facilitates the interaction between MAPs and microtubules, and thus promotes axon initiation by specifically stabilizing one neurite. Similar to the effect of global GSK3β inhibition, overexpression of phosphorylation-deficient CRMP2-Ser514Ala is sufficient to induce multiple axons during neuronal polarization. In addition, GSK3β-mediated phosphorylation of MAP1B may also contribute to microtubule dynamics (Trivedi et al., 2005).

Roles of Axin in Axon Formation and Outgrowth

After neurons reach their final destinations, the leading process develops into an apical dendrite and extends up to the pia,

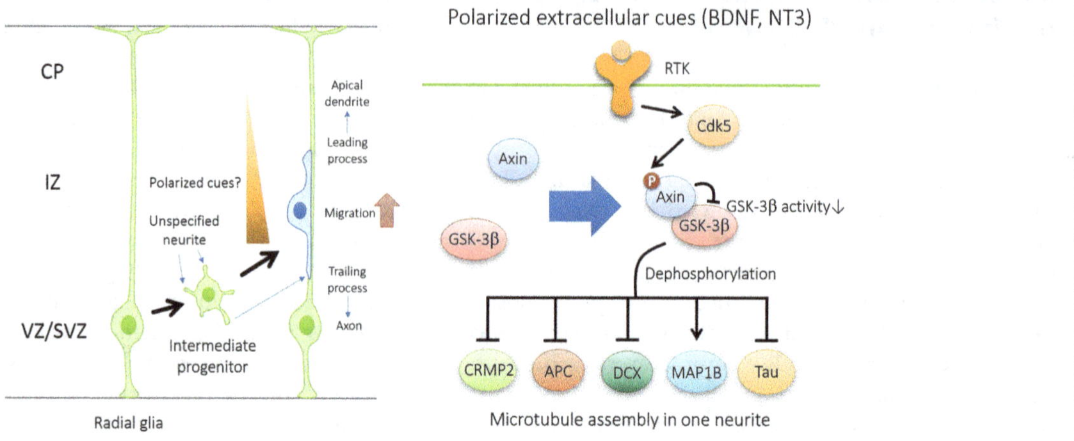

FIGURE 4 | Axin-GSK3β signaling regulates neuronal polarization during neuronal migration. In the presence of polarized extracellular cues such as brain-derived neurotrophic factor (BDNF) and NT3, Cdk5-dependent phosphorylation of Axin facilitates Axin-GSK3β interaction and local inhibition of GSK3β activity at the tip of nascent axon, and thus promotes microtubule assembly through the regulation of various microtubule-associated proteins, including CRMP2, APC, DCX, MAP1B, and Tau.

while the trailing process differentiates into an axon and grows toward the intermediate zone. Over time, the apical dendrite branches extensively and is accompanied by basal dendrites arborizing radially from the cell soma (Whitford et al., 2002). The axons pass vertically through the cortical plate and intermediate zone, sprout collaterals that arborize in specific intracortical layers, and bundle to form axonal tracts that project to intra- and subcortical areas (Hatanaka and Murakami, 2002). The projection targets determine the three basic subtypes of neurons: associative, commissural, and corticofugal, in which axons form connections within the cortex in the same hemisphere, opposite hemisphere, or away from the cortex, respectively (Molyneaux et al., 2007). Neurons in distinctive cortical and subcortical areas are functionally coordinated and integrated through their axonal projections to allow the proper cortical information processing. The patterns of axon projection and connection involve axon formation and extension, guidance, recognition of and targeting to specific areas, and elimination of inappropriate axon segments and branches. Among these processes, axon formation and extension are the most basic and are regulated by cytoskeletal reorganization.

Axon is initiated and facilitated by the extracellular cues. For example, TGF-β and its receptors specify the axon during brain development. TGF-β receptors are expressed in axons during embryonic development, and their receptor kinase activity is required for axon formation (Yi et al., 2010). The effect of TGF-β signaling on axon specification is mediated by the phosphorylation of Par6, a component of the Par3/Par6/aPKC complex. Neurotrophic factors such as brain-derived neurotrophic factor (BDNF) can also direct axon specification, because the first neurite contacting a BDNF stripe becomes the axon (Shelly et al., 2007). The effect of BDNF on axon specification requires the activation of the polarity-inducing kinase LKB1 via a cAMP-dependent protein kinase A pathway (Shelly et al., 2007). In another case, both BDNF and neurotrophin 3 stimulate the inhibition of GSK3β, resulting in the dephosphorylation of CRMP2, which consequently promotes axon outgrowth in cultured hippocampal neurons (Yoshimura et al., 2005).

Interestingly, recent evidence demonstrates that Axin plays an instrumental role in microtubule assembly and axonal transport in supporting axon formation and growth. Through Axin knockdown *in utero*, our laboratory demonstrated that the Cdk5-mediated phosphorylation of Axin contributes to axon formation through the inhibition of GSK3β *in vivo* (Fang et al., 2011). In particular, Cdk5 is activated through p35 to phosphorylate Axin at Thr485 in response to neurotrophins such as BDNF and neurotrophin 3 (NT-3). The phosphorylation of Axin enhances its interaction with GSK3β, which inhibits GSK3β activity, thereby increasing nonphosphorylated CRMP-2 and Tau in the growth cone (Fang et al., 2011). Non-phosphorylated CRMP-2 and Tau, which represents the active form, promotes microtubule assembly and stabilization to support the elongation of growing axons during development. Therefore, Axin expression and phosphorylation by Cdk5 are essential for axon formation and outgrowth through the regulation of microtubule dynamics (**Figure 5**). In addition to microtubule dynamics, efficient axonal transport requires Cdk5-mediated suppression of GSK3β, thereby preventing premature GSK3β-mediated cargo release (Morfini et al., 2004). Whether Cdk5 inhibits GSK3β by facilitating Axin-GSK3β interaction awaits further investigation.

Implications of Axin in Neurodevelopmental Disorders

As Axin is a multifaceted scaffold protein involved in diverse signaling pathways that regulate neural progenitor proliferation and differentiation, it is not surprising that its deregulation is associated with brain malformations such as micro- and

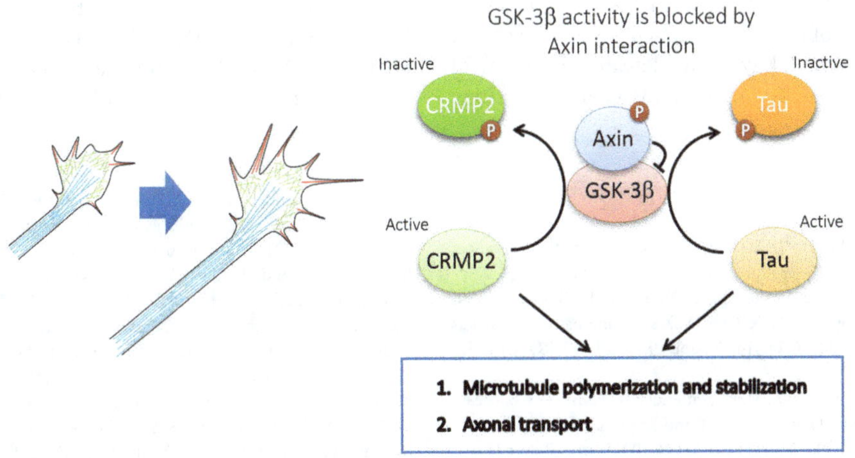

FIGURE 5 | Axin-GSK3β signaling promotes axon growth through microtubule assembly and axonal transport. GSK3β inactivation by Axin interaction maintains CRMP2 and Tau in active form and coordinates the local axon assembly at the growth cone and efficient axon growth.

macrocephaly. Notably, a previous study demonstrates that a mutation in the GSK3-binding domain of Axin results in the formation of small brains, mimicking human microcephaly (Heisenberg et al., 2001). Additional evidence in a human genetic study shows that the *Axin* gene is located in the same chromosomal region (16p13.3–12.1) as genetic mutations found in microcephaly patients (Kavaslar et al., 2000). Despite the lack of an Axin genetic mouse model, the recent development of *in utero* electroporation techniques have enabled the manipulation of Axin protein in neural progenitor cells during cerebral cortical development *in vivo* (Saito and Nakatsuji, 2001; Tabata and Nakajima, 2001). Accordingly, depletion or overexpression of Axin in the mouse neocortex results in premature and suppressed neuronal differentiation, which eventually lead to reduced and excessive numbers of cortical neurons at birth, respectively (Fang et al., 2013).

Axin is also implicated in the etiology of autism, a childhood-onset neurodevelopmental disorder characterized by disabilities in social interaction and communication as well as repetitive and compulsive behaviors. A postmortem study suggests that patients with autism often have increased neuronal density and number in the prefrontal cortex (McCaffery and Deutsch, 2005; Courchesne et al., 2011). We have recently generated a mouse model with enhanced neurogenesis by intraventricular injection of a tankyrase inhibitor, XAV939 (**Figure 1**; Huang et al., 2009). Injection of XAV939 transiently elevates the protein level of Axin in neural progenitors by preventing tankyrase-mediated protein degradation and consequently increases the number of upper-layer neurons in the developing mouse cortex without affecting astrogenesis or microglial reactivity (Fang et al., 2014). We demonstrated that enhanced neurogenesis leads to the overproduction of excitatory neurons, and impairs excitatory and inhibitory synaptic connection and balance. More importantly, these mice exhibit autism-like features, namely social interaction deficits in the three-chamber sociability test and compulsive behaviors such as increased self-grooming and marble burying (Fang et al., 2014). These results collectively illustrate a neurodevelopmental mechanism wherein enhanced neurogenesis and increased neuronal production result in autism-like features, hinting at the etiology of autism.

Concluding Remarks and Perspectives

Current evidence from several studies clearly indicates that Axin acts as a scaffold protein to integrate upstream signals while regulating various downstream interacting proteins involved in a wide array of cellular activities. Specifically, cytosolic Axin modulates downstream signaling of extracellular signals, including neurotrophins, WNT, Notch, and TGFβ. In addition, Axin enables efficient cytoskeletal reorganization and axon transport through GSK3β signaling and various MAPs. Moreover, nuclear Axin regulates gene expression by interacting with β-catenin and activating various neurogenic transcriptional factors. Therefore, Axin appears to be a master scaffold that modulates various developmental steps in the development of cerebral cortex.

After embryonic development, lifelong neurogenesis occurs in specific regions of the adult brain; various Axin-regulated signaling proteins such as GSK3β and β-catenin continue to play important roles in adult neurogenesis (Lie et al., 2005; Mao et al., 2009; Morales-Garcia et al., 2012). Therefore, it will be of interest to investigate how Axin regulates the proliferation and differentiation of adult neural stem cells and if enhancing Axin protein level improves adult neurogenesis, which is implicated in depression and neurodegenerative diseases such as Alzheimer's disease.

Acknowledgments

We apologize to the researchers whose studies could not be discussed or cited because of space limitations. We would like to thank Ka-Chun Lok for his help with preparing the figure and members of the Ip Laboratory for helpful discussions. This study was supported in part by the Hong Kong Research Grants Council Theme-based Research Scheme (T13-607/12R), the National Key Basic Research Program of China (2013CB530900), the Research Grants Council of Hong Kong SAR (HKUST660110, HKUST660610, HKUST660810, HKUST660110, HKUST661111, HKUST661212, and HKUST661013), the Innovation and Technology Fund for State Key Laboratory (ITCPT/17-9), and the SH Ho Foundation.

References

Ayala, R., Shu, T., and Tsai, L. H. (2007). Trekking across the brain: the journey of neuronal migration. *Cell* 128, 29–43. doi: 10.1016/j.cell.2006.12.021

Bilimoria, P. M., de la Torre-Ubieta, L., Ikeuchi, Y., Becker, E. B., Reiner, O., and Bonni, A. (2010). A JIP3-regulated GSK3beta/DCX signaling pathway restricts axon branching. *J. Neurosci.* 30, 16766–16776. doi: 10.1523/JNEUROSCI.1362-10.2010

Courchesne, E., Mouton, P. R., Calhoun, M. E., Semendeferi, K., Ahrens-Barbeau, C., Hallet, M. J., et al. (2011). Neuron number and size in prefrontal cortex of children with autism. *JAMA* 306, 2001–2010. doi: 10.1001/jama.2011.1638

Dulabon, L., Olson, E. C., Taglienti, M. G., Eisenhuth, S., McGrath, B., Walsh, C. A., et al. (2000). Reelin binds alpha3beta1 integrin and inhibits neuronal migration. *Neuron* 27, 33–44. doi: 10.1016/s0896-6273(00)00007-6

Ever, L., and Gaiano, N. (2005). Radial 'glial' progenitors: neurogenesis and signaling. *Curr. Opin. Neurobiol.* 15, 29–33. doi: 10.1016/j.conb.2005.01.005

Fang, W. Q., Chen, W. W., Fu, A. K., and Ip, N. Y. (2013). Axin directs the amplification and differentiation of intermediate progenitors in the developing cerebral cortex. *Neuron* 79, 665–679. doi: 10.1016/j.neuron.2013.06.017

Fang, W. Q., Chen, W. W., Jiang, L., Liu, K., Yung, W. H., Fu, A. K., et al. (2014). Overproduction of upper-layer neurons in the neocortex leads to autism-like features in mice. *Cell Rep.* 9, 1635–1643. doi: 10.1016/j.celrep.2014.11.003

Fang, W. Q., Ip, J. P., Li, R., Ng, Y. P., Lin, S. C., Chen, Y., et al. (2011). Cdk5-mediated phosphorylation of Axin directs axon formation during cerebral cortex development. *J. Neurosci.* 31, 13613–13624. doi: 10.1523/JNEUROSCI.3120-11.2011

Farkas, L. M., and Huttner, W. B. (2008). The cell biology of neural stem and progenitor cells and its significance for their proliferation versus differentiation during mammalian brain development. *Curr. Opin. Cell Biol.* 20, 707–715. doi: 10.1016/j.ceb.2008.09.008

Furuhashi, M., Yagi, K., Yamamoto, H., Furukawa, Y., Shimada, S., Nakamura, Y., et al. (2001). Axin facilitates Smad3 activation in the transforming growth factor beta signaling pathway. *Mol. Cell Biol.* 21, 5132–5141. doi: 10.1128/mcb.21.15.5132-5141.2001

Götz, M., and Huttner, W. B. (2005). The cell biology of neurogenesis. *Nat. Rev. Mol. Cell Biol.* 6, 777–788. doi: 10.1038/nrm1739

Götz, M., Malatesta, P., Hack, M. A., Hartfuss, E., Kettenmann, H., Klinkert, W., et al. (2003). Neuronal or glial progeny: regional differences in radial glia fate. *Neuron* 37, 751–764. doi: 10.1016/S0896-6273(03)00116-8

Guo, X., Ramirez, A., Waddell, D. S., Li, Z., Liu, X., and Wang, X. F. (2008). Axin and GSK3-control Smad3 protein stability and modulate TGF-signaling. *Genes Dev.* 22, 106–120. doi: 10.1101/gad.1590908

Hatanaka, Y., and Murakami, F. (2002). *In vitro* analysis of the origin, migratory behavior and maturation of cortical pyramidal cells. *J. Comp. Neurol.* 454, 1–14. doi: 10.1002/cne.10421

Heintz, N., Anthony, T. E., Klein, C., and Fishell, G. (2004). Radial glia serve as neuronal progenitors in all regions of the central nervous system. *Neuron* 41, 881–890. doi: 10.1016/s0896-6273(04)00140-0

Heisenberg, C. P., Houart, C., Take-Uchi, M., Rauch, G. J., Young, N., Coutinho, P., et al. (2001). A mutation in the Gsk3-binding domain of zebrafish Masterblind/Axin1 leads to a fate transformation of telencephalon and eyes to diencephalon. *Genes Dev.* 15, 1427–1434. doi: 10.1101/gad.194301

Huang, S. M., Mishina, Y. M., Liu, S., Cheung, A., Stegmeier, F., Michaud, G. A., et al. (2009). Tankyrase inhibition stabilizes axin and antagonizes Wnt signalling. *Nature* 461, 614–620. doi: 10.1038/nature08356

Hur, E. M., and Zhou, F. Q. (2010). GSK3 signalling in neural development. *Nat. Rev. Neurosci.* 11, 539–551. doi: 10.1038/nrn2870

Huttner, W. B., and Kosodo, Y. (2005). Symmetric versus asymmetric cell division during neurogenesis in the developing vertebrate central nervous system. *Curr. Opin. Cell Biol.* 17, 648–657. doi: 10.1016/j.ceb.2005.10.005

Inagaki, N., Chihara, K., Arimura, N., Ménager, C., Kawano, Y., Matsuo, N., et al. (2001). CRMP-2 induces axons in cultured hippocampal neurons. *Nat. Neurosci.* 4, 781–782. doi: 10.1038/90476

Johnson, G. V., and Stoothoff, W. H. (2004). Tau phosphorylation in neuronal cell function and dysfunction. *J. Cell Sci.* 117, 5721–5729. doi: 10.1242/jcs.01558

Kavaslar, G. N., Onengüt, S., Derman, O., Kaya, A., and Tolun, A. (2000). The novel genetic disorder microhydranencephaly maps to chromosome 16p13.3-12.1. *Am. J. Hum. Genet.* 66, 1705–1709. doi: 10.1086/302898

Kikuchi, A. (1999). Roles of Axin in the Wnt signalling pathway. *Cell. Signal.* 11, 777–788. doi: 10.1016/s0898-6568(99)00054-6

Kowalczyk, T., Pontious, A., Englund, C., Daza, R. A., Bedogni, F., Hodge, R., et al. (2009). Intermediate neuronal progenitors (basal progenitors) produce pyramidal-projection neurons for all layers of cerebral cortex. *Cereb. Cortex* 19, 2439–2450. doi: 10.1093/cercor/bhn260

Kriegstein, A. R., Noctor, S. C., Flint, A. C., Weissman, T. A., Wong, W. S., and Clinton, B. K. (2002). Dividing precursor cells of the embryonic cortical ventricular zone have morphological and molecular characteristics of radial glia. *J. Neurosci.* 22, 3161–3173.

Lie, D. C., Colamarino, S. A., Song, H. J., Désiré, L., Mira, H., Consiglio, A., et al. (2005). Wnt signalling regulates adult hippocampal neurogenesis. *Nature* 437, 1370–1375. doi: 10.1038/nature04108

Liu, W., Rui, H., Wang, J., Lin, S., He, Y., Chen, M., et al. (2006). Axin is a scaffold protein in TGF-beta signaling that promotes degradation of Smad7 by Arkadia. *EMBO J.* 25, 1646–1658. doi: 10.1038/sj.emboj.7601057

Luo, W., and Lin, S. C. (2004). Axin: a master scaffold for multiple signaling pathways. *Neurosignals* 13, 99–113. doi: 10.1159/000076563

Mao, Y., Ge, X., Frank, C. L., Madison, J. M., Koehler, A. N., Doud, M. K., et al. (2009). Disrupted in schizophrenia 1 regulates neuronal progenitor proliferation via modulation of GSK3beta/beta-catenin signaling. *Cell* 136, 1017–1031. doi: 10.1016/j.cell.2008.12.044

McCaffery, P., and Deutsch, C. K. (2005). Macrocephaly and the control of brain growth in autistic disorders. *Prog. Neurobiol.* 77, 38–56. doi: 10.1016/j.pneurobio.2005.10.005

Molyneaux, B. J., Arlotta, P., Menezes, J. R., and Macklis, J. D. (2007). Neuronal subtype specification in the cerebral cortex. *Nat. Rev. Neurosci.* 8, 427–437. doi: 10.1038/nrn2151

Morales-Garcia, J. A., Luna-Medina, R., Alonso-Gil, S., Sanz-Sancristobal, M., Palomo, V., Gil, C., et al. (2012). Glycogen synthase kinase 3 inhibition promotes adult hippocampal neurogenesis *in vitro* and *in vivo*. *ACS Chem. Neurosci.* 3, 963–971. doi: 10.1021/cn300110c

Morfini, G., Szebenyi, G., Brown, H., Pant, H. C., Pigino, G., DeBoer, S., et al. (2004). A novel CDK5-dependent pathway for regulating GSK3 activity and kinesin-driven motility in neurons. *EMBO J.* 23, 2235–2245. doi: 10.1038/sj.emboj.7600237

Morgan-Smith, M., Wu, Y., Zhu, X., Pringle, J., and Snider, W. D. (2014). GSK-3 signaling in developing cortical neurons is essential for radial migration and dendritic orientation. *Elife* 3:e02663. doi: 10.7554/elife.02663

Nadarajah, B., Brunstrom, J. E., Grutzendler, J., Wong, R. O., and Pearlman, A. L. (2001). Two modes of radial migration in early development of the cerebral cortex. *Nat. Neurosci.* 4, 143–150. doi: 10.1038/83967

Noctor, S. C., Martínez-Cerdeño, V., Ivic, L., and Kriegstein, A. R. (2004). Cortical neurons arise in symmetric and asymmetric division zones and migrate through specific phases. *Nat. Neurosci.* 7, 136–144. doi: 10.1038/nn1172

Pontious, A., Kowalczyk, T., Englund, C., and Hevner, R. F. (2008). Role of intermediate progenitor cells in cerebral cortex development. *Dev. Neurosci.* 30, 24–32. doi: 10.1159/000109848

Saito, T., and Nakatsuji, N. (2001). Efficient gene transfer into the embryonic mouse brain using *in vivo* electroporation. *Dev. Biol.* 240, 237–246. doi: 10.1006/dbio.2001.0439

Sekine, K., Kawauchi, T., Kubo, K., Honda, T., Herz, J., Hattori, M., et al. (2012). Reelin controls neuronal positioning by promoting cell-matrix adhesion via inside-out activation of integrin alpha5beta1. *Neuron* 76, 353–369. doi: 10.1016/j.neuron.2012.07.020

Shelly, M., Cancedda, L., Heilshorn, S., Sumbre, G., and Poo, M. M. (2007). LKB1/STRAD promotes axon initiation during neuronal polarization. *Cell* 129, 565–577. doi: 10.1016/j.cell.2007.04.012

Tabata, H., and Nakajima, K. (2001). Efficient *in utero* gene transfer system to the developing mouse brain using electroporation: visualization of neuronal migration in the developing cortex. *Neuroscience* 103, 865–872. doi: 10.1016/s0306-4522(01)00016-1

Trivedi, N., Marsh, P., Goold, R. G., Wood-Kaczmar, A., and Gordon-Weeks, P. R. (2005). Glycogen synthase kinase-3beta phosphorylation of MAP1B at Ser1260 and Thr1265 is spatially restricted to growing axons. *J. Cell Sci.* 118, 993–1005. doi: 10.1242/jcs.01697

Tsai, L. H., and Gleeson, J. G. (2005). Nucleokinesis in neuronal migration. *Neuron* 46, 383–388. doi: 10.1016/j.neuron.2005.04.013

Whitford, K. L., Dijkhuizen, P., Polleux, F., and Ghosh, A. (2002). Molecular control of cortical dendrite development. *Annu. Rev. Neurosci.* 25, 127–149. doi: 10.1146/annurev.neuro.25.112701.142932

Yi, J. J., Barnes, A. P., Hand, R., Polleux, F., and Ehlers, M. D. (2010). TGF-beta signaling specifies axons during brain development. *Cell* 142, 144–157. doi: 10.1016/j.cell.2010.06.010

Yoshimura, T., Kawano, Y., Arimura, N., Kawabata, S., Kikuchi, A., and Kaibuchi, K. (2005). GSK-3beta regulates phosphorylation of CRMP-2 and neuronal polarity. *Cell* 120, 137–149. doi: 10.1016/j.cell.2004.11.012

Zeng, L., Fagotto, F., Zhang, T., Hsu, W., Vasicek, T. J., Perry, W. L., et al. (1997). The mouse Fused locus encodes Axin, an inhibitor of the Wnt signaling pathway that regulates embryonic axis formation. *Cell* 90, 181–192. doi: 10.1016/s0092-8674(00)80324-4

Zumbrunn, J., Kinoshita, K., Hyman, A. A., and Näthke, I. S. (2001). Binding of the adenomatous polyposis coli protein to microtubules increases microtubule stability and is regulated by GSK3 beta phosphorylation. *Curr. Biol.* 11, 44–49. doi: 10.1016/s0960-9822(01)00002-1

15

Regulation of Cerebral Cortical Neurogenesis by the Pax6 Transcription Factor

Martine N. Manuel[†], *Da Mi*[†], *John O. Mason and David J. Price* *

Centre for Integrative Physiology, The University of Edinburgh, Edinburgh, UK

***Correspondence:**
David J. Price,
Centre for Integrative Physiology, The University of Edinburgh, Hugh Robson Building, George Square, Edinburgh EH8 9XD, UK
David.Price@ed.ac.uk

[†] *These authors have contributed equally to this work.*

Understanding brain development remains a major challenge at the heart of understanding what makes us human. The neocortex, in evolutionary terms the newest part of the cerebral cortex, is the seat of higher cognitive functions. Its normal development requires the production, positioning, and appropriate interconnection of very large numbers of both excitatory and inhibitory neurons. Pax6 is one of a relatively small group of transcription factors that exert high-level control of cortical development, and whose mutation or deletion from developing embryos causes major brain defects and a wide range of neurodevelopmental disorders. Pax6 is very highly conserved between primate and non-primate species, is expressed in a gradient throughout the developing cortex and is essential for normal corticogenesis. Our understanding of Pax6's functions and the cellular processes that it regulates during mammalian cortical development has significantly advanced in the last decade, owing to the combined application of genetic and biochemical analyses. Here, we review the functional importance of Pax6 in regulating cortical progenitor proliferation, neurogenesis, and formation of cortical layers and highlight important differences between rodents and primates. We also review the pathological effects of *PAX6* mutations in human neurodevelopmental disorders. We discuss some aspects of Pax6's molecular actions including its own complex transcriptional regulation, the distinct molecular functions of its splice variants and some of Pax6's known direct targets which mediate its actions during cortical development.

Keywords: proliferation, cell cycle, differentiation, neuronal fate, neurotransmitter fate, cortical lamination, BAF complex, Meis2

Introduction

The expansion of the cerebral cortex is a major hallmark of mammalian evolution, particularly in the primate lineages where it achieves its greatest complexity in humans (Martin, 1990). Despite great variation in size, there are many similarities in the structure and function of the cerebral cortex across all mammalian species. These similarities have encouraged neuroscientists to use relatively simple cortices, such as those of rodents, as models in which to investigate biological processes and mechanisms with likely relevance to humans. The strength of rodent models, in particular mice, derives in large part from the genetic and transgenic approaches that can be used to study molecular mechanisms. Much of the research described in this review comes from studies of mice and the view of cortical development and Pax6's role in that process presented here is strongly biased toward mouse corticogenesis. It is important to recognize, however, that significant differences exist between the developing and mature cortices of primate and non-primate species that are more than just differences of scale, and we shall highlight some of these. It is remarkable that many high-level regulatory genes such as *Pax6* are themselves extremely highly conserved between primates and non-primates although they influence and control aspects of cortical development that differ: for example, the amino acid sequences of human PAX6 and mouse Pax6 are identical (Ton et al., 1992) although Pax6's expression in primate embryos extends to cortical structures that do not exist in mice. This implies that evolutionary changes in the functions of these regulators have been achieved by changes in the mechanisms regulating their expression and in the ways in which the downstream molecular networks respond to them, but we know almost nothing about these evolutionary changes at a molecular level.

The cerebral cortex is derived from the dorsal component (or pallium) of the embryonic telencephalon, which is itself the anterior-most subdivision of the forebrain (Kiecker and Lumsden, 2005). The cerebral cortex can be further sub-divided into distinct regions, including the neocortex, a novel acquisition of mammals that has evolved between the phylogenetically older archicortex (comprising entorhinal cortex, retrosplenial cortex, subiculum, and hippocampus) and paleocortex (olfactory piriform cortex). The evolutionary expansion of the neocortex is thought to account for much of the increase in overall brain size and complexity in more advanced species (Krubitzer and Kaas, 2005; O'Leary et al., 2007). The neocortex (hereafter referred to simply as cortex) contains an extraordinarily large number of neurons arrayed in a six-layered sheet, with neurons in each layer organized into a complex network of local circuits and subcortical connections. In primates, some of these layers are subdivided in some cortical areas: for example, in primary visual cortex, layer 4 is subdivided into layers 4a, b, and c. The primate cortex is also characterized by an expansion of the superficial layers of the cortex, layers 2 and 3 (also known as the supragranular layers), which have an important function in the transfer of information between cortical areas. Increased intracortical information processing is likely to have contributed to heightened cognitive ability. In all mammals, the cortex comprises two major groups of neurons: the majority are excitatory glutamatergic projection neurons (70–80%), which exhibit a characteristic pyramidal morphology and extend axons to distant intracortical, subcortical, and subcerebral targets; a minority are inhibitory GABAergic non-pyramidal interneurons (25–30% in primates, 15–20% in rodents), which have short axons and project locally (Hendry et al., 1987; Beaulieu, 1993). An appropriate balance between the excitatory and inhibitory circuitry of the cortex is critical for its normal function.

Pax6 is a pivotal gene in CNS development. It is expressed when the major components of the developing CNS first emerge after neural tube closure and its expression patterns change considerably as major structures such as the cerebral cortex specialize and expand. Its expression plays a major role in the subsequent development of the regions that continue to express it. In this review we shall discuss how Pax6 plays critical roles in aspects of corticogenesis that include the early patterning of telencephalic subdivisions, control of cortical cell number, normal cortical layer formation and the development of the correct balance of excitatory and inhibitory neurons. We shall review what is known about the upstream control of *Pax6*'s transcription, the molecular basis of its functions and its actions on genes downstream of it and the cellular processes they regulate.

Corticogenesis in Rodents and Primates and the Cortical Expression of Pax6

The closure of the neural tube is accompanied by its disproportionate expansion anteriorly to generate the early forebrain. The earliest cortical progenitors undergo symmetric proliferative divisions at the ventricular surface to amplify a pool of progenitors, an increasing proportion of which then divide asymmetrically to regenerate progenitors and to produce other cell types including neurons.

In mouse, the generation of excitatory cortical neurons occurs between embryonic day 11 (E11) and E18 (Gillies and Price, 1993; Price et al., 1997; Levers et al., 2001). Their progenitors are located in one of two pallial germinal epithelia, namely the ventricular zone (VZ), which lies adjacent to the ventricles, and the subventricular zone (SVZ), which lies just above the VZ (**Figure 1**). The early symmetrically dividing cortical neuroepithelial cells (NECs) that each produce two daughter NECs per division and whose population rapidly expands laterally and radially, transform into another type of progenitor called, for historical reasons, radial glial cells (RGCs; **Figure 1**). RGCs, whose long processes span the neuroepithelium, have been known for a long time to provide guidance for migrating neurons (Levitt and Rakic, 1980; Rakic, 1988; Hatten, 2002; Tan and Shi, 2013). Despite having morphological and molecular features associated with glial cells, they are progenitors capable of generating other types of progenitor, neurons and glial cells (Malatesta et al., 2000, 2003; Miyata et al., 2001; Noctor et al., 2001; Skogh et al., 2001; Heins et al., 2002; Tan and Shi, 2013). RGCs constitute the majority of the VZ progenitor population. They are often referred to as apical progenitors (APs) due to the location of their cell body close to the ventricular or apical surface of the VZ, to which they extend a short process while sending a longer basal process radially to the pial surface of the cortex (Cameron and Rakic, 1991; Bentivoglio and Mazzarello, 1999; Tan and Shi, 2013). As they progress through the cell cycle, RGCs undergo interkinetic nuclear migration. Their nucleus migrates radially through the cytoplasm such that mitosis occurs at the apical ventricular surface and S-phase at a basal position in the VZ. While at early stages of corticogenesis RGCs predominantly self-renew via symmetric divisions, they progressively switch to asymmetric divisions, which produce one daughter RGC and one daughter cell with a heightened level of commitment (Noctor et al., 2001, 2004; Haydar et al., 2003; Huttner and Kosodo, 2005; Tan and Shi, 2013). The differentiating daughter cell either migrates radially to the pial surface and differentiates into a neuron or migrates to the

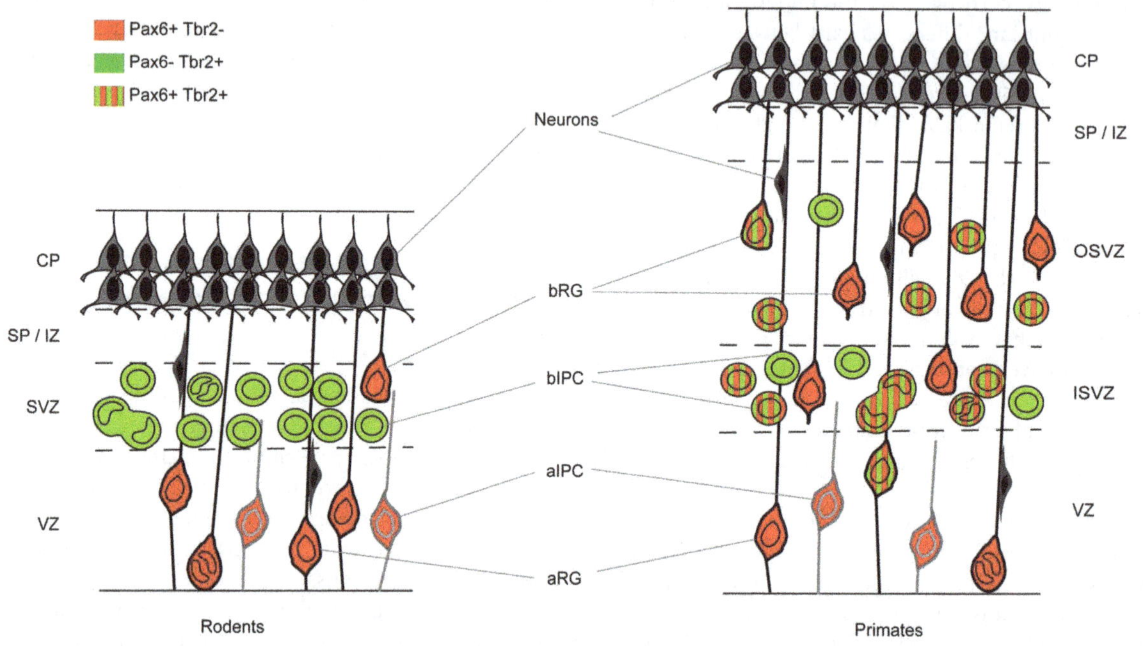

FIGURE 1 | Cortical germinal areas of rodents and primates. Coronal section through the developing cortex of a rodent and a primate showing progenitor types and whether they express Pax6 and/or Tbr2. CP, cortical plate; SP, subplate; IZ, intermediate zone; SVZ, subventricular zone; ISVZ, inner subventricular zone; OSVZ, outer subventricular zone; VZ, ventricular zone; aRG, apical radial glia; bRG, basal radial glia; aIPC, apical intermediate progenitor cell; bIPC, basal intermediate progenitor cell.

SVZ to become an intermediate progenitor cell (IPC), also called a basal progenitor (BP) or basal IPC (bIPC; **Figure 1**; Haubensak et al., 2004; Miyata et al., 2004; Noctor et al., 2004). BPs accumulate in the SVZ and divide mainly symmetrically to generate two neurons. It is thought that most cortical projection neurons are generated by BPs (Farkas and Huttner, 2008). In addition to RGCs, the VZ contains another smaller subpopulation of APs called short neural precursors (SNPs), also known as apical IPCs (aIPC; **Figure 1**). Unlike RGCs, aIPCs do not self-renew and only generate pairs of neurons via symmetric divisions (Gal et al., 2006; Tan and Shi, 2013).

Significant progress in understanding the mechanisms underlying corticogenesis has been made through analysis of gene expression in both progenitor cells and post-mitotic neurons. Such studies have revealed a crucial role for transcription factors (TFs) as molecular markers of distinct progenitor and neuron types and as key regulators of progenitor cell proliferation and cell fate decisions. At the onset of neurogenesis, TFs including Pax6, Emx2, and Tlx expressed in the cortical neuroepithelium function mainly to influence areal patterning and regulate progenitor cell proliferation (Bishop et al., 2000, 2002; Muzio et al., 2002; Muzio and Mallamaci, 2003; Stenman et al., 2003a,b; Hevner, 2006). As neurogenesis proceeds, a large number of TFs are involved in regulating the balance between progenitor cell proliferation and neuronal differentiation. Regulating this balance is essential for the generation of the correct proportions of different classes of neurons and subsequent circuit assembly.

During the neurogenic period in the mouse cortex, Pax6 is expressed by VZ APs in a high rostro-lateral to low caudo-medial gradient (**Figures 2** and **3**). As well as being graded spatially, the expression of Pax6 is also graded temporally, with highest levels present at the onset of corticogenesis. APs that give rise to BPs transiently express the proneural TF Neurogenin 2 (Ngn2; Britz et al., 2006). Pax6 is not expressed in BPs which are characterized by their expression of another TF, Tbr2, or in post-mitotic neurons which express Tbr1 (**Figure 1**; Englund et al., 2005). Thus a sequential Pax6 → Ngn2 → Tbr2 → Tbr1 expression correlates with the transition of APs to BPs to post-mitotic neurons.

In the macaque cortex, Rakic (1974) showed that cortical neurogenesis occurs between E45 and E100. Gestation in this species lasts 165 days and so cortical neurons are generated relatively earlier in gestation in primates than in rodents. The primate SVZ forms earlier and shows a much greater expansion than in rodents, becoming the predominant progenitor zone by mid-corticogenesis (Smart et al., 2002). It is split into the inner and outer SVZs separated by an inner fiber layer (Smart et al., 2002; Lukaszewicz et al., 2005; Zecevic et al., 2005; Fietz et al., 2010; Hansen et al., 2010; Florio and Huttner, 2014). The inner subventricular zone (ISVZ) contains mainly IPCs similar to those in the rodent SVZ whereas the outer subventricular zone (OSVZ) contains mainly basal RGCs (bRGCs) similar to the APs present in the rodent VZ (**Figure 1**). bRGCs undergo proliferative divisions and self renewing asymmetric divisions to generate one bRGC daughter cell and one IPC that can proliferate further (Fietz et al., 2010; Hansen et al., 2010; Florio and Huttner, 2014). bRGCs have

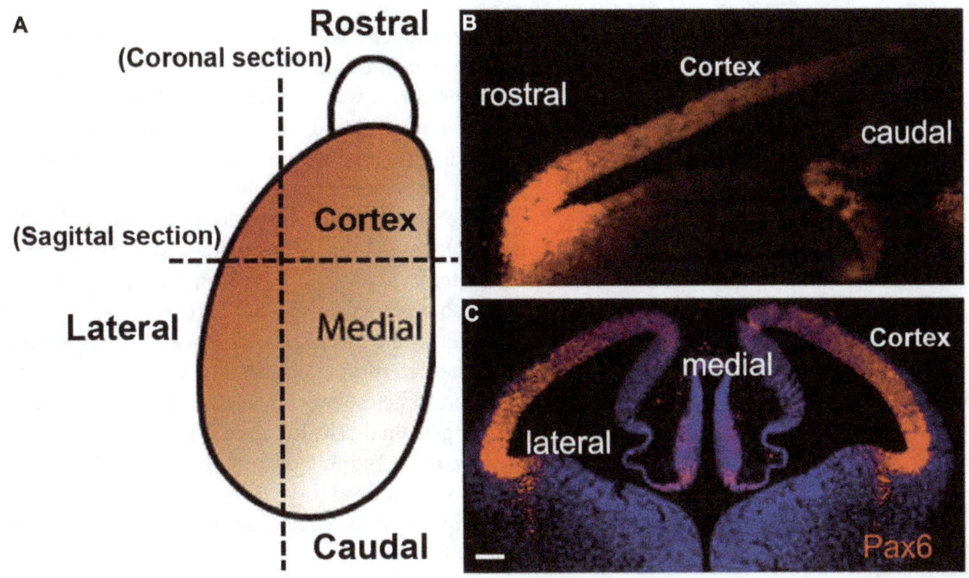

FIGURE 2 | The gradient expression pattern of Pax6 protein in the mouse developing cortex. (A) A schematic diagram shows the Pax6 protein (red) is normally expressed in a ^{high}rostrolateral to ^{low}caudomedial gradient in the developing cortex during early cortical development. **(B,C)** immunofluorescence staining for Pax6 protein in sagittal section **(B)** and coronal section **(C)** from E12.5 mouse WT embryos (scale bars, 100 μm).

also been observed in the rodent SVZ but, while they constitute about half of all progenitors present in the primate SVZ, they account for only a minute fraction of the SVZ progenitors in rodents (**Figure 1**). The OSVZ is the major source of supragranular layer neurons (Letinic et al., 2002; Lukaszewicz et al., 2005).

The sequential Pax6 → Ngn2 → Tbr2 → Tbr1 expression that correlates with the AP → BP → post-mitotic neuron transition in mice is not found during primate corticogenesis. In contrast to rodents, Pax6 is expressed by progenitors in the VZ, ISVZ, and OSVZ in primates (**Figure 3**; Fietz et al., 2010; Betizeau et al., 2013; Florio and Huttner, 2014) and many progenitors co-express Pax6 and Tbr2 (**Figure 1**). In the macaque, the majority of VZ progenitors (60–80%) express only Pax6 during early and mid-stages of corticogenesis (up to E79), but at later stages (after E79) 40% of them co-express Tbr2 (Betizeau et al., 2013; Florio and Huttner, 2014; **Figure 1**). In the ISVZ, 60–80% of progenitors co-express Pax6 and Tbr2, 5–30% express only Tbr2 and less than 15% express only Pax6. In the OSVZ, Pax6, and Tbr2 are co-expressed by 25–50% of progenitors while 20–35% express only Pax6 and 10–20% only Tbr2 (**Figure 1**; Betizeau et al., 2013; Florio and Huttner, 2014).

In mice, cortical GABAergic interneurons originate from distant germinal domains in the ganglionic eminences and follow tangential migratory routes to reach the developing cortex (Gelman and Marin, 2010). In primates, the origin of cortical interneurons is controversial. It has been proposed that while many interneurons have a ventral telencephalic origin, a significant fraction are produced in the progenitor layers of the cortex itself during the second half of corticogenesis (Letinic et al., 2002; Zecevic et al., 2005; Petanjek et al., 2008; Jakovcevski et al., 2011). However, a recent study by Hansen et al. (2013) found no evidence of interneuron production in the cortical wall. Instead, their analysis suggests that, as in rodents, the vast majority of human cortical interneurons are produced in the ganglionic eminences (Hansen et al., 2013).

In all mammalian species, the positions adopted by neurons migrating from the cortical progenitor zones to the overlying developing cortical plate (CP) are related to their birthdate. Each successive generation of newly born projection neurons bypasses earlier-born neurons and settles close to the pial edge of the CP. Thus, cortical layers (with the exception of layer 1) are formed in a deep-first superficial-last sequence (Angevine and Sidman, 1961; Berry and Rogers, 1965; Rakic, 1974; McConnell, 1995; Tan and Shi, 2013). When projection neurons arrive in their final laminar positions, they undergo terminal differentiation including elaboration of their dendrites and axons to establish connections and eventually form the cortical circuitry. Projection neurons in each layer tend to exhibit similar gene expression patterns, morphologies and organization of afferent and efferent connections (Stiles and Jernigan, 2010).

Human Brain Disorders Associated with *PAX6* Mutations

In humans, heterozygous loss-of-function mutations of *PAX6* cause sight-threatening congenital eye defects, typically including severe hypoplasia of the iris (aniridia) and retina. These mutations are also associated with a range of neurological and psychiatric conditions including nystagmus, impaired auditory processing and verbal working memory, autism, and mental retardation (Malandrini et al., 2001; Bamiou et al., 2004, 2007a,b; Davis et al., 2008; Hingorani et al., 2009; Maekawa et al.,

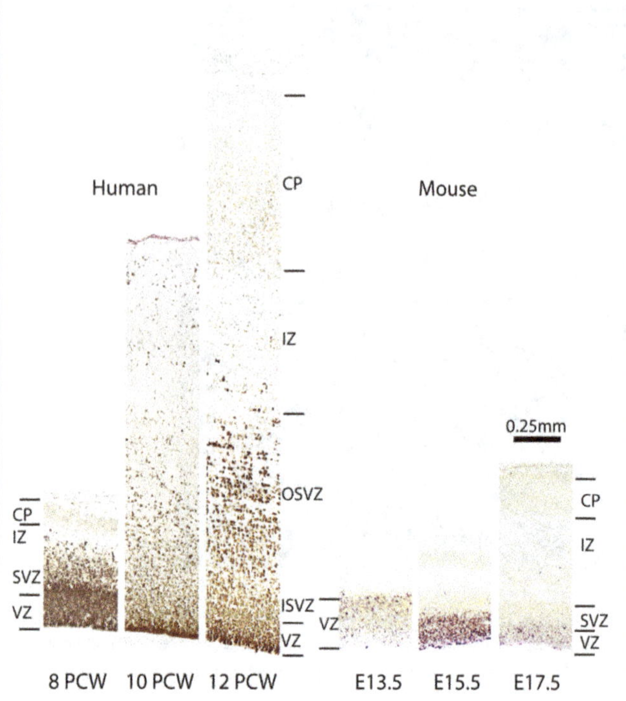

FIGURE 3 | Comparison of Pax6 expression in embryonic human and mouse cortex. Images from human cortices at 8, 10, and 12 post-coital weeks (PCWs) were generated using material from the Human Developmental Biology Resource (www.hdbr.org) as part of the HuDSeN (Kerwin et al., 2010) human gene expression spatial database (http://www.hudsen.org) based at Newcastle University. PAX6 is expressed in the ventricular zone (VZ) and subventricular zone (SVZ) at 8 PCW. The SVZ divides into an outer and an inner subventricular zone (OSVZ and ISVZ), both of which continue to express PAX6. In mice, Pax6 expression is confined almost exclusively to the VZ during corticogenesis, as shown here at embryonic days (E) 13.5, 15.5, and 17.5. Additional abbreviations: CP, cortical plate; IZ, intermediate zone.

2009). These conditions are linked to structural brain defects including reduced size of the corpus callosum and anterior commissure, abnormalities of the cerebral cortex and cerebellum and absence of the pineal gland (Sisodiya et al., 2001; Free et al., 2003; Mitchell et al., 2003; Bamiou et al., 2004, 2007b; Ellison-Wright et al., 2004).

Only four cases of children with mutations in both *PAX6* alleles (compound heterozygotes) have been reported (Glaser et al., 1994; Schmidt-Sidor et al., 2009; Solomon et al., 2009). Two of them survived past birth, one only for about 1 week (Glaser et al., 1994), the other until at least 4 years (Solomon et al., 2009). The former had anophthalmia, the latter microphthalmia, and both had numerous defects in the CNS including agenesis of the corpus callosum and microcephaly. Glaser et al. (1994) described a disturbed stratification of the cerebral cortex with heterotopic islands of germinal and ependymal cells, as well as focal polymicrogyria of the cerebral cortex. Two other cases were sibling fetuses with the pregnancies terminated at 21 and 23 weeks (Schmidt-Sidor et al., 2009). In both cases the brain was very small, filling only 1/3 of the cranial cavity, and displayed completely disorganized structures of the brain hemispheres and cerebellum. Microscopic analysis showed that the cerebral hemispheres contained an enormous amount of germinal matrix both in the inner parts and at the surface of the hemispheres. The cortex was very narrow with a paucity of cells with an irregular distribution of large neurons. The structure of the cortex was disturbed with a thick layer of germinal cells on its surface, a poorly defined marginal zone and no normal stratification. In the entire cortex the cells were mainly in clusters. The development of the white matter was also severely disturbed. The intermediate zone was absent. In several places of the cortex and also between clusters of neuroblasts inside the brain hemispheres there were fascicles of axons which did not form normal tracts. The heterotopia of germinal cells observed in the human compound heterozygotes (**Figure 4A**) are reminiscent of the clusters of germinal cells found in the intermediate zone of the cortex of *Pax6*$^{-/-}$ mouse embryos (**Figure 4B**; Caric et al., 1997). In these Pax6 mutant embryos it is thought that the clusters form as a consequence of a cell non-autonomous migration defect (Caric et al., 1997).

Structure and Transcriptional Regulation of the *Pax6* Locus

In both human and mouse, the *Pax6* gene has 16 exons distributed over a 30 kb genomic region including alternatively spliced exons *alpha* and 5a (Glaser et al., 1992; Williams et al., 1998; Kammandel et al., 1999; Plaza et al., 1999a; Xu et al., 1999b). Four transcription start sites have been identified in mouse *Pax6*, associated with the P_0, P_1, P_{alpha}, and P_4 promoters respectively (**Figure 5**; Kammandel et al., 1999; Xu et al., 1999b; Kleinjan et al., 2004; Morgan, 2004). Transcriptional regulation of the *Pax6* locus is particularly complex. A number of short-range regulatory elements have been identified in the vicinity of the *Pax6* coding region which control tissue-specific *Pax6* expression (**Figure 5**; Kammandel et al., 1999; Plaza et al., 1999b;

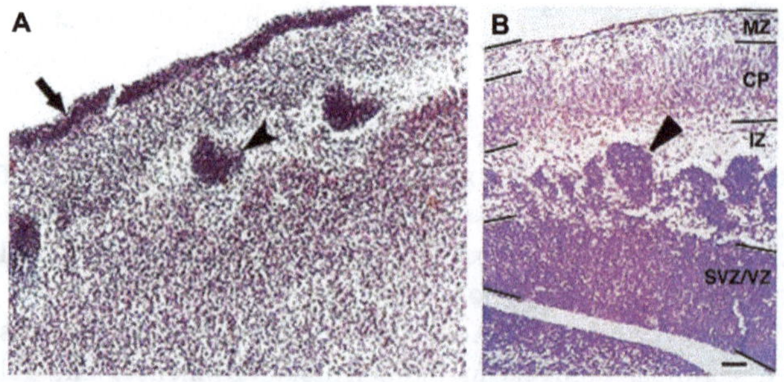

FIGURE 4 | Histology of *Pax6*$^{-/-}$ developing cortex in human and mouse. (A) Coronal section through the cortex of a fetus with a compound heterozygosity for two *PAX6* mutations showing a layer of germinal cells on the surface of the cortex (arrow) and heterotopia of germinal cells within the cortex (arrowhead). Photograph taken from Schmidt-Sidor et al. (2009). **(B)** Coronal section through the cortex of a *Pax6*$^{-/-}$ mutant mouse embryo showing clusters of germinal cells in the intermediate zone (arrowhead). Photograph from Caric et al. (1997).

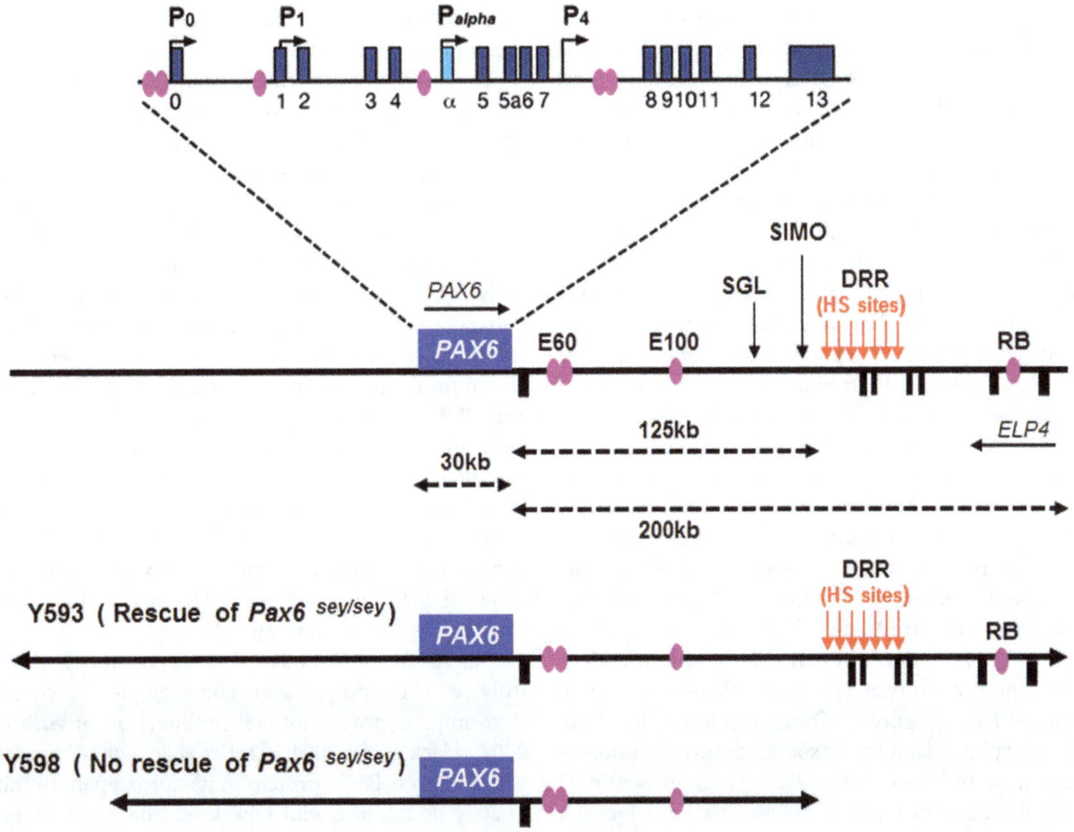

FIGURE 5 | Structure and transcriptional regulation of the *PAX6* locus. Schematic map of human chromosome 11p13 shows the locations of the PAX6 and ELP4 loci, which are in an antisense orientation relative to each other. The locations of PAX6 promoters (P0, P1, Pa, and P4) are indicated by black arrows. Blue rectangles indicate *PAX6* exons, while black rectangles below the line indicate *ELP4* exons. The known highly conserved regulatory elements, such as E60, E100 and RB, are indicated by purple ellipses. The breakpoints of the two distal-most aniridia-associated rearrangements are indicated by "SGL" and "SIMO." The location of the downstream regulatory region (DRR) is shown by red arrows. The known DNaseI hypersensitive sites (HS sites) within the DRR region are shown by red arrows. The schematic maps of YACs Y593 (420 kb) and Y589 (310 kb) are indicated. In transgenic mice, Y593, but not Y589, rescues the mouse *Sey* phenotype and homozygous *Sey* lethality.

Kleinjan et al., 2001, 2004; Griffin et al., 2002). Some of these elements exhibit overlapping tissue specificity, particularly in the eye, telencephalon and diencephalon, suggesting that they exert functions through cooperative interactions.

Although these short-range regulatory elements account for much of *Pax6*'s normal expression pattern in mice, genetic analyses in both humans and mice revealed that they are insufficient to drive the full pattern of *Pax6* expression, particularly in the eye and forebrain (Kim and Lauderdale, 2006; Kleinjan et al., 2006; McBride et al., 2011). The first evidence that PAX6 expression is influenced by distant regulatory elements located far downstream of *PAX6*'s coding exons came from studies of aniridia patients, a subset of which harbor chromosomal rearrangements whose breakpoints are located far downstream of the *PAX6* transcriptional unit (Fukushima et al., 1993; Fantes et al., 1995; Lauderdale et al., 2000; Kleinjan et al., 2001; Crolla and Van Heyningen, 2002). The most distant of these breakpoints, designated "SIMO," is located 124 kb downstream of the *PAX6* polyadenylation site (Fantes et al., 1995; Kleinjan et al., 2001; **Figure 5**). The functional importance of regulatory regions around distant breakpoints was confirmed by the finding that a yeast artificial chromosome (YAC) comprising 420 kb of the human *PAX6* coding sequence and flanking regions stretching beyond the SIMO breakpoint rescues the mouse *small eye* (*Sey*) phenotype, whereas a YAC transgene with 110 kb less DNA sequence at the 3′ end fails to rescue (Kleinjan et al., 2001). Subsequent analyses revealed the presence of essential 3′ distant regulatory elements within a 75 kb region termed the *PAX6* downstream regulatory region (DRR) located 3′ of the SIMO breakpoint (**Figure 5**; Schedl et al., 1996; Kleinjan et al., 2001; McBride et al., 2011). A number of other conserved regulatory elements, including E60, E100, and RB (**Figure 5**), located either upstream or downstream of the DRR region are thought to be crucial for the induction of *PAX6* expression in the eye and forebrain (Griffin et al., 2002; Kleinjan et al., 2002, 2006; Kim and Lauderdale, 2006; McBride et al., 2011).

We recently reported a detailed examination of a series of novel transgenic reporter mice lines, carrying versions of either the full length 420 kb YAC described above or truncated versions that lacked putative regulatory elements. The YAC transgenes were modified by the introduction of a tau-GFP reporter cassette into the first coding exon of *PAX6*, such that GFP expression marks cells in which the transgenes are expressed. We found that regulatory elements that lie outside the 420 kb YAC transgene are required for correct *PAX6* expression in sub-regions of the telencephalon and diencephalon, indicating that recapitulation of the full *PAX6* expression pattern requires even more elements than had previously been thought (Mi et al., 2013b).

The *Pax6* locus is subject to autoregulation – *Pax6* has been shown to regulate its own expression. Putative Pax6 binding sites have been identified in *Pax6* regulatory elements in several species. For example, in *Drosophila*, two intronic enhancer elements containing putative Pax6 binding sites mediate autoactivation of *eyeless* (a *Drosophila Pax6* homolog) in the nervous system and eye (Hauck et al., 1999). These elements may serve the same function in vertebrates as they exhibit significant sequence identity between *Drosophila* and vertebrate species (Chow et al., 1999). In addition, Pax6 directly interacts with putative Pax6-responsive elements within the head surface ectoderm-specific enhancer of mouse *Pax6*, positively regulating its own transcription (Aota et al., 2003). Similarly, Pax6 autoregulation in the forebrain was revealed through the identification of a highly conserved regulatory element (CE2) in intron 7 of mouse *Pax6* (**Figure 5**). Overexpressing either Pax6 or its alternative spliced isoform Pax6(5a) positively autoregulated expression of the endogenous *Pax6* locus in Neuro2D and NIH3T3 cell lines (Pinson et al., 2006). The *Pax6* locus is also subject to negative autoregulation, whereby Pax6 represses transcription of the *Pax6* locus, as shown in the developing telencephalon (Manuel et al., 2007). In summary, these studies highlight the fact that appropriate levels of Pax6 expression are regulated by both positive and negative autoregulation during development.

Pax6 Regulates Cell Cycle Length and Cell Cycle Exit

Generating the correct number of cortical neurons of the correct types involves changes in both the mode of division of cortical progenitors and length of their cell cycle. As discussed above, cortical progenitors switch progressively from proliferative symmetrical divisions to differentiative asymmetrical divisions during corticogenesis. At the same time, the length of the cell cycle in AP cells in mouse cortex increases from 8 h at the onset of neurogenesis (E10) to 18 h at the end (E18), largely due to lengthening of the G1 phase (Takahashi et al., 1993, 1995; Estivill-Torrus et al., 2002). Subsequent studies showed that G1 lengthening acts to promote the genesis of BP cells which have much longer cell cycle length (around 26 h in E14.5 mouse cortex) due to increase in the G1 length (Arai et al., 2011). In the macaque, AP cell cycle length is much longer than in rodents and it follows a different developmental course (Kornack and Rakic, 1998). It lengthens linearly from 23 h at E40 to 54 h at E60, then shortens linearly to 27 h by E80 (Kornack and Rakic, 1998). As the neurogenic period is 10 times longer than in rodents, macaque cortical progenitors undergo many more rounds of division even though the duration of the cell cycle is longer (Kornack and Rakic, 1998), generating a greater number of cortical cells and a larger cortex.

There is mounting evidence that TFs exert region-specific control of cortical progenitor cell cycle progression. Pax6 is one of a number of TFs that are expressed in distinct gradients across cortical areas (Zaki et al., 2003; Sansom and Livesey, 2009; Salomoni and Calegari, 2010; Georgala et al., 2011a) and several studies have implicated Pax6 in the temporal and spatial control of cell cycle duration in cortical progenitors. Loss of Pax6 during early cortical development (E12.5) in mice *in vivo* led to a shortening of the cell cycle of progenitors coupled with higher proportions of asymmetrical divisions, resulting in a temporary increase in the production of post-mitotic neurons (Warren et al., 1999; Estivill-Torrus et al., 2002; Walcher et al., 2013). Experiments with cultured *Pax6*$^{-/-}$ mutant cortical cells showed that they too exhibit accelerated proliferation, indicating that Pax6's effects on the cell cycle are cell autonomous (Estivill-Torrus et al., 2002). In contrast, at the mid-corticogenesis stage (E15.5) *Pax6*$^{-/-}$ progenitor cells proliferated more slowly than wild type controls, showing that the effects of Pax6 on the cell cycle of cortical progenitors are context-dependent.

Gain of function studies also support the idea that Pax6 controls cell cycle progression. For example, forced expression of Pax6 impairs progenitor cell proliferation *in vitro* (Heins et al., 2002; Hack et al., 2004; Cartier et al., 2006). In *PAX77* mice, which express PAX6 protein in its normal pattern but at approximately double the wild type level, there is a reduction in the number of proliferating progenitors in the rostral and central cortex, the areas where levels of Pax6 expression are normally highest (Manuel et al., 2007). Further, APs located in rostral cortical areas proliferate more slowly in these mice (Georgala et al., 2011a,b). Thus, both gain and loss of Pax6 function studies have revealed powerful context-specific effects of Pax6 on the cell cycle of progenitor cells in a variety of cortical areas and stages.

Early in corticogenesis, expression levels of Pax6 vary between different cortical regions but its expression levels become increasingly uniform with embryonic age (Mansouri et al., 1994; Stoykova and Gruss, 1994; Manuel et al., 2007). Some of the evidence cited above indicates that the actions of Pax6 on the cell cycle of cortical progenitors are associated with its expression levels. This assumption is strongly supported by our recent study in which cell cycle parameters were systematically examined in different cortical regions at different developmental stages using mouse models with either constitutive or conditional loss of Pax6 function (Mi et al., 2013a). During early corticogenesis (E12.5), when the Pax6 gradient is steepest, areas of highest expression correlate with regions where the cell cycle duration is longest (**Figure 6**). Loss of Pax6 causes shortening of the cell cycle only in these areas (**Figure 6**). In normal embryos at older ages, the Pax6 gradient becomes progressively more uniform across the cortex, as does cell cycle length, and loss of Pax6 causes shortening of the cell cycle in all areas (**Figure 6**; Mi et al., 2013a). Taken together, these studies indicate that Pax6 primarily exerts a repressive action on the cell cycle progression of cortical progenitors, and distinct expression levels of Pax6 confer

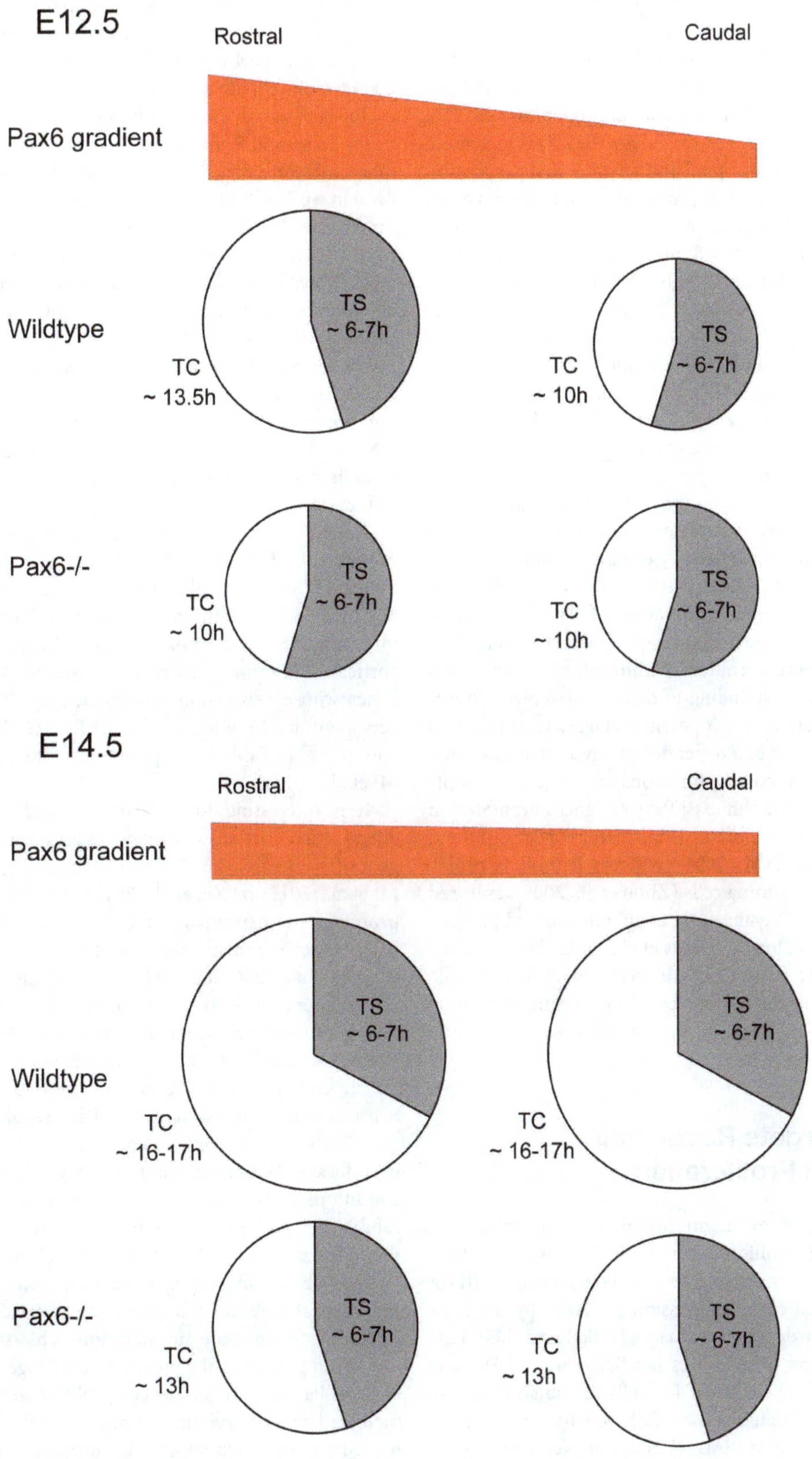

FIGURE 6 | Effect of loss of Pax6 on cortical progenitor cell cycle parameters. Diagram showing the cell cycle length and S-phase length of cortical progenitors at a rostral or caudal position in Wild type or *Pax6*$^{-/-}$ embryos. At E12.5 Pax6 is normally expressed in a high rostral to low caudal gradient and loss of Pax6 results in a shortening of the cell cycle rostrally with no effect on S-phase length. At E14.5 Pax6 is expressed in a flatter rostro-caudal gradient and loss of Pax6 causes a shortening of the cell cycle both rostrally and caudally while the S-phase length remains unaffected.

its region and age -specific role in regulating progenitor cell proliferation.

As well as regulating the length of the cell cycle in cortical progenitors, Pax6 is involved in the control of cell cycle exit. In the *Pax6*$^{sey/sey}$ mutant cortex, the number of progenitor cells that exit the cell cycle during early corticogenesis (E12.5) is increased, leading to a smaller progenitor pool and an increased proportion of newborn neurons (Estivill-Torrus et al., 2002; Quinn et al., 2007). A similar effect has been seen in the eye and the spinal cord, where loss of Pax6 caused precocious neuronal differentiation due to premature cell cycle exit (Philips et al., 2005; Bel-Vialar et al., 2007). Interestingly, a study using *PAX77* mice revealed that increasing Pax6 levels also causes an increase in the proportion of progenitor cells exiting the cell cycle during late corticogenesis (E15.5; Georgala et al., 2011b), indicating that there is no simple dosage-dependent relationship between Pax6 level and progenitor cell cycle exit rate. Recently, we found that loss of Pax6 led to fewer progenitors exiting the cell cycle at the PSPB (pallial–subpallial boundary) at E12.5, the area of the telencephalon where Pax6 expression is highest, contrasting with the previous finding that *Pax6*$^{-/-}$ cortical progenitors show increased cell cycle exit at E12.5 (Estivill-Torrus et al., 2002). It appears that, although a general function of Pax6 is to influence cell cycle exit, the exact nature of its effect depends on the molecular and cellular context within which it acts. This context may change corresponding to diverse Pax6 levels in different regions at different developmental stages. In support of this assumption, a number of independent analyses demonstrated that Pax6 exerts different control functions on progenitor proliferation in different cellular contexts: Pax6 enhances proliferation in the neural retina of vertebrates (Marquardt et al., 2001) and *Drosophila* (Dominguez et al., 2004), whereas it inhibits proliferation of human glioblastoma cells (Zhou et al., 2005), cultured corneal epithelial cells (Ouyang et al., 2006) and cortical progenitors in primary cell cultures (Heins et al., 2002; Haubst et al., 2004) as well as *in vivo* (Estivill-Torrus et al., 2002; Berger et al., 2007). Therefore, it is difficult to conclude a simple universally consistent role of Pax6 in the regulation of cell cycle exit.

Pax6 Direct Targets Regulating Progenitor Cell Proliferation

As described above, Pax6 is important for the regulation of cortical progenitor proliferation (Estivill-Torrus et al., 2002; Manuel et al., 2007; Quinn et al., 2007; Georgala et al., 2011b; Mi et al., 2013a,b). Cell cycle progression is driven by the concerted action of cyclin-dependent kinases (Cdks) and their activating partners, cyclins (Malumbres and Barbacid, 2005). Low levels of Cdk activity are sufficient for cells to transit from G1 into S phase, whereas high-levels of Cdk activity are required for the cell to undergo mitosis (Dehay and Kennedy, 2007; Kaldis and Richardson, 2012). During G1, cells integrate and respond to extracellular cues that either allow the cell to continue cycling or promote its withdrawal from the cell cycle and begin differentiation (Zetterberg et al., 1995). Progression through G1 is mainly driven by the activation of Cdk4/6 and their activating partners, D-type cyclins (Cyclin D1 and D2) as well as Cdk2 and its partner Cyclin E (Malumbres and Barbacid, 2001, 2005). Cdk activity is negatively regulated by members of the cyclin-dependent kinase inhibitors family (CKIs; Polyak et al., 1994; Sherr and Roberts, 1995; Vidal and Koff, 2000). The primary substrate of Cdks during G1 phase is the retinoblastoma protein (pRb). pRb acts as a repressor of E2F TFs through direct interaction. In quiescent cells, the activities of E2Fs are repressed through direct interaction with hypophosphorylated pRb. In cycling cells, mitogenic stimuli that elevate Cyclin levels promote pRb phosphorylation by Cyclin/Cdk complexes, which in turn prevents pRb from binding to E2Fs. Consequently, pRb/E2F complexes are dissociated and free E2Fs are now active and ready to drive the transcription of genes encoding proteins that are involved in G1 phase progression and DNA replication. Gene expression profiling studies showed that Pax6 is capable of regulating the expression of a number of cell cycle genes involved in G1 to S phase transition, such as *Cdk4, Cdk6, Ccnd1, Ccnd2, p27*^{kip1}, *Cdc6, Mcm3, Mcm5, Mcm6, Cdca2* and *Cdca7*, with many of them being repressed by Pax6 (Sansom et al., 2009; Mi et al., 2013a,b). These findings are in line with the notion that Pax6 mainly acts as an important regulator of progenitor cell proliferation during early cortical development as reviewed above. Among the cell cycle genes whose expression is regulated by Pax6, Pax6 direct targets identified to date include *Cdk4, Cdk6, Mcm3, Cdca2, Cdca7,* and p27^{kip1} (**Table 1**; Duparc et al., 2007; Sansom et al., 2009; Mi et al., 2013a,b).

It is interesting to note that in addition to its repressive effect, Pax6 can also activate expression of some cell cycle genes (Holm et al., 2007; Osumi et al., 2008; Sansom et al., 2009; Mi et al., 2013a,b; Xie et al., 2013). For example, Pax6 directly promotes the expression of *Cdk4* in neural stem cells in early cortical development (Sansom et al., 2009). This supports the concept that Pax6 has dual roles to both promote and inhibit cell proliferation in the developing cortex, possibly through the divergent functions of its DNA-binding subdomains (see below; Walcher et al., 2013). Using transcriptome analysis of the cortex in embryos with either gain and loss of Pax6 function, Sansom et al. (2009) showed that Pax6 regulates a core transcriptional network that controls cortical neural stem cell proliferation in a dosage-dependent manner. They found that under normal conditions *in vivo*, Pax6 has the potential to both promote and inhibit stem cell proliferation by exhibiting opposing effects on the expression of different sets of cell cycle genes, but when Pax6 levels are increased, as in transgenic cortex overexpressing Pax6, the neurogenic functions of Pax6 are dominant over its ability to promote proliferation. This study is in line with our finding that at the onset of corticogenesis, the repressive effect of Pax6 on progenitor cell proliferation and the Cdk/Cyclin mediated phosphorylation of pRb is localized to regions of cortex where Pax6 expression is normally highest, indicating a relationship between the level of Pax6 expression and its antiproliferative effect (Mi et al., 2013a). Given that Pax6 is expressed in a gradient during early cortical development, the dosage-dependent effects of Pax6 on cell proliferation are important in the context of understanding how the cerebral cortex becomes divided into regions with specific cytoarchitectures and functions.

Pax6 is an Intrinsic Determinant of Neuronal Fate in the Developing Cortex

The observations that Pax6 is specifically expressed by radial glial progenitor cells in the developing cortex and is required for them to acquire their normal morphology, gene expression pattern and cell cycle characteristics (Gotz et al., 1998), suggested that Pax6 may control their ability to generate neurons. To address this question, Heins et al. (2002) used a combination of loss and gain of function approaches. They found that cultured RGCs isolated from the developing cortex of *Pax6*$^{-/-}$ mutant mouse embryos generated half as many pure neuronal clones as RGCs from control embryos. Using a tau-GFP transgene to label and quantify neurons by fluorescence activated cell sorting (FACS), they showed that the number of neurons in the cortex of *Pax6*$^{-/-}$ mutant mouse embryos was reduced by half at E14.5 and by a third at E16.5 compared to controls, consistent with the previously reported thinner CP in *Pax6*$^{-/-}$ cortex (Schmahl et al., 1993). Forced expression of Pax6 in cells dissociated from E14 cortex or in astrocytes from postnatal cortex, via transduction of a retroviral vector containing full length Pax6 cDNA, resulted in a significant increase in the number of pure neuronal clones generated, demonstrating that Pax6 is an intrinsic determinant of neuronal fate in murine cortical progenitors (Heins et al., 2002). Mo and Zecevic (2008) showed that siRNA-mediated knockdown of Pax6 expression in cultured human fetal RGCs led to a significant decrease in the number of neurons produced, suggesting that the role of Pax6 in cortical neurogenesis is maintained from rodents to humans (Mo and Zecevic, 2008).

TABLE 1 | Genes that have been identified as direct Pax6 targets in the mouse developing cortex grouped according to the developmental process that they affect.

Process	Gene	Approach							Reference
		ChIP-chip	ChIP	Microarray	EMSA	Luciferase assay	Transgenic mice	qRT-PCR	
Cell fate specification	*Etv1 (Er81)*	X		X	X		X		Tuoc and Stoykova (2008a), Sansom et al. (2009)
	Olig2		X			X			Jang and Goldman (2011)
	Isl1	X		X					Sansom et al. (2009), Xie et al. (2013)
	Foxd1	X		X					Sansom et al. (2009)
Basal progenitor genesis	*Neurod1*	X		X					Sansom et al. (2009)
	Gadd45g	X		X					Sansom et al. (2009)
	Tbr2	X	X	X				X	Sansom et al. (2009), Tuoc et al. (2013a)
Neurogenesis	*Ngn2*	X		X	X		X		Scardigli et al. (2003), Sansom et al. (2009)
	Sox4	X		X					Sansom et al. (2009)
	Sox11		X	X					Ninkovic et al. (2013)
	Pou3f4		X	X					Ninkovic et al. (2013)
	Nfib		X	X					Ninkovic et al. (2013)
	Cux1		X		X			X	Tuoc et al. (2013a)
	Tle1		X		X			X	Tuoc et al. (2013a)
Cell cycle	*Cdk6*		X		X	X			Mi et al. (2013a)
	Cdk4	X		X					Sansom et al. (2009)
	Mcm3	X		X					Sansom et al. (2009)
	Cdca2	X		X					Sansom et al. (2009)
	Cdca7	X		X					Sansom et al. (2009)
	P27^{kip1}		X					X	Duparc et al. (2007)
Cell proliferation	*Pten*	X		X					Sansom et al. (2009)
	Cdh1	X		X					Sansom et al. (2009)
	Lix1	X		X					Sansom et al. (2009)
	Hmga2	X		X					Sansom et al. (2009)
	Fgfr1	X		X					Sansom et al. (2009)
Axonal transport	*Kif1b*	X		X		X			Xie et al. (2013)
Unknown	*Snca*	X		X					Xie et al. (2013)

Pax6 Confers both Regional and Neurotransmitter Fates

The mammalian CP comprises mainly glutamatergic neurons born in the cortical VZ and GABAergic interneurons (INs). In mouse, most INs are born in the medial ganglionic eminence (MGE; ~70%) with others coming from the caudal ganglionic eminence (CGE) and areas including the preoptic area (POA; Anderson et al., 2001; Wonders and Anderson, 2006; Fogarty et al., 2007; Gelman et al., 2009; Miyoshi et al., 2010). INs born in the LGE populate the olfactory bulb (OB) and the ventral telencephalon. Most cortical glutamatergic neurons and GABAergic interneurons are generated between E12.5 and E16.5. By E18.5, GABAergic INs are distributed throughout the cortex of wild type embryos. In contrast, the cortex of *Pax6*$^{-/-}$ mutant embryos contains large subpial ectopias composed of GABAergic INs (Kroll and O'Leary, 2005). These ectopias develop from E15.5 onward and express markers of LGE-derived INs, including Sp8, rather than markers of MGE-born INs, such as Lhx6. Their development parallels a progressive ventralization of the dorsal telencephalic VZ in *Pax6*$^{-/-}$ mutant embryos. At the start of neurogenesis (E12.5–E13.5) the most ventrolateral part of the *Pax6*$^{-/-}$ mutant cortex ectopically expresses the ventral telencephalic markers Ascl1 and Gsh2. As neurogenesis progresses ventral telencephalic identities extend dorsally such that by E14.5 most of the dorsal telencephalic VZ exhibits ventral characteristics. This progressive ventralization is accompanied by a dorsal shift in expression of markers of GABAergic INs such as Dlx1/2 and GAD67. Importantly, the INs that form the ectopias are derived from Emx1-expressing cortical progenitors which normally generate glutamatergic neurons, demonstrating that in *Pax6*$^{-/-}$ mutant mice, cortical progenitors are re-specified to generate GABAergic INs instead of glutamatergic neurons (Kroll and O'Leary, 2005).

Dlx1/2, Ascl1, and Gsh2 have been shown to promote GABAergic fate, such as the expression of Gad67 (Long et al., 2009a,b; Wang et al., 2013). Thus it is possible that Pax6 normally represses GABAergic identities in the cortex by blocking the expression of these TFs.

In *Pax6*$^{-/-}$ embryos, early born CP neurons are correctly specified as dorsal telencephalic neurons, expressing dorsal markers Math2 and Tbr1 (Schuurmans et al., 2004). They fail, however, to adopt a correct glutamatergic phenotype. Interestingly, these early born neurons are not GABAergic either (Schuurmans et al., 2004). Thus, during early corticogenesis, Pax6 participates in the specification of a correct glutamatergic phenotype but is not required to suppress GABAergic identities. Schuurmans et al. (2004) analyzed double mutants for Ngn1 and Ngn2, and showed that, during early stages of corticogenesis (E13.5), neurogenins are required to specify a glutamatergic, cortical phenotype, and repress GABAergic identities. Conversely, cortical neurons born at later stages of corticogenesis (E15.5) acquire a normal cortical and glutamatergic phenotype in *Ngn1*$^{-/-}$; *Ngn2*$^{-/-}$ double mutants whereas in *Pax6*$^{-/-}$ embryos and in mutants lacking the orphan nuclear receptor Tlx, they express reduced levels of cortical and glutamatergic markers, compared to controls, and instead acquire a subcortical, GABAergic phenotype (Schuurmans et al., 2004). This study shows that distinct genetic programs operate during early and late corticogenesis to specify cortical regional identity and neurotransmitter fate: neurogenins are required during early stages while Pax6 and Tlx are required during later stages of corticogenesis (Schuurmans et al., 2004).

Pax6 Confers Laminar Fate

Throughout corticogenesis, newborn neurons migrate to the CP in an inside-out sequence such that deep layers are formed first and superficial layers form later. The final laminar position and subtype of cortical projection neurons is dependent on the time at which progenitors exit the cell cycle. In *Pax6*$^{-/-}$ mutant embryos, the SVZ and superficial cortical layers are defective, as shown by absence of expression of Svet1 (which marks the SVZ and superficial layers), while the VZ and deep CP layers are unaffected, as shown by the expression of Otx1 (Tarabykin et al., 2001).

Examination of cortical lamination in *Ngn1*$^{-/-}$; *Ngn2*$^{-/-}$ mutants showed that the expression of markers of deep cortical layers is reduced (Tbr1, Er81) while markers of superficial layers are expressed normally, indicating that late-born cortical neurons are correctly specified (Schuurmans et al., 2004). In contrast, no defects are detected in the deeper cortical layers of *Pax6*$^{-/-}$, *Tlx*$^{-/-}$, or *Pax6*$^{-/-}$; *Tlx*$^{-/-}$ double mutants. Markers of upper layers, however, are downregulated in Pax6 and Tlx single mutants and completely lost in *Pax6*$^{-/-}$;*Tlx*$^{-/-}$ embryos suggesting that Pax6 and Tlx cooperate to specify the identity of late-born cortical neurons (Schuurmans et al., 2004).

Study of cortical lamination in *Pax6*$^{-/-}$ mutants is limited by the fact that they die perinatally while cortical neurons do not reach their final location until around postnatal day 8 (P8). Therefore, more recent studies on the role of Pax6 in cortical lamination have used conditional mutants in which *Pax6* is inactivated specifically in the cortex and at later stages of cortical development and which survive postnatally. When *Pax6* was deleted specifically in the cortex from the onset of corticogenesis, markers of superficial layers were either downregulated or lost completely (Tuoc et al., 2009). In contrast, when *Pax6* was deleted in RGCs after the generation of deep cortical layers (between E14.5 and E16.5) using an hGFAP-cre transgenic line, the specification and number of late born neurons was unaffected (Tuoc et al., 2009), leading to the conclusion that Pax6 is not required for the specification of late born cortical neurons and that the defects of superficial layers observed in *Pax6*$^{-/-}$ and *Pax6*cKO mutants are a result of earlier defects in RGC proliferation. In a more recent study, Georgala et al. (2011b) used an *Emx1-creErT2* transgenic line to remove Pax6 specifically in the cortex between E12.5 and E13.5, before superficial layer neurons are born. The resulting cKO mutant brains showed a dramatic reduction in the thickness of the superficial cortical layers, compared to control embryos. Late-born neurons were birth-dated by injecting BrdU at E15.5 and stained for expression of Cux1, a marker of upper layer (II to IV) pyramidal neurons. There was a substantial reduction in the number of E15.5 born neurons in the superficial cortical layers of the *Pax6-cKO* mutants and many fewer late-born neurons expressed Cux1 (Georgala et al., 2011b), indicating that Pax6 plays a crucial role in generation and specification of late born cortical neurons. Note that Pax6 protein was lost slightly earlier in the conditional mutants generated by Georgala et al. (2011b) than in those used by Tuoc et al. (2009), potentially explaining the difference in outcomes between the two studies.

Direct Transcriptional Targets of Pax6 Regulate Basal Progenitor Genesis, Neurogenesis, and Cell Fate Specification

Pax6 exerts many of its effects, at least in part, by directly regulating the expression of specific target genes (**Table 1**). As described above, work in the mouse has shown that Pax6 expressing APs that give rise to BPs transiently express the proneural TF Neurogenin 2 (Ngn2). BPs do not express Pax6 but do express the TF Tbr2. Loss of Pax6 function results in loss of Ngn2 expression in the cortical VZ and downregulation of Tbr2 in the SVZ (Stoykova et al., 2000; Toresson et al., 2000; Yun et al., 2001; Scardigli et al., 2003; Holm et al., 2007; Quinn et al., 2007; Sansom and Livesey, 2009), suggesting that the development of BPs is impaired. Conversely, Pax6 overexpression results in a marked increase in both Ngn2 and Tbr2 expression (Scardigli et al., 2003; Sansom and Livesey, 2009), each of which have been shown to be directly regulated by Pax6 (Scardigli et al., 2003; Sansom and Livesey, 2009; Tuoc et al., 2013a). Scardigli et al. (2003) showed that Pax6 directly binds and regulates the activity of the E1 enhancer of *Ngn2*, which regulates *Ngn2* expression in the cortex and the ventral spinal cord.

Another direct target that is positively regulated by Pax6 is the anti-neurogenic transcriptional co-repressor Tle1, a member of the Groucho/transducin-like enhancer of split (Gro/Tle) family (Sansom et al., 2009; Tuoc et al., 2013a). Gro/Tle proteins are expressed in proliferating neural progenitor cells where they promote maintenance of the undifferentiated state by inhibiting/delaying neuronal differentiation (Buscarlet and Stifani, 2007; Jennings and Ish-Horowicz, 2008).

Pax6 also directly inhibits the expression of Olig2 (Jang and Goldman, 2011), a TF critical for glial cell fate determination (Marshall et al., 2005). Olig2 is expressed in a subset of cells in the rat neonatal SVZ, which differentiate into glia. Forced expression of Pax6 in these Olig2+ cells, using a retrovirus, caused downregulation of Olig2 and a shift toward neuronal fate (Jang and Goldman, 2011). These authors showed that Pax6 can directly bind to Olig2's promoter and repress its activity.

Pax6 directly regulates markers of specific neuronal subtypes including Er81 and Cux1 (Tuoc and Stoykova, 2008a; Sansom et al., 2009; Tuoc et al., 2013a). Er81 is a TF expressed in cortical progenitors, in a rostrolateral-high to caudomedial-low gradient, and in a subset of pyramidal cells scattered through layer 5 (Yoneshima et al., 2006; Tuoc and Stoykova, 2008a). In the absence of Pax6, cortical progenitors do not express Er81 and the rostrolateral cortex lacks Er81 positive layer 5 neurons. Cux1 is a marker of upper layer (II to IV) pyramidal neurons and functions as a negative regulator of dendritic complexity for these neurons (Cubelos et al., 2010, 2014; Li et al., 2010). As mentioned above, loss of Pax6 results in a dramatic reduction of Cux1+ upper layer neurons, suggesting that the specification of late born neurons is impaired (Georgala et al., 2011b).

How does a single gene exert such a wide range of biological effects? Part of the answer to this question is suggested by the findings that the Pax6 protein contains two distinct DNA-binding domains, one of which is regulated by alternate splicing and that Pax6 is able to interact with a number of co-factors, which influence its activity. This issue is discussed in the next section.

Complexity of Pax6 DNA-Binding Properties and its Distinct Functions

Pax6 binds to target DNA sequences through one or both of two DNA-binding domains, the paired domain (PD) and the homeodomain (HD; Bertuccioli et al., 1996; Jun and Desplan, 1996; Sheng et al., 1997; Singh et al., 2000). Transcriptional regulation of Pax6 target genes is mediated by a carboxy terminal proline/serine/threonine (PST) rich transactivation domain (Singh et al., 1998, 2001; Tang et al., 1998; **Figure 7**).

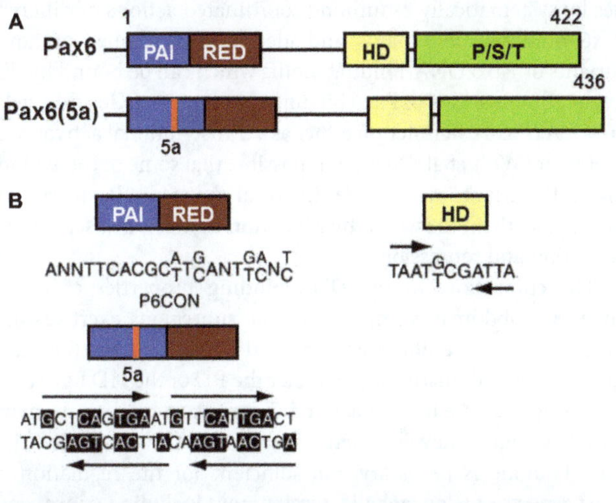

FIGURE 7 | Schematic representation of functional domains in Pax6 and Pax6(5a) and their "optimal" DNA binding sites. (A) Pax6 and Pax6(5a) differ in a 14 amino acid insertion in the PAI subdomain. **(B)** "Optimal" DNA-binding sites for Pax6 PD, PD5a and HD. P6CON and 5aCON sequences were generated by selection procedure (Epstein et al., 1994). P6CON is recognized by monomeric PD, while 5aCON contains four binding sites for PD5a that can bind up to four PD5a units. The "optimal" binding site of Pax6 HD is a dimer with typical HD binding sequences (ATTA/TAAT) separated by three nucleotides (G/T)CG (Czerny and Busslinger, 1995).

The PD is an evolutionarily conserved 128 amino acid DNA-binding domain shared by all members of the paired box (Pax) family of TFs (Pax1-Pax9; Chalepakis et al., 1992; Gruss and Walther, 1992). The Pax6 PD can be structurally and functionally separated into two independent DNA-binding globular helix-turn-helix subdomains, PAI and RED (Puschel et al., 1992; Czerny et al., 1993; Jun and Desplan, 1996; **Figure 7A**). The well-established DNA-binding motif for canonical Pax6 PD, known as P6CON, is a bipartite 20 base pair DNA sequence whose 5′-half is recognized by the PAI subdomain and 3′-half by the RED subdomain (Czerny et al., 1993; Epstein et al., 1994; **Figure 7A**). The crystal structure of the Pax6 PD – P6CON complex revealed direct interactions between both PAI and RED subdomains, the linker regions of PAI and RED subdomains and the N-terminal β-turn subdomain with individual bases and phosphate residues of cognate DNA (Czerny et al., 1993; Epstein et al., 1994; Xu et al., 1999a). Pax6 also contains an internal, paired-type HD (Czerny et al., 1999; Eberhard and Busslinger, 1999) which binds DNA in the form of a homodimer recognizing a symmetric binding site (Wilson et al., 1993; Eberhard and Busslinger, 1999; Mikkola et al., 2001; **Figure 7B**).

Although different Pax6 DNA-binding domains can independently bind to their "optimal" binding sites, using individual consensus binding motif to predict and confirm candidate Pax6-binding sites has proven to be very difficult (Shimoda et al., 2002; Visel et al., 2007; Wolf et al., 2009). Unlike sequence specific DNA-binding proteins which harbor only one DNA-binding domain, Pax6 exhibits increased DNA-binding complexity because of its multiple DNA-binding subdomains (PAI, RED, and HD) which can be used in varying combinations when binding to DNA (Cvekl et al., 2004; Grapp et al., 2009). A recent study further reinforced the complexity of Pax6 DNA-binding properties by systematically examining coordinated actions of different Pax6 binding subdomains and identified a number of novel variants of Pax6 DNA-binding motifs which can be bound by different combinations of Pax6 binding subdomains (Xie and Cvekl, 2011). As Pax6 can function either as a transcriptional activator or repressor (Wolf et al., 2009), it is possible that some of these binding motif variants may induce structural changes in Pax6 proteins that enable them to switch their function between transcriptional activation and repression.

The complexity of the DNA binding properties of different Pax6 subdomains implies that the subregions exert distinct functions during embryonic cortical development. Pax6 mutant mouse lines with disruption of either the PD or the HD have been used to investigate the impact of different Pax6 binding domains on telencephalic development. Haubst et al. (2004) showed that the PD alone is necessary and sufficient for the regulation of most aspects of telencephalic development including neurogenesis, progenitor cell proliferation, and patterning in the developing cortex. In contrast, HD-specific mutations affected only subtle aspects of telencephalic development, such as establishment of the PSPB, and had no obvious effect on neurogenesis or proliferation (Haubst et al., 2004). This suggests that the majority of Pax6's effects during telencephalic development are mediated by the PD with potentially different contributions by its subdomains. A recent study further dissected the roles of the different subdomains of the Pax6 PD during telencephalic development by examining mice with point mutations in its individual subdomains PAI and RED (Walcher et al., 2013). This showed that both PAI and RED act largely in a redundant manner in patterning of the telencephalon, with only the PAI mutation resulting in the ectopic expression of subpallial genes such as *Gsx2* and *Olig2* into the pallium, suggesting that RED subdomain on its own is not sufficient to regulate telencephalic patterning. In addition, neurogenesis was affected only by the PAI subdomain mutation, phenocopying the neurogenic defects observed in full $Pax6^{-/-}$ mutants. Strikingly, this study also revealed that subdomains of Pax6 PD have distinct roles in regulating cortical progenitor cell proliferation, with mutations affecting the PAI and RED subdomains respectively reducing and increasing the number of mitoses.

Alternatively Spliced Isoforms of Pax6 and their Functions

In addition to Pax6 and Pax6(5a) a number of other splice variants of Pax6 have been reported, named p43, p33 and p32, each of which is less abundant and mostly localized in the cytoplasm (Carriere et al., 1993; Jaworski et al., 1997; Pinson et al., 2006). The 14 amino acid insertion in Pax6(5a) destroys the DNA-binding capacity of the PAI subdomain, leaving the RED subdomain of the PD and the intact HD for DNA binding (Epstein et al., 1994; Kozmik et al., 1997). The PD in Pax6(5a) binds to a distinct DNA sequence from that bound by the canonical Pax6 PD, that has been named 5aCON (Epstein et al., 1994). Direct comparison of the DNA binding sites recognized by Pax6 PD and PD(5a) showed partial sequence homology between the 3' halves of P6CON and 5aCON (Epstein et al., 1994; Duncan et al., 1998, 2000). This homology allows Pax6 (which contains the canonical PD) to bind to both P6CON and 5aCON sites, whereas Pax6(5a) can only interact with the 5aCON site (Epstein et al., 1994).

The majority of published molecular studies have focused on Pax6, as it contains the canonical PD and appears to be more abundant than Pax6(5a) (Carriere et al., 1993; Richardson et al., 1995; Koroma et al., 1997). During early development, *Pax6* and *Pax6(5a)* transcripts are expressed in a ratio of 8:1 in the mouse forebrain, falling to 3:1 between E12.5 and E14.5 (Kozmik et al., 1997; Pinson et al., 2006). A reduced ratio between Pax6 and Pax6(5a) was also seen during chick retina development (Azuma et al., 2005). *PAX6* and *PAX6(5a)* transcripts are equally abundant in the human adult lens epithelium and cornea, as well as in monkey retina (Zhang et al., 2001). These findings raise the possibility that expression of the two main Pax6 isoforms are regulated in a tissue- and temporal-specific manner, thereby affecting which target genes they recognize.

Although Pax6 and Pax6(5a) are commonly co-expressed, there is evidence that they exert distinct functions during embryonic development. For example, overexpression of either Pax6 or Pax6(5a) in chick retina showed that both isoforms led to increased retinal progenitor cell proliferation, but Pax6(5a) induced ectopic differentiation of the retina to a stronger degree than Pax6 (Azuma et al., 2005). Similarly, Pax6(5a) strongly induces neural differentiation of murine embryonic stem cells *in vitro*, while Pax6 does not have such a strong effect (Shimizu et al., 2009). In the embryonic mouse forebrain, the different roles of the two Pax6 isoforms in regulation of cell proliferation and differentiation were also established from studies of Pax6 mutants. It was shown that mutations that abolish the binding property of the PD affect both proliferation and differentiation, while a PD(5a) mutation only affects proliferation and has no effect on cell fate/differentiation in mouse developing telencephalon (Haubst et al., 2004). In a more recent study, Pax6(5a) specific target genes were identified through microarray analyses of gene expression profiles in cell lines stably expressing either Pax6 or Pax6(5a) (Kiselev et al., 2012). This revealed that a number of genes involved in cell proliferation, differentiation, and migration are differentially regulated by Pax6 and Pax6(5a), providing a potential molecular basis by which Pax6 and Pax6(5a) could exert their distinct biological functions.

Co-Factors Influence Pax6's Direct Regulation of Target Genes Involved in Embryonic and Adult Neurogenesis

It is becoming clear that transcriptional regulation is highly dependent on the molecular and cellular context, one reason for which is that TFs do not act on their own but are dependent on interactions with other co-factors to exert their functions (Oikawa and Yamada, 2003; Westerman et al., 2003). These interactions introduce more specificity into the regulatory function of a given TF in a particular cellular context. A number co-factors that can interact with Pax6 have been identified. For example, Pax6 cooperates with Sox2 to target the lens-specific enhancer of the δ-*crystallin* gene (Kamachi et al., 2001); with MDIA to influence Pax6's functions in cerebellar granule cells (Tominaga et al., 2002); with Trim11 to mediate Pax6 degradation through the ubiquitin proteasome system (UPS) and modulate Pax6 transcriptional activity (Cooper and Hanson, 2005; Tuoc and Stoykova, 2008b). More recently, Brg1/Brm associated factors complex (BAF) and Meis2 have been identified as two new co-factors that affect Pax6's direct regulation of target genes expression, in turn regulating its role in both embryonic and adult neurogenesis (Ninkovic et al., 2013; Tuoc et al., 2013a,b; Agoston et al., 2014).

BAF Complex

A number of chromatin remodeling factors are known to play an important role during mammalian neural development, including the BAF complex (Ho et al., 2009a,b; Wu, 2012; Yip et al., 2012; Tuoc et al., 2013a,b). Interestingly, the function of the BAF complex in regulating neural development is dependent on its subunit composition. In mammals, BAF complexes contain two ATPase subunits Brg1 or Brm (Brahma), which are mutually exclusive and essential for remodeling activity, in combination with at least 15 different BAF (Brg1/Brm-associated factor) subunits (Ho et al., 2009a; Singhal et al., 2010). Certain BAF subunits have restricted expression patterns and thus could define tissue- or cell-type-specific BAF complexes. For example, the composition of BAF complexes in ES cells (esBAF) is defined by the incorporation of Brg1 but not Brm, BAF155 but not BAF170, and BAF60A but not BAF60C (**Figure 8**; Ho et al., 2009a,b). However, during the transition from ES cells to neural progenitors, the composition of BAF complexes is correspondingly changed, defining the neural progenitor specific BAF complex (npBAF; Lessard et al., 2007; Yan et al., 2008; Ho et al., 2009a). This process is accompanied by induction of BAF170 expression, replacing one of the BAF155 subunits and the recruitment of Brm as the ATP-ase subunit in the npBAF complex.

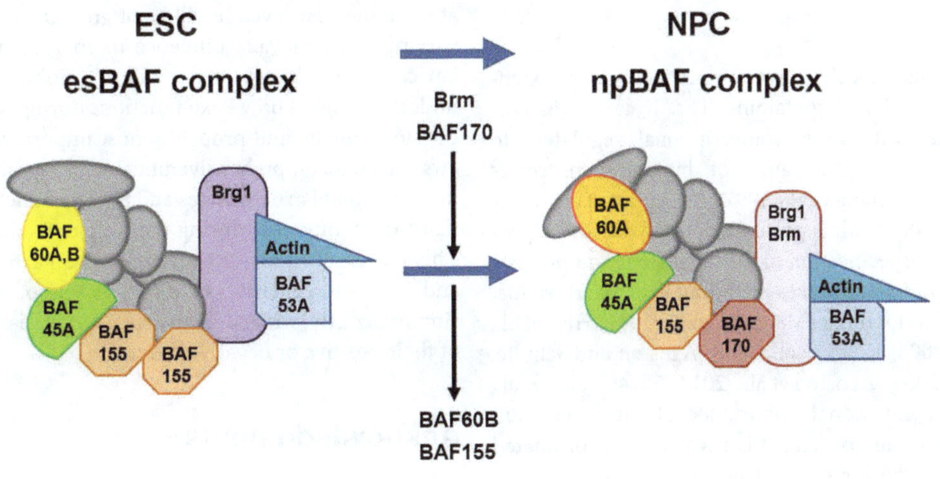

FIGURE 8 | Changes in subunit composition of BAF complexes during differentiation from ES cells to neural progenitor cells. BAF complexes undergo progressive changes in subunit composition during the transition from embryonic stem cells (ESCs) to neural progenitor cells (NPCs). The BAF complex in ESCs is called esBAF; in neuronal progenitors, npBAF. As ESCs differentiate into NPCs, The esBAF complexes incorporate Brm and BAF170, while excludes BAF60B and BAF155, thereby forming the neural progenitor-specific BAF (npBAF) complexes in NPCs.

In two recent studies, Tuoc et al. (2013a,b), described an elegant model in which time-specific binding of BAF subunits including BAF170, BAF155, and Brm-ATPase to Pax6 modulates the expression of Pax6 target genes (*Tbr2, Cux1,* and *Tle1*) involved in the specification and generation of BPs and upper layer neuronal fate in the developing cortex. Interestingly, this model involves competition between BAF170 and BAF155 subunits in the BAF complex, which modulates chromatin modifications and binding of the Pax6/REST co-repressor complex to Pax6 target genes, thereby affecting their expression. During early neurogenesis (E12.5 to E14.5), the presence of BAF170 in the Pax6-BAF complex prevents the euchromatin state (a lightly packed form of chromatin) of the Pax6 target genes *Tbr2, Cux1* and *Tle1*, limiting the ability of Pax6 to bind them, thereby inhibiting their expression and promoting direct neurogenesis (RGCs directly give rise to neurons) at this developmental stage. In contrast, after E14.5 the expression of BAF170 decreases, accompanied by enhanced expression of BAF155, leading to a relaxed chromatin state of the promoters of the Pax6 target genes mentioned above, thereby enhancing their expression and in turn promoting indirect neurogenesis (RGCs indirectly give rise to neurons through generating BPs). This study provides novel insight into the interaction between BAF complex and Pax6 in the generation of BPs and the mode of neurogenesis in the developing cortex. In another recent study, Ninkovic et al. (2013) showed that Pax6 directly interacts with Brg1-ATPase of the BAF complex to modulate expression of genes involved in neuronal fate specification in adult neural progenitors. This study indicated that direct interaction of Pax6 with the Brg1/BAF complex enhances the expression of Pax6 target neurogenic TFs including *Sox11, Nfib,* and *Pou3f4* which form a cross-regulatory network driving neurogenic fate during adult neurogenesis. This study improved our understanding of Pax6-mediated adult neurogenesis and shed light on molecular mechanisms underlying the function of Pax6 in cell fate specification and conversion.

Meis2

Meis2 belongs to the TALE (three amino acid loop extension) family of atypical HD-containing TFs. It can form heteromeric complexes with other transcriptional regulators to exert its functions during a range of biological processes (Moskow et al., 1995; Chang et al., 1997; Knoepfler et al., 1999; Moens and Selleri, 2006). Meis proteins control cell cycle progression and cell fate specification of different stem and progenitor cell types in a variety of tissues including liver, heart, retina, and brain during development (Mercader et al., 1999; Hisa et al., 2004; Bessa et al., 2008; Heine et al., 2008; Agoston and Schulte, 2009; Choe et al., 2009; Agoston et al., 2012, 2014; Paige et al., 2012). Recently the functional importance of Meis2 in adult neurogenesis has been discovered. It is involved in coordinated actions with Pax6 (Agoston et al., 2014). During mouse adult neurogenesis, Meis2 is strongly expressed in the SVZ and rostral migratory stream (RMS) and in a subset of OB interneurons (Agoston et al., 2014). Agoston et al. (2014) found that Meis2 can physically interact with Pax6 in cells in the SVZ and OB. This study also showed that the pro-neurogenic function of Pax6 in the adult SVZ requires direct interaction with Meis2. Meis2 has transcriptional activator function and Agoston et al. (2014) further confirmed that it acts as a Pax6 co-factor, binding to regulatory elements of the *Dcx* gene to promote its expression during adult SVZ neurogenesis.

Conclusion

The TF Pax6 is one of the most intensively studied high-level developmental regulators, playing crucial roles in brain development and implicated in disease. Numerous studies, including those from our group, have shown that in both humans and mice many abnormalities resulting from mutations in *PAX6/Pax6* are in the cerebral cortex, where they arise largely because Pax6 is required for spatio-temporal control of many biological processes including cortical stem and progenitor cell proliferation and differentiation, neurogenesis, cell and laminar fate specification, neuronal migration, axon guidance and cortical arealization during early corticogenesis. However, we are a long way from having a comprehensive knowledge of exactly how Pax6 exerts such complex actions. In particular, there are at least three major challenges toward improved understanding of Pax6 functions. First, how does such highly complex expression pattern of Pax6 come about? As described above, the transcriptional regulation of *Pax6* is particularly complex and involves both short-range and long-range control mechanisms. Future studies are required to gain better knowledge of tissue- and time-specific regulatory elements responsible for spatiotemporally and quantitatively correct expression of Pax6. Secondly, how does Pax6 expression level influence its functional outputs? Our studies along with others have shown that Pax6 expression levels are crucial for its functions such as regulating progenitor cell proliferation and differentiation, and that mutations affecting Pax6 protein levels cause neurodevelopmental disorders in both humans and mice. Now it is time to ask exactly how Pax6 levels influence its actions at the molecular level. It will be of great interest to examine how varying levels of Pax6 influence its molecular actions at different cell cycle phases, which will be critical to obtain a clearer understanding of how Pax6 functions during the dynamics of cell division. Finally and probably most importantly, we are still far away from a comprehensive understanding of the complex gene networks that Pax6 regulates and how these networks change spatially and temporally during the course of cortical development. This represents a major challenge since Pax6 likely exerts direct and indirect regulation of different sets of downstream genes simultaneously, with context-dependent variation in the strength of their positive or negative effects.

Acknowledgments

Research in the authors' laboratory was funded by the MRC (MR/J003662/1). Human embryonic and fetal material was provided by the Joint MRC/Wellcome Trust (grant # 099175/Z/12/Z) Human Developmental Biology Resource (www.hdbr.org).

References

Agoston, Z., Heine, P., Brill, M. S., Grebbin, B. M., Hau, A. C., Kallenborn-Gerhardt, W., et al. (2014). Meis2 is a Pax6 co-factor in neurogenesis and dopaminergic periglomerular fate specification in the adult olfactory bulb. *Development* 141, 28–38. doi: 10.1242/dev.097295

Agoston, Z., Li, N., Haslinger, A., Wizenmann, A., and Schulte, D. (2012). Genetic and physical interaction of Meis2, Pax3 and Pax7 during dorsal midbrain development. *BMC Dev. Biol.* 12:10. doi: 10.1186/1471-213X-12-10

Agoston, Z., and Schulte, D. (2009). Meis2 competes with the Groucho co-repressor Tle4 for binding to Otx2 and specifies tectal fate without induction of a secondary midbrain-hindbrain boundary organizer. *Development* 136, 3311–3322. doi: 10.1242/dev.037770

Anderson, S. A., Marin, O., Horn, C., Jennings, K., and Rubenstein, J. L. (2001). Distinct cortical migrations from the medial and lateral ganglionic eminences. *Development* 128, 353–363.

Angevine, J. B. Jr., and Sidman, R. L. (1961). Autoradiographic study of cell migration during histogenesis of cerebral cortex in the mouse. *Nature* 192, 766–768. doi: 10.1038/192766b0

Aota, S., Nakajima, N., Sakamoto, R., Watanabe, S., Ibaraki, N., and Okazaki, K. (2003). Pax6 autoregulation mediated by direct interaction of Pax6 protein with the head surface ectoderm-specific enhancer of the mouse Pax6 gene. *Dev. Biol.* 257, 1–13. doi: 10.1016/S0012-1606(03)00058-7

Arai, Y., Pulvers, J. N., Haffner, C., Schilling, B., Nüsslein, I., Calegari, F., et al. (2011). Neural stem and progenitor cells shorten S-phase on commitment to neuron production. *Nat. Commun.* 2, 154. doi: 10.1038/ncomms1155

Azuma, N., Tadokoro, K., Asaka, A., Yamada, M., Yamaguchi, Y., Handa, H., et al. (2005). The Pax6 isoform bearing an alternative spliced exon promotes the development of the neural retinal structure. *Hum. Mol. Genet.* 14, 735–745. doi: 10.1093/hmg/ddi069

Bamiou, D. E., Campbell, N. G., Musiek, F. E., Taylor, R., Chong, W. K., Moore, A., et al. (2007a). Auditory and verbal working memory deficits in a child with congenital aniridia due to a PAX6 mutation. *Int. J. Audiol.* 46, 196–202. doi: 10.1080/14992020601175952

Bamiou, D. E., Free, S. L., Sisodiya, S. M., Chong, W. K., Musiek, F., Williamson, K. A., et al. (2007b). Auditory interhemispheric transfer deficits, hearing difficulties, and brain magnetic resonance imaging abnormalities in children with congenital aniridia due to PAX6 mutations. *Arch. Pediatr. Adolesc. Med.* 161, 463–469. doi: 10.1001/archpedi.161.5.463

Bamiou, D. E., Musiek, F. E., Sisodiya, S. M., Free, S. L., Davies, R. A., Moore, A., et al. (2004). Deficient auditory interhemispheric transfer in patients with PAX6 mutations. *Ann. Neurol.* 56, 503–509. doi: 10.1002/ana.20227

Beaulieu, C. (1993). Numerical data on neocortical neurons in adult rat, with special reference to the GABA population. *Brain Res.* 609, 284–292. doi: 10.1016/0006-8993(93)90884-P

Bel-Vialar, S., Medevielle, F., and Pituello, F. (2007). The on/off of Pax6 controls the tempo of neuronal differentiation in the developing spinal cord. *Dev. Biol.* 305, 659–673. doi: 10.1016/j.ydbio.2007.02.012

Bentivoglio, M., and Mazzarello, P. (1999). The history of radial glia. *Brain Res. Bull.* 49, 305–315. doi: 10.1016/S0361-9230(99)00065-9

Berger, J., Berger, S., Tuoc, T. C., D'amelio, M., Cecconi, F., Gorski, J. A., et al. (2007). Conditional activation of Pax6 in the developing cortex of transgenic mice causes progenitor apoptosis. *Development* 134, 1311–1322. doi: 10.1242/dev.02809

Berry, M., and Rogers, A. W. (1965). The migration of neuroblasts in the developing cerebral cortex. *J. Anat.* 99, 691–709.

Bertuccioli, C., Fasano, L., Jun, S., Wang, S., Sheng, G., and Desplan, C. (1996). In vivo requirement for the paired domain and homeodomain of the paired segmentation gene product. *Development* 122, 2673–2685.

Bessa, J., Tavares, M. J., Santos, J., Kikuta, H., Laplante, M., Becker, T. S., et al. (2008). meis1 regulates cyclin D1 and c-myc expression, and controls the proliferation of the multipotent cells in the early developing zebrafish eye. *Development* 135, 799–803. doi: 10.1242/dev.011932 dev.011932

Betizeau, M., Cortay, V., Patti, D., Pfister, S., Gautier, E., Bellemin-Menard, A., et al. (2013). Precursor diversity and complexity of lineage relationships in the outer subventricular zone of the primate. *Neuron* 80, 442–457. doi: 10.1016/j.neuron.2013.09.032 S0896-6273(13)00863-5

Bishop, K. M., Goudreau, G., and O'leary, D. D. (2000). Regulation of area identity in the mammalian neocortex by Emx2 and Pax6. *Science* 288, 344–349. doi: 10.1126/science.288.5464.344

Bishop, K. M., Rubenstein, J. L., and O'leary, D. D. (2002). Distinct actions of Emx1, Emx2, and Pax6 in regulating the specification of areas in the developing neocortex. *J. Neurosci.* 22, 7627–7638.

Britz, O., Mattar, P., Nguyen, L., Langevin, L. M., Zimmer, C., Alam, S., et al. (2006). A role for proneural genes in the maturation of cortical progenitor cells. *Cereb. Cortex* 16(Suppl. 1), i138–i151. doi: 10.1093/cercor/bhj168

Buscarlet, M., and Stifani, S. (2007). The 'Marx' of Groucho on development and disease. *Trends Cell Biol.* 17, 353–361. doi: 10.1016/j.tcb.2007.07.002

Cameron, R. S., and Rakic, P. (1991). Glial cell lineage in the cerebral cortex: a review and synthesis. *Glia* 4, 124–137. doi: 10.1002/glia.440040204

Caric, D., Gooday, D., Hill, R. E., Mcconnell, S. K., and Price, D. J. (1997). Determination of the migratory capacity of embryonic cortical cells lacking the transcription factor Pax-6. *Development* 124, 5087–5096.

Carriere, C., Plaza, S., Martin, P., Quatannens, B., Bailly, M., Stehelin, D., et al. (1993). Characterization of quail Pax-6 (Pax-QNR) proteins expressed in the neuroretina. *Mol. Cell. Biol.* 13, 7257–7266. doi: 10.1128/MCB.13.12.7257

Cartier, L., Laforge, T., Feki, A., Arnaudeau, S., Dubois-Dauphin, M., and Krause, K. H. (2006). Pax6-induced alteration of cell fate: shape changes, expression of neuronal alpha tubulin, postmitotic phenotype, and cell migration. *J. Neurobiol.* 66, 421–436. doi: 10.1002/neu.20225

Chalepakis, G., Tremblay, P., and Gruss, P. (1992). Pax genes, mutants and molecular function. *J. Cell Sci. Suppl.* 16, 61–67. doi: 10.1242/jcs.1992.Supplement_16.8

Chang, C. P., Jacobs, Y., Nakamura, T., Jenkins, N. A., Copeland, N. G., and Cleary, M. L. (1997). Meis proteins are major in vivo DNA binding partners for wild-type but not chimeric Pbx proteins. *Mol. Cell. Biol.* 17, 5679–5687.

Choe, S. K., Lu, P., Nakamura, M., Lee, J., and Sagerstrom, C. G. (2009). Meis cofactors control HDAC and CBP accessibility at Hox-regulated promoters during zebrafish embryogenesis. *Dev. Cell* 17, 561–567. doi: 10.1016/j.devcel.2009.08.007

Chow, R. L., Altmann, C. R., Lang, R. A., and Hemmati-Brivanlou, A. (1999). Pax6 induces ectopic eyes in a vertebrate. *Development* 126, 4213–4222.

Cooper, S. T., and Hanson, I. M. (2005). A screen for proteins that interact with PAX6: C-terminal mutations disrupt interaction with HOMER3, DNCL1 and TRIM11. *BMC Genet.* 6:43. doi: 10.1186/1471-2156-6-43

Crolla, J. A., and van Heyningen, V. (2002). Frequent chromosome aberrations revealed by molecular cytogenetic studies in patients with aniridia. *Am. J. Hum. Genet.* 71, 1138–1149. doi: 10.1086/344396

Cubelos, B., Briz, C. G., Esteban-Ortega, G. M., and Nieto, M. (2014). Cux1 and Cux2 selectively target basal and apical dendritic compartments of layer II-III cortical neurons. *Dev. Neurobiol.* 75, 163–172. doi: 10.1002/dneu.22215

Cubelos, B., Sebastian-Serrano, A., Beccari, L., Calcagnotto, M. E., Cisneros, E., Kim, S., et al. (2010). Cux1 and Cux2 regulate dendritic branching, spine morphology, and synapses of the upper layer neurons of the cortex. *Neuron* 66, 523–535. doi: 10.1016/j.neuron.2010.04.038

Cvekl, A., Yang, Y., Chauhan, B. K., and Cveklova, K. (2004). Regulation of gene expression by Pax6 in ocular cells: a case of tissue-preferred expression of crystallins in lens. *Int. J. Dev. Biol.* 48, 829–844. doi: 10.1387/ijdb.041866ac

Czerny, T., and Busslinger, M. (1995). DNA-binding and transactivation properties of Pax-6: three amino acids in the paired domain are responsible for the different sequence recognition of Pax-6 and BSAP (Pax-5). *Mol. Cell. Biol.* 15, 2858–2871.

Czerny, T., Halder, G., Kloter, U., Souabni, A., Gehring, W. J., and Busslinger, M. (1999). twin of eyeless, a second Pax-6 gene of *Drosophila*, acts upstream of eyeless in the control of eye development. *Mol. Cell* 3, 297–307. doi: 10.1016/S1097-2765(00)80457-8

Czerny, T., Schaffner, G., and Busslinger, M. (1993). DNA sequence recognition by Pax proteins: bipartite structure of the paired domain and its binding site. *Genes Dev.* 7, 2048–2061. doi: 10.1101/gad.7.10.2048

Davis, L. K., Meyer, K. J., Rudd, D. S., Librant, A. L., Epping, E. A., Sheffield, V. C., et al. (2008). Pax6 3' deletion results in aniridia, autism and mental retardation. *Hum. Genet.* 123, 371–378. doi: 10.1007/s00439-008-0484-x

Dehay, C., and Kennedy, H. (2007). Cell-cycle control and cortical development. *Nat. Rev. Neurosci.* 8, 438–450. doi: 10.1038/nrn2097

Dominguez, M., Ferres-Marco, D., Gutierrez-Avino, F. J., Speicher, S. A., and Beneyto, M. (2004). Growth and specification of the eye are controlled independently by Eyegone and Eyeless in *Drosophila melanogaster*. *Nat. Genet.* 36, 31–39. doi: 10.1038/ng1281

Duncan, M. K., Cvekl, A., Li, X., and Piatigorsky, J. (2000). Truncated forms of Pax-6 disrupt lens morphology in transgenic mice. *Invest. Ophthalmol. Vis. Sci.* 41, 464–473.

Duncan, M. K., Haynes, J. I., Cvekl, A., and Piatigorsky, J. (1998). Dual roles for Pax-6: a transcriptional repressor of lens fiber cell-specific beta-crystallin genes. *Mol. Cell. Biol.* 18, 5579–5586.

Duparc, R. H., Abdouh, M., David, J., Lepine, M., Tetreault, N., and Bernier, G. (2007). Pax6 controls the proliferation rate of neuroepithelial progenitors from the mouse optic vesicle. *Dev. Biol.* 301, 374–387. doi: 10.1016/j.ydbio.2006.11.006

Eberhard, D., and Busslinger, M. (1999). The partial homeodomain of the transcription factor Pax-5 (BSAP) is an interaction motif for the retinoblastoma and TATA-binding proteins. *Cancer Res.* 59(Suppl. 7), 1716s–1724s.

Ellison-Wright, Z., Heyman, I., Frampton, I., Rubia, K., Chitnis, X., Ellison-Wright, I., et al. (2004). Heterozygous PAX6 mutation, adult brain structure and fronto-striato-thalamic function in a human family. *Eur. J. Neurosci.* 19, 1505–1512. doi: 10.1111/j.1460-9568.2004.03236.x

Englund, C., Fink, A., Lau, C., Pham, D., Daza, R. A., Bulfone, A., et al. (2005). Pax6, Tbr2, and Tbr1 are expressed sequentially by radial glia, intermediate progenitor cells, and postmitotic neurons in developing neocortex. *J. Neurosci.* 25, 247–251. doi: 10.1523/JNEUROSCI.2899-04.2005

Epstein, J., Cai, J., Glaser, T., Jepeal, L., and Maas, R. (1994). Identification of a Pax paired domain recognition sequence and evidence for DNA-dependent conformational changes. *J. Biol. Chem.* 269, 8355–8361.

Estivill-Torrus, G., Pearson, H., Van Heyningen, V., Price, D. J., and Rashbass, P. (2002). Pax6 is required to regulate the cell cycle and the rate of progression from symmetrical to asymmetrical division in mammalian cortical progenitors. *Development* 129, 455–466.

Fantes, J., Redeker, B., Breen, M., Boyle, S., Brown, J., Fletcher, J., et al. (1995). Aniridia-associated cytogenetic rearrangements suggest that a position effect may cause the mutant phenotype. *Hum. Mol. Genet.* 4, 415–422. doi: 10.1093/hmg/4.3.415

Farkas, L. M., and Huttner, W. B. (2008). The cell biology of neural stem and progenitor cells and its significance for their proliferation versus differentiation during mammalian brain development. *Curr. Opin. Cell Biol.* 20, 707–715. doi: 10.1016/j.ceb.2008.09.008

Fietz, S. A., Kelava, I., Vogt, J., Wilsch-Brauninger, M., Stenzel, D., Fish, J. L., et al. (2010). OSVZ progenitors of human and ferret neocortex are epithelial-like and expand by integrin signaling. *Nat. Neurosci.* 13, 690–699. doi: 10.1038/nn.2553 nn.2553

Florio, M., and Huttner, W. B. (2014). Neural progenitors, neurogenesis and the evolution of the neocortex. *Development* 141, 2182–2194. doi: 10.1242/dev.090571 141/11/2182

Fogarty, M., Grist, M., Gelman, D., Marin, O., Pachnis, V., and Kessaris, N. (2007). Spatial genetic patterning of the embryonic neuroepithelium generates GABAergic interneuron diversity in the adult cortex. *J. Neurosci.* 27, 10935–10946. doi: 10.1523/JNEUROSCI.1629-07.2007

Free, S. L., Mitchell, T. N., Williamson, K. A., Churchill, A. J., Shorvon, S. D., Moore, A. T., et al. (2003). Quantitative MR image analysis in subjects with defects in the PAX6 gene. *Neuroimage* 20, 2281–2290. doi: 10.1016/j.neuroimage.2003.07.001

Fukushima, Y., Hoovers, J., Mannens, M., Wakui, K., Ohashi, H., Ohno, T., et al. (1993). Detection of a cryptic paracentric inversion within band 11p13 in familial aniridia by fluorescence in situ hybridization. *Hum. Genet.* 91, 205–209. doi: 10.1007/BF00218257

Gal, J. S., Morozov, Y. M., Ayoub, A. E., Chatterjee, M., Rakic, P., and Haydar, T. F. (2006). Molecular and morphological heterogeneity of neural precursors in the mouse neocortical proliferative zones. *J. Neurosci.* 26, 1045–1056. doi: 10.1523/JNEUROSCI.4499-05.2006

Gelman, D. M., and Marin, O. (2010). Generation of interneuron diversity in the mouse cerebral cortex. *Eur. J. Neurosci.* 31, 2136–2141. doi: 10.1111/j.1460-9568.2010.07267.x

Gelman, D. M., Martini, F. J., Nobrega-Pereira, S., Pierani, A., Kessaris, N., and Marin, O. (2009). The embryonic preoptic area is a novel source of cortical GABAergic interneurons. *J. Neurosci.* 29, 9380–9389. doi: 10.1523/JNEUROSCI.0604-09.2009

Georgala, P. A., Carr, C. B., and Price, D. J. (2011a). The role of Pax6 in forebrain development. *Dev. Neurobiol.* 71, 690–709. doi: 10.1002/dneu.20895

Georgala, P. A., Manuel, M., and Price, D. J. (2011b). The generation of superficial cortical layers is regulated by levels of the transcription factor Pax6. *Cereb. Cortex* 21, 81–94. doi: 10.1093/cercor/bhq061

Gillies, K., and Price, D. J. (1993). The fates of cells in the developing cerebral cortex of normal and methylazoxymethanol acetate-lesioned mice. *Eur. J. Neurosci.* 5, 73–84. doi: 10.1111/j.1460-9568.1993.tb00207.x

Glaser, T., Jepeal, L., Edwards, J. G., Young, S. R., Favor, J., and Maas, R. L. (1994). PAX6 gene dosage effect in a family with congenital cataracts, aniridia, anophthalmia and central nervous system defects. *Nat. Genet.* 7, 463–471. doi: 10.1038/ng0894-463

Glaser, T., Walton, D. S., and Maas, R. L. (1992). Genomic structure, evolutionary conservation and aniridia mutations in the human PAX6 gene. *Nat. Genet.* 2, 232–239. doi: 10.1038/ng1192-232

Gotz, M., Stoykova, A., and Gruss, P. (1998). Pax6 controls radial glia differentiation in the cerebral cortex. *Neuron* 21, 1031–1044. doi: 10.1016/S0896-6273(00)80621-2

Grapp, M., Teichler, S., Kitz, J., Dibaj, P., Dickel, C., Knepel, W., et al. (2009). The homeodomain of PAX6 is essential for PAX6-dependent activation of the rat glucagon gene promoter: evidence for a PH0-like binding that induces an active conformation. *Biochim. Biophys. Acta* 1789, 403–412. doi: 10.1016/j.bbagrm.2009.02.001

Griffin, C., Kleinjan, D. A., Doe, B., and Van Heyningen, V. (2002). New 3' elements control Pax6 expression in the developing pretectum, neural retina and olfactory region. *Mech. Dev.* 112, 89–100. doi: 10.1016/S0925-4773(01)00646-3

Gruss, P., and Walther, C. (1992). Pax in development. *Cell* 69, 719–722. doi: 10.1016/0092-8674(92)90281-G

Hack, M. A., Sugimori, M., Lundberg, C., Nakafuku, M., and Gotz, M. (2004). Regionalization and fate specification in neurospheres: the role of Olig2 and Pax6. *Mol. Cell. Neurosci.* 25, 664–678. doi: 10.1016/j.mcn.2003.12.012 S1044743103003956

Hansen, D. V., Lui, J. H., Flandin, P., Yoshikawa, K., Rubenstein, J. L., Alvarez-Buylla, A., et al. (2013). Non-epithelial stem cells and cortical interneuron production in the human ganglionic eminences. *Nat. Neurosci.* 16, 1576–1587. doi: 10.1038/nn.3541

Hansen, D. V., Lui, J. H., Parker, P. R., and Kriegstein, A. R. (2010). Neurogenic radial glia in the outer subventricular zone of human neocortex. *Nature* 464, 554–561. doi: 10.1038/nature08845

Hatten, M. E. (2002). New directions in neuronal migration. *Science* 297, 1660–1663. doi: 10.1126/science.1074572

Haubensak, W., Attardo, A., Denk, W., and Huttner, W. B. (2004). Neurons arise in the basal neuroepithelium of the early mammalian telencephalon: a major site of neurogenesis. *Proc. Natl. Acad. Sci. U.S.A.* 101, 3196–3201. doi: 10.1073/pnas.0308600100

Haubst, N., Berger, J., Radjendirane, V., Graw, J., Favor, J., Saunders, G. F., et al. (2004). Molecular dissection of Pax6 function: the specific roles of the paired domain and homeodomain in brain development. *Development* 131, 6131–6140. doi: 10.1242/dev.01524

Hauck, B., Gehring, W. J., and Walldorf, U. (1999). Functional analysis of an eye specific enhancer of the eyeless gene in *Drosophila*. *Proc. Natl. Acad. Sci. U.S.A.* 96, 564–569. doi: 10.1073/pnas.96.2.564

Haydar, T. F., Ang, E. Jr., and Rakic, P. (2003). Mitotic spindle rotation and mode of cell division in the developing telencephalon. *Proc. Natl. Acad. Sci. U.S.A.* 100, 2890–2895. doi: 10.1073/pnas.04379691000437969100

Heine, P., Dohle, E., Bumsted-O'brien, K., Engelkamp, D., and Schulte, D. (2008). Evidence for an evolutionary conserved role of homothorax/Meis1/2 during vertebrate retina development. *Development* 135, 805–811. doi: 10.1242/dev.012088

Heins, N., Malatesta, P., Cecconi, F., Nakafuku, M., Tucker, K. L., Hack, M. A., et al. (2002). Glial cells generate neurons: the role of the transcription factor Pax6. *Nat. Neurosci.* 5, 308–315. doi: 10.1038/nn828

Hendry, S. H., Schwark, H. D., Jones, E. G., and Yan, J. (1987). Numbers and proportions of GABA-immunoreactive neurons in different areas of monkey cerebral cortex. *J. Neurosci.* 7, 1503–1519.

Hevner, R. F. (2006). From radial glia to pyramidal-projection neuron: transcription factor cascades in cerebral cortex development. *Mol. Neurobiol.* 33, 33–50. doi: 10.1385/MN:33:1:033

Hingorani, M., Williamson, K. A., Moore, A. T., and Van Heyningen, V. (2009). Detailed ophthalmologic evaluation of 43 individuals with PAX6 mutations. *Invest. Ophthalmol. Vis. Sci.* 50, 2581–2590. doi: 10.1167/iovs.08-2827

Hisa, T., Spence, S. E., Rachel, R. A., Fujita, M., Nakamura, T., Ward, J. M., et al. (2004). Hematopoietic, angiogenic and eye defects in Meis1 mutant animals. *EMBO J.* 23, 450–459. doi: 10.1038/sj.emboj.7600038

Ho, L., Jothi, R., Ronan, J. L., Cui, K., Zhao, K., and Crabtree, G. R. (2009a). An embryonic stem cell chromatin remodeling complex, esBAF, is an essential component of the core pluripotency transcriptional network. *Proc. Natl. Acad. Sci. U.S.A.* 106, 5187–5191. doi: 10.1073/pnas.0812888106

Ho, L., Ronan, J. L., Wu, J., Staahl, B. T., Chen, L., Kuo, A., et al. (2009b). An embryonic stem cell chromatin remodeling complex, esBAF, is essential for embryonic stem cell self-renewal and pluripotency. *Proc. Natl. Acad. Sci. U.S.A.* 106, 5181–5186. doi: 10.1073/pnas.0812889106

Holm, P. C., Mader, M. T., Haubst, N., Wizenmann, A., Sigvardsson, M., and Gotz, M. (2007). Loss- and gain-of-function analyses reveal targets of Pax6 in the developing mouse telencephalon. *Mol. Cell Neurosci.* 34, 99–119. doi: 10.1016/j.mcn.2006.10.008

Huttner, W. B., and Kosodo, Y. (2005). Symmetric versus asymmetric cell division during neurogenesis in the developing vertebrate central nervous system. *Curr. Opin. Cell Biol.* 17, 648–657. doi: 10.1016/j.ceb.2005.10.005

Jakovcevski, I., Mayer, N., and Zecevic, N. (2011). Multiple origins of human neocortical interneurons are supported by distinct expression of transcription factors. *Cereb. Cortex* 21, 1771–1782. doi: 10.1093/cercor/bhq245

Jang, E. S., and Goldman, J. E. (2011). Pax6 expression is sufficient to induce a neurogenic fate in glial progenitors of the neonatal subventricular zone. *PLoS ONE* 6:e20894. doi: 10.1371/journal.pone.0020894

Jaworski, C., Sperbeck, S., Graham, C., and Wistow, G. (1997). Alternative splicing of Pax6 in bovine eye and evolutionary conservation of intron sequences. *Biochem. Biophys. Res. Commun.* 240, 196–202. doi: 10.1006/bbrc.1997.7623

Jennings, B. H., and Ish-Horowicz, D. (2008). The Groucho/TLE/Grg family of transcriptional co-repressors. *Genome Biol.* 9, 205. doi: 10.1186/gb-2008-9-1-205gb

Jun, S., and Desplan, C. (1996). Cooperative interactions between paired domain and homeodomain. *Development* 122, 2639–2650.

Kaldis, P., and Richardson, H. E. (2012). When cell cycle meets development. *Development* 139, 225–230. doi: 10.1242/dev.073288

Kamachi, Y., Uchikawa, M., Tanouchi, A., Sekido, R., and Kondoh, H. (2001). Pax6 and SOX2 form a co-DNA-binding partner complex that regulates initiation of lens development. *Genes Dev.* 15, 1272–1286. doi: 10.1101/gad.887101

Kammandel, B., Chowdhury, K., Stoykova, A., Aparicio, S., Brenner, S., and Gruss, P. (1999). Distinct cis-essential modules direct the time-space pattern of the Pax6 gene activity. *Dev. Biol.* 205, 79–97. doi: 10.1006/dbio.1998.9128

Kerwin, J., Yang, Y., Merchan, P., Sarma, S., Thompson, J., Wang, X., et al. (2010). The HUDSEN Atlas: a three-dimensional (3D) spatial framework for studying gene expression in the developing human brain. *J. Anat.* 217, 289–299. doi: 10.1111/j.1469-7580.2010.01290.x

Kiecker, C., and Lumsden, A. (2005). Compartments and their boundaries in vertebrate brain development. *Nat. Rev. Neurosci.* 6, 553–564. doi: 10.1038/nrn1702

Kim, J., and Lauderdale, J. D. (2006). Analysis of Pax6 expression using a BAC transgene reveals the presence of a paired-less isoform of Pax6 in the eye and olfactory bulb. *Dev. Biol.* 292, 486–505. doi: 10.1016/j.ydbio.2005.12.041

Kiselev, Y., Eriksen, T. E., Forsdahl, S., Nguyen, L. H., and Mikkola, I. (2012). 3T3 cell lines stably expressing Pax6 or Pax6(5a)–a new tool used for identification of common and isoform specific target genes. *PLoS ONE* 7:e31915. doi: 10.1371/journal.pone.0031915

Kleinjan, D. A., Seawright, A., Childs, A. J., and Van Heyningen, V. (2004). Conserved elements in Pax6 intron 7 involved in (auto)regulation and alternative transcription. *Dev. Biol.* 265, 462–477. doi: 10.1016/j.ydbio.2003.09.011

Kleinjan, D. A., Seawright, A., Elgar, G., and Van Heyningen, V. (2002). Characterization of a novel gene adjacent to PAX6, revealing synteny conservation with functional significance. *Mamm. Genome* 13, 102–107. doi: 10.1007/s00335-001-3058-y

Kleinjan, D. A., Seawright, A., Mella, S., Carr, C. B., Tyas, D. A., Simpson, T. I., et al. (2006). Long-range downstream enhancers are essential for Pax6 expression. *Dev. Biol.* 299, 563–581. doi: 10.1016/j.ydbio.2006.08.060

Kleinjan, D. A., Seawright, A., Schedl, A., Quinlan, R. A., Danes, S., and Van Heyningen, V. (2001). Aniridia-associated translocations, DNase hypersensitivity, sequence comparison and transgenic analysis redefine the functional domain of PAX6. *Hum. Mol. Genet.* 10, 2049–2059. doi: 10.1093/hmg/10.19.2049

Knoepfler, P. S., Bergstrom, D. A., Uetsuki, T., Dac-Korytko, I., Sun, Y. H., Wright, W. E., et al. (1999). A conserved motif N-terminal to the DNA-binding domains of myogenic bHLH transcription factors mediates cooperative DNA binding with pbx-Meis1/Prep1. *Nucleic Acids Res.* 27, 3752–3761. doi: 10.1093/nar/27.18.3752

Kornack, D. R., and Rakic, P. (1998). Changes in cell-cycle kinetics during the development and evolution of primate neocortex. *Proc. Natl. Acad. Sci. U.S.A.* 95, 1242–1246. doi: 10.1073/pnas.95.3.1242

Koroma, B. M., Yang, J. M., and Sundin, O. H. (1997). The Pax-6 homeobox gene is expressed throughout the corneal and conjunctival epithelia. *Invest. Ophthalmol. Vis. Sci.* 38, 108–120.

Kozmik, Z., Czerny, T., and Busslinger, M. (1997). Alternatively spliced insertions in the paired domain restrict the DNA sequence specificity of Pax6 and Pax8. *EMBO J.* 16, 6793–6803. doi: 10.1093/emboj/16.22.6793

Kroll, T. T., and O'Leary, D. D. (2005). Ventralized dorsal telencephalic progenitors in Pax6 mutant mice generate GABA interneurons of a lateral ganglionic eminence fate. *Proc. Natl. Acad. Sci. U.S.A.* 102, 7374–7379. doi: 10.1073/pnas.0500819102

Krubitzer, L., and Kaas, J. (2005). The evolution of the neocortex in mammals: how is phenotypic diversity generated? *Curr. Opin. Neurobiol.* 15, 444–453. doi: 10.1016/j.conb.2005.07.003

Lauderdale, J. D., Wilensky, J. S., Oliver, E. R., Walton, D. S., and Glaser, T. (2000). 3' deletions cause aniridia by preventing PAX6 gene expression. *Proc. Natl. Acad. Sci. U.S.A.* 97, 13755–13759. doi: 10.1073/pnas.240398797

Lessard, J., Wu, J. I., Ranish, J. A., Wan, M., Winslow, M. M., Staahl, B. T., et al. (2007). An essential switch in subunit composition of a chromatin remodeling complex during neural development. *Neuron* 55, 201–215. doi: 10.1016/j.neuron.2007.06.019

Letinic, K., Zoncu, R., and Rakic, P. (2002). Origin of GABAergic neurons in the human neocortex. *Nature* 417, 645–649. doi: 10.1038/nature00779

Levers, T. E., Edgar, J. M., and Price, D. J. (2001). The fates of cells generated at the end of neurogenesis in developing mouse cortex. *J. Neurobiol.* 48, 265–277. doi: 10.1002/neu.1056

Levitt, P., and Rakic, P. (1980). Immunoperoxidase localization of glial fibrillary acidic protein in radial glial cells and astrocytes of the developing rhesus monkey brain. *J. Comp. Neurol.* 193, 815–840. doi: 10.1002/cne.901930316

Li, N., Zhao, C. T., Wang, Y., and Yuan, X. B. (2010). The transcription factor Cux1 regulates dendritic morphology of cortical pyramidal neurons. *PLoS ONE* 5:e10596. doi: 10.1371/journal.pone.0010596

Long, J. E., Cobos, I., Potter, G. B., and Rubenstein, J. L. (2009a). Dlx1&2 and Mash1 transcription factors control MGE and CGE patterning and differentiation through parallel and overlapping pathways. *Cereb. Cortex* 19(Suppl. 1), i96–i106. doi: 10.1093/cercor/bhp045bhp045

Long, J. E., Swan, C., Liang, W. S., Cobos, I., Potter, G. B., and Rubenstein, J. L. (2009b). Dlx1&2 and Mash1 transcription factors control striatal patterning and differentiation through parallel and overlapping pathways. *J. Comp. Neurol.* 512, 556–572. doi: 10.1002/cne.21854

Lukaszewicz, A., Savatier, P., Cortay, V., Giroud, P., Huissoud, C., Berland, M., et al. (2005). G1 phase regulation, area-specific cell cycle control, and cytoarchitectonics in the primate cortex. *Neuron* 47, 353–364. doi: 10.1016/j.neuron.2005.06.032

Maekawa, M., Iwayama, Y., Nakamura, K., Sato, M., Toyota, T., Ohnishi, T., et al. (2009). A novel missense mutation (Leu46Val) of PAX6 found in an autistic patient. *Neurosci. Lett.* 462, 267–271. doi: 10.1016/j.neulet.2009.07.021S0304-3940(09)00939-2

Malandrini, A., Mari, F., Palmeri, S., Gambelli, S., Berti, G., Bruttini, M., et al. (2001). PAX6 mutation in a family with aniridia, congenital ptosis, and mental retardation. *Clin. Genet.* 60, 151–154. doi: 10.1034/j.1399-0004.2001.600210.x

Malatesta, P., Hack, M. A., Hartfuss, E., Kettenmann, H., Klinkert, W., Kirchhoff, F., et al. (2003). Neuronal or glial progeny: regional differences in radial glia fate. *Neuron* 37, 751–764. doi: 10.1016/S0896-6273(03)00116-8

Malatesta, P., Hartfuss, E., and Gotz, M. (2000). Isolation of radial glial cells by fluorescent-activated cell sorting reveals a neuronal lineage. *Development* 127, 5253–5263.

Malumbres, M., and Barbacid, M. (2001). To cycle or not to cycle: a critical decision in cancer. *Nat. Rev. Cancer* 1, 222–231. doi: 10.1038/35106065

Malumbres, M., and Barbacid, M. (2005). Mammalian cyclin-dependent kinases. *Trends Biochem. Sci.* 30, 630–641. doi: 10.1016/j.tibs.2005.09.005

Mansouri, A., Stoykova, A., and Gruss, P. (1994). Pax genes in development. *J. Cell Sci. Suppl.* 18, 35–42. doi: 10.1242/jcs.1994.Supplement_18.5

Manuel, M., Georgala, P. A., Carr, C. B., Chanas, S., Kleinjan, D. A., Martynoga, B., et al. (2007). Controlled overexpression of Pax6 in vivo negatively autoregulates the Pax6 locus, causing cell-autonomous defects of late cortical progenitor proliferation with little effect on cortical arealization. *Development* 134, 545–555. doi: 10.1242/dev.02764

Marquardt, T., Ashery-Padan, R., Andrejewski, N., Scardigli, R., Guillemot, F., and Gruss, P. (2001). Pax6 is required for the multipotent state of retinal progenitor cells. *Cell* 105, 43–55. doi: 10.1016/S0092-8674(01)00295-1

Marshall, C. A., Novitch, B. G., and Goldman, J. E. (2005). Olig2 directs astrocyte and oligodendrocyte formation in postnatal subventricular zone cells. *J. Neurosci.* 25, 7289–7298. doi: 10.1523/JNEUROSCI.1924-05.2005

Martin, R. D. (1990). *Primate Origins and Evolution. A Phylogenetic Reconstruction.* London: Chapman & Hall.

McBride, D. J., Buckle, A., Van Heyningen, V., and Kleinjan, D. A. (2011). DNaseI hypersensitivity and ultraconservation reveal novel, interdependent long-range enhancers at the complex Pax6 cis-regulatory region. *PLoS ONE* 6:e28616. doi: 10.1371/journal.pone.0028616

McConnell, S. K. (1995). Strategies for the generation of neuronal diversity in the developing central nervous system. *J. Neurosci.* 15, 6987–6998.

Mercader, N., Leonardo, E., Azpiazu, N., Serrano, A., Morata, G., Martinez, C., et al. (1999). Conserved regulation of proximodistal limb axis development by Meis1/Hth. *Nature* 402, 425–429. doi: 10.1038/46580

Mi, D., Carr, C. B., Georgala, P. A., Huang, Y. T., Manuel, M. N., Jeanes, E., et al. (2013a). Pax6 exerts regional control of cortical progenitor proliferation via direct repression of Cdk6 and hypophosphorylation of pRb. *Neuron* 78, 269–284. doi: 10.1016/j.neuron.2013.02.012S0896-6273(13)00170-0

Mi, D., Huang, Y. T., Kleinjan, D. A., Mason, J. O., and Price, D. J. (2013b). Identification of genomic regions regulating Pax6 expression in embryonic forebrain using YAC reporter transgenic mouse lines. *PLoS ONE* 8:e80208. doi: 10.1371/journal.pone.0080208PONE-D-13-29798

Mikkola, I., Bruun, J. A., Holm, T., and Johansen, T. (2001). Superactivation of Pax6-mediated transactivation from paired domain-binding sites by dna-independent recruitment of different homeodomain proteins. *J. Biol. Chem.* 276, 4109–4118. doi: 10.1074/jbc.M008882200

Mitchell, T. N., Free, S. L., Williamson, K. A., Stevens, J. M., Churchill, A. J., Hanson, I. M., et al. (2003). Polymicrogyria and absence of pineal gland due to PAX6 mutation. *Ann. Neurol.* 53, 658–663. doi: 10.1002/ana.10576

Miyata, T., Kawaguchi, A., Okano, H., and Ogawa, M. (2001). Asymmetric inheritance of radial glial fibers by cortical neurons. *Neuron* 31, 727–741. doi: 10.1016/S0896-6273(01)00420-2

Miyata, T., Kawaguchi, A., Saito, K., Kawano, M., Muto, T., and Ogawa, M. (2004). Asymmetric production of surface-dividing and non-surface-dividing cortical progenitor cells. *Development* 131, 3133–3145. doi: 10.1242/dev.01173

Miyoshi, G., Hjerling-Leffler, J., Karayannis, T., Sousa, V. H., Butt, S. J., Battiste, J., et al. (2010). Genetic fate mapping reveals that the caudal ganglionic eminence produces a large and diverse population of superficial cortical interneurons. *J. Neurosci.* 30, 1582–1594. doi: 10.1523/JNEUROSCI.4515-09.201030/5/1582

Mo, Z., and Zecevic, N. (2008). Is Pax6 critical for neurogenesis in the human fetal brain? *Cereb. Cortex* 18, 1455–1465. doi: 10.1093/cercor/bhm181

Moens, C. B., and Selleri, L. (2006). Hox cofactors in vertebrate development. *Dev. Biol.* 291, 193–206. doi: 10.1016/j.ydbio.2005.10.032

Morgan, R. (2004). Conservation of sequence and function in the Pax6 regulatory elements. *Trends Genet.* 20, 283–287. doi: 10.1016/j.tig.2004.04.009S0168952504001076

Moskow, J. J., Bullrich, F., Huebner, K., Daar, I. O., and Buchberg, A. M. (1995). Meis1, a PBX1-related homeobox gene involved in myeloid leukemia in BXH-2 mice. *Mol. Cell Biol.* 15, 5434–5443.

Muzio, L., Dibenedetto, B., Stoykova, A., Boncinelli, E., Gruss, P., and Mallamaci, A. (2002). Emx2 and Pax6 control regionalization of the pre-neuronogenic cortical primordium. *Cereb. Cortex* 12, 129–139. doi: 10.1093/cercor/12.2.129

Muzio, L., and Mallamaci, A. (2003). Emx1, emx2 and pax6 in specification, regionalization and arealization of the cerebral cortex. *Cereb. Cortex* 13, 641–647. doi: 10.1093/cercor/13.6.641

Ninkovic, J., Steiner-Mezzadri, A., Jawerka, M., Akinci, U., Masserdotti, G., Petricca, S., et al. (2013). The BAF complex interacts with Pax6 in adult neural progenitors to establish a neurogenic cross-regulatory transcriptional network. *Cell Stem Cell* 13, 403–418. doi: 10.1016/j.stem.2013.07.002S1934-5909(13)00310-X

Noctor, S. C., Flint, A. C., Weissman, T. A., Dammerman, R. S., and Kriegstein, A. R. (2001). Neurons derived from radial glial cells establish radial units in neocortex. *Nature* 409, 714–720. doi: 10.1038/35055553

Noctor, S. C., Martinez-Cerdeno, V., Ivic, L., and Kriegstein, A. R. (2004). Cortical neurons arise in symmetric and asymmetric division zones and migrate through specific phases. *Nat. Neurosci.* 7, 136–144. doi: 10.1038/nn1172nn1172

Oikawa, T., and Yamada, T. (2003). Molecular biology of the Ets family of transcription factors. *Gene* 303, 11–34. doi: 10.1016/S0378-1119(02)01156-3

O'Leary, D. D., Chou, S. J., and Sahara, S. (2007). Area patterning of the mammalian cortex. *Neuron* 56, 252–269. doi: 10.1016/j.neuron.2007.10.010

Osumi, N., Shinohara, H., Numayama-Tsuruta, K., and Maekawa, M. (2008). Concise review: Pax6 transcription factor contributes to both embryonic and adult neurogenesis as a multifunctional regulator. *Stem Cells* 26, 1663–1672. doi: 10.1634/stemcells.2007-08842007-0884

Ouyang, J., Shen, Y. C., Yeh, L. K., Li, W., Coyle, B. M., Liu, C. Y., et al. (2006). Pax6 overexpression suppresses cell proliferation and retards the cell cycle in corneal epithelial cells. *Invest. Ophthalmol. Vis. Sci.* 47, 2397–2407. doi: 10.1167/iovs.05-1083

Paige, S. L., Thomas, S., Stoick-Cooper, C. L., Wang, H., Maves, L., Sandstrom, R., et al. (2012). A temporal chromatin signature in human embryonic stem cells identifies regulators of cardiac development. *Cell* 151, 221–232. doi: 10.1016/j.cell.2012.08.027S0092-8674(12)01058

Petanjek, Z., Dujmovic, A., Kostovic, I., and Esclapez, M. (2008). Distinct origin of GABA-ergic neurons in forebrain of man, nonhuman primates and lower mammals. *Coll. Antropol.* 32(Suppl. 1), 9–17.

Philips, G. T., Stair, C. N., Young Lee, H., Wroblewski, E., Berberoglu, M. A., Brown, N. L., et al. (2005). Precocious retinal neurons: Pax6 controls timing of differentiation and determination of cell type. *Dev. Biol.* 279, 308–321. doi: 10.1016/j.ydbio.2004.12.018

Pinson, J., Simpson, T. I., Mason, J. O., and Price, D. J. (2006). Positive autoregulation of the transcription factor Pax6 in response to increased levels of either of its major isoforms, Pax6 or Pax6(5a), in cultured cells. *BMC Dev. Biol.* 6:25. doi: 10.1186/1471-213X-6-25

Plaza, S., Aumercier, M., Bailly, M., Dozier, C., and Saule, S. (1999a). Involvement of poly (ADP-ribose)-polymerase in the Pax-6 gene regulation in neuroretina. *Oncogene* 18, 1041–1051. doi: 10.1038/sj.onc.1202406

Plaza, S., Saule, S., and Dozier, C. (1999b). High conservation of cis-regulatory elements between quail and human for the Pax-6 gene. *Dev. Genes Evol.* 209, 165–173. doi: 10.1007/s004270050240

Polyak, K., Lee, M. H., Erdjument-Bromage, H., Koff, A., Roberts, J. M., Tempst, P., et al. (1994). Cloning of p27Kip1, a cyclin-dependent kinase inhibitor and a potential mediator of extracellular antimitogenic signals. *Cell* 78, 59–66. doi: 10.1016/0092-8674(94)90572-X

Price, D. J., Aslam, S., Tasker, L., and Gillies, K. (1997). Fates of the earliest generated cells in the developing murine neocortex. *J. Comp. Neurol.* 377, 414–422. doi: 10.1002/(SICI)1096-9861(19970120)377:3<414::AID-CNE8>3.0.CO;2-5

Puschel, A. W., Gruss, P., and Westerfield, M. (1992). Sequence and expression pattern of pax-6 are highly conserved between zebrafish and mice. *Development* 114, 643–651.

Quinn, J. C., Molinek, M., Martynoga, B. S., Zaki, P. A., Faedo, A., Bulfone, A., et al. (2007). Pax6 controls cerebral cortical cell number by regulating exit from the cell cycle and specifies cortical cell identity by a cell autonomous mechanism. *Dev. Biol.* 302, 50–65. doi: 10.1016/j.ydbio.2006.08.035

Rakic, P. (1974). Neurons in rhesus monkey visual cortex: systematic relation between time of origin and eventual disposition. *Science* 183, 425–427. doi: 10.1126/science.183.4123.425

Rakic, P. (1988). Specification of cerebral cortical areas. *Science* 241, 170–176. doi: 10.1126/science.3291116

Richardson, J., Cvekl, A., and Wistow, G. (1995). Pax-6 is essential for lens-specific expression of zeta-crystallin. *Proc. Natl. Acad. Sci. U.S.A.* 92, 4676–4680. doi: 10.1073/pnas.92.10.4676

Salomoni, P., and Calegari, F. (2010). Cell cycle control of mammalian neural stem cells: putting a speed limit on G1. *Trends Cell Biol.* 20, 233–243. doi: 10.1016/j.tcb.2010.01.006

Sansom, S. N., Griffiths, D. S., Faedo, A., Kleinjan, D. J., Ruan, Y., Smith, J., et al. (2009). The level of the transcription factor Pax6 is essential for controlling the balance between neural stem cell self-renewal and neurogenesis. *PLoS Genet.* 5:e1000511. doi: 10.1371/journal.pgen.1000511

Sansom, S. N., and Livesey, F. J. (2009). Gradients in the brain: the control of the development of form and function in the cerebral cortex. *Cold Spring Harb. Perspect. Biol.* 1, a002519. doi: 10.1101/cshperspect.a002519

Scardigli, R., Baumer, N., Gruss, P., Guillemot, F., and Le Roux, I. (2003). Direct and concentration-dependent regulation of the proneural gene Neurogenin2 by Pax6. *Development* 130, 3269–3281. doi: 10.1242/dev.00539

Schedl, A., Ross, A., Lee, M., Engelkamp, D., Rashbass, P., Van Heyningen, V., et al. (1996). Influence of PAX6 gene dosage on development: overexpression causes severe eye abnormalities. *Cell* 86, 71–82. doi: 10.1016/S0092-8674(00)80078-1

Schmahl, W., Knoedlseder, M., Favor, J., and Davidson, D. (1993). Defects of neuronal migration and the pathogenesis of cortical malformations are associated with Small eye (Sey) in the mouse, a point mutation at the Pax-6-locus. *Acta Neuropathol. (Berl.)* 86, 126–135. doi: 10.1007/BF00334879

Schmidt-Sidor, B., Szymanska, K., Williamson, K., Van Heyningen, V., Roszkowski, T., Wierzba-Bobrowicz, T., et al. (2009). Malformations of the brain in two fetuses with a compound heterozygosity for two PAX6 mutations. *Folia Neuropathol.* 47, 372–382.

Schuurmans, C., Armant, O., Nieto, M., Stenman, J. M., Britz, O., Klenin, N., et al. (2004). Sequential phases of cortical specification involve Neurogenin-dependent and -independent pathways. *EMBO J.* 23, 2892–2902. doi: 10.1038/sj.emboj.7600278

Sheng, G., Thouvenot, E., Schmucker, D., Wilson, D. S., and Desplan, C. (1997). Direct regulation of rhodopsin 1 by Pax-6/eyeless in *Drosophila*: evidence for a conserved function in photoreceptors. *Genes Dev.* 11, 1122–1131. doi: 10.1101/gad.11.9.1122

Sherr, C. J., and Roberts, J. M. (1995). Inhibitors of mammalian G1 cyclin-dependent kinases. *Genes Dev.* 9, 1149–1163. doi: 10.1101/gad.9.10.1149

Shimizu, N., Watanabe, H., Kubota, J., Wu, J., Saito, R., Yokoi, T., et al. (2009). Pax6-5a promotes neuronal differentiation of murine embryonic stem cells. *Biol. Pharm. Bull.* 32, 999–1003. doi: 10.1248/bpb.32.999

Shimoda, Y., Tajima, Y., Osanai, T., Katsume, A., Kohara, M., Kudo, T., et al. (2002). Pax6 controls the expression of Lewis x epitope in the embryonic forebrain by regulating alpha 1,3-fucosyltransferase IX expression. *J. Biol. Chem.* 277, 2033–2039. doi: 10.1074/jbc.M108495200

Singh, S., Chao, L. Y., Mishra, R., Davies, J., and Saunders, G. F. (2001). Missense mutation at the C-terminus of PAX6 negatively modulates homeodomain function. *Hum. Mol. Genet.* 10, 911–918. doi: 10.1093/hmg/10.9.911

Singh, S., Stellrecht, C. M., Tang, H. K., and Saunders, G. F. (2000). Modulation of PAX6 homeodomain function by the paired domain. *J. Biol. Chem.* 275, 17306–17313. doi: 10.1074/jbc.M000359200

Singh, S., Tang, H. K., Lee, J. Y., and Saunders, G. F. (1998). Truncation mutations in the transactivation region of PAX6 result in dominant-negative mutants. *J. Biol. Chem.* 273, 21531–21541. doi: 10.1074/jbc.273.34.21531

Singhal, N., Graumann, J., Wu, G., Arauzo-Bravo, M. J., Han, D. W., Greber, B., et al. (2010). Chromatin-remodeling components of the BAF complex facilitate reprogramming. *Cell* 141, 943–955. doi: 10.1016/j.cell.2010.04.037S0092-8674(10)00491-5

Sisodiya, S. M., Free, S. L., Williamson, K. A., Mitchell, T. N., Willis, C., Stevens, J. M., et al. (2001). PAX6 haploinsufficiency causes cerebral malformation and olfactory dysfunction in humans. *Nat. Genet.* 28, 214–216. doi: 10.1038/90042

Skogh, C., Eriksson, C., Kokaia, M., Meijer, X. C., Wahlberg, L. U., Wictorin, K., et al. (2001). Generation of regionally specified neurons in expanded glial cultures derived from the mouse and human lateral ganglionic eminence. *Mol. Cell. Neurosci.* 17, 811–820. doi: 10.1006/mcne.2001.0973S1044-7431(01)90973-X

Smart, I. H., Dehay, C., Giroud, P., Berland, M., and Kennedy, H. (2002). Unique morphological features of the proliferative zones and postmitotic compartments of the neural epithelium giving rise to striate and extrastriate cortex in the monkey. *Cereb. Cortex* 12, 37–53. doi: 10.1093/cercor/12.1.37

Solomon, B. D., Pineda-Alvarez, D. E., Balog, J. Z., Hadley, D., Gropman, A. L., Nandagopal, R., et al. (2009). Compound heterozygosity for mutations in PAX6 in a patient with complex brain anomaly, neonatal diabetes mellitus, and microophthalmia. *Am. J. Med. Genet. A* 149A, 2543–2546. doi: 10.1002/ajmg.a.33081

Stenman, J., Yu, R. T., Evans, R. M., and Campbell, K. (2003a). Tlx and Pax6 co-operate genetically to establish the pallio-subpallial boundary in the embryonic mouse telencephalon. *Development* 130, 1113–1122. doi: 10.1242/dev.00328

Stenman, J. M., Wang, B., and Campbell, K. (2003b). Tlx controls proliferation and patterning of lateral telencephalic progenitor domains. *J. Neurosci.* 23, 10568–10576.

Stiles, J., and Jernigan, T. L. (2010). The basics of brain development. *Neuropsychol. Rev.* 20, 327–348. doi: 10.1007/s11065-010-9148-4

Stoykova, A., and Gruss, P. (1994). Roles of Pax-genes in developing and adult brain as suggested by expression patterns. *J. Neurosci.* 14, 1395–1412.

Stoykova, A., Treichel, D., Hallonet, M., and Gruss, P. (2000). Pax6 modulates the dorsoventral patterning of the mammalian telencephalon. *J. Neurosci.* 20, 8042–8050.

Takahashi, T., Nowakowski, R. S., and Caviness, V. S. Jr. (1993). Cell cycle parameters and patterns of nuclear movement in the neocortical proliferative zone of the fetal mouse. *J. Neurosci.* 13, 820–833.

Takahashi, T., Nowakowski, R. S., and Caviness, V. S. Jr. (1995). The cell cycle of the pseudostratified ventricular epithelium of the embryonic murine cerebral wall. *J. Neurosci.* 15, 6046–6057.

Tan, X., and Shi, S. H. (2013). Neocortical neurogenesis and neuronal migration. *Wiley Interdiscip. Rev. Dev. Biol.* 2, 443–459. doi: 10.1002/wdev.88

Tang, H. K., Singh, S., and Saunders, G. F. (1998). Dissection of the transactivation function of the transcription factor encoded by the eye developmental gene PAX6. *J. Biol. Chem.* 273, 7210–7221. doi: 10.1074/jbc.273.13.7210

Tarabykin, V., Stoykova, A., Usman, N., and Gruss, P. (2001). Cortical upper layer neurons derive from the subventricular zone as indicated by Svet1 gene expression. *Development* 128, 1983–1993.

Tominaga, T., Meng, W., Togashi, K., Urano, H., Alberts, A. S., and Tominaga, M. (2002). The Rho GTPase effector protein, mDia, inhibits the DNA binding ability of the transcription factor Pax6 and changes the pattern of neurite extension in cerebellar granule cells through its binding to Pax6. *J. Biol. Chem.* 277, 47686–47691. doi: 10.1074/jbc.M207539200M207539200

Ton, C. C., Miwa, H., and Saunders, G. F. (1992). Small eye (Sey): cloning and characterization of the murine homolog of the human aniridia gene. *Genomics* 13, 251–256. doi: 10.1016/0888-7543(92)90239-O

Toresson, H., Potter, S. S., and Campbell, K. (2000). Genetic control of dorsal-ventral identity in the telencephalon: opposing roles for Pax6 and Gsh2. *Development* 127, 4361–4371.

Tuoc, T. C., Boretius, S., Sansom, S. N., Pitulescu, M. E., Frahm, J., Livesey, F. J., et al. (2013a). Chromatin regulation by BAF170 controls cerebral cortical size and thickness. *Dev. Cell* 25, 256–269. doi: 10.1016/j.devcel.2013.04.005S1534-5807(13)00196-2

Tuoc, T. C., Narayanan, R., and Stoykova, A. (2013b). BAF chromatin remodeling complex: cortical size regulation and beyond. *Cell Cycle* 12, 2953–2959. doi: 10.4161/cc.2599925999

Tuoc, T. C., Radyushkin, K., Tonchev, A. B., Pinon, M. C., Ashery-Padan, R., Molnar, Z., et al. (2009). Selective cortical layering abnormalities and behavioral deficits in cortex-specific Pax6 knock-out mice. *J. Neurosci.* 29, 8335–8349. doi: 10.1523/JNEUROSCI.5669-08.2009

Tuoc, T. C., and Stoykova, A. (2008a). Er81 is a downstream target of Pax6 in cortical progenitors. *BMC Dev. Biol.* 8:23. doi: 10.1186/1471-213X-8-231471-213X-8-23

Tuoc, T. C., and Stoykova, A. (2008b). Trim11 modulates the function of neurogenic transcription factor Pax6 through ubiquitin-proteosome system. *Genes Dev.* 22, 1972–1986. doi: 10.1101/gad.47170822/14/1972

Vidal, A., and Koff, A. (2000). Cell-cycle inhibitors: three families united by a common cause. *Gene* 247, 1–15. doi: 10.1016/S0378-1119(00)00092-5

Visel, A., Bristow, J., and Pennacchio, L. A. (2007). Enhancer identification through comparative genomics. *Semin. Cell Dev. Biol.* 18, 140–152. doi: 10.1016/j.semcdb.2006.12.014

Walcher, T., Xie, Q., Sun, J., Irmler, M., Beckers, J., Ozturk, T., et al. (2013). Functional dissection of the paired domain of Pax6 reveals molecular mechanisms of coordinating neurogenesis and proliferation. *Development* 140, 1123–1136. doi: 10.1242/dev.082875140/5/1123

Wang, B., Long, J. E., Flandin, P., Pla, R., Waclaw, R. R., Campbell, K., et al. (2013). Loss of Gsx1 and Gsx2 function rescues distinct phenotypes in Dlx1/2 mutants. *J. Comp. Neurol.* 521, 1561–1584. doi: 10.1002/cne.23242

Warren, N., Caric, D., Pratt, T., Clausen, J. A., Asavaritikrai, P., Mason, J. O., et al. (1999). The transcription factor, Pax6, is required for cell proliferation and differentiation in the developing cerebral cortex. *Cereb. Cortex* 9, 627–635. doi: 10.1093/cercor/9.6.627

Westerman, B. A., Murre, C., and Oudejans, C. B. (2003). The cellular Pax-Hox-helix connection. *Biochim. Biophys. Acta* 1629, 1–7. doi: 10.1016/j.bbaexp.2003.08.002

Williams, S. C., Altmann, C. R., Chow, R. L., Hemmati-Brivanlou, A., and Lang, R. A. (1998). A highly conserved lens transcriptional control element from the Pax-6 gene. *Mech. Dev.* 73, 225–229. doi: 10.1016/S0925-4773(98)00057-4

Wilson, D., Sheng, G., Lecuit, T., Dostatni, N., and Desplan, C. (1993). Cooperative dimerization of paired class homeo domains on DNA. *Genes Dev.* 7, 2120–2134. doi: 10.1101/gad.7.11.2120

Wolf, L. V., Yang, Y., Wang, J., Xie, Q., Braunger, B., Tamm, E. R., et al. (2009). Identification of pax6-dependent gene regulatory networks in the mouse lens. *PLoS ONE* 4:e4159. doi: 10.1371/journal.pone.0004159

Wonders, C. P., and Anderson, S. A. (2006). The origin and specification of cortical interneurons. *Nat. Rev. Neurosci.* 7, 687–696. doi: 10.1038/nrn1954

Wu, J. I. (2012). Diverse functions of ATP-dependent chromatin remodeling complexes in development and cancer. *Acta Biochim. Biophys. Sin. (Shanghai)* 44, 54–69. doi: 10.1093/abbs/gmr099gmr099

Xie, Q., and Cvekl, A. (2011). The orchestration of mammalian tissue morphogenesis through a series of coherent feed-forward loops. *J. Biol. Chem.* 286, 43259–43271. doi: 10.1074/jbc.M111.264580

Xie, Q., Yang, Y., Huang, J., Ninkovic, J., Walcher, T., Wolf, L., et al. (2013). Pax6 interactions with chromatin and identification of its novel direct target genes in lens and forebrain. *PLoS ONE* 8:e54507. doi: 10.1371/journal.pone.0054507

Xu, H. E., Rould, M. A., Xu, W., Epstein, J. A., Maas, R. L., and Pabo, C. O. (1999a). Crystal structure of the human Pax6 paired domain-DNA complex reveals specific roles for the linker region and carboxy-terminal subdomain in DNA binding. *Genes Dev.* 13, 1263–1275. doi: 10.1101/gad.13.10.1263

Xu, P. X., Zhang, X., Heaney, S., Yoon, A., Michelson, A. M., and Maas, R. L. (1999b). Regulation of Pax6 expression is conserved between mice and flies. *Development* 126, 383–395.

Yan, Z., Wang, Z., Sharova, L., Sharov, A. A., Ling, C., Piao, Y., et al. (2008). BAF250B-associated SWI/SNF chromatin-remodeling complex is required to maintain undifferentiated mouse embryonic stem cells. *Stem Cells* 26, 1155–1165. doi: 10.1634/stemcells.2007-08462007-0846

Yip, D. J., Corcoran, C. P., Alvarez-Saavedra, M., Demaria, A., Rennick, S., Mears, A. J., et al. (2012). Snf2l regulates Foxg1-dependent progenitor cell expansion in the developing brain. *Dev. Cell* 22, 871–878. doi: 10.1016/j.devcel.2012.01.020S1534-5807(12)00054-8

Yoneshima, H., Yamasaki, S., Voelker, C. C., Molnar, Z., Christophe, E., Audinat, E., et al. (2006). Er81 is expressed in a subpopulation of layer 5 neurons in rodent and primate neocortices. *Neuroscience* 137, 401–412. doi: 10.1016/j.neuroscience.2005.08.075

Yun, K., Potter, S., and Rubenstein, J. L. (2001). Gsh2 and Pax6 play complementary roles in dorsoventral patterning of the mammalian telencephalon. *Development* 128, 193–205.

Zaki, P. A., Quinn, J. C., and Price, D. J. (2003). Mouse models of telencephalic development. *Curr. Opin. Genet. Dev.* 13, 423–437. doi: 10.1016/S0959-437X(03)00084-4

Zecevic, N., Chen, Y., and Filipovic, R. (2005). Contributions of cortical subventricular zone to the development of the human cerebral cortex. *J. Comp. Neurol.* 491, 109–122. doi: 10.1002/cne.20714

Zetterberg, A., Larsson, O., and Wiman, K. G. (1995). What is the restriction point? *Curr. Opin. Cell Biol.* 7, 835–842. doi: 10.1016/0955-0674(95)80067-0

Zhang, W., Cveklovam, K., Oppermann, B., Kantorow, M., and Cvekl, A. (2001). Quantitation of PAX6 and PAX6(5a) transcript levels in adult human lens, cornea, and monkey retina. *Mol. Vis.* 7, 1–5.

Zhou, Y. H., Wu, X., Tan, F., Shi, Y. X., Glass, T., Liu, T. J., et al. (2005). PAX6 suppresses growth of human glioblastoma cells. *J. Neurooncol.* 71, 223–229. doi: 10.1007/s11060-004-1720-4

16

Cellullar Insights into Cerebral Cortical Development: Focusing on the Locomotion Mode of Neuronal Migration

Takeshi Kawauchi [1, 2, 3*]

[1] Department of Physiology, Keio University School of Medicine, Tokyo, Japan, [2] Precursory Research for Embryonic Science and Technology (PRESTO), Japan Science and Technology Agency, Saitama, Japan, [3] Laboratory of Molecular Life Science, Institute of Biomedical Research and Innovation, Foundation for Biomedical Research and Innovation, Kobe, Japan

***Correspondence:**
Takeshi Kawauchi,
Laboratory of Molecular Life Science,
Institute of Biomedical Research and
Innovation, Foundation for Biomedical
Research and Innovation, 2-2
Minatojima-Minamimachi Chuo-ku,
Kobe 650-0047, Japan
takeshi-kawauchi@umin.ac.jp

The mammalian brain consists of numerous compartments that are closely connected with each other via neural networks, comprising the basis of higher order brain functions. The highly specialized structure originates from simple pseudostratified neuroepithelium-derived neural progenitors located near the ventricle. A long journey by neurons from the ventricular side is essential for the formation of a sophisticated brain structure, including a mammalian-specific six-layered cerebral cortex. Neuronal migration consists of several contiguous steps, but the locomotion mode comprises a large part of the migration. The locomoting neurons exhibit unique features; a radial glial fiber-dependent migration requiring the endocytic recycling of N-cadherin and a neuron-specific migration mode with dilation/swelling formation that requires the actin and microtubule organization possibly regulated by cyclin-dependent kinase 5 (Cdk5), Dcx, $p27^{kip1}$, Rac1, and POSH. Here I will introduce the roles of various cellular events, such as cytoskeletal organization, cell adhesion, and membrane trafficking, in the regulation of the neuronal migration, with particular focus on the locomotion mode.

Keywords: microtubule, actin cytoskeleton, endocytosis, JNK, Rab5, Rab11, Rab7, Rap1

Introduction

The brain is divided into many compartments, such as nuclei, layered structures, and cortical areas, allowing highly organized role allocations. The systematically allocated neuronal populations are generated from spatially restricted regions, the ventricular, and subventricular zones. Therefore, a long-distance migration from the ventricular side to the final destination is essential for constructing a functional brain. In line with this, defects in neuronal migration are associated with various neurological disorders (Gleeson and Walsh, 2000; Kawauchi and Hoshino, 2008). Several types of cortical malformations, including lissencephaly, double cortex syndrome (subcortical band heterotopia) and periventricular heterotopia (PVH), are thought to result from neuronal migration defects. These cortical malformations are frequently associated with intellectual disability and intractable epilepsy (Francis et al., 2006; Moon and Wynshaw-Boris, 2013; Reiner and Sapir, 2013; Lian and Sheen, 2015). *Lis1, Dcx, Filamin A, ArfGEF2, Arx, Reelin,* and several *Tubulin* genes (*TUBA1A, TUBA8, TUBB2B, TUBB3, TUBB5,* and *TUBG1)* are identified as causative genes for these cortical malformations (des Portes et al., 1998; Fox et al., 1998; Gleeson et al., 1998; Hong et al., 2000; Kitamura et al., 2002; Kato et al., 2004; Sheen et al., 2004; Keays et al., 2007; Abdollahi et al., 2009; Reiner and Sapir, 2013; Bahi-Buisson et al., 2014; Magen et al., 2015) (**Figures 1A,B**). Furthermore, suppression of genes related to dyslexia (e.g., *DCDC2, KIAA0319*), autism spectrum disorder (ASD) (e.g., *Auts2, CNTNAP2*) and schizophrenia (e.g., *SDCCAG8*) disturbs neuronal migration, although it is unclear whether the neuronal migration defect is the main cause of the pathogenesis of these neurological and psychiatric disorders (Hannula-Jouppi et al., 2005; Kamiya et al., 2005; Meng et al., 2005; Paracchini et al., 2006; Wang et al., 2006; Kähler et al., 2008; Peñagarikano et al., 2011; O'roak et al., 2012; Zhang et al., 2013a; Hori et al., 2014; Insolera et al., 2014; La Fata et al., 2014) (**Figure 1B**). Interestingly, in addition to these genes, several environmental factors, such as stress and inflammation, are also associated with cortical development, including neuronal migration (Stolp et al., 2012; Hashimoto-Torii et al., 2014; Ishii and Hashimoto-Torii, 2015).

In the developing cerebral cortex, neuronal migration consists of several contiguous steps (Nadarajah and Parnavelas, 2002; Cooper, 2014; Takano et al., 2015) (**Figure 1A**). Newly generated neurons exhibit multipolar morphology in the lower part of the intermediate zone. The multipolar neurons form an axon and a leading process almost coincidentally with retraction of other processes. The bipolar-shaped neurons are called "locomoting neurons," which migrate along radial glial fibers with unique morphological changes (the locomotion mode of neuronal migration) (**Figure 2A**). At the final phase of neuronal migration, they switch over from the "locomotion" into a "terminal translocation."

Most studies so far have focused on the mechanisms of the morphological changes at the early phase of neuronal migration, including the multipolar-to-bipolar transition (Kawauchi and Hoshino, 2008; Heng et al., 2010). One reason is that many cortical malformation-related gene products are involved in the multipolar-to-bipolar transition. Second, the acquirement of neuronal polarity, a key step of neuronal maturation, occurs nearly simultaneously with the multipolar-bipolar transition. Third, suppression of cytoskeletal proteins or kinases often leads to defects in the early phase of migration due to the occurrence of various morphological changes at this stage.

In contrast to the early phase of migration, our knowledge of the locomotion mode is relatively poor. However, recent morphological and cell biological analyses have uncovered unique features of locomoting neurons. In this review, I will introduce recent advances in the molecular and cellular biology of neuronal migration with particular focus on the locomotion mode.

The Early Phase of Neuronal Migration

Several steps of the early phase of neuronal migration, including the multipolar-to-bipolar transition, are required for the formation of the morphologies of the locomoting neurons. The formation of a leading process requires c-jun N-terminal kinase (JNK) (Kawauchi et al., 2003). Filamin A (FLNA), an actin-binding protein, is also involved in the early phase of migration, possibly including the leading process formation (Nagano et al., 2004). Knockdown of Lis1, a regulator of the dynein complex, a microtubule minus end-directed motor, suppresses the multipolar-bipolar transition (Tsai et al., 2005). FLNA and Lis1 have been identified as causative genes for PVH and lissencephaly, respectively, and both knockout of FLNA and Lis1 heterodeficiency show neuronal migration defects (Hirotsune et al., 1998; Zhang et al., 2013b).

In addition, many other molecules are reported to regulate the formation of multipolar morphology (e.g., Cdk5, $p27^{kip1}$, Arx, Rab5) (Kawauchi et al., 2006, 2010; Friocourt et al., 2008; Friocourt and Parnavelas, 2010) and multipolar-to-bipolar transition (e.g., Cdk5, PHF6, FMRP) (Ohshima et al., 2007; Zhang et al., 2013a; La Fata et al., 2014; Franzoni et al., 2015) at the early phase of migration (**Figure 1A**).

The Locomotion Mode of Neuronal Migration

The locomotion mode of neuronal migration covers the largest part of the neuronal journey, and is therefore a main contributor to proper neuronal positioning (Rakic, 2006; Nishimura et al., 2010). As described above, however, analysis of molecular mechanisms underlying the locomotion mode is difficult, because in many cases, neurons with defects in cytoskeletal proteins or kinases also show abnormalities early in neuronal migration prior to starting the locomotion (or no phenotypes). However, recent advances in *in vivo* cell biological approaches and novel technologies have uncovered several molecules regulating the unique features of the locomotion mode of neuronal migration. For example, a novel method, the *ex vivo* chemical inhibitor technique, that allows us to directly analyze molecules involved in the locomotion mode, has recently been established (Nishimura et al., 2010). Using this technique, Cdk5 and Src family kinases were shown to regulate the locomotion mode (Nishimura et al., 2010).

The locomotion mode of neuronal migration displays two major characteristics, a radial glial fiber-dependent migration and a neuron-specific unique migration mode with dilation/swelling formation and nuclear elongation (Rakic, 1972; Bellion et al., 2005; Schaar and McConnell, 2005) (**Figure 2**). In the next subsections, I will introduce the morphological, molecular, and cellular mechanisms of these unique characters of the locomotion mode.

A Unique Migration Mode with Dilation/Swelling Formation

Locomoting neurons exhibit distinct migration features (Bellion et al., 2005; Schaar and McConnell, 2005; Nishimura et al., 2014). (1) Locomoting neurons extend a leading process and form a cytoplasmic dilation (also referred as to "swelling" especially in tangentially migrating interneurons) at the proximal region of a leading process. (2) The nucleus in the locomoting neurons becomes elongated to enter the cytoplasmic dilation (**Figure 2**).

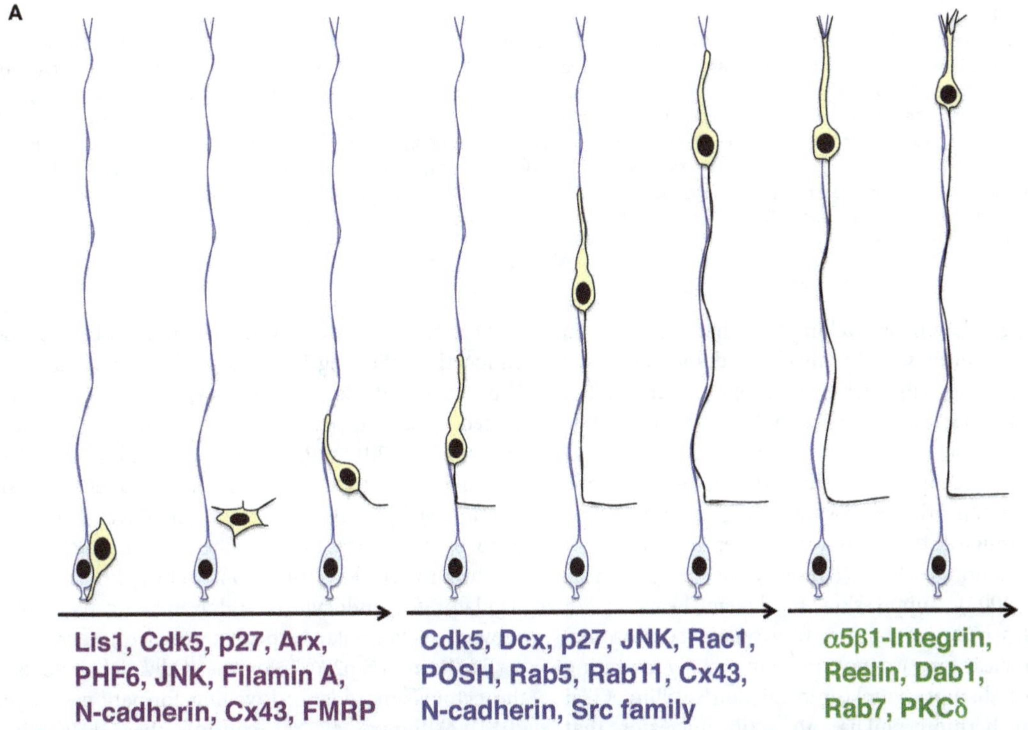

B

Molecule	Molecular and cellular function	Related brain disease
Lis1	Regulator for dynein motor	Lissencephaly, Millar-Dicker sydrome
Dcx	Microtubule binding and stabilizing	Lissencephaly, Subcortical band heterotopia
Filamin A	Actin binding and crosslinking	Periventricular heterotopia
ArfGEF2	Membrane trafficking	Periventricular heterotopia, Microcephaly
Reelin	Extracellular protein, Rap1 and Integrin activation	Lissencephaly, Schizophrenia, ASD
Cdk5	Signaling molecule, Cytoskelatal regulation	Lissencephaly
Tubulins*	Component of microtubules	Lissencephaly, Microcephaly
Arx	Transcription factor	Epilepsy, Lissencephaly, Intellectual disability
Dcdc2	DCX family, Involvement of ciliary functions (?)	Dyslexia
DYX1C1	Regulation of Dynein assembly and ciliary motility	Dyslexia (?)
KIAA0319	Single transmembrane protein	Dyslexia
ROBO1	Single transmembrane protein, Slit receptor	Dyslexia
Auts2	Transcriptional activation, Cytoskeletal regulation	ASD
CNTNAP2	Transmembrane protein, K^+ channel clustering	ASD, Epilepsy
Tbr1	Transcription factor	ASD
SDCCAG8	Regulation of centrosomal properties and function	Schizophrenia, Intellectual disability
Disc1	Ndel1/Dynein regulation, Wnt/GSK3β signal	Schizophrenia (?)
MDGA1	GPI-anchored immunoglobulin superfamily	Schizophrenia
PHF6	Binding to PAF1 transcription elongation complex	Intellectual disability (Börjeson-Forssman-Lehmann syndrome)
FMRP	mRNA binding, Regulation of translation	Intellectual disability (fragile X syndrome), ASD

* Tubulins: TUBA1A, TUBA8, TUBB2B, TUBB3, TUBB5 and TUBG1 (see Bahi-Buisson et al.)

FIGURE 1 | Molecules involved in the multi-step modes of neuronal migration and its related neurological disorders. (A) Immature neurons (light yellow cells), generated from radial glial progenitors (light blue cells) near the ventricle, migrate toward the pial surface. At the early phase of neuronal migration (the left three migrating neurons), many cytoskeletal-regulatory proteins (e.g., Lis1 and Filamin A), kinases (e.g., Cdk5 and JNK), and other proteins (e.g., p27^{kip1} and N-cadherin)

(Continued)

FIGURE 1 | Continued
are required for proper morphological changes of migrating neurons (Kawauchi and Hoshino, 2008; Lickiss et al., 2012; Kawauchi, 2014). Interestingly, some of these molecules are also involved in neurological disorders, such as Börjeson-Forssman-Lehmann syndrome (for PHF6) (Zhang et al., 2013a; Franzoni et al., 2015), Fragile X syndrome (for FMRP) (La Fata et al., 2014) and lissencephaly (for Lis1, Cdk5, and Arx) (Friocourt and Parnavelas, 2010; Reiner and Sapir, 2013; Magen et al., 2015). Subsequently, neurons undergo the locomotion mode of neuronal migration (the middle three migrating neurons). Cdk5 and its substrates, Dcx, and p27^{kip1}, control the dilation/swelling formation during the locomotion. POSH and Rac1 are also required for the dilation/swelling formation. N-cadherin and its regulation by Rab5- and Rab11-dependent endocytic recycling play important roles in radial glial fiber-dependent migration of the locomoting neurons. At the final phase of migration, neurons undergo the terminal translocation mode (the right two migrating neurons). The Reelin-Dab1-C3G-Rap1-Talin-Integrin pathway regulates the terminal translocation. PKCδ is also required for the terminal translocation. **(B)** Molecules involved in neuronal migration-related brain diseases.

The cytoplasmic dilation or swelling was first identified in 2005 as a migrating neuron-specific subcellular domain, because not only other migrating cells, such as neutrophils, keratocytes, and fibroblasts, but also static neurons do not form a cytoplasmic dilation/swelling (Bellion et al., 2005; Schaar and McConnell, 2005). Electron microscopy studies show that the cytoplasmic dilation/swelling contains the centrosome, Golgi apparatus, and microtubules. Although the centrosome frequently is a part of the cytoplasmic dilation/swelling (Bellion et al., 2005; Schaar and McConnell, 2005), suppression of dynein heavy chain or Lis1, both of which are known to regulate centrosomal positioning and nuclear forward movement in radially migrating neurons, does not disrupt cytoplasmic dilation/swelling (Tsai et al., 2007). Furthermore, mDia, an actin nucleator that acts as a downstream effector of RhoA, regulates centrosomal positioning, and nuclear translocation in tangentially migrating GABAergic interneurons. However, mDia deficiency does not impair the cytoplasmic dilation/swelling formation (Shinohara et al., 2012).

In contrast to RhoA, another Rho family small GTPase, Rac1 and its binding protein, POSH, are required for the formation of cytoplasmic dilation/swelling in cortical excitatory neurons (Yang et al., 2012). Suppression of Rac1 by the expression of the dominant negative mutant, shRNA-mediated knockdown, or gene targeting, disturbs neuronal migration (Kawauchi et al., 2003; Chen et al., 2007; Govek et al., 2011; Yang et al., 2012). Although Rac1 promotes the activity of JNK, which is known to regulate leading process morphology and neuronal migration (Kawauchi et al., 2003), JNK1-suppressing neurons are able to form the cytoplasmic dilation/swelling. The area of the cytoplasmic dilation/swelling is not significantly different between control and JNK1-knockdown neurons, although the morphologies of the cytoplasmic dilation/swelling in the JNK1-knockdown neurons are rough and irregular in part (Nishimura et al., 2014). Therefore, Rac1 and POSH are believed to control the formation of cytoplasmic dilation/swelling mainly in a JNK1-independent manner.

Considering that abundant microtubules are observed in the cytoplasmic dilation/swelling, microtubule-regulatory proteins may be involved in the formation of this subcellular domain. In fact, it has been reported that Dcx (previously known as Doublecortin) and its upstream kinase, Cdk5, are required for the formation of the cytoplasmic dilation/swelling (Nishimura et al., 2014). Interestingly, both *Dcx* and *Cdk5* are known as causative genes for lissencephaly (Gleeson et al., 1998; des Portes et al., 1998; Magen et al., 2015).

Dcx controls not only microtubule polymerization but also endocytic trafficking (Francis et al., 1999; Gleeson et al., 1999; Yap et al., 2012; Yap and Winckler, 2015), and clathrin-coated pits are observed in cytoplasmic dilation/swelling (Shieh et al., 2011). Pharmacological inhibition of microtubule polymerization (nocodazole treatment) or endocytosis (dynasore treatment) by using the *ex vivo* chemical inhibitor technique, disturbs the formation of the cytoplasmic dilation/swelling (Nishimura et al., 2014). Consistently, knockdown of Rab5, a regulator for endocytosis and trafficking to early endosomes, shows defects similar to the dynasore treatment.

Furthermore, p27^{kip1}, another Cdk5 substrate, is required for the cytoplasmic dilation/swelling formation (Nishimura et al., 2014). Although p27^{kip1} controls the G1 length in the cell cycle and promotes cell cycle exit, p27^{kip1} also plays a role in actin reorganization through suppression of RhoA activity and activation of an actin-binding protein, Cofilin, in the multipolar processes of neurons at the early phase of migration (Kawauchi et al., 2006, 2013). In addition, p27^{kip1} is required for the tangential migration of cortical GABAergic interneurons via microtubule organization (Godin et al., 2012). However, it is still unclear which downstream event(s) (the regulation of actin or microtubule or something else) is important for the cytoplasmic dilation/swelling formation in the locomoting neurons.

Nuclear Elongation and Forward Movement

After the formation of the cytoplasmic dilation/swelling, the nucleus elongates, and moves into the newly formed dilation. This nuclear elongation is closely coupled with the cytoplasmic dilation/swelling formation. In fact, suppression of Cdk5, Dcx, p27^{kip1}, Rab5, microtubule polymerization, or endocytosis perturbs the nuclear elongation as well as dilation/swelling formation during the locomotion mode (Nishimura et al., 2014). Interestingly, however, knockdown of JNK, which does not affect the area of the cytoplasmic dilation/swelling, suppresses the nuclear elongation, suggesting that Cdk5 and JNK, both of which promote microtubule dynamics (Kawauchi et al., 2003, 2005), have different roles in the locomotion mode of migration (Nishimura et al., 2014).

The elongated nuclei are surrounded by perinuclear cage-like microtubules, which contain abundant tyrosinated tubulins, components of dynamic microtubules (Rivas and Hatten, 1995; Schaar and McConnell, 2005; Umeshima et al., 2007). The regulation of microtubule dynamics is known to require Cdk5 and JNK activities (Kawauchi et al., 2005). Cdk5 phosphorylates focal adhesion kinase (FAK) at Ser732, and

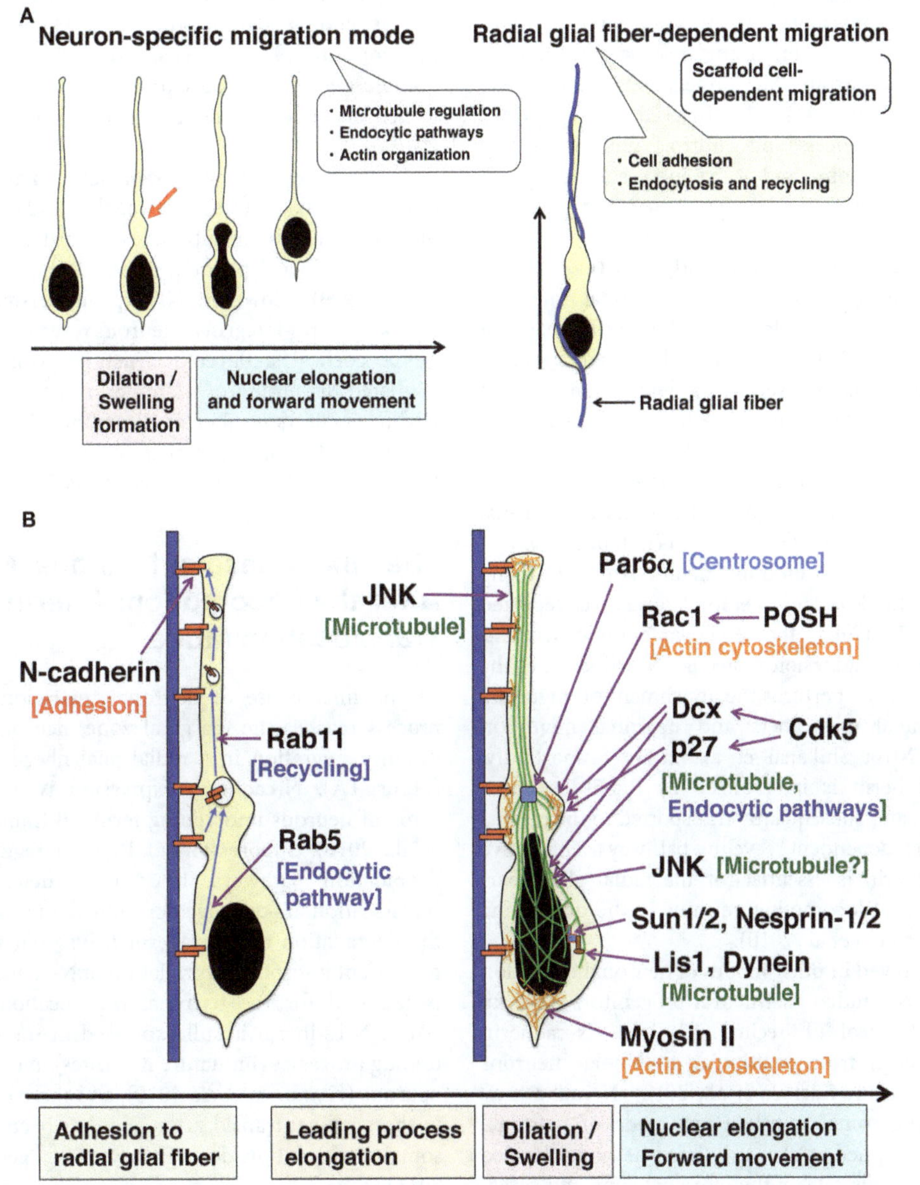

FIGURE 2 | Two unique features of the locomotion mode of neuronal migration. (A) Locomoting neurons exhibit a neuron-specific migration feature (left) and a scaffold cell-dependent migration (right). Locomoting neurons form a cytoplasmic dilation/swelling at the proximal region of a leading process, and subsequently, the nucleus shows an elongated morphology and moves into the dilation/swelling (left). Locomoting neurons also show a scaffold cell-dependent migration. They attach to and migrate along the neural progenitor-derived radial glial fibers (right). **(B)** Cellular events regulating two unique features of the locomotion mode of neuronal migration. N-cadherin is involved in the adhesion to radial glial fibers. Endocytic recycling of N-cadherin is required for the forward movement of neurons. JNK controls the leading process formation possibly through the regulation of microtubule dynamics. Par6α is localized at centrosomes and regulates perinuclear cage-like microtubules. Both POSH-Rac1 and Cdk5-Dcx pathways are required for the formation of cytoplasmic dilation/swelling. Another Cdk5 substrate, $p27^{kip1}$ also plays an important role in cytoplasmic dilation/swelling formation. Furthermore, Cdk5, Dcx, $p27^{kip1}$ as well as JNK are involved in the nuclear elongation in the locomoting neurons. Lis, Dynein, SUN1/2, Nesprin-1/2, and Myosin II regulate the nuclear forward movement. See the main text for more details.

Ser732-phosphorylated FAK is localized on the perinuclear cage-like microtubules (Xie et al., 2003). Cdk5 deficiency or expression of the Ser732-nonphosphorylatable mutant of FAK (S732A) disturbs the nuclear elongation in migrating neurons. It is also known that overexpression of Par6α, which is localized at the centrosome, disrupts the perinuclear cage (Solecki et al., 2004).

The forward movement of the nuclei (nucleokinesis) requires Lis1- and dynein-mediated motor activity (see the following excellent reviews: Tsai and Gleeson, 2005; Marín et al., 2010). SUN1/2 and Nesprin-1/2, which are localized at the inner and outer membranes of the nuclear envelope, respectively, connect the nucleus to the dynein complex on microtubules in the locomoting neurons (Zhang et al., 2009). In addition, actomyosin-mediated contractility at the posterior end of the cell is known to play an important role in the nuclear forward movement (Schaar and McConnell, 2005; Martini and Valdeolmillos, 2010). Myosin II is also observed at the proximal region of the leading process and controls the coordinated movement of the centrosome and soma in cerebellar granule neurons (Solecki et al., 2009).

A Radial Glial Fiber-dependent Migration

Another feature of the locomotion mode of neuronal migration is migration on other cells, called a scaffold cell-dependent migration (Kawauchi, 2012) (**Figure 2A**). It has been suggested that Astrotactin (Astn1) is involved in the interaction between migrating neurons and Bergmann glial fibers (Adams et al., 2002). Treatment with antibodies against Astn1, but not N-cadherin and L1-CAM, inhibits the attachment of cultured cerebellar granule neurons to astroglia and glia-guided neuronal migration (Stitt and Hatten, 1990; Fishell and Hatten, 1991).

The discovery that the locomoting neurons migrate along radial glial fibers in the developing cerebral cortex was reported in 1972 (Rakic, 1972). Unlike the cerebellar granule neurons, suppression of a cell-cell adhesion molecule, N-cadherin, in the developing cerebral cortex perturbs the attachment of migrating neurons to the radial glial fibers and neuronal migration (Kawauchi et al., 2010; Shikanai et al., 2011). Importantly, a portion of N-cadherin is internalized by Rab5-dependent endocytic pathways, and subsequently transported to the plasma membrane via Rab11-dependent recycling pathways. This active transport of N-cadherin is essential for the radial glial fiber-dependent migration of locomoting neurons in the developing cerebral cortex (Kawauchi et al., 2010).

N-cadherin is involved in other modes of neuronal migration and adhesions between radial glial neural progenitors (Solecki, 2012). Under the control of Reelin and Rap1, N-cadherin regulates the transition from multipolar to bipolar neurons (Jossin and Cooper, 2011; Gärtner et al., 2012). N-cadherin is also required for the somal translocation mode of neuronal migration, which is applied to the early-born neurons (Franco et al., 2011). Cajal-Retzius cells in the marginal zone and somal translocating neurons express immunoglobulin-like adhesion molecules, Nectin-1 and Nectin-3, respectively, and Nectin-3 upregulates N-cadherin to promote the somal translocation mode in early corticogenesis (Gil-Sanz et al., 2013). Interestingly, N-cadherin has also been implicated for a role in the tangential migration of cortical interneurons (Luccardini et al., 2013, 2015).

In addition to N-cadherin, other cell adhesion molecules, such as Connexin 43 (Cx43), Cx26, and JAM-C, have been shown to control neuronal migration. Cx43 and Cx26, gap junction proteins, stabilize a leading process on the radial glial fibers via enhancement of cell-cell adhesion, rather than formation of an aqueous channel (Elias et al., 2007). FAK promotes the assembly of Cx26 at contact sites between the locomoting neurons and radial glial fibers (Valiente et al., 2011). Interestingly, Cx43 is also involved in the formation of multipolar morphologies at the early phase of neuronal migration (Liu et al., 2012). Cx43 upregulates $p27^{kip1}$, which controls the multipolar morphologies through actin reorganization (Kawauchi et al., 2006). JAM-C and its binding adaptor protein, Pard3, are localized at the tight junctions in epithelial cells. However, in migrating cerebellar granule neurons, Pard3A promotes the recruitment of JAM-C to neuron-neuron or neuron-glial cell contacts (Famulski et al., 2010).

Integrin heterodimers are mainly involved in cell-to-extra cellular matrix adhesion (Kawauchi, 2012). It has been reported that treatment with antibodies against β1-integrin suppresses radial glial fiber-dependent neuronal migration *in vitro* (Anton et al., 1999). However, NEX promoter-mediated conditional knockout of β1-integrin in neurons revealed no migration defects in the cortical six-layered structures, while Nestin promoter-mediated disruption of β1-integrin in both neurons and radial glial progenitors resulted in disorganization of radial glial fibers and cortical laminae, similar to type II-lissencephaly (Graus-Porta et al., 2001; Belvindrah et al., 2007).

The Final Phase of Neuronal Migration After the Locomotion: A Terminal Translocation Mode

At the final phase of neuronal migration when the leading process reaches the marginal zone, neurons undergo a short-distance migration in a radial glial fiber-independent manner (**Figure 1A**). N-cadherin expression is decreased at the cell soma of neurons undergoing terminal translocation (Kawauchi et al., 2010). Suppression of Rab7, a regulator for lysosomal degradation pathways, leads to a defect in the terminal translocation. Taken together with the involvement of Rab7 in the degradation of N-cadherin *in vitro*, it suggests that Rab7-dependent lysosomal degradation of N-cadherin at the cell soma is required for the terminal translocation (Kawauchi et al., 2010). N-cadherin is still expressed in the distal region of the leading processes (immature dendrites) in terminal translocating neurons (Kawauchi et al., 2010), and therefore might play a role in the terminal translocation as it has been reported to control somal translocation during early corticogenesis (Franco et al., 2011).

Additionally, involvement of other cell adhesion molecules, such as α5β1-integrin, a receptor for fibronectin, and L1-CAM, and Protein kinase C delta (PKCδ) has been reported (Nishimura et al., 2010; Sekine et al., 2012; Tonosaki et al., 2014) (**Figure 1A**). Suppression of either α5-integrin or β1-integrin perturbs terminal translocation (Sekine et al., 2012). Reelin-mediated activation of Rap1 promotes the recruitment of Talin to the plasma membrane, which activates the Integrin heterodimers possibly through direct binding to the cytoplasmic region of β1-integrin (Sekine et al., 2012). As described above, Reelin also enhances the activation of Rap1 during the early phase of neuronal migration (Jossin and Cooper, 2011). Recent studies have revealed that two guanine-nucleotide exchange factors (GEFs), C3G, and RapGEF2, differentially activate Rap1 at the final or early phases of migration, respectively (Ye et al., 2014). However, defects in the multipolar-to-bipolar transition have been reported in C3G-knockout brains (Voss et al., 2008), suggesting that C3G may also be required for the early phase of neuronal migration.

Conclusion

From the 1990's, several key molecules involved in neuronal migration, such as Lis1, Dcx, FLNA, and Reelin, have been identified mainly by the use of molecular genetics. Furthermore, recent *in vivo* and *ex vivo* cell biological techniques, including *in vivo* electroporation, slice culture methods, time-lapse imaging and electron microscopy analyses, have uncovered essential roles for dynamic regulation of cytoskeleton and cell adhesion in neuronal migration. In the locomoting neurons, the formation of dilation/swelling requires proper regulation of microtubules, actin cytoskeleton, and endocytic pathways (**Figure 2**). Another feature of locomotion, a radial glial fiber-dependent migration, depends on the membrane trafficking-mediated remodeling of the cell adhesion complex (**Figure 2**). Thus, molecular pieces, identified from molecular genetics and *in vivo* electroporation, begin to take shape. However, the spatio-temporal regulation of these cellular events remains unclear. Furthermore, the dynamic behavior of each endosome in migrating neurons in cortical slices remains to be observed. Continual technological advances in *in vivo* cell biology and related research fields will shed light on unsolved questions to help us better understand the whole picture of cerebral cortical development.

Acknowledgments

The author thanks Dr. Ruth T. Yu for critical reading of the manuscript. Research in the author's group is supported by research grants from the JST PRESTO and the JSPS KAKENHI (26290015 and 26110718).

References

Abdollahi, M. R., Morrison, E., Sirey, T., Molnar, Z., Hayward, B. E., Carr, I. M., et al. (2009). Mutation of the variant alpha-tubulin TUBA8 results in polymicrogyria with optic nerve hypoplasia. *Am. J. Hum. Genet.* 85, 737–744. doi: 10.1016/j.ajhg.2009.10.007

Adams, N. C., Tomoda, T., Cooper, M., Dietz, G., and Hatten, M. E. (2002). Mice that lack astrotactin have slowed neuronal migration. *Development* 129, 965–972. Available online at: http://dev.biologists.org/content/129/4/965.long

Anton, E. S., Kreidberg, J. A., and Rakic, P. (1999). Distinct functions of alpha3 and alpha(v) integrin receptors in neuronal migration and laminar organization of the cerebral cortex. *Neuron* 22, 277–289. doi: 10.1016/S0896-6273(00)81089-2

Bahi-Buisson, N., Poirier, K., Fourniol, F., Saillour, Y., Valence, S., Lebrun, N., et al. (2014). The wide spectrum of tubulinopathies: what are the key features for the diagnosis? *Brain* 137, 1676–1700. doi: 10.1093/brain/awu082

Bellion, A., Baudoin, J. P., Alvarez, C., Bornens, M., and Metin, C. (2005). Nucleokinesis in tangentially migrating neurons comprises two alternating phases: forward migration of the Golgi/centrosome associated with centrosome splitting and myosin contraction at the rear. *J. Neurosci.* 25, 5691–5699. doi: 10.1523/JNEUROSCI.1030-05.2005

Belvindrah, R., Graus-Porta, D., Goebbels, S., Nave, K. A., and Muller, U. (2007). Beta1 integrins in radial glia but not in migrating neurons are essential for the formation of cell layers in the cerebral cortex. *J. Neurosci.* 27, 13854–13865. doi: 10.1523/JNEUROSCI.4494-07.2007

Chen, L., Liao, G., Waclaw, R. R., Burns, K. A., Linquist, D., Campbell, K., et al. (2007). Rac1 controls the formation of midline commissures and the competency of tangential migration in ventral telencephalic neurons. *J. Neurosci.* 27, 3884–3893. doi: 10.1523/JNEUROSCI.3509-06.2007

Cooper, J. A. (2014). Molecules and mechanisms that regulate multipolar migration in the intermediate zone. *Front. Cell. Neurosci.* 8:386. doi: 10.3389/fncel.2014.00386

des Portes, V., Pinard, J. M., Billuart, P., Vinet, M. C., Koulakoff, A., Carrié, A., et al. (1998). A novel CNS gene required for neuronal migration and involved in X-linked subcortical laminar heterotopia and lissencephaly syndrome. *Cell* 92, 51–61. doi: 10.1016/S0092-8674(00)80898-3

Elias, L. A., Wang, D. D., and Kriegstein, A. R. (2007). Gap junction adhesion is necessary for radial migration in the neocortex. *Nature* 448, 901–907. doi: 10.1038/nature06063

Famulski, J. K., Trivedi, N., Howell, D., Yang, Y., Tong, Y., Gilbertson, R., et al. (2010). Siah regulation of Pard3A controls neuronal cell adhesion during germinal zone exit. *Science* 330, 1834–1838. doi: 10.1126/science.1198480

Fishell, G., and Hatten, M. E. (1991). Astrotactin provides a receptor system for CNS neuronal migration. *Development* 113, 755–765.

Fox, J. W., Lamperti, E. D., Eksioglu, Y. Z., Hong, S. E., Feng, Y., Graham, D. A., et al. (1998). Mutations in filamin 1 prevent migration of cerebral cortical neurons in human periventricular heterotopia. *Neuron* 21, 1315–1325. doi: 10.1016/S0896-6273(00)80651-0

Francis, F., Koulakoff, A., Boucher, D., Chafey, P., Schaar, B., Vinet, M. C., et al. (1999). Doublecortin is a developmentally regulated, microtubule-associated protein expressed in migrating and differentiating neurons. *Neuron* 23, 247–256. doi: 10.1016/S0896-6273(00)80777-1

Francis, F., Meyer, G., Fallet-Bianco, C., Moreno, S., Kappeler, C., Socorro, A. C., et al. (2006). Human disorders of cortical development: from past to present. *Eur. J. Neurosci.* 23, 877–893. doi: 10.1111/j.1460-9568.2006.04649.x

Franco, S. J., Martinez-Garay, I., Gil-Sanz, C., Harkins-Perry, S. R., and Muller, U. (2011). Reelin regulates cadherin function via Dab1/Rap1 to control neuronal migration and lamination in the neocortex. *Neuron* 69, 482–497. doi: 10.1016/j.neuron.2011.01.003

Franzoni, E., Booker, S. A., Parthasarathy, S., Rehfeld, F., Grosser, S., Srivatsa, S., et al. (2015). miR-128 regulates neuronal migration, outgrowth and intrinsic excitability via the intellectual disability gene Phf6. *Elife* 4:e04263. doi: 10.7554/eLife.04263

Friocourt, G., Kanatani, S., Tabata, H., Yozu, M., Takahashi, T., Antypa, M., et al. (2008). Cell-autonomous roles of ARX in cell proliferation and neuronal migration during corticogenesis. *J. Neurosci.* 28, 5794–5805. doi: 10.1523/JNEUROSCI.1067-08.2008

Friocourt, G., and Parnavelas, J. G. (2010). Mutations in ARX Result in Several Defects Involving GABAergic Neurons. *Front. Cell. Neurosci.* 4:4. doi: 10.3389/fncel.2010.00004

Gärtner, A., Fornasiero, E. F., Munck, S., Vennekens, K., Seuntjens, E., Huttner, W. B., et al. (2012). N-cadherin specifies first asymmetry in developing neurons. *EMBO J.* 31, 1893–1903. doi: 10.1038/emboj.2012.41

Gil-Sanz, C., Franco, S. J., Martinez-Garay, I., Espinosa, A., Harkins-Perry, S., and Muller, U. (2013). Cajal-Retzius cells instruct neuronal migration by coincidence signaling between secreted and contact-dependent guidance cues. *Neuron* 79, 461–477. doi: 10.1016/j.neuron.2013.06.040

Gleeson, J. G., Allen, K. M., Fox, J. W., Lamperti, E. D., Berkovic, S., Scheffer, I., et al. (1998). Doublecortin, a brain-specific gene mutated in human X-linked lissencephaly and double cortex syndrome, encodes a putative signaling protein. *Cell* 92, 63–72. doi: 10.1016/S0092-8674(00)80899-5

Gleeson, J. G., Lin, P. T., Flanagan, L. A., and Walsh, C. A. (1999). Doublecortin is a microtubule-associated protein and is expressed widely by migrating neurons. *Neuron* 23, 257–271. doi: 10.1016/S0896-6273(00)80778-3

Gleeson, J. G., and Walsh, C. A. (2000). Neuronal migration disorders: from genetic diseases to developmental mechanisms. *Trends Neurosci.* 23, 352–359. doi: 10.1016/S0166-2236(00)01607-6

Godin, J. D., Thomas, N., Laguesse, S., Malinouskaya, L., Close, P., Malaise, O., et al. (2012). p27(Kip1) Is a microtubule-associated protein that promotes microtubule polymerization during neuron migration. *Dev. Cell* 23, 729–744. doi: 10.1016/j.devcel.2012.08.006

Govek, E. E., Hatten, M. E., and van Aelst, L. (2011). The role of Rho GTPase proteins in CNS neuronal migration. *Dev. Neurobiol.* 71, 528–553. doi: 10.1002/dneu.20850

Graus-Porta, D., Blaess, S., Senften, M., Littlewood-Evans, A., Damsky, C., Huang, Z., et al. (2001). Beta1-class integrins regulate the development of laminae and folia in the cerebral and cerebellar cortex. *Neuron* 31, 367–379. doi: 10.1016/S0896-6273(01)00374-9

Hannula-Jouppi, K., Kaminen-Ahola, N., Taipale, M., Eklund, R., Nopola-Hemmi, J., Kaariainen, H., et al. (2005). The axon guidance receptor gene ROBO1 is a candidate gene for developmental dyslexia. *PLoS Genet.* 1:e50. doi: 10.1371/journal.pgen.0010050

Hashimoto-Torii, K., Torii, M., Fujimoto, M., Nakai, A., El Fatimy, R., Mezger, V., et al. (2014). Roles of heat shock factor 1 in neuronal response to fetal environmental risks and its relevance to brain disorders. *Neuron* 82, 560–572. doi: 10.1016/j.neuron.2014.03.002

Heng, J. I., Chariot, A., and Nguyen, L. (2010). Molecular layers underlying cytoskeletal remodelling during cortical development. *Trends Neurosci.* 33, 38–47. doi: 10.1016/j.tins.2009.09.003

Hirotsune, S., Fleck, M. W., Gambello, M. J., Bix, G. J., Chen, A., Clark, G. D., et al. (1998). Graded reduction of Pafah1b1 (Lis1) activity results in neuronal migration defects and early embryonic lethality. *Nat. Genet.* 19, 333–339. doi: 10.1038/1221

Hong, S. E., Shugart, Y. Y., Huang, D. T., Shahwan, S. A., Grant, P. E., Hourihane, J. O., et al. (2000). Autosomal recessive lissencephaly with cerebellar hypoplasia is associated with human RELN mutations. *Nat. Genet.* 26, 93–96. doi: 10.1038/79246

Hori, K., Nagai, T., Shan, W., Sakamoto, A., Taya, S., Hashimoto, R., et al. (2014). Cytoskeletal regulation by AUTS2 in neuronal migration and neuritogenesis. *Cell Rep.* 9, 2166–2179. doi: 10.1016/j.celrep.2014.11.045

Insolera, R., Shao, W., Airik, R., Hildebrandt, F., and Shi, S. H. (2014). SDCCAG8 regulates pericentriolar material recruitment and neuronal migration in the developing cortex. *Neuron* 83, 805–822. doi: 10.1016/j.neuron.2014.06.029

Ishii, S., and Hashimoto-Torii, K. (2015). Impact of prenatal environmental stress on cortical development. *Front. Cell. Neurosci.* 9:207. doi: 10.3389/fncel.2015.00207

Jossin, Y., and Cooper, J. A. (2011). Reelin, Rap1 and N-cadherin orient the migration of multipolar neurons in the developing neocortex. *Nat. Neurosci.* 14, 697–703. doi: 10.1038/nn.2816

Kähler, A. K., Djurovic, S., Kulle, B., Jönsson, E. G., Agartz, I., Hall, H., et al. (2008). Association analysis of schizophrenia on 18 genes involved in neuronal migration: MDGA1 as a new susceptibility gene. *Am. J. Med. Genet. B Neuropsychiatr. Genet.* 147B, 1089–1100. doi: 10.1002/ajmg.b.30726

Kamiya, A., Kubo, K., Tomoda, T., Takaki, M., Youn, R., Ozeki, Y., et al. (2005). A schizophrenia-associated mutation of DISC1 perturbs cerebral cortex development. *Nat. Cell Biol.* 7, 1167–1178. doi: 10.1038/ncb1328

Kato, M., Das, S., Petras, K., Kitamura, K., Morohashi, K., Abuelo, D. N., et al. (2004). Mutations of ARX are associated with striking pleiotropy and consistent genotype-phenotype correlation. *Hum. Mutat.* 23, 147–159. doi: 10.1002/humu.10310

Kawauchi, T. (2012). Cell adhesion and its endocytic regulation in cell migration during neural development and cancer metastasis. *Int. J. Mol. Sci.* 13, 4564–4590. doi: 10.3390/ijms13044564

Kawauchi, T. (2014). Cdk5 regulates multiple cellular events in neural development, function and disease. *Dev. Growth Differ.* 56, 335–348. doi: 10.1111/dgd.12138

Kawauchi, T., Chihama, K., Nabeshima, Y., and Hoshino, M. (2003). The *in vivo* roles of STEF/Tiam1, Rac1 and JNK in cortical neuronal migration. *EMBO J.* 22, 4190–4201. doi: 10.1093/emboj/cdg413

Kawauchi, T., Chihama, K., Nabeshima, Y., and Hoshino, M. (2006). Cdk5 phosphorylates and stabilizes p27kip1 contributing to actin organization and cortical neuronal migration. *Nat. Cell Biol.* 8, 17–26. doi: 10.1038/ncb1338

Kawauchi, T., Chihama, K., Nishimura, Y. V., Nabeshima, Y., and Hoshino, M. (2005). MAP1B phosphorylation is differentially regulated by Cdk5/p35, Cdk5/p25, and JNK. *Biochem. Biophys. Res. Commun.* 331, 50–55. doi: 10.1016/j.bbrc.2005.03.132

Kawauchi, T., and Hoshino, M. (2008). Molecular pathways regulating cytoskeletal organization and morphological changes in migrating neurons. *Dev. Neurosci.* 30, 36–46. doi: 10.1159/000109850

Kawauchi, T., Sekine, K., Shikanai, M., Chihama, K., Tomita, K., Kubo, K., et al. (2010). Rab GTPases-dependent endocytic pathways regulate neuronal migration and maturation through N-cadherin trafficking. *Neuron* 67, 588–602. doi: 10.1016/j.neuron.2010.07.007

Kawauchi, T., Shikanai, M., and Kosodo, Y. (2013). Extra-cell cycle regulatory functions of cyclin-dependent kinases (CDK) and CDK inhibitor proteins contribute to brain development and neurological disorders. *Genes Cells* 18, 176–194. doi: 10.1111/gtc.12029

Keays, D. A., Tian, G., Poirier, K., Huang, G. J., Siebold, C., Cleak, J., et al. (2007). Mutations in alpha-tubulin cause abnormal neuronal migration in mice and lissencephaly in humans. *Cell* 128, 45–57. doi: 10.1016/j.cell.2006.12.017

Kitamura, K., Yanazawa, M., Sugiyama, N., Miura, H., Iizuka-Kogo, A., Kusaka, M., et al. (2002). Mutation of ARX causes abnormal development of forebrain and testes in mice and X-linked lissencephaly with abnormal genitalia in humans. *Nat. Genet.* 32, 359–369. doi: 10.1038/ng1009

La Fata, G., Gartner, A., Dominguez-Iturza, N., Dresselaers, T., Dawitz, J., Poorthuis, R. B., et al. (2014). FMRP regulates multipolar to bipolar transition affecting neuronal migration and cortical circuitry. *Nat. Neurosci.* 17, 1693–1700. doi: 10.1038/nn.3870

Lian, G., and Sheen, V. L. (2015). Cytoskeletal proteins in cortical development and disease: actin associated proteins in periventricular heterotopia. *Front. Cell. Neurosci.* 9:99. doi: 10.3389/fncel.2015.00099

Lickiss, T., Cheung, A. F., Hutchinson, C. E., Taylor, J. S., and Molnár, Z. (2012). Examining the relationship between early axon growth and transcription factor expression in the developing cerebral cortex. *J. Anat.* 220, 201–211. doi: 10.1111/j.1469-7580.2011.01466.x

Liu, X., Sun, L., Torii, M., and Rakic, P. (2012). Connexin 43 controls the multipolar phase of neuronal migration to the cerebral cortex. *Proc. Natl. Acad. Sci. U.S.A.* 109, 8280–8285. doi: 10.1073/pnas.1205880109

Luccardini, C., Hennekinne, L., Viou, L., Yanagida, M., Murakami, F., Kessaris, N., et al. (2013). N-cadherin sustains motility and polarity of future cortical interneurons during tangential migration. *J. Neurosci.* 33, 18149–18160. doi: 10.1523/JNEUROSCI.0593-13.2013

Luccardini, C., Leclech, C., Viou, L., Rio, J. P., and Métin, C. (2015). Cortical interneurons migrating on a pure substrate of N-cadherin exhibit fast synchronous centrosomal and nuclear movements and reduced ciliogenesis. *Front. Cell. Neurosci.* 9:286. doi: 10.3389/fncel.2015.00286

Magen, D., Ofir, A., Berger, L., Goldsher, D., Eran, A., Katib, N., et al. (2015). Autosomal recessive lissencephaly with cerebellar hypoplasia is associated with a loss-of-function mutation in CDK5. *Hum. Genet.* 134, 305–314. doi: 10.1007/s00439-014-1522-5

Marín, O., Valiente, M., Ge, X., and Tsai, L. H. (2010). Guiding neuronal cell migrations. *Cold Spring Harb. Perspect. Biol.* 2:a001834. doi: 10.1101/cshperspect.a001834

Martini, F. J., and Valdeolmillos, M. (2010). Actomyosin contraction at the cell rear drives nuclear translocation in migrating cortical interneurons. *J. Neurosci.* 30, 8660–8670. doi: 10.1523/JNEUROSCI.1962-10.2010

Meng, H., Smith, S. D., Hager, K., Held, M., Liu, J., Olson, R. K., et al. (2005). DCDC2 is associated with reading disability and modulates neuronal development in the brain. *Proc. Natl. Acad. Sci. U.S.A.* 102, 17053–17058. doi: 10.1073/pnas.0508591102

Moon, H. M., and Wynshaw-Boris, A. (2013). Cytoskeleton in action: lissencephaly, a neuronal migration disorder. *Wiley Interdiscip. Rev. Dev. Biol.* 2, 229–245. doi: 10.1002/wdev.67

Nadarajah, B., and Parnavelas, J. G. (2002). Modes of neuronal migration in the developing cerebral cortex. *Nat. Rev. Neurosci.* 3, 423–432. doi: 10.1038/nrn845

Nagano, T., Morikubo, S., and Sato, M. (2004). Filamin A and FILIP (Filamin A-Interacting Protein) regulate cell polarity and motility in neocortical subventricular and intermediate zones during radial migration. *J. Neurosci.* 24, 9648–9657. doi: 10.1523/JNEUROSCI.2363-04.2004

Nishimura, Y. V., Sekine, K., Chihama, K., Nakajima, K., Hoshino, M., Nabeshima, Y., et al. (2010). Dissecting the factors involved in the locomotion mode of neuronal migration in the developing cerebral cortex. *J. Biol. Chem.* 285, 5878–5887. doi: 10.1074/jbc.M109.033761

Nishimura, Y. V., Shikanai, M., Hoshino, M., Ohshima, T., Nabeshima, Y., Mizutani, K., et al. (2014). Cdk5 and its substrates, Dcx and p27kip1, regulate cytoplasmic dilation formation and nuclear elongation in migrating neurons. *Development* 141, 3540–3550. doi: 10.1242/dev.111294

Ohshima, T., Hirasawa, M., Tabata, H., Mutoh, T., Adachi, T., Suzuki, H., et al. (2007). Cdk5 is required for multipolar-to-bipolar transition during radial neuronal migration and proper dendrite development of pyramidal neurons in the cerebral cortex. *Development* 134, 2273–2282. doi: 10.1242/dev.02854

O'roak, B. J., Vives, L., Fu, W., Egertson, J. D., Stanaway, I. B., Phelps, I. G., et al. (2012). Multiplex targeted sequencing identifies recurrently mutated genes in autism spectrum disorders. *Science* 338, 1619–1622. doi: 10.1126/science.1227764

Paracchini, S., Thomas, A., Castro, S., Lai, C., Paramasivam, M., Wang, Y., et al. (2006). The chromosome 6p22 haplotype associated with dyslexia reduces the expression of KIAA0319, a novel gene involved in neuronal migration. *Hum. Mol. Genet.* 15, 1659–1666. doi: 10.1093/hmg/ddl089

Peñagarikano, O., Abrahams, B. S., Herman, E. I., Winden, K. D., Gdalyahu, A., Dong, H., et al. (2011). Absence of CNTNAP2 leads to epilepsy, neuronal migration abnormalities, and core autism-related deficits. *Cell* 147, 235–246. doi: 10.1016/j.cell.2011.08.040

Rakic, P. (1972). Mode of cell migration to the superficial layers of fetal monkey neocortex. *J. Comp. Neurol.* 145, 61–83. doi: 10.1002/cne.901450105

Rakic, P. (2006). A century of progress in corticoneurogenesis: from silver impregnation to genetic engineering. *Cereb. Cortex* 16(Suppl. 1), i3–i17. doi: 10.1093/cercor/bhk036

Reiner, O., and Sapir, T. (2013). LIS1 functions in normal development and disease. *Curr. Opin. Neurobiol.* 23, 951–956. doi: 10.1016/j.conb.2013.08.001

Rivas, R. J., and Hatten, M. E. (1995). Motility and cytoskeletal organization of migrating cerebellar granule neurons. *J. Neurosci.* 15, 981–989.

Schaar, B. T., and McConnell, S. K. (2005). Cytoskeletal coordination during neuronal migration. *Proc. Natl. Acad. Sci. U.S.A.* 102, 13652–13657. doi: 10.1073/pnas.0506008102

Sekine, K., Kawauchi, T., Kubo, K., Honda, T., Herz, J., Hattori, M., et al. (2012). Reelin controls neuronal positioning by promoting cell-matrix adhesion via inside-out activation of integrin alpha5beta1. *Neuron* 76, 353–369. doi: 10.1016/j.neuron.2012.07.020

Sheen, V. L., Ganesh, V. S., Topcu, M., Sebire, G., Bodell, A., Hill, R. S., et al. (2004). Mutations in ARFGEF2 implicate vesicle trafficking in neural progenitor proliferation and migration in the human cerebral cortex. *Nat. Genet.* 36, 69–76. doi: 10.1038/ng1276

Shieh, J. C., Schaar, B. T., Srinivasan, K., Brodsky, F. M., and McConnell, S. K. (2011). Endocytosis regulates cell soma translocation and the distribution of adhesion proteins in migrating neurons. *PLoS ONE* 6:e17802. doi: 10.1371/journal.pone.0017802

Shikanai, M., Nakajima, K., and Kawauchi, T. (2011). N-cadherin regulates radial glial fiber-dependent migration of cortical locomoting neurons. *Commun. Integr. Biol.* 4, 326–330. doi: 10.4161/cib.4.3.14886

Shinohara, R., Thumkeo, D., Kamijo, H., Kaneko, N., Sawamoto, K., Watanabe, K., et al. (2012). A role for mDia, a Rho-regulated actin nucleator, in tangential migration of interneuron precursors. *Nat. Neurosci.* 15, 373–380. doi: 10.1038/nn.3020

Solecki, D. J. (2012). Sticky situations: recent advances in control of cell adhesion during neuronal migration. *Curr. Opin. Neurobiol.* 22, 791–798. doi: 10.1016/j.conb.2012.04.010

Solecki, D. J., Model, L., Gaetz, J., Kapoor, T. M., and Hatten, M. E. (2004). Par6alpha signaling controls glial-guided neuronal migration. *Nat. Neurosci.* 7, 1195–1203. doi: 10.1038/nn1332

Solecki, D. J., Trivedi, N., Govek, E. E., Kerekes, R. A., Gleason, S. S., and Hatten, M. E. (2009). Myosin II motors and F-actin dynamics drive the coordinated movement of the centrosome and soma during CNS glial-guided neuronal migration. *Neuron* 63, 63–80. doi: 10.1016/j.neuron.2009.05.028

Stitt, T. N., and Hatten, M. E. (1990). Antibodies that recognize astrotactin block granule neuron binding to astroglia. *Neuron* 5, 639–649. doi: 10.1016/0896-6273(90)90218-5

Stolp, H., Neuhaus, A., Sundramoorthi, R., and Molnár, Z. (2012). The long and the short of it: gene and environment interactions during early cortical development and consequences for long-term neurological disease. *Front. Psychiatry* 3:50. doi: 10.3389/fpsyt.2012.00050

Takano, T., Xu, C., Funahashi, Y., Namba, T., and Kaibuchi, K. (2015). Neuronal polarization. *Development* 142, 2088–2093. doi: 10.1242/dev.114454

Tonosaki, M., Itoh, K., Umekage, M., Kishimoto, T., Yaoi, T., Lemmon, V. P., et al. (2014). L1cam is crucial for cell locomotion and terminal translocation of the Soma in radial migration during murine corticogenesis. *PLoS ONE* 9:e86186. doi: 10.1371/journal.pone.0086186

Tsai, J. W., Bremner, K. H., and Vallee, R. B. (2007). Dual subcellular roles for LIS1 and dynein in radial neuronal migration in live brain tissue. *Nat. Neurosci.* 10, 970–979. doi: 10.1038/nn1934

Tsai, J. W., Chen, Y., Kriegstein, A. R., and Vallee, R. B. (2005). LIS1 RNA interference blocks neural stem cell division, morphogenesis, and motility at multiple stages. *J. Cell Biol.* 170, 935–945. doi: 10.1083/jcb.200505166

Tsai, L. H., and Gleeson, J. G. (2005). Nucleokinesis in neuronal migration. *Neuron* 46, 383–388. doi: 10.1016/j.neuron.2005.04.013

Umeshima, H., Hirano, T., and Kengaku, M. (2007). Microtubule-based nuclear movement occurs independently of centrosome positioning in migrating neurons. *Proc. Natl. Acad. Sci. U.S.A.* 104, 16182–16187. doi: 10.1073/pnas.0708047104

Valiente, M., Ciceri, G., Rico, B., and Marín, O. (2011). Focal adhesion kinase modulates radial glia-dependent neuronal migration through connexin-26. *J. Neurosci.* 31, 11678–11691. doi: 10.1523/JNEUROSCI.2678-11.2011

Voss, A. K., Britto, J. M., Dixon, M. P., Sheikh, B. N., Collin, C., Tan, S. S., et al. (2008). C3G regulates cortical neuron migration, preplate splitting and radial glial cell attachment. *Development* 135, 2139–2149. doi: 10.1242/dev.016725

Wang, Y., Paramasivam, M., Thomas, A., Bai, J., Kaminen-Ahola, N., Kere, J., et al. (2006). DYX1C1 functions in neuronal migration in developing neocortex. *Neuroscience* 143, 515–522. doi: 10.1016/j.neuroscience.2006.08.022

Xie, Z., Sanada, K., Samuels, B. A., Shih, H., and Tsai, L. H. (2003). Serine 732 phosphorylation of FAK by Cdk5 is important for microtubule organization, nuclear movement, and neuronal migration. *Cell* 114, 469–482. doi: 10.1016/S0092-8674(03)00605-6

Yang, T., Sun, Y., Zhang, F., Zhu, Y., Shi, L., Li, H., et al. (2012). POSH localizes activated Rac1 to control the formation of cytoplasmic dilation of the leading process and neuronal migration. *Cell Rep.* 2, 640–651. doi: 10.1016/j.celrep.2012.08.007

Yap, C. C., Vakulenko, M., Kruczek, K., Motamedi, B., Digilio, L., Liu, J. S., et al. (2012). Doublecortin (DCX) mediates endocytosis of neurofascin independently of microtubule binding. *J. Neurosci.* 32, 7439–7453. doi: 10.1523/JNEUROSCI.5318-11.2012

Yap, C. C., and Winckler, B. (2015). Adapting for endocytosis: roles for endocytic sorting adaptors in directing neural development. *Front. Cell. Neurosci.* 9:119. doi: 10.3389/fncel.2015.00119

Ye, T., Ip, J. P., Fu, A. K., and Ip, N. Y. (2014). Cdk5-mediated phosphorylation of RapGEF2 controls neuronal migration in the developing cerebral cortex. *Nat. Commun.* 5, 4826. doi: 10.1038/ncomms5826

Zhang, C., Mejia, L. A., Huang, J., Valnegri, P., Bennett, E. J., Anckar, J., et al. (2013a). The X-linked intellectual disability protein PHF6 associates with the PAF1 complex and regulates neuronal migration in the mammalian brain. *Neuron* 78, 986–993. doi: 10.1016/j.neuron.2013.04.021

Zhang, J., Neal, J., Lian, G., Hu, J., Lu, J., and Sheen, V. (2013b). Filamin A regulates neuronal migration through brefeldin A-inhibited guanine exchange factor 2-dependent Arf1 activation. *J. Neurosci.* 33, 15735–15746. doi: 10.1523/JNEUROSCI.1939-13.2013

Zhang, X., Lei, K., Yuan, X., Wu, X., Zhuang, Y., Xu, T., et al. (2009). SUN1/2 and Syne/Nesprin-1/2 complexes connect centrosome to the nucleus during neurogenesis and neuronal migration in mice. *Neuron* 64, 173–187. doi: 10.1016/j.neuron.2009.08.018

17

Real-Time Imaging of bHLH Transcription Factors Reveals their Dynamic Control in the Multipotency and Fate Choice of Neural Stem Cells

Itaru Imayoshi[1,2,3,4*], *Fumiyoshi Ishidate*[3] *and Ryoichiro Kageyama*[2,3,5*]

[1] The Hakubi Center, Kyoto University, Kyoto, Japan, [2] Laboratory of Growth Regulation, Institute for Virus Research, Kyoto University, Kyoto, Japan, [3] World Premier International Research Initiative–Institute for Integrated Cell-Material Sciences, Kyoto University, Kyoto, Japan, [4] Precursory Research for Embryonic Science and Technology, Japan Science and Technology Agency, Saitama, Japan, [5] Core Research for Evolutional Science and Technology, Japan Science and Technology Agency, Saitama, Japan

***Correspondence:**
*Itaru Imayoshi,
The Hakubi Center, Institute for Virus Research, Kyoto University, Shogoin-Kawahara 53, Sakyo-ku, Kyoto 606-8507, Japan
iimayosh@virus.kyoto-u.ac.jp;
Ryoichiro Kageyama,
Institute for Virus Research, Kyoto University, Shogoin-Kawahara, Sakyo-ku, Kyoto 606-8507, Japan
rkageyam@virus.kyoto-u.ac.jp*

The basic-helix-loop-helix (bHLH) transcription factors Ascl1/Mash1, Hes1, and Olig2 regulate the fate choice of neurons, astrocytes, and oligodendrocytes, respectively; however, these factors are coexpressed in self-renewing multipotent neural stem cells (NSCs) even before cell fate determination. This fact raises the possibility that these fate determination factors are differentially expressed between self-renewing and differentiating NSCs with unique expression dynamics. Real-time imaging analysis utilizing fluorescent proteins is a powerful strategy for monitoring expression dynamics. Fusion with fluorescent reporters makes it possible to analyze the dynamic behavior of specific proteins in living cells. However, it is technically challenging to conduct long-term imaging of proteins, particularly those with low expression levels, because a high-sensitivity and low-noise imaging system is required, and very often bleaching of fluorescent proteins and cell toxicity by prolonged laser exposure are problematic. Furthermore, to analyze the functional roles of the dynamic expression of cellular proteins, it is essential to image reporter fusion proteins that are expressed at comparable levels to their endogenous expression. In this review, we introduce our recent reports about the dynamic control of bHLH transcription factors in multipotency and fate choice of NSCs, focusing on real-time imaging of fluorescent reporters fused with bHLH transcription factors. Our imaging results indicate that bHLH transcription factors are expressed in an oscillatory manner by NSCs, and that one of them becomes dominant during fate choice. We propose that the multipotent state of NSCs correlates with the oscillatory expression of several bHLH transcription factors, whereas the differentiated state correlates with the sustained expression of a single bHLH transcription factor.

Keywords: bHLH, neural stem cells, oscillation, fluorescent protein, imaging

Introduction

Neural stem cells (NSCs) are multipotent and self-renewable cells that can give rise to neurons, astrocytes, and oligodendrocytes (Fishell and Kriegstein, 2003; Götz and Huttner, 2005; Kriegstein and Alvarez-Buylla, 2009). During brain development, basic helix-loop-helix (bHLH) transcription factors play pivotal roles in the self-renewal of NSCs and fate determination of neurons, astrocytes, and oligodendrocytes (Bertrand et al., 2002; Ross et al., 2003; Meijer et al., 2012; Wilkinson et al., 2013; Imayoshi and Kageyama, 2014a). bHLH transcription factors, such as Hesl and Hes5, regulate the self-renewal of NSCs as downstream effectors of Notch signaling, whereas proneural bHLH transcription factors, such as Ascl1 and Neurogl/2, promote neuronal differentiation. Other bHLH transcription factors, e.g., Oligl and Olig2, regulate oligodendrocyte differentiation. However, in addition to Hesl/Hes5, some bHLH fate determination factors, such as Ascl1 and Olig2, are also known to have roles in NSC maintenance or proliferation. In addition, Hesl induces astrocyte formation at later stages. Currently, it is not understood completely how these various and sometimes opposing functions of each bHLH transcription factor in the self-renewal and fate-choice events of NSCs are achieved (Vasconcelos and Castro, 2014; Imayoshi and Kageyama, 2014a,b). We previously found that transcription of some bHLH genes is differentially controlled in NSCs and differentiating cells (Shimojo et al., 2008). Therefore, we decided to analyze the expression dynamics of bHLH transcription factors in more detail.

Heterogeneous Expression of bHLH Transcription Factors in Cultured NSCs

NSCs can be cultured in an undifferentiated state *in vitro*. For instance, in the presence of epidermal growth factor and basic fibroblast growth factor, NSCs can be expanded from enzymatically dissociated brain tissues in a monolayer condition (NS cell culture) (Conti et al., 2003). NSCs can reportedly be established from brains at various stages, from embryos to adults. Furthermore, the purity of these cultures is very high; more than 99% of cells express NSC marker proteins, such as Nestin. Cultured NSCs also express bHLH transcription factors, including Hesl, Ascl1, and Olig2 (Imayoshi et al., 2013a).

In actively-dividing and self-renewing NS cells, Hesl, Ascl1, and Olig2 bHLH transcription factors are expressed (**Figure 1A**). Compared with the homogeneous expression of Sox2, which is a member of the high-mobility-group transcription factor family, the expression of all three bHLH transcription factors is variable among cells, indicating their dynamic expression (**Figure 1A**) (Imayoshi et al., 2013b). In order to elucidate the heterogeneous expression of bHLH transcription factors, we adopted a real-time imaging strategy to monitor the expression dynamics of bHLH proteins in cultured NSCs.

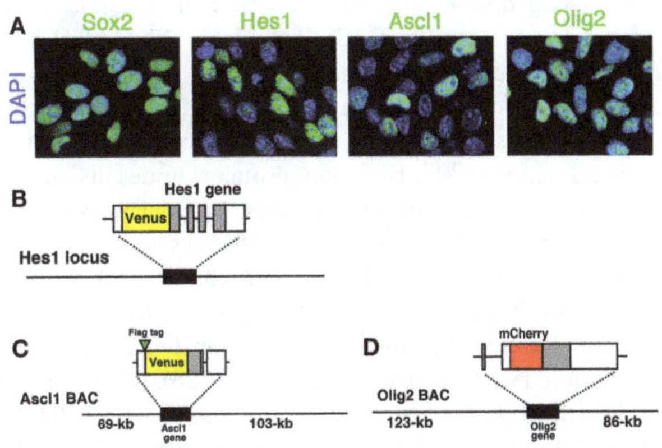

FIGURE 1 | Expression of bHLH factors in NS cells and fluorescent reporter-bHLH fusion constructs. (A) Self-renewing NS cells were immunostained with anti-Sox2, anti-Hes1, anti-Ascl1, and anti-Olig2 antibodies. Hes1, Ascl1, and Olig2 expression levels were variable while another NSC-specific factor, Sox2, was expressed at a relatively constant level. **(B)** Venus-Hes1 fusion knock-in mouse strain. **(C)** Venus-Ascl1 fusion BAC Tg mouse strain. **(D)** mCherry-Olig2 fusion BAC Tg mouse strain. Coding regions of bHLH factors are shown in gray. The pictures and graphs of this figure are reprinted from Supplementary Figures S1C,E; S2A; S6A–D of Imayoshi et al. (2013b).

Fluorescent Reporter-fusion Knock-in or Bacterial Artificial Chromosome (BAC) Transgenic (Tg) Strategy for Monitoring Protein Expression Dynamics of bHLH Transcription Factors

Fusion reporter constructs are used to monitor the expression dynamics of proteins of interest in living cells (**Figures 1B–D**) (Miyawaki, 2011; Imayoshi et al., 2013a). In addition to fluorescent reporter proteins, bioluminescent reporters, such as luciferase, are also effective. One advantage of the reporter-fusion strategy is that the half-life and cellular localization of proteins basically depend on the fused target protein, at least in the case of bHLH transcription factors. Most bHLH transcription factors have very short half-lives, such as ~20 min, and therefore reporter-bHLH fusion proteins are also very unstable.

In order to analyze precisely the fine expression dynamics of bHLH transcription factors, it is necessary that reporter-bHLH fusion proteins are expressed under the control of their original promoter/enhancer sequences. One of the reliable ways to mimic the original regulation of bHLH gene expression is the knock-in strategy (Imayoshi et al., 2013a,b). By homologous recombination in embryonic stem cells, a reporter coding sequence is inserted into the N− or C− terminus of a bHLH gene so that the reporter-bHLH fusion protein is expressed from the original bHLH gene locus. As far as we know, the reporter-bHLH fusion protein is functional and, in most cases, the allele carrying the knocked-in fusion reporter functions as normally as the wild-type allele. Another strategy to express reporter-bHLH fusion proteins optimally is the generation of Tg mice with a BAC. Using homologous recombination in *Escherichia coli*, we can edit and modify BACs (Lee et al., 2001). BACs can contain very long DNA sequences, such as ~200-kb. Therefore, by utilizing BAC clones with the promoter/enhancer sequences of a bHLH gene, it is possible to make transgene constructs designed to express reporter-bHLH fusion proteins under its original regulatory elements. From the Tg mouse founder lines carrying BAC transgene constructs, we can choose ones with a transgene copy number of only one by Southern blotting or real-time PCR analysis. These one-copy BAC Tg mice work as reporter strains for real-time imaging of the expression dynamics of bHLH transcription factors (Imayoshi et al., 2013b). One concsern regarding the reporter-fusion BAC Tg mouse strategy is that the number of functional bHLH gene alleles is increased from two to three. Ideally, reporter expression should be analyzed in a heterozygous-mutant background of the target gene by crossing with a mouse strain harboring a null allele. However, at least in the case of bHLH transcription factors, such as Hes1, Ascl1, or Olig2, the addition of the reporter-fusion transgenes dose not apparently affect the normal development of the nervous system (Imayoshi et al., 2013b).

As far as we know, the N-terminal fusion of a reporter proteins in both knock-in and BAC Tg mice shows better results than for a C-terminal fusion. The fluorescence or bioluminescence of a reporter protein is brighter when it is fused to the N-terminus than to the C-terminus of bHLH transcription factors. This is probably because translation starts from the N-terminus, so a reporter protein located at the N-terminus starts to work earlier during its expression.

For quantitative live-imaging of fluorescent reporters, we established NS cell cultures from each knock-in or BAC Tg mouse strain (Imayoshi et al., 2013b). In fluorescent protein-bHLH fusion reporter mice, Venus-Hes1 fusion knock-in, Venus-Ascl1 fusion BAC Tg, and mCherry-Olig2 fusion BAC Tg mouse strains (**Figures 1B–D**), the expression levels of fusion proteins and endogenous bHLH proteins were highly correlated to each other in cultured NSCs (Imayoshi et al., 2013b). Therefore, we conducted real-time imaging of fluorescent protein-bHLH fusion reporters in cultured NSCs with confocal fluorescence microscopy.

Real-time Imaging of Fluorescent Reporter-fusion bHLH Proteins with Confocal Fluorescent Microscopy

For real-time imaging of fluorescent proteins with low expression levels, it is important to prepare a highly sensitive and low-noise imaging system. As we mentioned earlier, the mRNA and protein of most bHLH transcription factors have very short half-lives (e.g., ~20 min): therefore, the reporter-bHLH fusion proteins are also very unstable (Imayoshi et al., 2013a,b). We can measure the decay time of reporter-bHLH fusion products by pharmacologically blocking the synthesis of new cellular proteins with cycloheximide. Indeed, the reporter activity of bHLH-fusion products are decayed with the same time course as the original bHLH proteins (data not shown). Furthermore, in cultured NSCs derived from knock-in or BAC Tg mice, reporter-bHLH fusion proteins are expressed from a limited number of gene alleles. Therefore, the fluorescent signals of reporter-bHLH fusion proteins in NSCs are very dim and sometimes invisible by simple observation through ocular lenses.

To acquire these very weak fluorescent signals, we utilized a confocal microscope equipped with a highly sensitive detector (Imayoshi et al., 2013b). In some cases, the fluorescent signal intensity of reporter-bHLH fusion proteins is much weaker than that of the autofluorescence of cultured NSCs. To overcome this problem, a spectral imaging technique is very effective. Spectral imaging and linear unmixing has become an important tool in confocal fluorescence microscopy to discriminate between fluorescent signals with overlapping spectral characteristics. For example, when cultured NSCs are illuminated with a 514-nm argon laser, the autofluorescent signal appears at approximately 560 nm. Real signals from Venus-Hes1 or Venus-Ascl1 fusion proteins are observed approximately 530 nm, and their intensity is weaker than the autofluorescence of NSCs. However, when the fluorescent signals are acquired with a spectral GaAsP array detector, specific Venus-bHLH signals can be separated from autofluorescence by applying linear unmixing algorithms.

In addition to the highly sensitive and spectral imaging techniques, imaging systems should be optimized for low-noise and reliable quantitative analysis. As the fluorescent signal intensity of reporter-bHLH fusion proteins is very weak, contamination with noise signals impairs the reliable quantitative analysis of the expression dynamics of bHLH transcription factors. To prevent bleaching the fluorescent reporters and avoid photodamage to NSCs by the excitation lasers, the sensitivity of the imaging system is again critically important. Bleaching of the reporters impairs the reliability of the imaging results. During long-term continuous imaging, laser power should be as small as possible, because NSCs are delicate and very sensitive to exogenous perturbations, including photodamage by exposure to a strong laser.

Oscillatory Expression of bHLH Transcription Factors in Multipotent NSCs

NS cell cultures established from Venus-Hes1 fusion knock-in, Venus-Ascl1 fusion BAC Tg, and mCherry-Olig2 fusion BAC Tg mouse strains were used for real-time imaging with confocal fluorescence microscopy. This analysis revealed that the fluorescent fusion reporter proteins with Hes1, Ascl1, or Olig2 exhibited dynamic expression changes in NS cells (**Supplementary Movies 1–3**), as observed in the bioluminescence imaging experiments with luciferase-bHLH fusion reporters (Imayoshi et al., 2013b). By quantitative analysis of single cells, the levels of Hes1 and Ascl1 proteins seem to oscillate with a 2–3-h period (**Figures 2A,B**), while Olig2 oscillates with a longer period, such as 5–8 h (**Figure 2C**) (Imayoshi et al., 2013b). Although fluorescent reporter-bHLH proteins showed dynamic expression changes, oscillatory expression was observed more clearly in the bioluminescence imaging experiments with luciferase-bHLH fusion reporters.

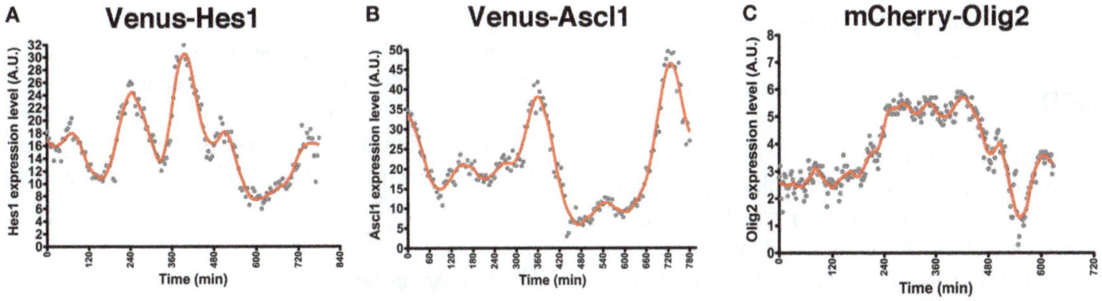

FIGURE 2 | Oscillatory expression of bHLH factors in NSCs. NS cell cultures were prepared from Venus-Hes1 knock-in mice **(A)**, Venus-Ascl1 BAC Tg mice **(B)**, or mCherry-Olig2 BAC Tg mice **(C)**. **(A–C)** Examples of quantification of each fusion protein dynamics in self-renewing NSCs. The graphs of this figure are reprinted from Supplementary Figures S8C; S11G; S12D of Imayoshi et al. (2013b).

Especially, the peak amplitude during signal changes was larger in the case of luciferase-bHLH fusion reporters (Imayoshi et al., 2013b), which is partly because the protein maturation time of luciferase is more rapid than that of fluorescent proteins, such as Venus and mCherry. Our observations revealed that, in actively dividing and multipotent NSCs, bHLH transcription factors are expressed in an oscillatory manner.

The oscillatory expression of bHLH transcription factors raised the possibility that NSCs may change their fate preferences over time. Indeed, when cultured NSCs are sorted by their expression levels of each bHLH transcription factor, their differentiation preferences are correlated with bHLH expression levels (Imayoshi et al., 2013b). For instance, Hes1-high NSCs preferentially differentiate into astrocytes, whereas Ascl1-high and Olig2-high NSCs preferentially differentiate into neurons and oligodendrocytes, respectively. These results suggest that different expression levels of bHLH transcription factors bias the fate choices of NSCs. However, such transient high expression of bHLH transcription factors may not be sufficient for cell fate determination, because these NSCs are still multipotent. Thus, we analyzed how the expression of these bHLH transcription factors changes during cell fate choice.

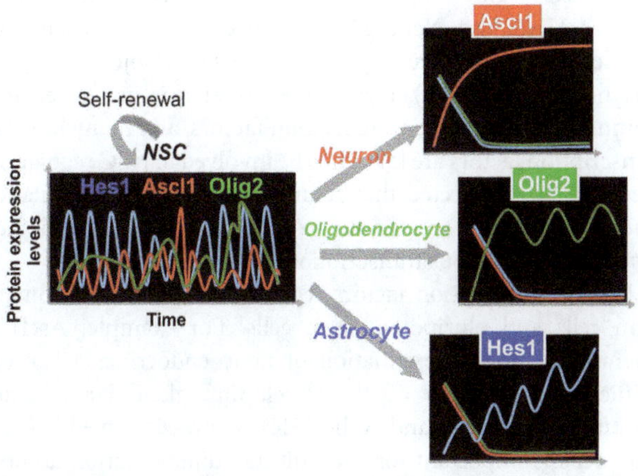

FIGURE 3 | Expression dynamics of bHLH factors in multipotency and cell fate choice. In multipotent NSCs, the levels of Hes1 and Ascl1 oscillate with periods of 2–3 h, while that of Olig2 oscillates with a period of 5–8 h. By contrast, during cell fate choice, one of the bHLH factors is expressed in a sustained manner, while the others are repressed.

Expression Dynamics of bHLH Transcription Factors in Multipotency and Fate Choice

In contrast to oscillatory expression of multiple bHLH transcription factors in self-renewing NSCs, one of the bHLH transcription factors is expressed in a sustained manner during cell fate choice, while the others are repressed (**Figure 3**) (Imayoshi et al., 2013b). For instance, we found that the transient down-regulation of Hes1 expression and the concomitant up-regulation of Ascl1 before cell division bias NSCs toward a neuronal fate choice, and the sustained expression of Ascl1 after cell division irreversibly determines neuronal fate (**Figure 3**). During astrocyte and oligodendrocyte differentiation, the expression of Hes1 and Olig2 is upregulated, respectively, although they still oscillate. However, even during the trough phases, both Hes1 and Olig2 levels are higher than they are in NSCs, indicating that Hes1 and Olig2 expression continues in a sustained manner during astrocyte and oligodendrocyte differentiation (**Figure 3**). When Hes1 or Olig2 becomes dominant, the expression of the other two factors is downregulated. These results indicate that Hes1, Ascl1, and Olig2 are expressed in an oscillatory manner in multipotent NSCs, and that one of them becomes dominant during cell fate choice (Imayoshi et al., 2013b).

From these analyses, we propose the following model: the oscillatory expression of multiple bHLH transcription factors is correlated with the multipotent and self-renewable state of NSCs, whereas the sustained expression of a selected bHLH transcription factor regulates fate determination (**Figure 3**) (Imayoshi et al., 2013b; Imayoshi and Kageyama, 2014a,b). To validate this model, we applied a new optogenetic method (photo-activatable Gal4/UAS system) to manipulate artificially the expression patterns of bHLH transcription factors using blue light illumination, showing that oscillatory expression activates the proliferation of NSCs, whereas sustained expression induces cell fate determination. Detailed results are reviewed elsewhere (Imayoshi et al., 2013b; Imayoshi and Kageyama, 2014a,b).

Conclusion

Previous reports have shown some evidence that the bHLH transcription factors Hesl, Ascl1, and Olig2 have multiple functions, such as NSC proliferation, self-renewal, and differentiation. Of course, protein modifications and/or partner co-factor variation may be involved in these different activities of bHLH transcription factors in a complex manner, but our studies revealed that oscillatory versus sustained expression dynamics also contribute to these different functions. More generally, our studies indicated that expression patterns, rather than simply the expression levels, of various transcription factors regulate whether stem cells proliferate or differentiate. In addition to Hesl, Ascl1, and Olig2, other bHLH transcription factors, such as Hes5 and Neurog2, are expressed in an oscillatory manner in NSCs or neural precursor cells (Shimojo et al., 2008; Imayoshi et al., 2013b). Dynamic expression is not necessarily confined to bHLH-type transcription factors, and many kinds of transcription factors are known to be involved in NSC regulation: therefore, it is expected that future imaging and manipulation studies will unveil the unique expression dynamics and their significance of various transcription factors in NSCs.

bHLH transcription factors regulate other kinds of somatic stem cells and pluripotent stem cells. For example, Ascl1 is essential for the differentiation of neuroendocrine cells from epithelial progenitors of the developing glandular stomach (Kokubu et al., 2008), and cyclical Hes1 expression in embryonic stem cells is important for their diverse differentiation abilities (Kobayashi et al., 2009). Therefore, the dynamic control of bHLH transcription factors, including their oscillatory expression, may regulate many regulatory processes of other kinds of stem cells.

Our studies suggest the importance and future possibilities of imaging techniques for the analysis of the expression dynamics of endogenous proteins at the single-cell level by coupling with various cellular events, such as cell cycle progression and cell differentiation (Miyawaki, 2011; Isomura and Kageyama, 2014). Under the current situation in developmental biology in which many biological processes start to be understood from the viewpoint of systems biology or single-cell biology (Levine et al., 2013; Sanchez and Golding, 2013; Zenobi, 2013), it is expected to become even more important to image subcellular localization and expression dynamics over time at a high resolution while keeping the original expression levels of target proteins.

Acknowledgments

This work was supported by research grants from the Ministry of Education, Culture, Sports, Science and Technology of Japan (MEXT) and Japan Science and Technology Agency (JST): Grant-in-Aid for Scientific Research on Young Scientists (A) (JSPS 24680035; 15H05570) (II), Challenging Exploratory Research (JSPS 26640011) (II), Innovative Areas (JSPS 26117511; 15H01489) (II), and the JST PRESTO program (II). We also thank the supports by the Human Frontier Science Program, the Nakajima Foundation, the Suzuken Memorial Foundation, the Mochida Memorial Foundation, the Sumitomo Foundation, the Senri Life Science Foundation, the Uehara Memorial Foundation, The Waksman Foundation of Japan INC, the Research Foundation for Pharmaceutical Sciences, the Cell Science Research Foundation, the Brain Science Research Foundation, and Platform for Dynamic Approaches to Living System from the MEXT.

Supplementary Material

Supplementary Movie 1 | Venus-Hes1 expression in self-renewing NSCs. Time in h and min is indicated. Related to **Figure 2A**.

Supplementary Movie 2 | Venus-Ascl1 expression in self-renewing NSCs. Time in hr min, and sec is indicated. Related to **Figure 2B**.

Supplementary Movie 3 | mCherry-Olig2 expression in self-renewing NSCs. Time in hr min, and sec is indicated. Related to **Figure 2C**.

References

Bertrand, N., Castro, D. S., and Guillemot, F. (2002). Proneural genes and the specification of neural cell types. *Nat. Rev. Neurosci.* 3, 517–530. doi: 10.1038/nrn874

Conti, L., Pollard, S. M., Gorba, T., Reitano, E., Toselli, M., Biella, G., et al. (2003). Niche-independent symmetrical self-renewal of a mammalian tissue stem cell. *PLoS Biol.* 3:e283. doi: 10.1371/journal.pbio.0030283

Fishell, G., and Kriegstein, A. R. (2003). Neurons from radial glia: the consequences of asymmetric inheritance. *Curr. Opin. Beurobiol.* 13, 34–41. doi: 10.1016/S0959-4388(03)00013-8

Götz, M., and Huttner, W. B. (2005). The cell biology of neurogenesis. *Nat. Rev. Cell Biol.* 6, 777–788. doi: 10.1038/nrm1739

Imayoshi, I., Isomura, A., Harima, Y., Kawaguchi, K., Kori, H., Miyachi, H., et al. (2013b). Oscillatory control of factors determining multipotency and fate in mouse neural progenitors. *Science* 342, 1203–1208. doi: 10.1126/science.1242366

Imayoshi, I., and Kageyama, R. (2014a). bHLH factors in self-renewal, multipotency, and fate choice of neural progenitor cells. *Neuron* 82, 9–23. doi: 10.1016/j.neuron.2014.03.018

Imayoshi, I., and Kageyama, R. (2014b). Oscillatory control of bHLH factors in neural progenitors. *Trends Neurosci.* 37, 531–538. doi: 10.1016/j.tins.2014.07.006

Imayoshi, I., Shimojo, H., Sakamoto, M., Ohtsuka, T., and Kageyama, R. (2013a). Genetic visualization of notch signaling in mammalian neurogenesis. *Cell Mol. Life Sci.* 70, 2045–2057. doi: 10.1007/s00018-012-1151-x

Isomura, A., and Kageyama, R. (2014). Ultradian oscillations and pulses: coordinating cellular responses and cell fate decisions. *Development.* 141, 3627–3636. doi: 10.1242/dev.1 04497

Kobayashi, T., Mizuno, H., Imayoshi, I., Furusawa, C., Shirahige, K., and Kageyama, R. (2009). The cyclic gene Hes1 contributes to diverse differentiation responses of embryonic stem cells. *Genes Dev.* 23, 870–875. doi: 10.1101/gad.18 23109

Kokubu, H., Ohtsuka, T., and Kageyama, R. (2008). Mash1 is required for neuroendocrine cell development in the glandular stomach. *Genes Cells* 13, 41–51. doi: 10.1111/j.1365-2443.2007.01146.x

Kriegstein, A., and Alvarez-Buylla, A. (2009). The glial nature of embryonic and adult neural stem cells. *Annu. Rev. Neurosci.* 32, 149–184. doi: 10.1146/annurev.neuro.051508.135600

Lee, E. C., Yu, D., Martinez de Velasco, J., Tessarollo, L., Swing, D. A., Court, D. L., et al. (2001). A highly efficient Escherichia coli-based chromosome engineering system adapted for recombinogenic targeting and subcloning of BAC DNA. *Genomics* 73, 56–65. doi: 10.1006/geno.2000.6451

Levine, J. H., and Lin, Y., and Elowitz, M. B. (2013). Functional roles of pulsing in genetic circuits. *Science* 342, 1193–1200. doi: 10.1126/science.1239999

Meijer, D. H., Kane, M. F., Mehta, S., Liu, H., Harrington, E., Taylor, C. M., et al. (2012). Separated at birth? The functional and molecular divergence of OLIG1 and OLIG2. *Nat. Rev. Neurosci.* 13, 819–831. doi: 10.1038/nrn3386

Miyawaki, A. (2011). Proteins on the move: insights gained from fluorescent protein technologies. *Nat. Rev. Mol. Cell Biol.* 12, 656–668. doi: 10.1038/nrm3199

Ross, S. E., Greenberg, M. E., and Stiles, C. D. (2003). Basic helix-loop-helix factors in cortical development. *Neuron* 39, 13–25. doi: 10.1016/S0896-6273(03)00365-9

Sanchez, A., and Golding, I. (2013). Genetic determinants and cellular constraints in noisy gene expression. *Science* 342, 1188–1193. doi: 10.1126/science.1242975

Shimojo, H., Ohtsuka, T., and Kageyama, R. (2008). Oscillations in notch signaling regulate maintenance of neural progenitors. *Neuron* 58, 52–64. doi: 10.1016/j.neuron.2008.02.014

Vasconcelos, F. F., and Castro, D. S. (2014). Transcriptional control of vertebrate neurogenesis by the proneural factor Ascl1. *Front. Cell Neurosci.* 8:412. doi: 10.3389/fncel.2014.00412

Wilkinson, G., Dennis, D., and Schuurmans, C. (2013). Proneural genes in neocortical development. *Neuroscience* 253, 256–273. doi: 10.1016/j.neuroscience.2013.08.029

Zenobi, R. (2013). Single-cell metabolomics: analytical and biological perspectives. *Science* 342:1243259. doi: 10.1126/science.1243259

18

The Role of the Extracellular Matrix in Neural Progenitor Cell Proliferation and Cortical Folding During Human Neocortex Development

Katherine R. Long[1,2]* *and Wieland B. Huttner*[3]*

[1]*Centre for Developmental Neurobiology, Institute of Psychiatry, Psychology and Neuroscience, King's College London, London, United Kingdom,* [2]*MRC Centre for Neurodevelopmental Disorders, King's College London, London, United Kingdom,* [3]*Max Planck Institute of Molecular Cell Biology and Genetics, Dresden, Germany*

***Correspondence:**
Katherine R. Long
katie.long@kcl.ac.uk
Wieland B. Huttner
huttner@mpi-cbg.de

Extracellular matrix (ECM) has long been known to regulate many aspects of neural development in many different species. However, the role of the ECM in the development of the human neocortex is not yet fully understood. In this review we discuss the role of the ECM in human neocortex development and the different model systems that can be used to investigate this. In particular, we will focus on how the ECM regulates human neural stem and progenitor cell proliferation and differentiation, how the ECM regulates the architecture of the developing human neocortex and the effect of mutations in ECM and ECM-associated genes in neurodevelopmental disorders.

Keywords: extracelluar matrix, human, neocortex, development, neural progenitor

INTRODUCTION

The human brain has long been known to contain a large amount of extracellular matrix (ECM) and ECM-associated molecules (Sanes, 1983, 1989). In the adult, this equates to roughly 20% of the total brain volume, but during fetal development, it is double that amount, at roughly 40% (Jovanov Milošević et al., 2014). Given its abundance, it is a little surprising that we do not fully understand the role of the ECM in the development of the neocortex. In fact, we do not yet know exactly which ECM components are expressed throughout development. We have learnt a lot about the role of ECM in neural development from many different animal and *in vitro* model systems (expertly reviewed elsewhere; Bandtlow and Zimmermann, 2000; Zimmermann and Dours-Zimmermann, 2008; Marthiens et al., 2010; Barros et al., 2011; Franco and Müller, 2011; Long and Huttner, 2019; Amin and Borrell, 2020). This includes roles in neural progenitor proliferation, differentiation, morphology, axonal and dendritic elongation and connectivity, neuronal migration and cortical folding. It has also been suggested that the ECM can create functional microdomains within the developing neocortex, for example by regulating the diffusion of signalling factors, restricting them to a discrete area, or by altering the migration route of newborn neurons (Dityatev et al., 2010). However, much of this data has been generated in animal models and it remains unclear how much can be extrapolated to human neocortex development. Major differences have been reported for human and non-human primate neocortex development in comparison to mouse development. For example, RNA-sequencing studies have revealed important differences in ECM expression between the developing human neocortex compared to the embryonic mouse neocortex (Fietz et al., 2012; Miller et al., 2014; Florio et al., 2015). One of the most striking of these differences is that significantly more ECM is expressed in the human fetal neocortex (Fietz et al., 2012).

This raises the question as to whether this ECM has played an important role in the evolution of the human neocortex.

In this review, we will discuss the role of the ECM in human and non-human primate neocortex development, focusing on neural progenitors, neocortical tissue architecture and neurodevelopmental disorders.

ECM AND NEURAL PROGENITORS

ECM and ECM receptors have long been known to regulate the behaviour of neural progenitor cells (NPCs; Loulier et al., 2009; Radakovits et al., 2009; Fietz et al., 2010; Barros et al., 2011; Long et al., 2016; Long and Huttner, 2019; Amin and Borrell, 2020). However, compared to the large volume of evidence of ECM function in animal models, the data in human and non-human primate neocortex is limited.

ECM Expression and Function

The RNA sequencing studies described above have suggested that many ECM components and receptors are expressed in the developing human neocortex (**Figure 1**; Fietz et al., 2012; Miller et al., 2014; Florio et al., 2015). This includes the major family of ECM receptors, the integrins (Hynes, 2002). Downstream of the integrins lie many important signalling pathways already known to regulate aspects of neural development, including PI3-kinase and Akt for cell survival, ERK and CyclinD1 for proliferation, and cdc42 and rac for cell migration (Hynes, 2002). The role of these factors, and others such as integrin-linked kinase and focal adhesion kinase, have been well studied in animal models (Beggs et al., 2003; Niewmierzycka et al., 2005; Tsuda et al., 2010; Valiente et al., 2011; Long et al., 2016), but less is known about their function in the developing human neocortex. However, more is known about the integrins themselves. In particular, integrins alpha 6 and beta 1 are known to be markers of human neural stem cells (NSCs; Hall et al., 2006). This integrin combination is able to bind to two of the main families of ECM components, the laminins and the collagens.

The most well-known of the laminins is laminin-111, which is highly expressed in both early mouse and human neocortex but is down-regulated later in development (Barros et al., 2020). The roles of laminins in mouse neocortex development are highly varied (Haubst et al., 2006; Loulier et al., 2009; Radakovits et al., 2009; Güven et al., 2020), but their roles in human neocortex development are yet to be fully investigated. Current evidence has shown that plating human NSCs onto laminin *in vitro* promotes both neurogenesis of the NSCs and then neurite outgrowth from the newborn neurons (Flanagan et al., 2006; Ma et al., 2008). However, in contrast, laminin has also been shown to promote the proliferation of human NSCs (Flanagan et al., 2006; Hall et al., 2008). Indeed, laminin-derived peptides, such as RGD, can promote both NSC proliferation and differentiation *in vitro* (Li et al., 2014), suggesting the function of laminins is highly complex and may be context-dependent, as seen in the mouse neocortex (Haubst et al., 2006; Loulier et al., 2009; Radakovits et al., 2009; Güven et al., 2020).

Other ECM components have also been reported to promote proliferation of human NSCs/NPCs, such as collagen IV (Hubert et al., 2009) and heparan sulphate proteoglycans (HSPGs; Oikari et al., 2016; Yu et al., 2017). However, as with laminins, these ECM components have also been implicated in neural differentiation (Oikari et al., 2016; Okolicsanyi et al., 2018). HSPGs are part of the proteoglycan family, which also includes the chondroitin sulphate proteoglycans, syndecans and glypicans. They have been shown to regulate several aspects of neural development, particularly neuronal migration (Bandtlow and Zimmermann, 2000; Ishii and Maeda, 2008; Maeda, 2015). The majority of these findings have been reported in 2D *in vitro* experiments using human NSCs/NPCs, but very few studies have investigated their function within an intact tissue environment. As ECM components often interact with each other and the surrounding tissue, their functions may differ between these simplified 2D environments and the complex 3D environment of the neocortex.

To address this, several studies have focused on understanding the specific network of ECM components that are important for human neocortex development. Fietz and colleagues showed that multiple ECM components were more highly expressed in the developing human neocortex compared to mouse (**Figure 1**; Fietz et al., 2012). This was particularly so in regions of the cortical wall that contained highly proliferative progenitors. In the mouse neocortex, this was the ventricular zone, which contains proliferative apical progenitors (APs). Within these APs, ECM was more highly expressed in proliferative progenitors in comparison to progenitors about to undergo differentiative divisions (Arai et al., 2011). However, in the human neocortex, ECM expression was not only high in the ventricular zone but was also high in both the inner and outer subventricular zones, which contain proliferative basal progenitors (BPs; Fietz et al., 2012). This suggested a pro-proliferative role of the ECM in the developing neocortex. Further analysis indicated the regulation of this ECM could be controlled by the transcription factor SOX9. SOX9 was found to only be expressed in mouse APs but was expressed in both APs and BPs in the human fetal neocortex (Güven et al., 2020). Additionally, SOX9 over-expression in the embryonic mouse neocortex resulted in an increase in BP proliferation and increased ECM expression (Güven et al., 2020).

This proliferative role of the ECM is further supported by the expression and activation of integrins in BPs. Integrin alpha v beta 3 is more highly expressed in the proliferative human BPs compared to the less proliferative mouse BPs (Stenzel et al., 2014), consistent with the above reports of higher ECM expression in the former cells (Fietz et al., 2012; Miller et al., 2014; Florio et al., 2015). When integrin alpha v beta 3 was activated in the embryonic mouse neocortex, by addition of a function-activating antibody, this increased BP proliferation (Stenzel et al., 2014). Integrin beta 1 activation is also important for human BP proliferation, as blocking integrin beta 1 function in human fetal neocortex slice cultures decreased BP proliferation (Kalebic et al., 2019). The expression and function of integrins in human BPs is thought to be important for the interaction of these cells with their pro-proliferative ECM environment, enabling their increased proliferative capacity compared to BPs in the mouse. Human BPs have a more complex morphology in comparison to mouse, with more variation and a higher number of radial processes. These processes contain integrins that are able to interact with the surrounding ECM. Therefore, the more radial processes, the more pro-proliferative signals the BP can receive from the ECM environment (Kalebic et al., 2019; Kalebic and Huttner, 2020).

Models to Study ECM

A major reason for our limited knowledge of the role of the ECM in human and non-human primate neocortex development is the difficulty in modelling primate neocortex development. There are several options currently available, including the use of primary tissue or the generation of 2D and 3D models, notably brain organoids, from embryonic and induced pluripotent stem cells (ESCs and iPSCS). Primary tissue studies have provided valuable insight, as described above (Kalebic et al., 2019) and in the following section in more detail (Long et al., 2018). This includes the use of primary tissue to study ECM expression patterns (Fietz et al., 2012; Jovanov Milošević et al., 2014; Miller et al., 2014; Florio et al., 2015; Long et al., 2018) and the use of *ex vivo* tissue culture techniques to study the role of the ECM in an intact human tissue environment (Long et al., 2018; Kalebic et al., 2019; Eigel et al., 2021). However, access to this tissue is limited, making the 2D and 3D models from ESCs and iPSCs an attractive alternative for many researchers.

Using these 2D and 3D models comes with many clear advantages. They allow the study of human and non-human primate cells, and recent protocols have shown early neocortex development can be recapitulated relatively well in these *in vitro* systems (Mason and Price, 2016; Jabaudon and Lancaster, 2018; Heide et al., 2018; Kanton et al., 2019; Kyrousi and Cappello, 2019; Molnár et al., 2019). However, how these cells are cultured may have a significant effect on the investigation of ECM function in these models. For example, the ECM generated *in vitro* by human iPSC-derived NPCs is different in 2D cultures compared to 3D culture systems (**Figure 2**). The ECM is more similar to the *in vivo* composition when iPSC-derived NPCs are culture in 3D neurospheres than 2D systems, containing more proteoglycans and fewer basement membrane components (**Figure 2**; Simão et al., 2018). When these cells are grown as more complex cerebral organoids, the ECM composition expressed by the APs is indeed more similar to those of APs in the human fetal neocortex (Camp et al., 2015). This includes the ECM components collagen IV alpha 5, laminin alpha 1 and brevican, and the ECM receptors integrin alpha 6 and beta 8.

Additionally, the non-neuronal cells within the organoids also express ECM found in the fetal neocortex, including decorin, lumican, and collagen I alpha 2 (Camp et al., 2015). This data would suggest that 3D *in vitro* models, such as cerebral organoids, are better suited for the study of the role of ECM in neocortex development. However, although these 3D culture systems promote expression of some ECM components, there are still many that are not expressed that may play important roles. These include those secreted from cell types not present in these organoids, such as the blood vessels and meninges. It would be interesting to investigate how the addition of the ECM generated by these cells affects the development of such cerebral organoids.

One way to study the entire ECM network in 3D cell-based models is to use ECM extracted from primary tissue. Human iPSCs grown on ECM secreted by NPCs increased the expression of neuronal genes, such as tubulin beta 3, in comparison to ECM secreted by ESCs (Yan et al., 2015). ECM extracted from adult human brain tissue promoted increased laminin deposition in cerebral organoids, increased proliferation of APs and increased neural production (Cho et al., 2021). It would be interesting to investigate the effect of ECM extracted from fetal neocortex tissue using this model, as it is highly likely to differ in composition to the adult ECM extract used in this study.

How the ECM composition can direct the neurogenesis of iPSC-derived NPCs is yet to be determined. In addition to the known signalling functions of ECM, such as activation of integrins, the stiffness and elasticity of the matrix can also alter neurogenesis. Human iPSCs grown in softer ECM matrices differentiate into neuroectoderm and generate neurons, unlike iPSCs grown on stiffer matrices (Keung et al., 2012). This raises an interesting issue when comparing 2D and 3D *in vitro* models, as 3D models will inherently generate environments that are softer than 2D cultures grown on glass or plastic. How stiffness changes in these culture systems and how this compares to tissue will be important to determine the different roles of distinct ECM compositions in human neocortex development.

ECM AND NEOCORTEX TISSUE ARCHITECTURE

The expression and function of ECM have also been studied in human fetal neocortex tissue. ECM expression appears to be dynamic, with changes in the cortical wall over the course of development. For example, hyaluronic acid expression levels change with the laminar structure of the subplate between 13 and 21 post-conception weeks (Kostović et al., 2019). Temporal and spatial changes in ECM expression could have a major impact on the development of the neocortex and has been hypothesised to affect the folding of the cortical plate (van Essen, 2020). This could occur in several ways, including mechanical forces and neuronal migration.

ECM composition has already been shown to affect the stiffness of human fetal neocortex slice cultures, as removing specific ECM components (hyaluronic acid) using enzymatic degradation (by hyaluronidases) resulted in reduced stiffness (Long et al., 2018). In addition, cortical folding could be induced in these human fetal neocortex slice cultures by adding the ECM components Hyaluronan And Proteoglycan Link Protein 1 (HAPLN1), lumican, and collagen I (**Figure 3**; Long et al., 2018). This ECM-induced folding was also replicated in sliced neocortical organoids (Qian et al., 2020). In the primary tissue, the ECM-induced folding required an increase in ECM stiffness prior to the fold formation, resulting in a specific pattern of stiffer ECM at the gyrus of the fold and softer ECM in the sulcus (**Figure 3**; Long et al., 2018). Although tissue and ECM mechanics are hypothesised to regulate cortical folding (Karlinski and Reiner, 2018), this ECM-induced folding also required ERK signalling downstream of the hyaluronic acid receptor CD168 (Long et al., 2018),

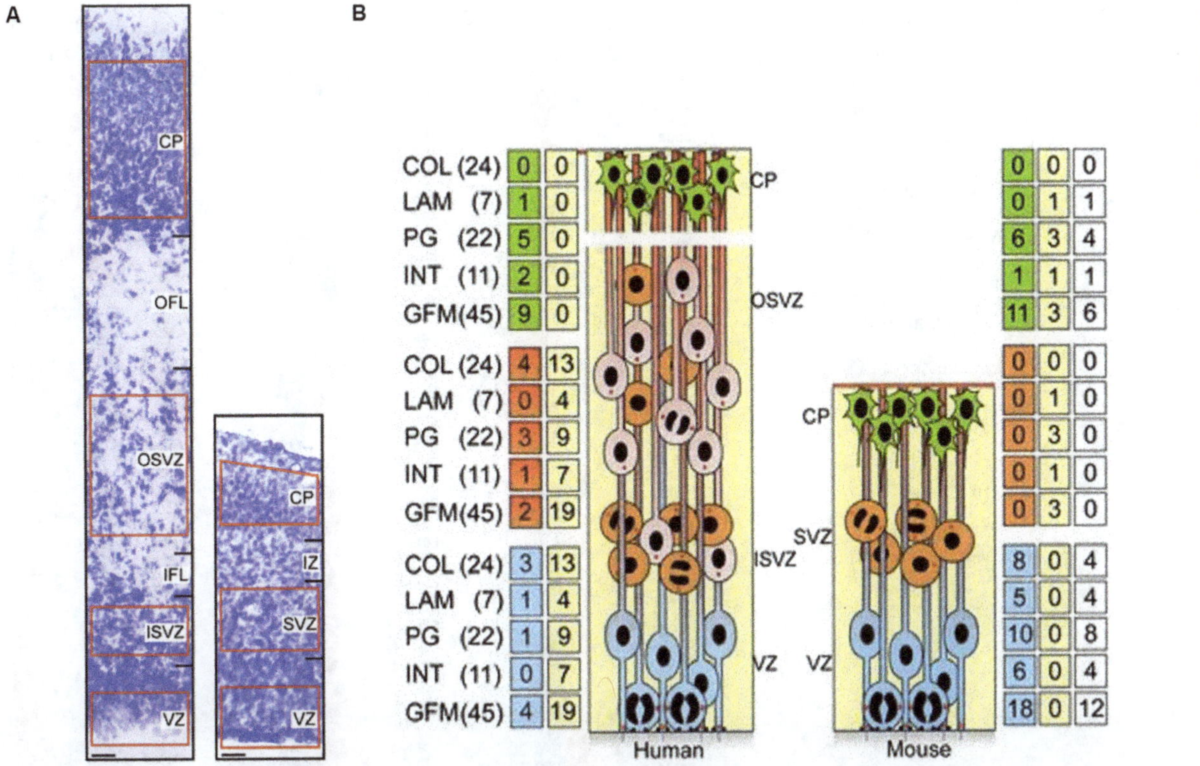

FIGURE 1 | Increased expression of extracellular matrix (ECM) components in the proliferative zones of the human fetal neocortex compared to the embryonic mouse neocortex. **(A)** Nissl staining of the cortical wall of a 15 post-conception week (pcw) human fetal neocortex (left) and of an embryonic day (E) 14.5 embryonic mouse neocortex (right). Scale bars represent 20 μm. The areas used for transcriptomic analysis are highlighted in red. The different zones of the cortical wall are labelled as ventricular zone (VZ), subventricular zone (SVZ), inner SVZ (ISVZ), outer SVZ (OSVZ), inner fibre layer (IFL), outer fibre layer (OFL), intermediate zone (IZ) and cortical plate (CP). **(B)** Schematic illustrating the major cell types within the developing cortical wall (APs = blue, BPs = orange and red, neurons = green) and the distribution of ECM and ECM-associated components within these areas. The major families of ECM components are the collagens (COL), laminins (LAM), proteoglycans (PG), integrins (INT) and growth factors/morphogens (GFM). Numbers in parentheses indicate the total numbers of genes within each family. Numbers in the green/red/blue boxes indicate the number of genes overexpressed in the adjacent area. Numbers in the yellow boxes indicate the number of genes that are overexpressed in more than one human or mouse zone. Numbers in the white boxes indicate the number of genes that are overexpressed in both humans and mice. The cells within the zones are: APs are located within the VZ in both mice and humans, BPs are located in the SVZ in mice, and within the ISVZ and OSVZ in humans, neurons are located in the CP in both species. Adapted from Fietz et al. (2012).

suggesting the role of ECM in cortical folding and tissue morphology will require both mechanical changes and signalling *via* ECM receptors.

ECM composition was also hypothesised to affect the migration of neurons. In the mouse, the majority of glutamatergic neuronal migration in the cortex is thought to occur radially, with neurons migrating along the radial glia scaffold up to the cortical plate. However, tangential migration of glutamatergic neurons has been observed in the developing macaque cortex (Cortay et al., 2020) and is thought to be important for cortical folding (van Essen, 2020). It has been hypothesised that ECM could direct this migration by providing directional cues or a scaffold for the neurons to migrate along. ECM components and receptors could also alter the morphology of the newborn neurons, as over-expression of integrin alpha 9 in human NPCs increased the outgrowth of neurites *in vitro* when grown on tenascin-C and when grafted into newborn rat cortex (Forbes and Andrews, 2019). Increased processes may be important for the interaction with the ECM environment, as discussed above for BPs (Kalebic et al., 2019).

ECM, once expressed, can be present in tissues for a long period of time (Brückner et al., 1998; Zimmermann and Dours-Zimmermann, 2008; Ewald, 2020). Therefore, the removal of ECM components at the right time is also important for neocortex development. Modulation of the ECM, such as degradation by metalloproteases (MMPs), has been reported throughout neocortex development. MMP2 has been shown to modulate the ECM deposited by growing microvessels within the early fetal human neocortex (Girolamo et al., 2004). This could impact neuronal migration, as BPs are reported to attach their basal process to blood vessel ECM later in neocortex development (Nowakowski et al., 2016), altering the scaffold of cell processes newborn neurons are able to migrate along. This builds a complex picture of ECM deposition and modulation that may help direct the migration of neurons and eventually determine the shape of the developing neocortex.

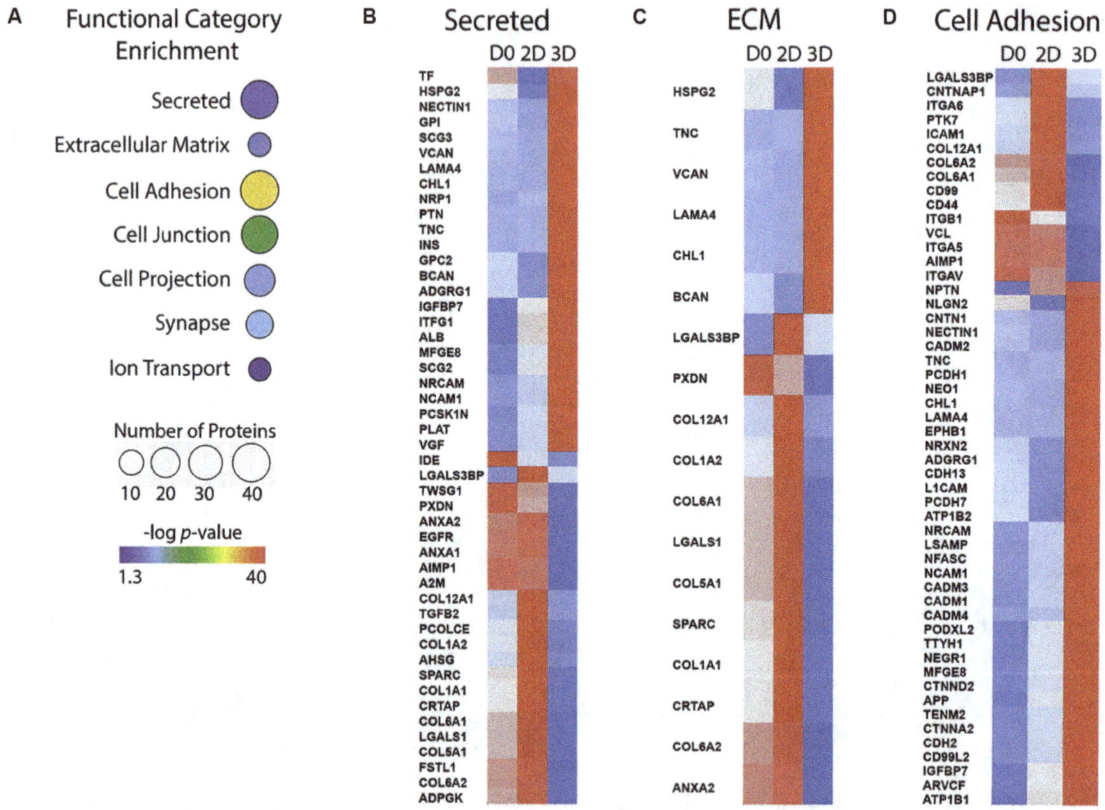

FIGURE 2 | ECM components expressed differ between 2D and 3D *in vitro* cultures of human iPSCs undergoing differentiation to NPCs. **(A)** Functional categories that are significantly over-represented in 3D iPSC to NPC differentiation, selected from proteomic analysis of 2D and 3D cultures. The number of proteins is indicated by sphere size, the *p*-value is indicated by colour. **(B–D)** Heatmaps showing protein abundance profile at day 0 (D0) of culture, day 30 of 2D culture (2D) and day 30 of 3D culture (3D). *Z* scores are colour-coded from blue (downregulation) to red (upregulation). Secreted proteins **(B)**, ECM **(C)** and cell adhesion protein **(D)** categories are shown. Adapted from Simão et al. (2018). iPSC, induced pluripotent stem cell; NPC, neural progenitor cell.

ECM AND NEURODEVELOPMENTAL DISORDERS

It can be difficult to study the function of the ECM in human neurodevelopment, despite the recent advances in human cell- and tissue-based culture models. However, a lot has been learnt about the normal function of the ECM in neocortex development from various neurodevelopmental disorders. There are many mutations in ECM genes, or genes affecting ECM function, that lead to neurodevelopmental disorders, with RELN (for the protein Reelin) being one the most well-known examples.

Reelin is an ECM glycoprotein (Hynes and Naba, 2012) secreted by several cell types, including the Cajal Retzius cells, early in the human fetal cortex (D'Arcangelo et al., 1995; Meyer et al., 2002). Mutations in the human gene RELN are linked to various neurodevelopmental disorders, including schizophrenia, bipolar disorder, and autism spectrum disorder (Ishii and Maeda, 2008; Lakatosova and Ostatnikova, 2012). RELN mutations are also known to cause type I lissencephaly, with abnormal lamination of the cortical plate and a loss of cortical folding (**Figure 4A**; Hong et al., 2000). The mechanisms underlying this malformation have been elucidated in mouse models (Hong et al., 2000; Fatemi, 2001; Rice and Curran, 2001; Pérez-Martínez et al., 2012; Sekine et al., 2012; Hirota and Nakajima, 2017; Mizukami et al., 2018), which show that Reelin is important for directing the migration of newborn neurons and the correct positioning of these neurons in the cortical plate.

The role of ECM in neuronal migration disorders is relatively common. Patients with another type of lissencephaly, cobblestone lissencephaly, also have mutations in genes that alter ECM function. In particular, the enzymes POMT1/2 that glycosylate the ECM receptor alpha-dystroglycan have been found in patients with cobblestone lissencephaly (**Figure 4B**; Devisme et al., 2012) and in Walker-Warburg syndrome (De Bernabé et al., 2002; Van Reeuwijk et al., 2005). Mutations in the genes that encode for the laminin subunits beta 2 and gamma 2 (LAMB2 and LAMC2) have also been associated with disorganisation of the cortical layers, similar to cobblestone lissencephaly (Radner et al., 2013), as have mutations in the laminin subunit beta 1 (LAMB1; Radmanesh et al., 2013). These mutations are thought to lead to these disorders *via* disruption of the pial basement membrane, which lies at the top of the cortical plate. This disruption enables migrating neurons to bypass their usual stop signals, migrating above the cortical

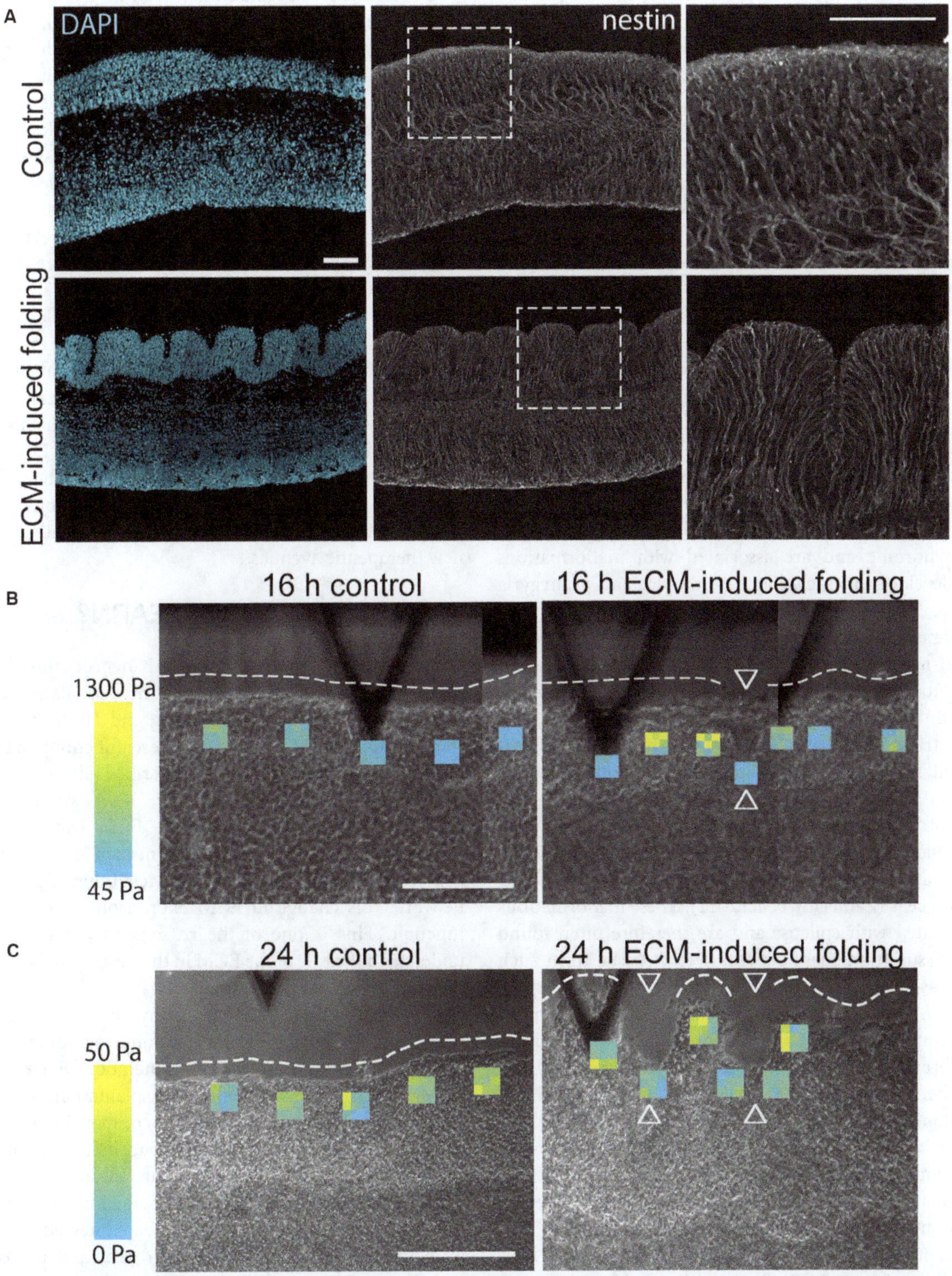

FIGURE 3 | ECM can induce folding and changes in ECM stiffness in human fetal neocortex *ex vivo* cultures. **(A)** Images showing a 13 gestation week (GW) human fetal neocortex after 24 h of *ex vivo* culture in the control condition (upper panels) or after the addition of the ECM components HAPLN1, lumican and collagen I (lower panels), with DAPI staining (blue) and immunofluorescence for the radial glial process marker nestin (grey). The addition of these ECM components induced the folding of the cortical plate. White dashed boxes delineate areas shown in the panels on the right. Scale bar represents 50 μm. **(B,C)** Images showing atomic force microscopy of 13 GW human fetal neocortex after 16 h (**B**, folding ongoing) or 24 h (**C**, folding complete) of *ex vivo* culture in control conditions (left panels) or after the addition of the ECM components HAPLN1, lumican and collagen I (right panels, ECM-induced folding). Each heatmap square shows nine Young's modulus values in the position the measurement was taken (see the range of values from blue (lowest) to yellow (highest)). White dashed lines outline the unfolded or folded CP surface; arrowheads indicate sulci. The stiffest measurements (yellow) are found in the forming gyri compared to the softer measurements (blue) in the forming sulci. Scale bar represents 200 μm. Adapted from Long et al. (2018).

plate and creating a bumpy, cobblestone-like appearance (Radner et al., 2013).

Mutations in laminin subunits are also linked to another folding disorder, polymicrogyria, characterised by an excess of shallower folds on the cortical surface. LAMC3 mutations have been found in patients with a developmental delay in the occipital cortex and focal areas of polymicrogyria (Barak et al., 2011). This laminin subunit was found to be highly expressed in the cortical plate at 20 post-conception weeks (pcw) human fetal cortex, with lower expression levels in the ventricular and inner and outer subventricular zones. This expression peaked around mid-gestation and was maintained until 12 months postnatally, coinciding with the peak of dendritogenesis and the generation of the majority of the cortical folds (Barak et al., 2011).

ECM has also been linked to other aspects of cortex shape during development and neurodevelopmental disorders, with several mutations in the collagen family found in patients. Mutations in collagen IV alpha 1 (COL4A1) have been linked to porencephaly, the development of a cavity in the cortex filled with cerebrospinal fluid (Hubert et al., 2009). COL18A1 mutations have also been found in patients with Knobloch syndrome and are associated with malformations of cortical development including heterotopias and pachygyria (Hubert et al., 2009). Both of these malformations are the result of abnormal neuronal migration, resulting in neurons clustering in abnormal layers in the cortical wall. Finally, COL1A1 and COL2A1 mutations have been associated with hydrocephaly, characterised by increased cerebrospinal fluid pressure and enlarged ventricles (Hubert et al., 2009). Together, this suggests an important role of ECM in shaping the developing human neocortex.

Many neurodevelopmental abnormalities are linked to much more focal malformations of cortical development, such as the abnormal lamination of neurons or dysmorphic neuronal cells, called balloon cells (Zamecnik et al., 2012). These malformations can be associated with epilepsy and are therefore often found in resected tissue from these patients. When tissue from such resections was examined, changes in the extracellular space were observed. These included an increase in the expression of the ECM components tenascin-C, tenascin-R, versican, and a decrease in brevican expression (Zamecnik et al., 2012).

Finally, there is also evidence that the modulation of the ECM in the developing neocortex is important for its development. Mutations in the enzyme neurotrypsin, a serine protease that degrades agrin, are linked to intellectual disability in a small number of patients (Molinari et al., 2002). Agrin is expressed during fetal neocortex development and is thought to help regulate synaptic function and be important for memory later on in life (Molinari et al., 2002). Several other ECM components are also known to have a vital role in perineuronal nets, which are also important for synaptic function (Barros et al., 2011; De Luca and Papa, 2016; Sorg et al., 2016; Miyata and Kitagawa, 2017). Perineuronal nets are lattice-like ECM structures that surround the synapses of certain neurons, including several interneurons (Sorg et al., 2016). They are predominately made up of chondroitin sulfate proteoglycans, tenascin, hyaluronan, and proteoglycan link proteins and hyaluronic acid (Sorg et al., 2016).

Impairment of perineuronal nets, in particular the enzyme that modifies them (matrix metalloproteinase-9), has been linked to several neurodevelopmental disorders, including fragile X syndrome, autism spectrum disorder, and epilepsy (Reinhard et al., 2015; Rogers et al., 2018; Wen et al., 2018). It has also been suggested that neuronal activity could feed back and modulate ECM expression surrounding neurons too (Lazarevich et al., 2020). As synaptic pruning occurs over the first few years of life in humans and non-human primates (Hensch, 2004), the ability to modulate the ECM that regulates synapse formation and stabilisation is vital to ensure this happens correctly (Gundelfinger et al., 2010).

There is growing evidence for the role of ECM in neurodevelopmental disorders, with more and more mutations in genes affecting ECM function discovered in patients. However, whilst we can associate the ECM with the cortical abnormalities detected, we still do not understand the mechanisms underlying them. Understanding the normal function of ECM in human neocortex development is an important step that would enable us to uncover how altering its functions leads to the malformations observed in these patients, potentially opening up new therapeutic avenues.

WHAT ELSE CAN WE LEARN?

Many of the functions of the ECM in neocortex development have been uncovered using animal models (Barros et al., 2011; Faissner and Reinhard, 2015; Long and Huttner, 2019), but it remains unclear how many of these functions are conserved in humans. However, as we described above in the "ECM and Neural Progenitors" section, RNA sequencing studies have revealed key differences in ECM expression between these models and the developing human neocortex. As ECM components often interact with each other, functioning as a network, this change in ECM expression is likely to affect its function. This is one of the reasons why it is important we understand the role of the ECM in the development of the human neocortex.

Another reason is that many of the findings from development can be useful for understanding the role of the ECM in injury and neurodegeneration. For example, how ECM expression changes upon transplantation of iPSC-derived cells into the adult brain, how ECM composition is altered upon injury, and how this change may impact inflammation and repair (Roll and Faissner, 2014), which are all key issues for future research. ECM and ECM modulators are known to be expressed by reactive astrocytes but can also be expressed at lower levels by neurons, oligodendrocytes, microglia, and the cells of the vasculature. These include chondroitin sulphate proteoglycans, associated with the inhibition of axonal outgrowth, and heparan sulphate proteoglycans, associated with the promotion of axonal outgrowth. The balance of these two ECM families is vital for the repair of the adult neocortex (Roll and Faissner, 2014). Understanding their roles in human neocortex development could provide important information about this balance in the adult, informing and potentially improving current avenues for therapeutic options.

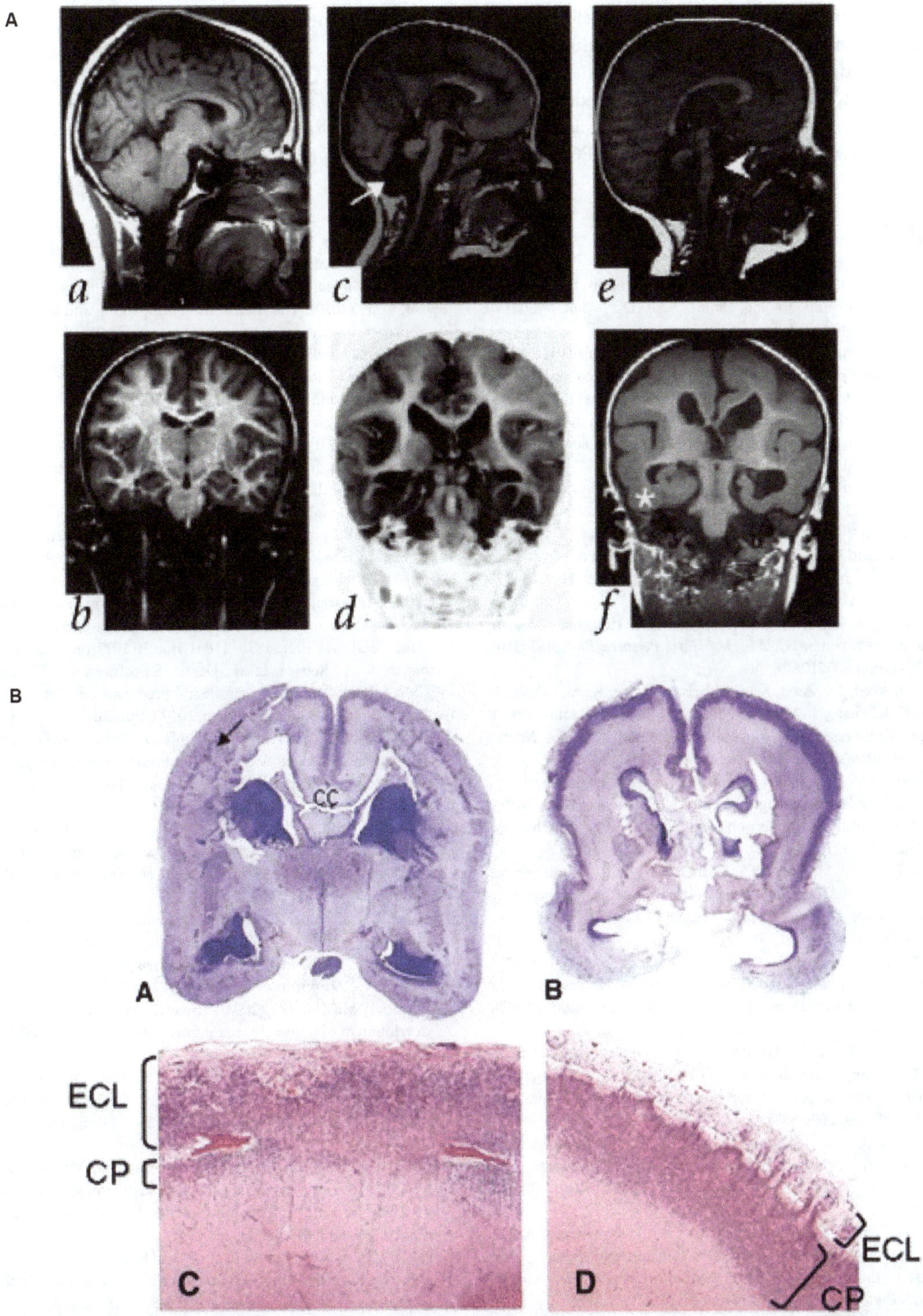

FIGURE 4 | Lissencephaly in patients with mutations in ECM and ECM-associated genes. **(A)** Parasagittal (upper panels) and coronal (lower panels) MRI from patients with a normally developing brain (*a,b*), and two patients with lissencephaly associated with RELN mutations (*c,d*; *e,f*). Note the thickened cortex and reduced folding present. Adapted from Hong et al. (2000). **(B)** Images showing examples of cobblestone lissencephaly in a 19 pcw fetus with a POMT1 mutation (**A,C**, left panels) and 26 pcw fetus with a POMGNT1 mutation (**B,D**, right panels). The top panels show whole-mount sections of the brain. Arrow indicates impoverished cortical plate in the top left panel. The lower panels show higher magnification images of the cortical plate from these fetuses. Note the reduced size of the cortical plate (CP) and the thickened extracortical layer (ECL) in the lower left panel, but the thin ECL in the lower right panel. CC indicates the corpus callosum. Adapted from Devisme et al. (2012).

We therefore still have a lot to learn about the role of the ECM in human and non-human primate neocortex development. It is clear that ECM components are involved in almost every aspect of neocortex development, but exactly what ECM is expressed when and where is not yet known. Understanding these dynamics and the differences between species will be an important step forward in understanding how ECM shapes human neocortex development and the role it has played in the evolution of the human brain.

AUTHOR CONTRIBUTIONS

KL and WH wrote the manuscript. All authors contributed to the article and approved the submitted version.

REFERENCES

Amin, S., and Borrell, V. (2020). The extracellular matrix in the evolution of cortical development and folding. *Front. Cell Dev. Biol.* 8:604448. doi: 10.3389/fcell.2020.604448

Arai, Y., Pulvers, J. N., Haffner, C., Schilling, B., Nüsslein, I., Calegari, F., et al. (2011). Neural stem and progenitor cells shorten S-phase on commitment to neuron production. *Nat. Commun.* 2:154. doi: 10.1038/ncomms1155

Bandtlow, C. E., and Zimmermann, D. R. (2000). Proteoglycans in the developing brain: new conceptual insights for old proteins. *Physiol. Rev.* 80, 1267–1290. doi: 10.1152/physrev.2000.80.4.1267

Barak, T., Kwan, K. Y., Louvi, A., Demirbilek, V., Saygi, S., Tüysüz, B., et al. (2011). Recessive LAMC3 mutations cause malformations of occipital cortical development. *Nat. Genet.* 43, 590–594. doi: 10.1038/ng.836

Barros, D., Amaral, I. F., and Pêgo, A. P. (2020). Laminin-inspired cell-instructive microenvironments for neural stem cells. *Biomacromolecules* 21, 276–293. doi: 10.1021/acs.biomac.9b01319

Barros, C. S., Franco, S. J., and Müller, U. (2011). Extracellular matrix: functions in the nervous system. *Cold Spring Harb. Perspect. Biol.* 3:a005108. doi: 10.1101/cshperspect.a005108

Beggs, H. E., Schahin-Reed, D., Zang, K., Goebbels, S., Nave, K. A., Gorski, J., et al. (2003). FAK deficiency in cells contributing to the basal lamina results in cortical abnormalities resembling congenital muscular dystrophies. *Neuron* 40, 501–514. doi: 10.1016/s0896-6273(03)00666-4

Brückner, G., Bringmann, A., Härtig, W., Köppe, G., Delpech, B., and Brauer, K. (1998). Acute and long-lasting changes in extracellular-matrix chondroitin-sulphate proteoglycans induced by injection of chondroitinase ABC in the adult rat brain. *Exp. Brain Res.* 121, 300–310. doi: 10.1007/s002210050463

Camp, J. G., Badsha, F., Florio, M., Kanton, S., Gerber, T., Wilsch-Bräuninger, M., et al. (2015). Human cerebral organoids recapitulate gene expression programs of fetal neocortex development. *Proc. Natl. Acad. Sci. U S A* 112, 15672–15677. doi: 10.1073/pnas.1520760112

Cho, A.-N., Jin, Y., An, Y., Kim, J., Choi, Y. S., Lee, J. S., et al. (2021). Microfluidic device with brain extracellular matrix promotes structural and functional maturation of human brain organoids. *Nat. Commun.* 12:4730. doi: 10.1038/s41467-021-24775-5

Cortay, V., Delaunay, D., Patti, D., Gautier, E., Doerflinger, N., Giroud, P., et al. (2020). Radial migration dynamics is modulated in a laminar and area-specific manner during primate corticogenesis. *Front. Cell Dev. Biol.* 8:588814. doi: 10.3389/fcell.2020.588814

D'Arcangelo, G., Miao, G. G., Chen, S. C., Soares, H. D., Morgan, J. I., and Curran, T. (1995). A protein related to extracellular matrix proteins deleted in the mouse mutant reeler. *Nature* 374, 719–723. doi: 10.1038/374719a0

De Bernabé, D. B. V., Currier, S., Steinbrecher, A., Celli, J., Van Beusekom, E., Van der Zwaag, B., et al. (2002). Mutations in the O-mannosyltransferase gene POMT1 give rise to the severe neuronal migration disorder walker-warburg syndrome. *Am. J. Hum. Genet.* 71, 1033–1043. doi: 10.1086/342975

De Luca, C., and Papa, M. (2016). Looking inside the matrix: perineuronal nets in plasticity, maladaptive plasticity and neurological disorders. *Neurochem. Res.* 41, 1507–1515. doi: 10.1007/s11064-016-1876-2

Devisme, L., Bouchet, C., Gonzalès, M., Alanio, E., Bazin, A., Bessières, B., et al. (2012). Cobblestone lissencephaly: neuropathological subtypes and correlations with genes of dystroglycanopathies. *Brain* 135, 469–482. doi: 10.1093/brain/awr357

Dityatev, A., Seidenbecher, C. I., and Schachner, M. (2010). Compartmentalization from the outside: the extracellular matrix and functional microdomains in the brain. *Trends Neurosci.* 33, 503–512. doi: 10.1016/j.tins.2010.08.003

Eigel, D., Schuster, R., Männel, M.J., Thiele, J., Panasiuk, M. J., Andreae, L. C., et al. (2021). Sulfonated cryogel scaffolds for focal delivery in ex-vivo brain tissue cultures. *Biomaterials* 271:120712. doi: 10.1016/j.biomaterials.2021.120712

Ewald, C. Y. (2020). The matrisome during aging and longevity: a systems-level approach toward defining matreotypes promoting healthy aging. *Gerontology* 66, 266–274. doi: 10.1159/000504295

Faissner, A., and Reinhard, J. (2015). The extracellular matrix compartment of neural stem and glial progenitor cells. *Glia* 63, 1330–1349. doi: 10.1002/glia.22839

Fatemi, S. H. (2001). Reelin mutations in mouse and man: from reeler mouse to schizophrenia, mood disorders, autism and lissencephaly. *Mol. Psychiatry* 6, 129–133. doi: 10.1038/sj.mp.4000129

Fietz, S. A., Kelava, I., Vogt, J., Wilsch-Bräuninger, M., Stenzel, D., Fish, J. L., et al. (2010). OSVZ progenitors of human and ferret neocortex are epithelial-like and expand by integrin signaling. *Nat. Neurosci.* 13, 690–699. doi: 10.1038/nn.2553

Fietz, S. A., Lachmann, R., Brandl, H., Kircher, M., Samusik, N., and Schröder, R. (2012). Transcriptomes of germinal zones of human and mouse fetal neocortex suggest a role of extracellular matrix in progenitor self-renewal. *Proc. Natl. Acad. Sci. U S A* 109, 11836–11841. doi: 10.1073/pnas.1209647109

Flanagan, L. A., Rebaza, L. M., Derzic, S., Schwartz, P. H., and Monuki, E. S. (2006). Regulation of human neural precursor cells by laminin and integrins. *J. Neurosci. Res.* 83, 845–856. doi: 10.1002/jnr.20778

Florio, M., Albert, M., Taverna, E., Namba, T., Brandl, H., Lewitus, E., et al. (2015). Human-specific gene ARHGAP11B promotes basal progenitor amplification and neocortex expansion. *Science* 347, 1465–1470. doi: 10.1126/science.aaa1975

Forbes, L. H., and Andrews, M. R. (2019). Grafted human iPSC-derived neural progenitor cells express integrins and extend long-distance axons within the developing corticospinal tract. *Front. Cell. Neurosci.* 13:26. doi: 10.3389/fncel.2019.00026

Franco, S. J., and Müller, U. (2011). Extracellular matrix functions during neuronal migration and lamination in the mammalian central nervous system. *Dev. Neurobiol.* 71, 889–900. doi: 10.1002/dneu.20946

Girolamo, F., Virgintino, D., Errede, M., Capobianco, C., Bernardini, N., Bertossi, M., et al. (2004). Involvement of metalloprotease-2 in the development of human brain microvessels. *Histochem. Cell Biol.* 122, 261–270. doi: 10.1007/s00418-004-0705-x

Gundelfinger, E. D., Frischknecht, R., Choquet, D., and Heine, M. (2010). Converting juvenile into adult plasticity: a role for the brain's extracellular matrix. *Eur. J. Neurosci.* 31, 2156–2165. doi: 10.1111/j.1460-9568.2010.07253.x

Güven, A., Kalebic, N., Long, K. R., Florio, M., Vaid, S., Brandl, H., et al. (2020). Extracellular matrix-inducing Sox9 promotes both basal progenitor proliferation and gliogenesis in developing neocortex. *eLife* 9:e49808. doi: 10.7554/eLife.49808

Hall, P. E., Lathia, J. D., Caldwell, M. A., and Ffrench-Constant, C. (2008). Laminin enhances the growth of human neural stem cells in defined culture media. *BMC Neurosci.* 9:71. doi: 10.1186/1471-2202-9-71

Hall, P. E., Lathia, J. D., Miller, N. G. A., Caldwell, M. A., and ffrench-Constant, C. (2006). Integrins are markers of human neural stem cells. *Stem Cells* 24, 2078–2084. doi: 10.1634/stemcells.2005-0595

Haubst, N., Georges-Labouesse, E., De Arcangelis, A., Mayer, U., and Götz, M. (2006). Basement membrane attachment is dispensable for radial glial cell fate and for proliferation, but affects positioning of neuronal subtypes. *Development* 133, 3245–3254. doi: 10.1242/dev.02486

Heide, M., Huttner, W. B., and Mora-Bermúdez, F. (2018). Brain organoids as models to study human neocortex development and evolution. *Curr. Opin. Cell Biol.* 55, 8–16. doi: 10.1016/j.ceb.2018.06.006

Hensch, T. K. (2004). Critical period regulation. *Annu. Rev. Neurosci.* 27, 549–579. doi: 10.1146/annurev.neuro.27.070203.144327

Hirota, Y., and Nakajima, K. (2017). Control of neuronal migration and aggregation by reelin signaling in the developing cerebral cortex. *Front. Cell Dev. Biol.* 5:40. doi: 10.3389/fcell.2017.00040

Hong, S. E., Shugart, Y. Y., Huang, D. T., Al Shahwan, S., Grant, P. E., Hourihane, J. O. B., et al. (2000). Autosomal recessive lissencephaly with cerebellar hypoplasia is associated with human RELN mutations. *Nat. Genet.* 26, 93–96. doi: 10.1038/79246

Hubert, T., Grimal, S., Carroll, P., and Fichard-Carroll, A. (2009). Collagens in the developing and diseased nervous system. *Cell. Mol. Life Sci.* 66, 1223–1238. doi: 10.1007/s00018-008-8561-9

Hynes, R. O. (2002). Integrins: bidirectional, allosteric signaling machines. *Cell* 110, 673–687. doi: 10.1016/s0092-8674(02)00971-6

Hynes, R. O., and Naba, A. (2012). Overview of the matrisome--an inventory of extracellular matrix constituents and functions. *Cold Spring Harb. Perspect. Biol.* 4:a004903. doi: 10.1101/cshperspect.a004903

Ishii, M., and Maeda, N. (2008). Oversulfated chondroitin sulfate plays critical roles in the neuronal migration in the cerebral cortex. *J. Biol. Chem.* 283, 32610–32620. doi: 10.1074/jbc.M806331200

Jabaudon, D., and Lancaster, M. (2018). Exploring landscapes of brain morphogenesis with organoids. *Development* 145:dev172049. doi: 10.1242/dev.172049

Jovanov Milošević, N., Judaš, M., Aronica, E., and Kostovic, I. (2014). Neural ECM in laminar organization and connectivity development in healthy and diseased human brain. *Prog. Brain Res.* 214, 159–178. doi: 10.1016/B978-0-444-63486-3.00007-4

Kalebic, N., Gilardi, C., Stepien, B., Wilsch-Bräuninger, M., Long, K. R., Namba, T., et al. (2019). Neocortical expansion due to increased proliferation of basal progenitors is linked to changes in their morphology. *Cell Stem Cell* 24, 535–550.e9. doi: 10.1016/j.stem.2019.02.017

Kalebic, N., and Huttner, W. B. (2020). Basal progenitor morphology and neocortex evolution. *Trends Neurosci.* 43, 843–853. doi: 10.1016/j.tins.2020.07.009

Kanton, S., Boyle, M. J., He, Z., Santel, M., Weigert, A., Sanchís-Calleja, F., et al. (2019). Organoid single-cell genomic atlas uncovers human-specific features of brain development. *Nature* 574, 418–422. doi: 10.1038/s41586-019-1654-9

Karlinski, M., and Reiner, O. (2018). Unfolding the folds: how the biomechanics of the extracellular matrix contributes to cortical gyrification. *Opera Medica Physiol.* 4, 63–70. doi: 10.20388/omp2018.001.0058

Keung, A. J., Asuri, P., Kumar, S., and Schaffer, D. V. (2012). Soft microenvironments promote the early neurogenic differentiation but not self-renewal of human pluripotent stem cells. *Integr. Biol. (Camb).* 4, 1049–1058. doi: 10.1039/c2ib20083j

Kostović, I., Išasegi, I. Z., and Krsnik, Z. (2019). Sublaminar organization of the human subplate: developmental changes in the distribution of neurons, glia, growing axons and extracellular matrix. *J. Anat.* 235, 481–506. doi: 10.1111/joa.12920

Kyrousi, C., and Cappello, S. (2019). Using brain organoids to study human neurodevelopment, evolution and disease. *Wiley Interdiscip. Rev. Dev. Biol.* 9:e347. doi: 10.1002/wdev.347

Lakatosova, S., and Ostatnikova, D. (2012). Reelin and its complex involvement in brain development and function. *Int. J. Biochem. Cell Biol.* 44, 1501–1504. doi: 10.1016/j.biocel.2012.06.002

Lazarevich, I., Stasenko, S., Rozhnova, M., Pankratova, E., Dityatev, A., and Kazantsev, V. (2020). Activity-dependent switches between dynamic regimes of extracellular matrix expression. *PLoS One* 15:e0227917. doi: 10.1371/journal.pone.0227917

Li, X., Liu, X., Josey, B., Chou, C. J., Tan, Y., Zhang, N., et al. (2014). Short laminin peptide for improved neural stem cell growth. *Stem Cells Transl. Med.* 3, 662–670. doi: 10.5966/sctm.2013-0015

Long, K. R., and Huttner, W. B. (2019). How the extracellular matrix shapes neural development. *Open Biol.* 9:180216. doi: 10.1098/rsob.180216

Long, K., Moss, L., Laursen, L., Boulter, L., and ffrench-Constant, C. (2016). Integrin signalling regulates the expansion of neuroepithelial progenitors and neurogenesis *via* Wnt7a and decorin. *Nat. Commun.* 7:10354. doi: 10.1038/ncomms10354

Long, K. R., Newland, B., Florio, M., Kalebic, N., Langen, B., Kolterer, A., et al. (2018). Extracellular matrix components HAPLN1, lumican and collagen I cause hyaluronic acid-dependent folding of the developing human neocortex. *Neuron* 99, 702–719.e6. doi: 10.1016/j.neuron.2018.07.013

Loulier, K., Lathia, J. D., Marthiens, V., Relucio, J., Mughal, M. R., Tang, S.-C., et al. (2009). beta1 integrin maintains integrity of the embryonic neocortical stem cell niche. *PLoS Biol.* 7:e1000176. doi: 10.1371/journal.pbio.1000176

Ma, W., Tavakoli, T., Derby, E., Serebryakova, Y., Rao, M. S., and Mattson, M. P. (2008). Cell-extracellular matrix interactions regulate neural differentiation of human embryonic stem cells. *BMC Dev. Biol.* 8:90. doi: 10.1186/1471-213X-8-90

Maeda, N. (2015). Proteoglycans and neuronal migration in the cerebral cortex during development and disease. *Front. Neurosci.* 9:98. doi: 10.3389/fnins.2015.00098

Marthiens, V., Kazanis, I., Moss, L., Long, K., and ffrench-Constant, C. (2010). Adhesion molecules in the stem cell niche – more than just staying in shape?. *J. Cell Sci.* 123, 1613–1622. doi: 10.1242/jcs.054312

Mason, J. O., and Price, D. J. (2016). Building brains in a dish: prospects for growing cerebral organoids from stem cells. *Neuroscience* 334, 105–118. doi: 10.1016/j.neuroscience.2016.07.048

Meyer, G., Perez-Garcia, C. G., Abraham, H., and Caput, D. (2002). Expression of p73 and reelin in the developing human cortex. *J. Neurosci.* 22, 4973–4986. doi: 10.1523/JNEUROSCI.22-12-04973.2002

Miller, J. A., Ding, S.-L., Sunkin, S. M., Smith, K. A., Ng, L., Szafer, A., et al. (2014). Transcriptional landscape of the prenatal human brain. *Nature* 508, 199–206. doi: 10.1038/nature13185

Miyata, S., and Kitagawa, H. (2017). Formation and remodeling of the brain extracellular matrix in neural plasticity: roles of chondroitin sulfate and hyaluronan. *Biochim. Biophys. Acta Gen. Subj.* 1861, 2420–2434. doi: 10.1016/j.bbagen.2017.06.010

Mizukami, T., Ikeda, K., Shimanaka, Y., Korogi, K., Zhou, C., Takase, H., et al. (2018). Reelin deficiency leads to aberrant lipid composition in mouse brain. *Biochem. Biophys. Res. Commun.* 505, 81–86. doi: 10.1016/j.bbrc.2018.09.089

Molinari, F., Rio, M., Meskenaite, V., Encha-Razavi, F., Augé, J., Bacq, D., et al. (2002). Truncating neurotrypsin mutation in autosomal recessive nonsyndromic mental retardation. *Science* 298, 1779–1781. doi: 10.1126/science.1076521

Molnár, Z., Clowry, G. J., Šestan, N., Alzu'bi, A., Bakken, T., Hevner, R. F., et al. (2019). New insights into the development of the human cerebral cortex. *J. Anat.* 235, 432–451. doi: 10.1111/joa.13055

Niewmierzycka, A., Mills, J., St-Arnaud, R., Dedhar, S., and Reichardt, L. F. (2005). Integrin-linked kinase deletion from mouse cortex results in cortical lamination defects resembling cobblestone lissencephaly. *J. Neurosci.* 25, 7022–7031. doi: 10.1523/JNEUROSCI.1695-05.2005

Nowakowski, T. J., Pollen, A. A., Sandoval-Espinosa, C., and Kriegstein, A. R. (2016). Transformation of the radial glia scaffold demarcates two stages of human cerebral cortex development. *Neuron* 91, 1219–1227. doi: 10.1016/j.neuron.2016.09.005

Oikari, L. E., Okolicsanyi, R. K., Qin, A., Yu, C., Griffiths, L. R., and Haupt, L. M. (2016). Cell surface heparan sulfate proteoglycans as novel markers of human neural stem cell fate determination. *Stem Cell Res.* 16, 92–104. doi: 10.1016/j.scr.2015.12.011

Okolicsanyi, R. K., Oikari, L. E., Yu, C., Griffiths, L. R., and Haupt, L. M. (2018). Heparan sulfate proteoglycans as drivers of neural progenitors derived from human mesenchymal stem cells. *Front. Mol. Neurosci.* 11:134. doi: 10.3389/fnmol.2018.00134

Pérez-Martínez, F. J., Luque-Río, A., Sakakibara, A., Hattori, M., Miyata, T., and Luque, J. M. (2012). Reelin-dependent ApoER2 downregulation uncouples newborn neurons from progenitor cells. *Biol. Open* 1, 1258–1263. doi: 10.1242/bio.20122816

Qian, X., Su, Y., Adam, C. D., Deutschmann, A. U., Pather, S. R., Goldberg, E. M., et al. (2020). Sliced human cortical organoids for modeling distinct cortical layer formation. *Cell Stem Cell* 26, 766–781.e9. doi: 10.1016/j.stem.2020.02.002

Radakovits, R., Barros, C. S., Belvindrah, R., Patton, B., and Müller, U. (2009). Regulation of radial glial survival by signals from the meninges. *J. Neurosci.* 29, 7694–7705. doi: 10.1523/JNEUROSCI.5537-08.2009

Radmanesh, F., Caglayan, A. O., Silhavy, J. L., Yilmaz, C., Cantagrel, V., Omar, T., et al. (2013). Mutations in LAMB1 cause cobblestone brain malformation without muscular or ocular abnormalities. *Am. J. Hum. Genet.* 92, 468–474. doi: 10.1097/j.jcrs.0000000000000867

Radner, S., Banos, C., Bachay, G., Li, Y. N., Hunter, D. D., Brunken, W. J., et al. (2013). β2 and γ3 laminins are critical cortical basement membrane components: ablation of Lamb2 and Lamc3 genes disrupts cortical lamination and produces dysplasia. *Dev. Neurobiol.* 73, 209–229. doi: 10.1002/dneu.22057

Reinhard, S. M., Razak, K., and Ethell, I. M. (2015). A delicate balance: role of MMP-9 in brain development and pathophysiology of neurodevelopmental disorders. *Front. Cell. Neurosci.* 9:280. doi: 10.3389/fncel.2015.00280

Rice, D. S., and Curran, T. (2001). Role of the reelin signaling pathway in central nervous system development. *Annu. Rev. Neurosci.* 24, 1005–1039. doi: 10.1146/annurev.neuro.24.1.1005

Rogers, S. L., Rankin-Gee, E., Risbud, R. M., Porter, B. E., and Marsh, E. D. (2018). Normal development of the perineuronal net in humans; in patients with and without epilepsy. *Neuroscience* 384, 350–360. doi: 10.1016/j.neuroscience.2018.05.039

Roll, L., and Faissner, A. (2014). Influence of the extracellular matrix on endogenous and transplanted stem cells after brain damage. *Front. Cell. Neurosci.* 8:219. doi: 10.3389/fncel.2014.00219

Sanes, J. R. (1983). Roles of extracellular matrix in neural development. *Annu. Rev. Physiol.* 45, 581–600. doi: 10.1146/annurev.ph.45.030183.003053

Sanes, J. R. (1989). Extracellular matrix molecules that influence neural development. *Annu. Rev. Neurosci.* 12, 491–516. doi: 10.1146/annurev.ne.12.030189.002423

Sekine, K., Kawauchi, T., Kubo, K., Honda, T., Herz, J., Hattori, M., et al. (2012). Reelin controls neuronal positioning by promoting cell-matrix adhesion *via* inside-out activation of integrin α5β1. *Neuron* 76, 353–369. doi: 10.1016/j.neuron.2012.07.020

Simão, D., Silva, M. M., Terrasso, A. P., Arez, F., Sousa, M. F. Q., Mehrjardi, N. Z., et al. (2018). Recapitulation of human neural microenvironment signatures in iPSC-derived NPC 3D differentiation. *Stem Cell Rep.* 11, 552–564. doi: 10.1016/j.stemcr.2018.06.020

Sorg, B. A., Berretta, S., Blacktop, J. M., Fawcett, J. W., Kitagawa, H., Kwok, J. C. F., et al. (2016). Casting a wide net: role of perineuronal nets in neural plasticity. *J. Neurosci.* 36, 11459–11468. doi: 10.1523/JNEUROSCI.2351-16.2016

Stenzel, D., Wilsch-Bräuninger, M., Wong, F. K., Heuer, H., and Huttner, W. B. (2014). Integrin αvβ3 and thyroid hormones promote expansion of progenitors in embryonic neocortex. *Development* 141, 795–806. doi: 10.1242/dev.101907

Tsuda, S., Kitagawa, T., Takashima, S., Asakawa, S., Shimizu, N., Mitani, H., et al. (2010). FAK-mediated extracellular signals are essential for interkinetic nuclear migration and planar divisions in the neuroepithelium. *J. Cell Sci.* 123, 484–496. doi: 10.1242/jcs.057851

Valiente, M., Ciceri, G., Rico, B., and Marin, O. (2011). Focal adhesion kinase modulates radial glia-dependent neuronal migration through connexin-26. *J. Neurosci.* 31, 11678–11691. doi: 10.1523/JNEUROSCI.2678-11.2011

van Essen, D. C. (2020). A 2020 view of tension-based cortical morphogenesis. *Proc. Natl. Acad. Sci. U S A* 117, 32868–32879. doi: 10.1073/pnas.2016830117

Van Reeuwijk, J., Janssen, M., Van Den Elzen, C., Beltran-Valero De Bernabé, D., Sabatelli, P., Merlini, L., et al. (2005). POMT2 mutations cause α-dystroglycan hypoglycosylation and walker-warburg syndrome. *J. Med. Genet.* 42, 907–912. doi: 10.1136/jmg.2005.031963

Wen, T. H., Binder, D. K., Ethell, I. M., and Razak, K. A. (2018). The perineuronal 'safety' net? Perineuronal net abnormalities in neurological disorders. *Front. Mol. Neurosci.* 11:270. doi: 10.3389/fnmol.2018.00270

Yan, Y., Martin, L. M., Bosco, D. B., Bundy, J. L., Nowakowski, R. S., Sang, Q. X. A., et al. (2015). Differential effects of acellular embryonic matrices on pluripotent stem cell expansion and neural differentiation. *Biomaterials* 73, 231–242. doi: 10.1016/j.biomaterials.2015.09.020

Yu, C., Griffiths, L. R., and Haupt, L. M. (2017). Exploiting heparan sulfate proteoglycans in human neurogenesis-controlling lineage specification and fate. *Front. Integr. Neurosci.* 11:28. doi: 10.3389/fnint.2017.00028

Zamecnik, J., Homola, A., Cicanic, M., Kuncova, K., Marusic, P., Krsek, P., et al. (2012). The extracellular matrix and diffusion barriers in focal cortical dysplasias. *Eur. J. Neurosci.* 36, 2017–2024. doi: 10.1111/j.1460-9568.2012.08107.x

Zimmermann, D. R., and Dours-Zimmermann, M. T. (2008). Extracellular matrix of the central nervous system: from neglect to challenge. *Histochem. Cell Biol.* 130, 635–653. doi: 10.1007/s00418-008-0485-9

Permissions

All chapters in this book were first published by Frontiers; hereby published with permission under the Creative Commons Attribution License or equivalent. Every chapter published in this book has been scrutinized by our experts. Their significance has been extensively debated. The topics covered herein carry significant findings which will fuel the growth of the discipline. They may even be implemented as practical applications or may be referred to as a beginning point for another development.

The contributors of this book come from diverse backgrounds, making this book a truly international effort. This book will bring forth new frontiers with its revolutionizing research information and detailed analysis of the nascent developments around the world.

We would like to thank all the contributing authors for lending their expertise to make the book truly unique. They have played a crucial role in the development of this book. Without their invaluable contributions this book wouldn't have been possible. They have made vital efforts to compile up to date information on the varied aspects of this subject to make this book a valuable addition to the collection of many professionals and students.

This book was conceptualized with the vision of imparting up-to-date information and advanced data in this field. To ensure the same, a matchless editorial board was set up. Every individual on the board went through rigorous rounds of assessment to prove their worth. After which they invested a large part of their time researching and compiling the most relevant data for our readers.

The editorial board has been involved in producing this book since its inception. They have spent rigorous hours researching and exploring the diverse topics which have resulted in the successful publishing of this book. They have passed on their knowledge of decades through this book. To expedite this challenging task, the publisher supported the team at every step. A small team of assistant editors was also appointed to further simplify the editing procedure and attain best results for the readers.

Apart from the editorial board, the designing team has also invested a significant amount of their time in understanding the subject and creating the most relevant covers. They scrutinized every image to scout for the most suitable representation of the subject and create an appropriate cover for the book.

The publishing team has been an ardent support to the editorial, designing and production team. Their endless efforts to recruit the best for this project, has resulted in the accomplishment of this book. They are a veteran in the field of academics and their pool of knowledge is as vast as their experience in printing. Their expertise and guidance has proved useful at every step. Their uncompromising quality standards have made this book an exceptional effort. Their encouragement from time to time has been an inspiration for everyone.

The publisher and the editorial board hope that this book will prove to be a valuable piece of knowledge for researchers, students, practitioners and scholars across the globe.

List of Contributors

Elise Peyre and Carla G. Silva
GIGA-Neurosciences, University of Liège, Liège, Belgium
Interdisciplinary Cluster for Applied Genoproteomics (GIGA-R), University of Liège, Liège, Belgium

Laurent Nguyen
GIGA-Neurosciences, University of Liège, Liège, Belgium
Interdisciplinary Cluster for Applied Genoproteomics (GIGA-R), University of Liège, Liège, Belgium
Wallon Excellence in Lifesciences and Biotechnology, University of Liège, Liège, Belgium

Jeremy N. Pulvers
Sydney Medical Program, University of Sydney, Sydney, Australia

Nathalie Journiac and Jeannette Nardelli
U1141 Inserm, Paris, France
Université Paris Diderot, Sorbonne Paris Cité, UMRS 1141, Paris, France

Yoko Arai
Institut Jacques Monod, CNRS UMR 7592, Université Paris Diderot, Sorbonne Paris Cité, Paris, France
Centre for Interdisciplinary Research in Biology (CIRB), Collège de France, CNRS UMR 7241/INSERM U1050, PSL Research University, Paris, France
Department of Evolutionary Genetics, Max Planck Institute for Evolutionary Anthropology (MPG), Leipzig, Germany
Max Planck Institute of Molecular Cell Biology and Genetics, Dresden, Germany

Heiko J. Luhmann
Institute of Physiology, University Medical Center Mainz, Mainz, Germany

Camilla Luccardini, Claire Leclech, Lucie Viou, Jean-Paul Rio and Christine Métin
INSERM, UMR-S839, Paris, France
Sorbonne Universités, UPMC University Paris 06, UMR-S839, Paris, France
Institut du Fer à Moulin, Paris, France

Elena Taverna
Centre for Interdisciplinary Research in Biology (CIRB), Collège de France, CNRS UMR 7241/INSERM U1050, PSL Research University, Paris, France
Department of Evolutionary Genetics, Max Planck Institute for Evolutionary Anthropology (MPG), Leipzig, Germany

Gewei Lian and Volney L. Sheen
Department of Neurology, Beth Israel Deaconess Medical Center and Harvard Medical School, Boston, MA, USA

Giulia Quattrocolo, Keagan Dunville and Maximiliano José Nigro
Center for Neural Computation, Egil and Pauline Braathen and Fred Kavli Center for Cortical Microcircuits, Kavli Institute for Systems Neuroscience, Norwegian University of Science and Technology, Trondheim, Norway

Seiji Ishii
Center for Neuroscience Research, Children's National Medical Center, Children's Research Institute, Washington, DC, USA

Kazue Hashimoto-Torii
Center for Neuroscience Research, Children's National Medical Center, Children's Research Institute, Washington, DC, USA
Department of Pediatrics, Pharmacology and Physiology, School of Medicine and Health Sciences, The George Washington University, Washington, DC, USA
Department of Neurobiology, School of Medicine, Kavli Institute for Neuroscience, Yale University, New Haven, CT, USA

Andi H. Hansen, Christian Duellberg, Christine Mieck, Martin Loose and Simon Hippenmeyer
Institute of Science and Technology Austria, Klosterneuburg, Austria

Chan Choo Yap and Bettina Winckler
Department of Neuroscience, University of Virginia, Charlottesville, VA, USA

Aslam Abbasi Akhtar
Board of Governors Regenerative Medicine Institute, Cedars-Sinai Medical Center, Los Angeles, CA, USA
Department of Biomedical Sciences, Cedars-Sinai Medical Center, Los Angeles, CA, USA

Joshua J. Breunig
Board of Governors Regenerative Medicine Institute, Cedars-Sinai Medical Center, Los Angeles, CA, USA
Department of Biomedical Sciences, Cedars-Sinai Medical Center, Los Angeles, CA, USA
Samuel Oschin Comprehensive Cancer Institute, Cedars-Sinai Medical Center, Los Angeles, CA, USA

Julio L. Sampaio, Michaela Wilsch-Bräuninger, Andreas W. Ettinger, Christiane Haffner and Wieland B. Huttner
Max Planck Institute of Molecular Cell Biology and Genetics, Dresden, Germany

Yanyan Sun, Zhen Tang and Na Hu
Department of Pediatrics, The Third Xiangya Hospital of Central South University, Changsha, China

Mingyan Hei and Bo Wang
Neonatal Center, Beijing Children's Hospital, Capital Medical University, Beijing, China

Zhihui Fang
Department of Nuclear Medicine, The Second Xiangya Hospital of Central South University, Changsha, China

Tao Ye, Amy K. Y. Fu and Nancy Y. Ip
Division of Life Science, Molecular Neuroscience Center and State Key Laboratory of Molecular Neuroscience, The Hong Kong University of Science and Technology, Hong Kong, China

Martine N. Manuel, Da Mi, John O. Mason and David J. Price
Centre for Integrative Physiology, The University of Edinburgh, Edinburgh, UK

Takeshi Kawauchi
Department of Physiology, Keio University School of Medicine, Tokyo, Japan
Precursory Research for Embryonic Science and Technology (PRESTO), Japan Science and Technology Agency, Saitama, Japan
Laboratory of Molecular Life Science, Institute of Biomedical Research and Innovation, Foundation for Biomedical Research and Innovation, Kobe, Japan

Itaru Imayoshi
The Hakubi Center, Kyoto University, Kyoto, Japan
Laboratory of Growth Regulation, Institute for Virus Research, Kyoto University, Kyoto, Japan
World Premier International Research Initiative-Institute for Integrated Cell-Material Sciences, Kyoto University, Kyoto, Japan
Precursory Research for Embryonic Science and Technology, Japan Science and Technology Agency, Saitama, Japan

Fumiyoshi Ishidate
World Premier International Research Initiative-Institute for Integrated Cell-Material Sciences, Kyoto University, Kyoto, Japan

Ryoichiro Kageyama
Laboratory of Growth Regulation, Institute for Virus Research, Kyoto University, Kyoto, Japan
World Premier International Research Initiative-Institute for Integrated Cell-Material Sciences, Kyoto University, Kyoto, Japan
Core Research for Evolutional Science and Technology, Japan Science and Technology Agency, Saitama, Japan

Katherine R. Long
Centre for Developmental Neurobiology, Institute of Psychiatry, Psychology and Neuroscience, King's College London, London, United Kingdom
MRC Centre for Neurodevelopmental Disorders, King's College London, London, United Kingdom

Index

www.ingramcontent.com/pod-product-compliance
Lightning Source LLC
LaVergne TN
LVHW082218200926
848484LV00008B/2274